COMA AND IMPAIRED CONSCIOUSNESS

NOTICE

COMA AND IMPAIRED CONSCIOUSNESS: A CLINICAL PERSPECTIVE

EDITORS

G. Bryan Young, M.D.

Professor of Neurology
Department of Clinical Neurological Sciences
Victoria Hospital, University of Western Ontario
London, Ontario, Canada

Allan H. Ropper, M.D.

Professor of Neurology, Tufts University School of Medicine
Chief, Neurology Service
St. Elizabeth's Medical Center
Boston, Massachusetts

Charles F. Bolton, M.D.

Professor of Neurology
Department of Clinical Neurological Sciences
Victoria Hospital, University of Western Ontario
London, Ontario, Canada

McGraw-Hill
HEALTH PROFESSIONS DIVISION

New York   St. Louis   San Francisco   Auckland   Bogotá
Caracas   Lisbon   London   Madrid   Mexico City   Milan   Montreal
New Delhi   San Juan   Singapore   Sydney   Tokyo   Toronto

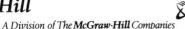

McGraw-Hill

A Division of The McGraw·Hill Companies

COMA AND IMPAIRED CONSCIOUSNESS: A CLINICAL PERSPECTIVE

Copyright © 1998 by The McGraw-Hill Companies, Inc. All rights reserved.
Printed in the United States of America. Except as permitted under the
United States Copyright Act of 1976, no part of this publication may be
reproduced or distributed in any form or by any means, or stored in a data
base or retrieval system, without the prior written permission of the publisher.

1234567890 DOC DOC 9987

ISBN 0-07-072371-0

This book was set in Times Roman by Keyword Publishing Services Ltd.
The editors were Joseph Hefta and Peter McCurdy.
The production supervisor was Catherine Saggese.
The cover designer was Robert Freese.
R. R. Donnelley & Son Company was printer and binder.

This book is printed on acid-free paper.

Cataloging-in-Publication data is on file for this title at the Library of Congress.

About the cover: The PET images are from a study of activity in the midbrain reticular formation and the
thalamic intralaminar nuclei in which participants were given tasks which demanded attention and quick
reaction times. From S. Kinomura, J. Larsson, B. Gulyás, P. E. Roland, *Science* **271**, 512 (1996). Reprinted
with the permission of the author and publisher.

CONTENTS

CONTRIBUTORS

Charles F. Bolton, M.D., F.R.C.P.C.
Professor of Neurology
Department of Clinical Neurological Sciences
University of Western Ontario
London, Ontario, Canada
(Chapter 11)

Debra A. DeRubeis, M.D.
Department of Clinical Neurological Sciences
University of Western Ontario
London, Ontario, Canada
(Chapter 13)

Rocco V. Gerace, M.D., F.R.C.P.C.
Professor
Department of Emergency Medicine
University of Western Ontario
London, Ontario, Canada
(Chapters 16, 19)

William A. McCauley, M.D., F.R.C.P.C.
Assistant Professor
Department of Emergency Medicine
University of Western Ontario
London, Ontario, Canada
(Chapter 19)

Richard J. Moulton, M.D., F.R.C.S.C.
Associate Professor of Neurosurgery
Department of Surgery
University of Toronto
Toronto, Ontario, Canada
(Chapter 6)

Allan H. Ropper, M.D.
Professor of Neurology
Tufts University School of Medicine
Chief, Division of Neurology
St. Elizabeth's Hospital, Boston, Massachusetts
(Chapter 4)

Paul R. Steacy, B.A., LL.B.
Attorney, London, Ontario, Canada
(Chapter 24)

Christopher G. Wherrett, M.D., F.R.C.P.C.
Assistant Professor
Department of Anesthesia
University of Ottawa
Ottawa, Ontario, Canada
(Chapter 16)

Eelco F. M. Wijdicks, M.D., Ph.D., F.A.C.P.
Associate Professor of Neurology
Mayo Medical School
and
Co-Director, Neurology-Neurosurgery
Intensive Care Unit
Senior Associate Consultant
Department of Neurology
Mayo Clinic and Mayo Foundation
Rochester, Minnesota
(Chapters 5, 17, 19, 20, 21)

G. Bryan Young, M.D., F.R.C.P.C.
Professor of Neurology
Department of Clinical Neurological Sciences
University of Western Ontario
London, Ontario, Canada
(Chapters 1, 2, 3, 7, 8, 9, 10, 12, 13, 14, 15, 17, 18, 19, 22, 23, 24)

FOREWORD

Few situations in clinical practice are more challenging than the arrival in the emergency room of a patient out of touch with his or her environment. Whether the condition is one of confusion, of mild stupor, or deep coma, the physician is deprived of the most useful instrument available to a medical practitioner: the history of the illness obtained from the alert and helpful patient. The physician becomes a detective and is confronted with the epitome of medical problem-solving. Relatives, friends, or even strangers who come with the patient may make the resolution of the mystery fairly simple. They may recount that he or she has been previously in the emergency department because of an epileptic condition, or has been pulled from an overturned vehicle, or was found under a tree on a golf course in a thunderstorm, or had been spraying an orchard all week with toxic pesticides.

The causes of stupor or coma are so many as to unnerve physicians who have not themselves "been there before." Fortunately for medical practitioners and nurses in emergency rooms and intensive care units, for family physicians, internists, pediatricians, neurologists, neurosurgeons, for physicians training in all specialties and certified specialists who wish to hone their skills, Drs. Bryan Young, Allan Ropper, and Charles Bolton have all been there before for some decades. They have been on neurological wards in Boston and London, Ontario. They have been in the hustle and bustle of emergency rooms and intensive care units with their eyes and ears open. They have consulted with their colleagues on medical, surgical, obstetric, and pediatric wards and have solved many of the clinical problems presented in this collation of their collective experiences.

The arrival of Plum and Posner's monograph on *Stupor and Coma* 40 years ago cast a very bright light on the physical diagnosis of the stuporous and comatose patient. This new work takes us a step further and presents an orderly and readable survey of the majority of the conditions, and their mechanisms which bring confused and unconscious patients to hospital.

Any practitioner who will be asked why a patient is unconscious, asked how to plan the appropriate investigation, and asked what emergency treatment to initiate, will be grateful for the fact that three colleagues from two neighboring countries have made it much easier for all of us to seek these answers.

H. J. M. BARNETT, M.D.
Scientist, The John P. Robarts Research Institute
Professor Emeritus,
The University of Western Ontario

PREFACE

Medical and lay persons have long been fascinated by coma. The roots of this captivation apparently derive from a perception that coma is the polar opposite of the sentient human state, penultimate only to death, its closest companion. For the physician, the sensational and conspicuous alteration in the normal state of awareness is the phenomenon that attracts most attention at the bedside. The term "coma" is derived from Comus of Greek mythology, a guardian of banquets that included wine. The altered behavior ("comic" has a similar derivation) and impairment of consciousness produced by alcohol were thus recognized in antiquity as manifestations of a toxic encephalopathy (as the authors can attest). The ancients must also have appreciated that there is a spectrum of impairment of consciousness from too much wine, ranging from whimsical and slightly disinhibited behavior to an unresponsive sleep-like state. These variable and multidimensional aspects of consciousness have recently been rediscovered. It is now legitimate to address the mystery of man's consciousness on a number of fronts. But as modern philosophers draw increasingly on cognitive and neural sciences, intellectual artifices that define consciousness run into interminable trouble. They and others become bogged down in the study of *apperception* that is closely tied to sensory perception and in relating the aggregated perceived properties of an object and self-awareness as a sensation to the firing of groups of neurons, as detected by modern electrophysiological and functional neuroimaging technology.

For the neurologist the problem is, fortunately, simpler. The deeply unresponsive patient, beyond a state of sleep and lacking any cerebral response to the world, is comatose. Some engine of the brain maintains what we call the mind, and this is continuously active throughout life, much the same as the respiratory centers of the medulla. This "driving force," to some extent, assures that we are the same person when we wake as when we went to sleep. It imparts to man the state of being awake and allows for his interaction with the extrapersonal world and for thinking. The failure of this managerial function is easy to recognize when all derived behaviors falter, i.e., coma.

There has been a surprising absence of books on coma, even though impaired consciousness remains a common and challenging problem in clinical medicine. It is encountered in the home, at the roadside, and in the emergency rooms, intensive care units, and wards of modern hospitals. Plum and Posner's classical monograph, *Stupor and Coma*, was last published nearly two decades ago, and much has transpired since: the increased numbers and availability of street drugs, newer medical treatments with neurologic complications, novel infections, the recognition of the effects of systemic inflammation and other generalized illnesses on brain function, and new insights into head trauma and anoxic-ischemic encephalopathy.

Clinical evaluation is still of great importance, often yielding the specific diagnosis. However, new techniques have allowed more exquisite assessments of cerebral structure and function in the comatose patient, for diagnostic, monitoring, and prognostic purposes. Evidence-based clinical research has provided better guidelines for the determination of prognosis and the planning of management. The application of ethical principles to disorders of the brain has been clarified and refined. These reasons justify the compilation of a new book on coma and related impairments of consciousness. We give due respect to Plum and Posner's *Stupor and Coma* and acknowledge a debt for the interest the book created for us as students and for the seminal precepts it codified for medicine, particularly the notion of herniations as the causes of coma. The second reason for publishing our book is to present a different view of the clinical system of impaired consciousness that is not so dependent on pathologic findings.

Coma and Impaired Consciousness: A Clinical Perspective is written by clinicians for clinicians as a comprehensive review and update of coma and derangements of consciousness, meant thereby to be accessible without declining to the simplicity of a handbook. The first section addresses the concepts underlying the state of coma and outlines the major causative syndromes, gives a clinical approach to each, and illustrates the investigations that are useful in certain circumstances. The numerous structural causes of coma are then considered. This is followed by sections on inflammatory, metabolic, and toxic conditions that diminish consciousness. The syndromes of transient impairment are considered separately, followed by a consideration of the clinical contexts in which we encounter patients. We conclude with the ever-present ethical concerns that influence management. Throughout, we take a practical attitude, giving a consensus or evidence-based approach from the latest literature, but offering our own perspectives when personal experience has something to contribute. This approach is meant to make the book immediately useful not only to neurologists and neurosurgeons, but also to internists, pediatricians, intensivists, emergency ward doctors, and investigators interested in coma and its constituent features.

We hope and trust the book will be of use to those on the "front lines" of medical care and a resource to students of the brain.

G.B.Y., A.H.R., C.F.B
London, Ontario and Boston

ACKNOWLEDGMENTS

The editors wish to thank the following individuals for inspiration and assistance: Michael Aminoff, Leo Assis, Warren Blume, Stephan Brudzinski, Merrill Edmonds, Andrew Gibson, John Girvin, Ingrid Hutchinson, Kenneth Jordan, Michael Kovacs, Donald Lee, Andrea Lozosky, David Nicolle, Susan Pigott, David Ramsay, Robert Reed, Frank Rutledge, Dwight Stewart, Jeanne Teitelbaum, and Jane Upfold. We are also grateful to Tara Cassidy and Joel Herring for much of the artwork.

Charles Bolton and Allan Ropper are particularly appreciative of the efforts of Bryan Young. As can be seen, he has been responsible for writing the majority of the book. His many hours of thorough, painstaking work are greatly appreciated.

COMA AND IMPAIRED CONSCIOUSNESS

Part 1

CONSCIOUSNESS, MAJOR SYNDROMES, AND APPROACH

Chapter 1
CONSCIOUSNESS

G. Bryan Young

Consciousness is far from being unitary.
E. Bisiach, 1991[1]

William James defined consciousness as awareness of oneself (or one's own cognitive experience) and the environment.[2] This apparently simple definition belies complex brain functions that are still incompletely resolved. There are several conceptual levels of consciousness, as the term has been used in medical and other writings:[3]

- "Crude consciousness" or alertness: this allows only for a state of behavioral alertness and wake and sleep cycles. Alertness is the opposite of coma, an unarousable unconscious state. An "awake" individual may or may not be aware of self or the environment.

- "Phenomenal consciousness": this is where the brain registers internal or external phenomena without this mode of processing demanding attention or entering into cognitive awareness and decision-making. There is, therefore, an awareness in the brain, but this is not apparent to the individual at the time.

- "Access consciousness": this is where there is directed attention, with cognitive awareness and decision making. This "higher level" consciousness includes either self-awareness, external awareness, or both, and most closely matches the intent of William James' definition. However, within this higher level of consciousness there are *components* that require further discussion.

- The philosophic "highest level" or *philosophia perennis* of nondimensional awareness of the harmony of the universe.[4]

CONCEPTS OF CONSCIOUSNESS

Strehler and others propose that consciousness has a number of discrete, if interrelated, qualities and components:[5-10] The following are abstracted from their writings:

1. Consciousness is an active process with multiple components.

2. Wakefulness or alertness is a precondition for consciousness.

3. There is the capacity for self-awareness, i.e., awareness of (at least some of) one's own cognition and mental processes.

4. There is perceived sensation, expressed symbolically, of internal and external stimuli on the person. Such perception is processed in an orderly fashion; the perceptions are prioritized for attention. There is a focusing of attention on some items and exclusion or filtering of others. "Motivation," an internal drive, underlies much of the selectivity process,

5. A small number of events can be held in the active (working) memory and are used in minute-to-minute decisions and actions. This is intimately related to attention.

6. Memories can be recovered and displayed, along with their spatial and temporal ordering, i.e., the brain can relate remembered

events to each other in time and space. Memories are often invoked when processing information for its relevance.

7. A decision-making capacity exists for action, dependent on the attention directed to particular parts of sensory or motor input. Motivation is involved with prioritizing and choosing behavior, after processing information.

8. Cognition or thought, traditionally at the "highest level" of cognitive functioning (e.g., deductive reasoning), involves the synthesis of the various components listed above. There is the potential to store conscious experience and cognitive conclusions in the long-term memory. This is necessary for consciousness to be useful to the individual, e.g., in planning and higher level behavior.

In summary, most definitions of consciousness recognize complex and multifaceted functions resting on basic alertness and awareness. In addition, consciousness is a function of the brain that, like breathing, is active throughout the healthy life of the individual. Furthermore, an adequate explanation of consciousness must explain unconsciousness as observed by the physician in clinical situations.

In the following discussion, the development of ideas of consciousness and the components of consciousness are discussed according to the disciplines that gave form to principal concepts. Early thoughts on consciousness came from philosophers, who still contribute to our thinking on this elusive topic. Psychologists and psychiatrists, based on their practical experience with patients, and experimental models, added another dimension. Insights of basic scientists awaited the technologic advances and experimental studies that are discussed separately.

Philosophic, Psychologic, and Psychiatric Contributions

John Locke defined consciousness as "the perception of what goes on in a man's own mind."[11] While this definition of consciousness as an internal state of awareness is appealing in its brevity and simplicity, it does not reveal the content, mechanism, or definition of the "mind." Early philosophers considered that there was a duality of mind and body or mind and physical reality (pluralism).

Rene Descartes equated personhood with the capacity for active thought: "*Cogito, ergo sum*" (I think, therefore, I am).[12] However, he realized that there must be a physical basis or location of self in the body. He settled on the pineal gland, since it was a strategically placed, deep midline structure that could receive information from both sides of the body without bias, and serve as the place of communion with the soul.[12] This localization may have been influenced by the earlier galenistic concept that the brain was organized into three midline chambers that received and processed incoming sensory information.[13] Descartes proposed that visual images are projected from both eyes to the pineal gland, where they are fused into a single true image that is viewed by the soul.[14] Although this now seems primitive, Descartes' thinking was a step beyond the aristotelian view of sensory information entering a "black box" of the body, where it was viewed.[14] At least, Descartes conceived of a transfer of information within the nervous system. This was likely the first attempt to solve the "binding problem," i.e., the conversion of the physiologic activity of the brain into conscious awareness or perception.[15]

The relationship between mind and body is not resolved to everyone's satisfaction. That such a relationship exists is exemplified by the expressions of the will that are carried out by the body. Early concepts of the mind as a nonphysical entity that mysteriously interacted with the body, or a "ghost in a machine", have been a philosophic stumbling block.[16,17] A recent attempt to explain the mind-body relationship using quantum mechanics faces the same problem of relating what is apparently immaterial to actual structures.[18]

Attempts at holism, or fusing the mind and body, have utilized introspection and combined philosophic, psychologic, and neurophysiologic approaches.[19] These will be reviewed subsequently.

The subjective nature of conscious experience is difficult to clarify. Although sentience, thought, and reason form important components of consciousness, there are other constituents. Early philosophers, including Kant and Jaspers, concluded that there were factors beyond knowledge that made up consciousness: awareness of self and the human quality in others; subjectivity or personal interpretation of knowledge; feelings and emotions; nonverbal or unexpressed "deep" emotions or feelings that play a role in our makeup and behavior.[20] William James and his disciples favored a unified approach in which mental activity, including consciousness, arose from brain activity. James viewed consciousness as a function of knowing. This philosophic view has generally prevailed, although a conceptual separation of mind and body persisted in some circles.

Early attempts at reaching a definition of consciousness relied on introspective methods, but experimenters could not agree upon fundamental observations. Because of the inability of workers to reach a consensus, the behaviorist school felt that consciousness was not amenable to study.

Psychologists and psychiatrists overlapped with and succeeded the philosophers in conceptualizing consciousness, a "subconscious," and the nature of the mind. The view of William James that consciousness was the product of brain function and that the mind and body were not separable was adopted.[21] This allowed the pursuit of mental functions on a more concrete basis.

Two opposing psychologic theories of the mind arose: the "structuralist" and "functionalist" schools. The structuralist school, led by Tichener, held that the mind was formed of three basic elements, all of which could be disclosed by careful introspection:

1. *Sensations*: properties included (a) quality (e.g., the "blueness" of light), (b) intensity (the strength of the sensation or image), (c) duration (the time the sensation or image lasts), (d) vividness or contrast between foreground and background, and (e) extensity (the extent of the image or sensation).

2. *Memories or images*: these could have similar properties as sensations.

3. *"Feelings"*: emotional reactions that accompanied sensations or images.

Problems that have been raised with the structuralist view include: (1) How can attention be fully explained? (2) Some mental processes, cognitive higher order reasoning, emotions, and psychopathology could not be addressed by structuralist principles and methods such as introspection. Some mental operations are apparently effortless, e.g., the effortless recall of the name of an object. Some highly abstracted processes may also be free of "processing capacity" as measured by interference with other mental activities. This suggests that some complex mental operations that alter behavior go on at a level that is not apparent to the "self" at a "conscious" level.

James argued that consciousness has the following properties: (1) it is personal, i.e., unique to the individual; (2) it is an "ever-changing" stream rather than a static entity; (3) it is continuous, rather than divided into elements as the structuralists would have it; and (4) it is selective, i.e., the human mind can only attend or concentrate upon a limited number of entities in the sea of stimuli that bombard the nervous system. Rosenfield later amplified these statements: (1) self-referential mechanisms are the basis of consciousness and of an individual's knowledge; (2) memory is vital to the meaningful interpretation of the present; and (3) a conscious perception is a product integrated from past and present experience.[7]

Although each school had appealing aspects, numerous hypotheses (e.g., concerning the origin of emotions) could not be adequately addressed or tested in the early years.

Freudian ideas occupy a special place in the evolution of concepts of consciousness. Although controversy exists about Freud's theories, a central notion is that one is not aware of all that is within his/her mind, implying specifically that some mental activity is "subconscious" or "unconscious."[22] Such unconscious mental activity is felt, nonetheless, to play a role in motivated behavior. The unconscious contents of the mind can be probed using psychoanalysis and hypnosis.

That such an unconscious component of the mind exists is still debated. Certainly, this use of the term "unconscious" has a wholly different meaning than the clinical absence of waking behavior.

Sartre, the French existentialist philosopher, vigorously opposed Freud's central tenet that there is much that is hidden from conscious awareness.[23] Sartre viewed all mental processes as accessible to the conscious mind, but considered that the limited capacity of language prevented the recounting of some experiences. This appears to be a semantic position. Both Freud and Sartre believed that unexpressed mental processes formed part of the psyche of the individual and helped to determine behavior, sometimes expressed symbolically."[24]

Basic and Clinical Neuroscience Contributions

Insights provided by basic scientists awaited the advances in technology. Although it was generally accepted that the brain was responsible for alertness, consciousness, memory, emotion, and behavior, it was not until the development of the compound microscope that the cellular (neuronal) basis of brain function was appreciated. By the end of the nineteenth century, a more precise cellular examination of the brain was possible, culminating in the work of Ramón y Cajal that laid the foundation for the neuron theory of Waldeyer in 1891.[25–27] The neuron theory related brain function to individual signaling elements, the neurons, which communicated with other neurons through synapses.

Neurophysiologists then demonstrated the electrical component of neuronal functioning.[28,29] This paralleled the discovery of a chemical component of brain function. Drugs interacted with receptors on nerve cells; hence, naturally occurring chemical ligands were likely present.[30,31]

A nodal point in the understanding of consciousness occurred when Moruzzi and Magoun produced electroencephalogram (EEG) arousal by stimulation of the brainstem reticular formation rostral to the midpons.[32] This system, including its rostral projection, was termed the "ascending reticular activating system" (ARAS) (Fig. 1-1). The relation of this system to consciousness per se is further discussed in the subsequent section on "Alertness." Although alertness and higher functions are discussed separately, their strong interrelation is illustrated by recent neurophysiologic data. Munk and colleagues showed that activation of the midbrain reticular formation, important in arousal and vigilance, enhances the stimulus-specific synchronization of neuronal discharges in the visual cortex of cats.[33] Thus, there is an interaction of the alerting and sensory processing systems in the brain. Further, there is a variation in the "augmenting response," an enhanced response of the cortex to electrical stimulation of the ventrolateral nucleus of the thalamus, depending on the activity state of the animal.[34] This enhanced response is reduced if the animal is vigilant and exploring, but is accentuated during idle behavior. This, again, suggests an interaction of vigilance and different processing roles of the cortex and subcortical structures.

Another electrophysiologic phenomenon, the gamma or "40-Hz rhythm," is produced by thalamocortical circuits during attention and sensory processing tasks that require attention and the "binding" of processed sensory information with memory, attention, and motor responses.[35] This rhythm is synchronous across various regions linking thalamocortical networks, as well as the hippocampus and neocortex. It has been proposed that such coherent rhythms allow a timing reference that fosters simultaneous or parallel brain activity in a networked rather than purely hierarchic fashion.[35] In this way, for example, all modalities of an object held in the memory can be appreciated.

Sensory processing has been examined using computer averaging techniques. Ruddell and Hua examined the "recognition potential" from the midline parietal region when bilingual Chinese subjects concentrated on detecting either Chinese or English words.[36] When subjects attended English words, a recognition potential (P3, at about 300 ms) occurred only when English words were shown. There was no response to Chinese words. The reverse applied to the conscious detection of Chinese words. The latency for

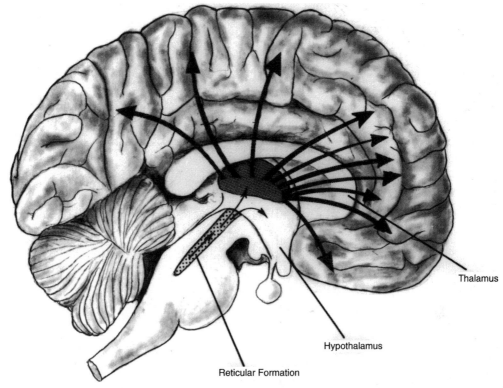

Figure 1-1

The ascending reticular activating system (ARAS), shown as a network beginning in the rostral brainstem tegmentum and projecting to the thalamus and then to the cerebral cortex, with weighting towards the anterior aspect.

the P3 component was longer for English than Chinese words, suggesting that the English words took longer to process. The findings support the concept that attention and processing have categoric specificity in the human brain.

Neuroscientists argue that the "black box" of brain function needs to be opened and probed to determine how neurons function individually and collectively in order to understand awareness. The focusing on sensory processing, especially visual awareness, has led to further understanding of some brain operations directly relevant to consciousness and to proposals that consciousness is the experience of midlevel sensory processing.[10]

Hebb, a neurophysiologist, inspired much of the progress in neurophysiologic research and

cybernetic modeling of the brain activity involved in the processing of information. This has been succinctly stated in "Hebb's rule"[37]:

> *When an axon of a cell A is near enough to excite a cell B and repeatedly and persistently takes part in firing it, some growth process or metabolic change takes place in one or both cells such that A's efficiency, as one of the cells firing B, is increased.*

Cybernetics has allowed some limited computer-modeling insights into brain functions, respecting Hebb's rule. "Neural network" computer systems differ from most computers in that (1) they can be "taught"; (2) they are able to weigh incoming information in order to make decisions;

and (3) they "degrade gracefully" (instead of "crashing" like standard computers, they continue to function, but not as well). By weighting the strength of connections, analogous to strengthening synaptic connections in the brain, computers are trained to recognize certain patterns. When well trained, they can correctly judge the nature of the information, even if only part of it is presented. Neural nets thus can "remember." The back-propagation of neural nets allows checking and polishing of a graded output, similar to that of the brain. Properties that emerge from such systems, admittedly simplistic compared with the brain, give some insights into brain processing.

Although consciousness is far from being completely understood, important components are recognized and reviewed below.

COMPONENTS OF CONSCIOUSNESS

Alertness (Crude Consciousness)

Alertness, also called "crude consciousness," the arousal component or wakefulness, is dependent on the upper brainstem and diencephalon. The ARAS (see above) ascends the brainstem tegmentum, from the midpons extending rostrally, through the midline and intralaminar (formerly called "nonspecific") nuclei of the thalamus (Figs. 1-1 and 1-2), to the cerebral cortex (Fig. 1-3).

Figure 1-2

The thalamus. The intralaminar nuclei are important components of the reticular formation. The reticular nucleus, a thin gray matter sheet over the thalamus, performs a gating function in controlling projections from the thalamus to the cerebral cortex. (Redrawn from Kandel ER, Schwartz JH, Jessell TM, Principles of Natural Science, *3rd ed. New York, Elsevier, 1991, with permission.)*

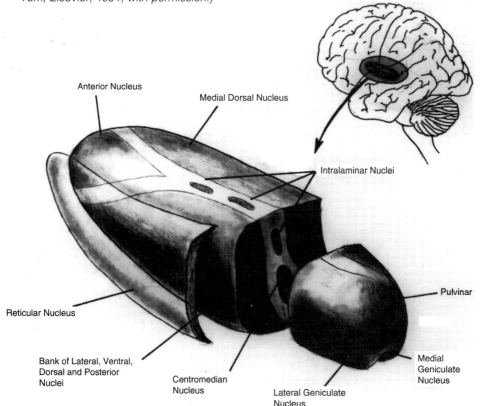

Anterior Nucleus

Medial Dorsal Nucleus

Intralaminar Nuclei

Pulvinar

Reticular Nucleus

Bank of Lateral, Ventral, Dorsal and Posterior Nuclei

Centromedian Nucleus

Lateral Geniculate Nucleus

Medial Geniculate Nucleus

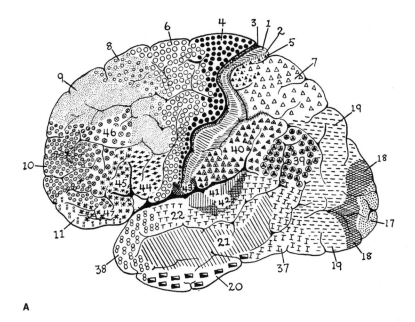

A

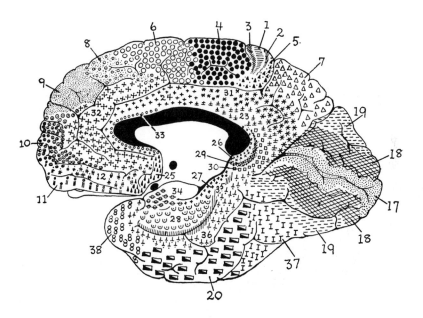

B

Figure 1-3
The cerebral cortex, with the Brodmann cytoarchitechtonic numbered areas shown;
A. convexity surface and B. *medial surface. (From Brodmann K,* Vergleichende Lokalisa-
tion lehre der Grosshirnrinde in ihren Prinzipien dargestelt auf Grund des Zellenbaues.
Leipzig, JA Barth, 1909, p 324.)

The ARAS was thought to be composed of an undifferentiated collection of neurons in these regions, with extensive internal connections and projections, both rostrally and caudally. Further studies on the morphology, connections, and neurochemistry of separate cell groups in these regions revealed that they have distinct properties, as well as being components of the arousal "system." Discrete regions of the brainstem reticular formation project to several thalamic nuclei besides the midline and intralaminar group, and have connections to motor and other centers.[38] For example, the midbrain reticular formation has connections with the zona incerta, as well as with lateral thalamic nuclei.[38] Subsequent clarification by Nauta and Whitlock[39] and Scheibel and Scheibel[40] revealed that the dorsal leaf of the ascending reticular projection goes to the "nonspecific" thalamic nuclei, but there is also a ventral leaf that runs lateral and ventral through the subthalamus and hypothalamus and goes ventral to the thalamic reticular nucleus. Axons of cells of the nonspecific thalamic nuclei perforate the reticular nucleus and continue rostrally as the inferior thalamic peduncle. Another component runs back to the tegmental level.

The thalamic reticular nucleus (Fig. 1-2) performs a key role in gating reticular activity and allowing feedback to the brainstem centers that play a role in arousal and alertness. The reticular thalamic nucleus receives projections from the brainstem reticular formation and large regions of the cerebral cortex, and projects mainly to the brainstem reticular formation and the superior colliculus. With activation or stimulation of the mesencephalic reticular formation, the reticular thalamic nucleus is inhibited; this reduces the tonic inhibition that the reticular nucleus exerts on thalamic relay nuclei. Sensory information is then transmitted to the cerebral cortex for further processing.[41] This gating function should be thought of as a network of "neural portals" that are capable of individually or collectively regulating information flow to the cortex.[42] Thalamic gating is also influenced by feedback from the prefrontal cortex, allowing selection of certain stimuli and disallowing others from reaching the

cortex for further processing.[43] This is likely relevant for attention and concentration, in which selection is an important component.

Early studies by physiologists and anatomists suggested that the thalamic midline and intralaminar, or "nonspecific," nuclei, identified as part of the reticular activating system, did not project directly to the cerebral cortex, but to specific thalamic nuclei that did have a cortical projection.[44] The nonspecific thalamic nuclei receive cholinergic innervation from the brainstem that probably modulates the activity of the basal ganglia-thalamocortical system.[45] In addition, the individual nuclei in this group receive specific sets of afferents and project to particular parts of the cerebral cortex and striatum.[45] Thus, the more rostral portion of the ARAS is also not a diffuse, homogenous network, but consists of interconnected specific and distinct neuronal groupings, with individual as well as collective functions.

The discovery of the ARAS led to the belief that the center for consciousness had been found. It was soon realized, however, that consciousness and awareness could not be totally assigned to this structure. As Penfield stated:[46]

> It would be absurd to suppose that central integration could take place without implication and employment of cortical areas selected appropriately to the needs of the organization that faces the brain mechanism. To suppose that centrencephalic integration is possible without utilization of the cortex would be to return to the thinking of Descartes and to enthrone again a spiritual homunculus in some area as the nearby pineal gland. It would be equally absurd to consider that the reticular formation is functionally separate from the cortex.

At the same time, the interactive role of the cortex and subcortical structures must be recognized. The complex interactions of the rostral brainstem reticular formation, the thalamus, other subcortical structures, and the cortex probably allow for alertness, awareness, and the selection of attention depending on the importance (e.g., danger, needs, or cognitive values) at the time.[47]

The electrophysiologic differences among conscious wakefulness, coma, sleep, and the state produced by general anesthesia imply that there are basic differences in neuronal functional activities in these conditions. More recent electrophysiologic studies indicate that there are three fundamentally distinct, naturally occurring, or physiologic states of consciousness: the awake state, rapid-eye-movement (REM) or paradoxical sleep, and slow-wave sleep.[48] Unlike coma, there is the capacity to respond to external stimuli in each of these. In sleep, however, the responsiveness to external stimuli is reduced. In slow-wave sleep, this reduced responsiveness to afferent stimuli is reflected in reduced cortical-thalamic evoked responses in the primary sensory cortices.[49] In REM sleep and wakefulness, such early cortical sensory components are preserved, because thalamic inhibition is tonically reduced.[48] In REM sleep, however, further sensory processing of such cortical responses is markedly reduced compared with wakefulness.[48] In REM sleep, the brain appears to be more "self-absorbed" in its own intrinsic activity, perhaps the playback of memories in active dreaming. In wakefulness, cerebral cortical activity is more readily modified towards processing and attending to input from stimuli from the outside world.[48]

More recent physiologic-anatomic information on the alertness or vigilance component of attention comes from studies using positron emission tomography (PET) with measures of regional cerebral blood flow and metabolism. Kinomura and colleagues studied a group of normal volunteers in the awake-relaxed state and during reaction-time tests in which vigilance and attention were increased.[50] There were significant regional increases in blood flow above baseline during the attention-enhanced tasks. The structures affected included the midbrain reticular formation and the region of the thalamic intralaminar nuclei, as well as a diffuse increase in metabolic activity occurring across the cerebral cortex. These increases are independent of the type of sensory modality for the test and the initiation of motor activity.

Neurochemistry of Alertness

The neurotransmitters in the arousal system constitute the "wet physiology" that relates to the "dry physiology" and anatomy just reviewed. The principal neurotransmitter systems relevant to arousal are cholinergic, monoaminergic, and GABA-nergic.

Cholinergic System Cholinergic pathways play a contributory role in arousal and alertness as components of the ARAS (Fig. 1-4). Cholinergic activation of the thalamus facilitates thalamocortical transmission by decreasing the tonic inhibition of the thalamic reticular nucleus.[51] Cholinergic input into the medial structures of the diencephalon and basal forebrain is also involved in emotional arousal.[52,53] The cholinergic cell bodies in the pontomesencephalic reticular formation probably mediate this effect. The desynchronized arousal response on the EEG, a hallmark of arousal and heightened alertness, shows a positive correlation with the amount of acetylcholine released, and is abolished by cholinergic antagonists.[54,55] This cortical effect relates to enhanced activity in the projection to the cortex from the nucleus basalis of Meynert.[55] Also, the cholinergic septal projection to the hippocampus is essential for the hippocampal theta rhythm, which is present during exploratory activity and vigilance in animals.[56]

There are, however, a variety of very different functions in different parts of the cholinergic "system." Pontomesencephalic cholinergic cells release acetylcholine in the basal forebrain and directly affect cholinergic neurons in the basal nuclear complex.[57] Further, increased cholinergic activity in the pontine tegmental cholinergic system has been found to accompany unconsciousness caused by concussion.[58,59] A number of rostral structures project to the pontine tegmental nucleus of Gudden.[60] Increased cholinergic activity at this site may contribute to reduced level of alertness, by rostral projections, and to atonia, by descending connections.

Monoaminergic Systems The role of the monoaminergic (noradrenergic, dopaminergic,

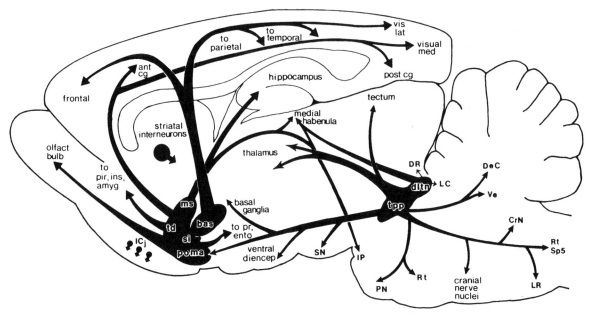

Figure 1-4

Cholinergic pathways, shown in a diagrammatic, generic mammalian brain, play a contributory role in arousal and alertness as components of the ARAS. The basal forebrain complex [medial septal nucleus (ms), diagonal band nuclei (td), substantia innominata (si), and magnocellular preoptic field (poma)] projects to the entire neocortex and allocortex (including hippocampi). The pontomesencephalic complex [pedunculo-pontine (tpp) and laterodorsal (dltn)] tegmental nuclei have ascending projections to the diencephalon, especially the thalamus, and descending pathways to the pontine and medullary reticular formations. (From Cooper et al,[65] with permission.)

and serotonergic) systems in consciousness and higher functions is incompletely understood.

Noradrenergic System Cell bodies are located in the locus ceruleus in the medulla and the lateral tegmental nuclei in the pons and medulla (Fig. 1-5). The locus ceruleus projects to sensory nuclei in the brainstem and diencephalon, especially the dorsal thalamus. Fibers are also sent to the hypothalamus, the basal forebrain, especially the hippocampus, and the neocortex. The lateral tegmental nuclei play a comparatively small role in cerebral function; their projections are mainly to brainstem nuclei and the spinal cord.

Stimulation of the locus ceruleus by sensory inputs leads to burst-firing of neurons in the nucleus. This, in turn, leads to activation of β-adrenergic receptors in the hippocampus, enhancing excitation, though increasing cyclic adenosine monophosphate (AMP) formation and thus inhibiting calcium-mediated potassium conductance. The effect is the opposite in the neocortex, where the activation of α-adrenergic receptors causes the neurons to become hyperpolarized and decrease their rate of spontaneous firing. The net effect is to assist in attending to sudden contrasting or adverse stimuli and to increase the relative response to stimulus-specific stimuli.[61]

Destruction of the locus ceruleus in experimental animals is followed by a modest increase in sleep, but there is no chronic effect on arousal or the EEG.[62]

Figure 1-5
The noradrenergic system. Cell bodies are located in the locus ceruleus (LC) in the medulla and the lateral tegmental nuclei in the pons and medulla. The locus ceruleus projects to the cerebral cortex (CTX), thalamus (TH), sensory nuclei in the brainstem (BS), the pretectal (PT) and tectal (T) areas, and the cerebellum (CER). (From Cooper et al,[65] with permission.)

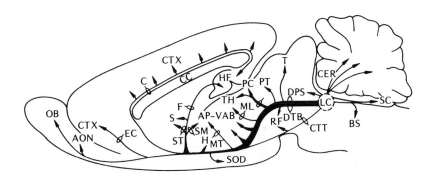

Dopaminergic System The majority of the cell bodies are in the ventral brainstem tegmentum (Fig. 1-6). Projections are grouped into the neostriatal (involved in motor function) and the mesolimbic and mesocortical pathways. The effects of amphetamines (enhanced dopaminergic activity) and antipsychotic drugs (blocked dopaminergic activity) provide some evidence that the dopaminergic system plays a role in cognitive function. There is little evidence that dopamine plays a role

Figure 1-6
The dopaminergic system. The majority of the cell bodies are in the ventral brainstem tegmentum (A8, A9 and A10). Projections are grouped into the neostriatal (involved in motor function) and the mesolimbic and mesocortical pathways. (From Cooper et al,[65] with permission.)

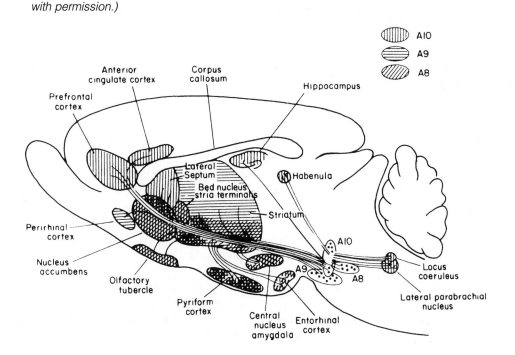

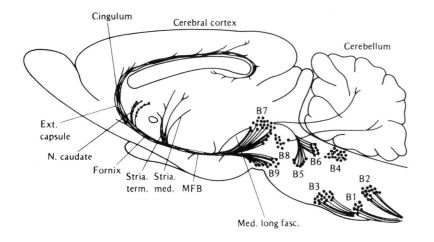

Figure 1-7
The serotonergic system. The cell bodies located in the midline raphe nuclei of the brainstem tegmentum project through the median forebrain bundle to the cerebral cortex and the limbic system, including the pyriform cortex, hypothalamus, hippocampus, and the diencephalon. (From Cooper et al,[65] with permission.)

in arousal, but dopaminergic agonists may produce remarkable improvement in *responsiveness* in certain patients with akinetic mutism, as discussed in the next chapter.

Serotonergic System   The cell bodies located in the midline raphe nuclei of the brainstem tegmentum project through the median forebrain bundle to the cerebral cortex and the limbic system, including the pyriform cortex, hypothalamus, hippocampus, and the diencephalon (Fig. 1-7). Serotonin probably has a net inhibitory function on these neurons: activation of serotonin class 2 (HT2) receptors opens potassium channels, producing neuronal hyperpolarization. Spoont has proposed that the serotonergic system has a stabilizing role in information processing: it inhibits interference when such processing is ongoing.[63] Only signals that are of sufficient intensity and relevance can interfere. In conditions of serotonin deficiency, e.g., alcohol withdrawal, the animal or human is distractible, impulsive, and overreacts. The rostral projection of the serotonergic pathway is also involved in sleep: stimulation inhibits the phasic portion of REM sleep. After destruction of the raphe nucleus, there is insomnia, likely due to the failure of inhibition of waking stimuli.[64] This is typically transient; serotonin appears to have a modulatory role in the wake-sleep cycle.

GABA-nergic Neurons   Neurons that synthesize gamma-aminobutyric acid (GABA) are widely distributed in the central nervous system (CNS). The GABA functions as an inhibitory neurotransmitter in the cerebral cortex, thalamus, basal ganglia, cerebellum, and spinal cord.[65] The physiologic role of GABA in arousal or consciousness is uncertain. Inhibition directly or indirectly allows a "sculpturing" and selecting of information for processing.[66] Nonphysiologic increases in GABA-nergic activity are produced by barbiturates or exogenous or endogenous "ozepines" that facilitate the binding of GABA to its receptor (linked, in turn, to the chloride channel) or that directly act on the GABA receptor (i.e., anesthetic barbiturates, such as thiopental and pentobarbital).[67] This activity is produced in the rostral part of the ARAS. Such actions can produce a marked decrease in alertness and concentration that is blocked by the antagonist flumazenil (see Chap. 18)

Glutamic and Aspartic Acid   Glutamic and aspartic acid are amino acid neurotransmitters that are synthesized in the cortex. They play a key role in the excitatory synaptic activity in the cortex, in corticofugal projections, and in at least some thalamocortical afferent connections.[68] Receptors for glutamate, at least, are of two principal types: a rapidly acting fast type or AMPA (alpha-amino-3-hydroxy-5-methyl-4-isoxazole propionic acid)/

kainate receptor and a slower-responding NMDA (*N*-methyl-D-aspartate) receptor that produces a more sustained depolarization. Although these neurotransmitters probably do not play a role in arousal, they constitute a principal material for cortical-cortical communication.

Peptides and Other Chemicals A complex mixture of peptides, which may function as neuro-transmitters or neuromodulators, exists in the cerebral cortex. These include: vasoactive intestinal polypeptide, cholecystokinin, somatostatin, neuro-peptide Y, and peptides that also serve elsewhere as hormones or releasing factors. In addition, there are receptors, and usually endogenous ligands, for opiates, benzodiazepine-like substances, adeno-sine, and other substances. Their role concerning cortical functions is still unclear, but it is probable that their disturbances or imbalances can signifi-cantly alter cortical function.

Combined Neurochemical Deficits The com-bination of cholinergic and serotonergic receptor blockade produces a global dementia in the rat that mimics decortication, a much more profound effect than that produced by either deficit alone.[69] Although arousal and crude consciousness are intact, the animals are incapable of acquiring and retaining appropriate responses to the environ-ment, e.g., sequential organized behavior.

Anatomic-Pathologic Observations

It has long been known that lesions in various brain regions affect consciousness and alertness. These lesions usually have both local and remote effects: no brain region operates in isolation; dysfunction in one region produces derangement in the function of other regions, even to the point of transsynaptic degeneration in some instances.[70,71] Most knowl-edge concerning humans comes from well-studied cases of stroke. (These are likely more valid than cases of tumor or other disorders in which there is less complete tissue destruction and fewer local effects.) Prior to the advent of magnetic resonance imaging (MRI), the only reliable anatomic infor-mation came from postmortem examinations.

However, high resolution and functional MRI can now reveal areas of infarction or dysfunction in regions of the brainstem that were not reliably examined with computed tomographic (CT) scans and earlier imaging techniques. Observations during the acute phase after stroke are emphasized, but it should be kept in mind that clinical dis-turbances generally do not remain static: patients rarely remain in coma if they survive for many months or years. Wake and sleep cycles usually return or there may be various degrees of respon-siveness or reactivity to the environment.

Brainstem and Diencephalic Disorders Most of the coma-producing ischemic strokes involving the brainstem are related to occlusion of the basilar artery. Chase and colleagues, Kaada and coworkers and Wilkus and colleagues each reported a single case of coma in which the most rostral lesion involved the midpontine tegmentum at the level of the trigeminal outflow.[72-74] The paramedian pontine tegmentum was involved in each case, with minimal damage to tegmental parts of the brainstem more rostrally. Cases selectively involving the basis pontis typically produce the "locked-in" syndrome, in which the patient retains consciousness, but is quadriplegic with severe pseudobulbar palsy below the level of the lesion.[75] The patient retains vertical eye movements that may serve as the only means of communication or behavioral expression. Furthermore, the EEG is essentially normal, with wake and sleep activity and normal posteriorly situated alpha activity that is blocked by eye opening.[76]

Midbrain Coma-producing lesions of the mid-brain are almost invariably associated with thalamic or pontine tegmental damage, or more widespread damage to the cerebral cortex.[71,77] Extensive bilateral destructive lesions of the mid-brain tegmentum and thalamus consistently eliminate the capacity for alerting, however.[78] Transections of the brainstem at the midbrain level result in permanent coma in animals.[79]

Strehler argues that the superior colliculus is an important integrating center for consciousness.[5] The superior colliculus receives afferents from many areas of the cerebral cortex, including the visual, limbic, auditory, and vestibular systems. It projects to the pulvinar of the thalamus, which, in turn, communicates with various cortical regions involved in memory and stored motor and sensory programs.[5] The superior colliculus contains multimodal neurons that might integrate inputs from various sensory pathways and synthesize a three-dimensional map of personal and extrapersonal space.[80]

In humans, the frontal lobe or inferior parietal lobule participate in the prioritization of information and the direction of conscious attention; therefore, these roles cannot be assigned entirely to the superior colliculus. Another argument against the superior colliculus being the main "consciousness center" or "center of self-awareness" is that animals whose superior colliculi are destroyed surgically or chemically are not unconscious.[81] (Since self-awareness cannot be readily assessed in animals, it would be valuable to assess a human with similar restricted lesions.) In attention, the role of the superior colliculus is intimately related to eye movements to the object of interest. If eye movement is *not* made during directed attention, the superior colliculus is silent.[82] Thus, the superior collicular activity is not essential for attention. Furthermore, it is unlikely that the superior colliculi are important in visual awareness as the information transfer from the visual cortex does not use the intertectal commissure connecting the superior colliculi.

Thalamus Among patients with thalamic lesions, only those with bilateral dorsal paramedian lesions have shown coma or impaired arousal responses.[83–87] Conversely, not all patients with bilateral paramedian thalamic lesions are in coma.[88] When coma does occur, it is almost never permanent if the person survives for several weeks or more. Coma-producing lesions often also involve the rostral midbrain, manifested by Parinaud syndrome or paralysis of vertical gaze, especially upgaze.[89] In a clinical-pathologic study of patients with thalamic infarcts, impaired consciousness was a feature in all five of those with bilateral paramedian infarcts. The intralaminar,

parafascicular, medial dorsal, and ventral portions of the centromedian nuclei were affected, but lesions extended into the paramedian midbrain tegmentum in three cases.[87] The mammillothalamic tract was interrupted at least unilaterally in three cases and bilaterally in one. In one case, there was bilateral involvement of the subthalamic and hypothalamic region.

Severe neurologic deficits are almost universal in patients with bilateral paramedian thalamic-rostral midbrain infarction.[85,87,90] These include a permanent, amnestic dementia with impaired attention and apathy.[91,92] Lesions of the thalamus of the dominant hemisphere, usually the left, may produce a persistent verbal amnesia.[93] Right-sided thalamic injuries are sometimes associated with impaired attention and spatial memory, as well as confusion, hallucinations, or delirium.[94]

Cerebral Hemispheres There is surprisingly inconclusive evidence that diffuse cerebral cortical dysfunction in humans causes coma. It is probably not reasonable to base conclusions on experimental studies in animals, especially lower nonprimates, as the relative functions of the cerebral cortex may differ from those of humans. In human cases, dysfunction is rarely, if ever, purely cortical. Lesions often involve other sites. In addition, dysfunction of the cortex has profound influences on numerous subcortical regions; loss of this influence may impair their function by "diaschisis," described below.[70]

Diaschisis was developed as an hypothesis to explain the recovery of function after an insult to the brain. Von Monakow[95] described the four main components of diaschisis:

1. Damage to one brain area can, by loss of excitation, produce loss of function in regions adjacent to, or remote from, but connected to the primary site of damage ... may be regarded as a "shock" confined to distinct nervous structures ....

2. Diaschisis is a clinical diagnosis whose presumptive mechanism was loss of excitation to intact regions (rather than inhibition).

3. Diaschisis undergoes gradual regression in well-defined phases, such that the resolution will parallel resumption of function in areas of diaschisis.

4. The "wave of diaschisis" follows neuroanatomical pathways spreading from the site of injury. There are three kinds:

a. Diaschisis cortico-spinalis: progression from a motor cortex injury to the spinal cord along the pyramidal tracts.

b. Diaschisis commissuralis: functional contralateral cortical depression via axons of the corpus callosum following injury to the cortex of one hemisphere.

c. Diaschisis associativa: intracortical fiber-mediated depression of function in intact cortical areas neighboring the locus of injury.

There is some support for diaschisis with thalamic lesions: EEG and PET studies show slowing and decreased metabolism, respectively, in large cortical areas after lesions of the thalamus.[96,97] At least for the EEG, this involves primarily the intralaminar, medial dorsal, ventral anterior, and reticular nuclei. Thalamic lesions in animals and humans also induce mild contralateral cortical metabolic depression that likely relates to transcallosal effects of second-order neurons.[98]

The evidence is incomplete for transcallosal diaschisis.[99] However:

1. A lesion in the brain may cause transient retrograde reactions in, e.g., the locus ceruleus, to cause widespread dysfunction in the projection of that nucleus.

2. Experimentally, right middle cerebral artery ischemia causes transcallosal physiologic changes. The depressed noradrenaline may play a role.

For regions of ipsilateral cerebral cortex the evidence is controversial.[70] There are, however, subcortical effects of cerebral cortical lesions: for example, frontal lesions produce hypometabolism in the pallidum and several other structures, an effect that is reversed by amphetamine.

Clinically, one not infrequently observes that acute, unilateral, especially left or dominant, cerebral dysfunction produces transient coma or unresponsiveness. Serefetinides and colleagues found that, following left internal carotid artery injections of amobarbital, patients became globally unresponsive.[100] Similarly, patients with large left middle cerebral artery territory damage often have reduced arousal; in contrast, this is infrequent in patients with nondominant hemisphere lesions of comparable size and territory.[101,102] These observations have not been subjected to rigorous study.

Attention

Moscovitch has defined attention as "a control process that enables the individual to select, from a number of alternatives, the task he will perform or the stimulus he will process, and the cognitive strategy he will adopt to carry out these operations."[103] As a prerequisite, the individual must be awake and alert. Attention's main features include directivity and selectivity of mental processes.

There is a close physiologic, relationship among alertness, attention, and perception. Stimulation of the ARAS facilitates the ability to perceive differences between competing stimuli.[33] In addition, the brain can attenuate sensory input that is not novel or relevant. For example, in *habituation*, the amplitude of evoked cerebral responses to continued, repetitive, monotonous stimuli is reduced compared with the initial response. This attenuated response is found not only at the cortex but also all the way down to the receptor level. The "lower centers" are likely affected by inhibitory pathways from the brainstem reticular formation. Conversely, repeated stimuli that are relevant (e.g., flashes of light or tone pips that the individual is instructed to count) are associated with a constant or even enhanced response. It seems likely that a central analyzer or comparator weights the relevance and novelty of stimuli to determine whether they should be inhibited, maintained, or facilitated.

Structures involved in attention have been studied with microelectrode recordings in animal models and with PET scans and functional MRI.[104] Using these methods, it has been found that the frontal lobes, especially the anterior cingulate gyrus, are involved in a wide range of activities involving attention and discrimination of stimuli requiring making choices of response.[105,106] Specific coinvolved regions varied with different tasks. These include the left frontal language areas when subjects define nouns, and the pre-striate (visual association) areas when a response to a color is required. In addition, different regions of the anterior cingulate cortex are activated in oculomotor, manual, or speech tasks, as measured with PET studies.[107] The *degree* of activation of the anterior cingulate is proportional to the complexity and novelty of the task, and decreases with practice. The anterior cingulate region is thus involved in higher order motor control of a large number of tasks. It may, by means of its connections, be the most likely site of "critically effective neurons," proposed by Eccles, that are related to conscious-ness, decision making, and will.[108]

Closely related to the anterior cingulate's role in directing tasks is the role of the dorsolateral prefrontal cortex in "working memory." Working memory involves short-term retention of a limited number of items that are held in consciousness for immediate use with ongoing tasks. Lesions of this region produce impaired performance of delayed recognition tasks, tasks in which the individual has to determine the relative recency of various stimuli, as well as exercises involving frequency estimates and self-ordered recall.[109,110] It appears that frontal lesions do not cause classic amnesia as described below, but can affect attentional and organiza-tional steps that are required for later processing in long-term memory.

The parietal regions are also important in tasks that involve attention. The right parietal lobe is concerned with attention to both visual fields, while the left is more restricted to the right visual field.[111] The pulvinar of the thalamus is also involved in selecting information for attention.[105]

Unilateral lesions of the mesencephalic tegmentum can result in neglect of contralateral hemispace, possibly because of diminished "activa-tion" of more rostral structures.[112] The reticular thalamic nucleus performs a gating function on sensory relay or "activation" of the cerebral cortex. Mesencephalic lesions may prevent the deactiva-tion of the reticular nucleus, so that its inhibitory tone prevails.

Lesions of the thalamic relay nuclei or the primary sensory areas cause sensory loss rather than neglect. Dysfunction of polymodal sensory areas, especially that in the inferior parietal lobule, produces profound neglect of contralateral hemi-space.[113,114] This area is a region of convergence of multiple sensory inputs and has limbic connections. It thus serves as an important cerebral center for sensory attention.

The dorsolateral prefrontal region has im-portant connections that underlie its roles in atten-tion and intention: multimodal sensory areas (including the inferior parietal lobule), the cingu-late gyrus (part of the limbic system), the basal ganglia and subcortical thalamic nuclei that are components of the ARAS [especially the centro-median and parafascicular (CM-Pf) nuclei], and projections of brainstem neurotransmitter pathways.[115] Motor inattention results from lesions of the dorsolateral frontal region. Watson and colleagues showed that such lesions prevent a motor response to a stimulus in contralateral hemi-space, even though the monkey was trained to make a response with the limb contralateral to the stimulus or ipsilateral to the lesion (i.e., it could not be explained by weakness). Akinetic mutism, a condition in which the animal appears awake, but does not respond to stimuli, can be produced by lesions of the CM-Pf nuclei.[112]

An individual can be awake yet show impair-ment of consciousness if attention is seriously compromised. This can range from the acute con-fusional state through "akinetic mutism" to the "persistent vegetative state," also known as "coma vigil."[116] This is discussed in detail in the next chapter.

Even if the posterior aspects of the hemi-spheres are functioning well enough for the initial processing of, for example, visual information, inattention prevents full appreciation of its signifi-cance (e.g., comprehension of a written passage) and often precludes the initiation of a response or the ability to act other than reflexly. A separate type of abnormal attention is that in which the patient is unable to change the "mind set" sufficiently to attend and adjust to a changing paradigm (e.g., the Wisconsin card-sorting test), so that the patient perseverates (inappropriately continues) in the same task.[110,117]

Attention in the domain of the visual system has been extensively studied. The three main structures are the frontal eye fields, the posterior parietal cortex, and the superior colliculi. When a monkey makes a saccadic eye movement towards an object of interest, neurons in these three areas discharge prior to the movement.[118] This only occurs when the object is of interest and lies in the receptive field. If the animal has to attend to a large visual stimulus (e.g., a fading light source) towards which it does *not* make an eye movement, only neurons in the posterior parietal region fire; those in the frontal eye field and the superior colliculus remain silent.[82] Thus, those neurons in the posterior parietal region are dissociated from the eye movement associated with visual attention. The frontal eye fields and superior colliculus are involved in the motor aspect of attentional activity.

Macroelectrophysiologic studies using EEG and evoked responses also give insight into attentional mechanisms. A 40-Hz cortical rhythm has been described with attention (alluded to earlier and further discussed below).[119] Surface negative shifts in electric potentials are found over the frontal sagittal region in response to attention to stimuli of various modalities (visual, auditory, or somatic).[120] Knight and colleagues found an asymmetry in this response, in that the right frontal lobe was involved with stimuli from either side, while the left frontal lobe only attended to stimuli from the right hemispace.[121] The P300 potential is a positive DC shift that occurs approximately 300 ms after the detection of a novel stimulus to which the subject has been instructed to attend. Although the P300 lies over the parietal cortex, it is likely generated deep to it.[122] Halgren and colleagues have localized its origin to the vicinity of the hippocampus, based on reversals of polarity in this region.[123] However, since polarity reversals have also been noted in the thalamus and

periaqueductal gray matter, it is likely that several regions are coactivated to produce the P300 or produce different potentials of similar latency.[124]

Some general observations on the neurochemical basis for attention are of interest. The dopaminergic system is important in attentional responses. Marshall and colleagues have shown that damage to the nigrostriatal projection, especially the caudate-putamen dopaminergic terminals or receptors, produces behavioral inattention to contralateral stimuli in the rat.[125] The noradrenergic system is important in maintaining attention on a task or stimulus. Rats with bilateral damage to the locus ceruleus–forebrain projection are more easily distracted than control rats while performing a motor task.[126] The right frontal lobe of primates receives an important projection from the locus ceruleus; the posterior visual areas involved in visual attention also have noradrenergic input.[105]

In summary, brain structures that are required to generate attention are the anterior cingulate gyrus, the dorsolateral prefrontal cortex, the inferior parietal lobule, the CM-Pf thalamic nuclei, the thalamic reticular nucleus, the reticular formation of the midbrain tegmentum, and (possibly) the superior colliculus. Connections of the inferior parietal lobule and frontal regions with the limbic system (especially the cingulate gyrus) and projection pathways of the subcortical noradrenergic systems are also involved.

Sensation and Perception

Sensation involves the awareness of something happening to the individual as a result of a stimulus acting on a sensory receptor.[8] The five traditional primary sensory modalities are visual, auditory, somatosensory, olfactory, and gustatory. However, there are others, including a vestibular sense of movement, visceral sensations, etc. Sensations have pathways of conduction in the CNS and primary cerebral cortical receiving areas. All but olfactory sensation have a thalamic relay. Sensations have temporal (timing relative to the present) and spatial (reflecting the part of the body affected) characteristics and are modality-specific (e.g., visual sensation is distinct from somatosensory stimulation, even if both refer to the same extra-personal object). Humphrey argues that sensation is possible because of reverberating central circuits that allow the sensation to be retained in the brain.[8] Sensations can be then linked with memory and affect to allow recognition and appreciation of their significance. Humphrey maintains that sensation is the fundamental, universal essence of consciousness and can occur without higher order cognitive reasoning (*Sentio, ergo sum:* I feel, therefore, I exist).[8]

Perception involves the appropriate processing of sensory information, allowing a concept of what is happening in the external world.[8] Attention forms a component of perception, in that it accounts for the selection and directed concentration on processing certain information with the exclusion of other competing stimuli or data. Many higher order activities take place in the CNS without conscious perception. Thus, in the studies of Hubel and Wiesel, hypercomplex cells in the visual cortex could be identified by their functional properties while animals were under general anesthesia.[127] Resultant behavior may not always be consciously directed or driven.

Sensation and perception appear to be parallel but interdependent activities.[8] Sensation is necessary to allow for conscious appreciation. Usually, perception will override sensation when both are present, such that we are less aware of what is happening to ourselves than our interpretation of what is happening in the outside world.

Conscious sensation and perception require alertness and a focusing of attention or concentration. What system is devoted to the selective activity manifested in awareness?

It is instructive to review sensory processing in the brain, then the insights given from lesions, followed by sensorimotor integration.

Sensory Processing

The visual system (Fig. 1-8) is the best understood sensory processing system. This begins at the retina, which is functionally organized into concentric receptive fields. "On center" fields produce maximal discharge of ganglion cells when the light stimulus fills the inner part of the field. A circular zone surrounding this region causes inhibition of firing. Obversely, fields with "off center" and "on surround" also exist. There are different types and sizes of receptive fields, e.g., fields with sustained or transient trains of discharges. This arrangement simplifies the response patterns from the millions of retinal neurons to a few basic ones.

The projections from the retina to the hypothalamus represent the next organizational level after the retina itself. The response to illumination regulates the secretion of melatonin. This does not involve the geniculate pathways or cerebral cortex. Such activity goes on below conscious awareness, but does allow the organism to adapt wake and sleep cycles to changes in environmental illumination.

A parallel lower level system of visual processing requires the integrity of the extrageniculate nuclei, allowing the pupillary light reflex, the photic blink reflex, and opticokinetic nystagmus. This system, like the hypothalamic projection, functions in comatose patients. Neither system's activity achieves conscious awareness, but both have some protective value for the organism.

The primary visual area, area 17 or V1, contains neurons that respond to oriented bars of light. Sensory information then fans out through cortical-cortical connections from the primary sensory cortex to association cortex. In the visual system, over 25 visual areas have been identified.[128] The information appears to flow in separate but interacting series of connections from the primary to secondary visual areas and then to higher levels of processing. In general, information is processed by (1) converging feedforward projections from lower to higher levels (this allows for abstraction or separation of certain common properties of visual information); (2) recruitment of lateral connections within the cortex, to compensate for any loss of input from certain cells; and (3) synchronization of neuronal responses and tagging of lower level cell activity by re-entrant signals from higher levels (this activity may play a role in the perceptual

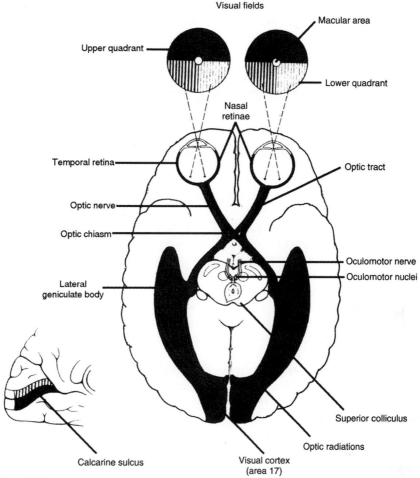

Figure 1-8

The visual pathways from the ventral surface of the brain. The visual fields of each eye are depicted by the circles. The images are inverted and reversed in the eyes. This theme is carried posteriorly. Information regarding the left visual field is conveyed to the right occipital region (see inset), with the dorsal part being represented in the dorsal bank of the calcarine sulcus. (Redrawn from Carpenter MB, Sutin J, Human Neuroanatomy, 8th ed, Baltimore, Williams and Wilkins, 1983, with permission.)

separation of an object in motion from its background).[129]

There are both forward and backward interconnections between the various regions; i.e., the system is not a one-way hierarchic system from primary sensory cortex to other regions without considerable interaction involved in processing. Serial (hierarchic) and parallel processing of information both occur.

Perception

The next level still does not involve conscious awareness, but can alter behavioral responses. Lesions that destroy or isolate the primary visual cortex, but spare the extrageniculostriate and the extrastriate cortical areas, allow some reactions to "unseen" visual stimuli. This is referred to as "blindsight."[130] Such individuals can make accurate projections into a visual field for which there is no sensation of vision, but deny conscious awareness of the existence of the object in extrapersonal space. Experimentally, responses in the hemianopic field interfere with simultaneous stimuli applied to the intact field; in "forced choice" paradigms, the responses are better than chance. Thus, there is an effect on conscious activity even though the stimuli do not achieve conscious perception.

Higher levels of visual processing do achieve conscious perception. The lowest level of perception appears to be the appreciation of "qualia" or certain discrete properties, such as wavelength of light (color) or luminance intensity.[131] There is at least an awareness of this, even though it is a crude or fundamental perception, requiring integrity of the visual pathway up to and including the primary visual cortex, also called V1 or area 17.[132] At this level, however, there is no "object vision." Object vision involves the ability to segment the image into background and foreground and to fuse the impressions into shapes and objects. Patients who cannot do this are suffering from apperceptive visual agnosia and usually have lesions involving the extrastriate cortex bordering on, but sparing V1 and V2. Formulating background from fore-around, or grouping parts of images, and higher ordering visual processes rest on the integrity of qualia as serial processing, according to Stoerig, who argues that there are no cases of visual agnosia with intact qualia perception.[131] There is a dissociation, however, from some primary visual defects, i.e., some qualia may be missing.

The effects of occipital lesions further our understanding of the relative roles of these regions in visual perception. For example, cortical color blindness results from lesions of a discrete part of area 19; a lesion in area 19 may also lead to reduced perception of movement (akinetopsia). Thus, area 19 is intimately involved in the appreciation of color and movement. It is, however, more difficult to decide whether color and movement are "perceived" there.

The next level of conscious vision is that of object recognition, a complex process involving the primary visual cortex, visual association areas, and reciprocal connections with memory stores.[133] It is likely that meaning and significance are given to parallel and serially processed sensory information by feedback and feedforward connections involving multiple hierarchic levels.

Temporal aspects of awareness are worth considering before proceeding. Awareness without detection occurs with central somatosensory thalamic stimulation in humans. Libet and colleagues report that thalamic stimulation usually must last over 500 ms to achieve conscious detection, even though subjects can indicate that they were stimulated in a forced choice paradigm.[134] There is an intermediate state of partial awareness with some stimuli of under 500 ms; the transition from detection without awareness to detection with awareness is not an abrupt change. This somewhat variable temporal threshold may have some value with respect to attending to stimuli that last longer and are more important for behavioral decision making. Longer duration stimuli are processed to greater degrees.

The awareness of time itself is dependent on the growth and decay of perceptions and stored abstractions in the memory.[135] Since time, 500 ms or longer, is required for perception, the awareness of the present is likely to be an averaged series of very recent events from the immediate past.

Individuals with lesions in certain cortical areas may have selective associative agnosias. Agnosias are failures of perception, despite preservation of at least some sensation. A good example is prosopagnosia, the failure to recognize faces with which the patient was familiar. Such lesions usually involve the inferior temporal regions. Even though the patient knows the image is a face and can discriminate it from the background, he/she is unable to recognize the individual. There is still debate as to the level of dysfunction, i.e., does the problem lie with (1) basic sensations and early processing (e.g., perception of simple forms); (2) synthesizing sensations to produce a *Gestalt* or concept; or (3) linking sensations to stored memories?[136] For example, larger lesions affecting multiple prestriate regions bilaterally may cause a visual agnosia such as simultagnosia, in which the patient cannot synthesize the information into a general shape (e.g., a hamburger), but may perceive lines and/or parts of the object.

As an aside, it is worth discussing the somewhat related "neglect syndromes," in which there is loss of conscious awareness of primary sensory stimuli in the presence of intact sensory pathways. These are most common in parietal or frontal lesions. Unilateral neglect with nondominant parietal lesions can extend from the person to extrapersonal space. The person may fail to wash the left side of the body, to comb the hair or shave on the left side, and may wear a glove only on the right hand. There may be decreased associated movements of the left limbs for simple tasks, even though there is no paresis.[137] This disordered "body image" may relate to an interruption of sensory processing that moves from primary sensations to hierarchic processing in the parietal and frontal lobes. The highest level of modeling of self and extrapersonal space is reflected in goals and behavior. Presumably, neglect as described above relates to disrupted processing at an intermediate level.[138]

The next phase of processing involves the *use* that is made of the visual information, or perceptual-motor integration. Examples include verbally describing what is seen, reading aloud, or hitting a ball with a bat. This relies on the integrity of pathways and structures that link vision, memory, and motor systems, as discussed below.

Perceptual-Motor Integration

Stimulus processing refers to various learning paradigms that can function independently of each other, e.g., different memory systems for different sensory inputs.[139] Patients with right parietal lesions characteristically show reduced awareness of visual stimuli presented to the contralateral hemifield, especially if a competing stimulus is simultaneously presented in the hemifield on the side of the lesion. In one tachistoscopic study in which stimuli were flashed separately or simultaneously onto both hemifields, patients often neglected the left-field stimulus when they *verbally* reported their experience. However, when they

registered their observations *manually* (by pressing buttons), they reported the left-field stimuli significantly less than with verbal reporting.[140] Thus, it appears that there are different pathways or mechanisms for sensorimotor integration.

Neglect also shows a spatial continuum rather than abrupt transitions. Patients with nondominant lesions tend to bisect a horizontal line at a point to the right of center. If a mirror is used so that movements appear to be in the opposite direction, the error rate decreases, especially in patients with right frontal lesions. Perceptual and premotor processing are probably both involved in performing this task. A further distinction between the perceptual and premotor components of a task was shown by a test in which the images were reversed by using a mirror, so that the lines on the left of the midline were projected to the left cerebrum. When subjects were asked to cross out lines, some crossed out lines projected to the left hemisphere, but they performed the act in the left side of hemispace. These individuals had parietal perceptual problems, while those who could not operate in left hemispace and crossed out lines on the opposite side had premotor deficits. Such directional "hypokinesia" is a feature of lesions affecting the frontal lobe or basal ganglia.[141]

The Issue of Self-Awareness

The mechanisms for *self-awareness* of one's own perceptions of the external environment, one's own body and, more introspectively, of one's own thoughts have not been adequately explained, but there is now hope for a more scientific approach through the study of perception, discussed above.[10]

Numerous models have been proposed. The "Cartesian theater," a limited-capacity mechanism in which personal experiences are represented in the brain and then viewed, still allows a "mind-brain dichotomy." Further, a "single locus of awareness" has not been adequately supported by anatomic or physiologic studies. (As Posner points out, the anterior cingulate gyrus comes closest to this when it comes to attention.[105]) Instead of a "center," parallel processing of information is performed by a network of numerous interconnected modular processors across vast regions of cerebral cortex; these have also reciprocal connections with subcortical structures. To formulate a unifying hypothesis, Kinsbourne proposed a "dominant neuronal action pattern" or "dominant focus": the phenomenon represented by the most widespread coded neuronal activity is the one that achieves consciousness at that time.[142] Some phenomena, e.g., pain, may have a powerful overriding influence. A dominant focus is one that drives other regions in synchronous neuronal firing or rhythms. If this reaches a critical size, it is perceived as consciousness.

A "limited-capacity system" may allow for the limited amount of information we can attend to and hold in the working memory at any one time. Working memory, probably a frontal lobe function, is a very short-term memory that allows us to perform acts in continuity.[143] Baars proposes that the brain works in a manner similar to "global workspace" computer models, allowing competition of a number of parallel processes.[144] The selected activities achieve conscious awareness. He proposes that the reticular activating system of the brainstem and the reticular nucleus of the thalamus are examples of biologic systems that work on this principle; these together, plus other systems, e.g., cortical parietal and temporal regions, may be necessary and sufficient for this model.

While networking of brain regions is necessary, aspects of self-awareness are probably not diffusely and homogeneously distributed throughout the brain. Lesions of the frontal, inferior parietal, and superior temporal regions disturb the integration of cognitive and affective components of awareness. The recognition and awareness of *parts* of one's self or the environment may be seriously compromised, at least acutely, by nondominant parietal lesions that are often accompanied by hemianopsia, disorientation, mood disorder, and impaired abstract reasoning.[145] Lesions of primary sensory areas in themselves usually do not cause such loss of awareness of the body, space, or of the deficit itself. Lesions of multimodal processing regions are probably key regions.[146]

Motivational System

Motivation refers to underlying drives that help determine behavior, once the person or animal has attended to the stimulus and assessed its significance relevant to competing internal or external factors. The motivational system of the brain relates, at least in part, to emotions and is closely allied to crude consciousness, perception, goal-directed activity, and responses to the environment. The hypothalamus plays a major role in the outward expressions that we use as indicators of emotion: autonomic phenomena and some display behaviors. This small diencephalic structure receives afferents from various parts of the brain, including other components of the limbic system (both the amygdala-diencephalon and hippocampal-forniceal-mammillary subdivisions), the cerebral cortex, and the reticular formation. The hypothalamus is also sensitive to the internal milieu of the body and is largely responsible for maintaining homeostasis through endocrine, autonomic, and motivational behavior. The diverse functions of the hypothalamus are related to the "final pathways" for various activities of importance to the organism. Such phenomena can be produced by direct stimulation or ablation of parts of the hypothalamus, but these are not accompanied by subjective emotional experiences.[147] Thus, the hypothalamus is hardly the key structure for the production of emotional motivation or "emotional cognition."[148]

More important structures in the generation of internal feelings and motivation are the amygdala, hippocampus, and associated limbic structures. The hippocampus and amygdala on each side of the brain receive parallel-convergent projections from the various sensory systems. The hippocampus consolidates the information into the memory and accesses stores of recent memory in the neocortex.[149] The amygdala, by its connections with various cortical structures, gives the sensory information an affective and experiential tone, as well as the "expression" of emotion through its connections with the hypothalamus.[150] Other limbic structures also play a role in emotional experience and behavior. Lesions of the posterior insula cause "pain asymboli," in which painful stimuli are not emotionally perceived or acted upon.[151] This may relate to a disruption in the multisynaptic connections between the limbic system and the neocortex.

Thus, "emotional cognition," including motivation, depends upon a network of structures, limbic and nonlimbic, and neurotransmitter systems, and cannot be isolated to a single, independent entity.

MEMORY

Memory has numerous links to other aspects of brain function that help to determine awake behavior and provides references used in decision-making. Memory consists of certain mental processes that are involved in information storage and retrieval. An individual without memory would not be considered to be "unconscious," in that alertness is preserved and he/she interacts with the environment in a responsive manner. However, an important component of mental activity, that which allows the linking of past and present, is missing. Memory is vital to the meaningful interpretation of the present. Full appreciation depends on matching the present experience with even a short-term representation.[152] The person without a current memory is "isolated in a single moment of being, with a moat of lacuna of forgetting all around him.... He is man without past (or future), stuck in a constantly changing, meaningless moment."[153]

Memory functions consist of: (1) *Input*: this includes sensory processing, short-term storage, acquisition processes (encoding, elaborating, establishing associations, etc.), and long-term storage. The latter is what we commonly think of as memory, i.e., a knowledge base of well-established and stored material from any time in the past. (2) *Output*: this comprises retrieval and recital of the learned material.

Memory can be classified in different ways. One classification includes declarative memory (memory that is directly accessible to conscious retrieval, manipulation, and expression, e.g., verbal and non-verbal learned facts re: the multiplication table and recognition of objects, respectively), dependent on hippocampal function for retention and/or recall, and procedural memory (usually learned motor skills and some conditioned responses), likely dependent on extrahippocampal sites.[154]

In discussing the anatomy of declarative memory, we shall concentrate on the structures involved in the ongoing storage and encoding of memory. Damage to these regions is manifest principally by anterograde amnesia, i.e., the inability to lay down new, declarative, long-term memories. Two principal structural units have long been recognized: the hippocampal system and the diencephalic or medial dorsal thalamic system.

Hippocampal System

Several clinical studies have documented that bilateral damage to the mesial temporal structures leads to permanent loss of the ability to commit new declarative material to long-term memory storage. The most notable is that of patient H.M. who, in 1953, had bilateral resection of the most rostral 8 cm of both medial temporal lobes to control seizures.[155] This resulted in severe global anterograde amnesia that has persisted to this day. Interestingly, his memories from before age 16, the time of onset of his seizures, are preserved. Thus, the hippocampi appear to play a more important role in the acquisition of new memories than in the recall of older stored memory.

One of the most precise localizations for a vital part of the medial temporal region is the case reported by Zola-Morgan et al.[156] This patient had suffered a cardiac arrest, followed by a profound amnestic syndrome in which he could not lay down new memories. He died several years later and was found to have selective damage to the CA1 region of the hippocampus bilaterally (see Fig. 1-9), as the only damaged limbic structure.

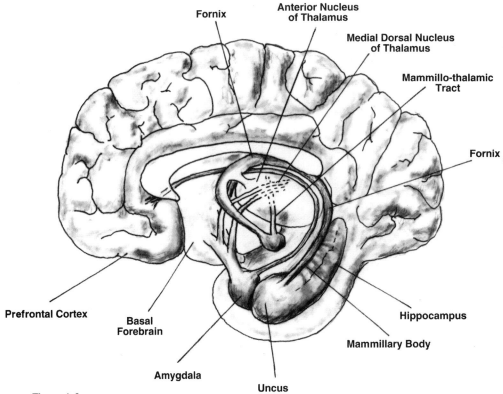

Figure 1-9

The principal components of the limbic system. The amygdala projects to the magno-cellular part of the medial dorsal nucleus of the thalamus, which also receives an input from the orbital surface of the frontal lobe. The hippocampus projects by way of the fornix to the mammillary body which, in turn, communicates with the anterior thalamic nucleus via the mammillothalamic tract.

Diencephalon

The prototypic clinical disorder for thalamic amnesia is Korsakoff syndrome, in which there is a loss of anterograde declarative memory. Other less consistent features include confabulation and a polyneuropathy. It has been shown that the condition is due to a deficiency of thiamine.[157] Victor and colleagues observed that the medial dorsal nuclei of the thalamus and the mammillary bodies were consistently necrotic in patients with amnesia.[157] However, some patients who were not amnestic had only mammillary body necrosis. Thus, it appeared that the medial dorsal nuclei of the thalamus were the key structures responsible for the memory loss. This has been supported by other cases of tumors or strokes in which a memory defect has occurred with damage to the medial dorsal thalamus, sparing the mammillary bodies.[158–160] The mammillothalamic tract is often involved with these lesions. Other neighboring structures in the dorsal medial thalamus, e.g., the parataenial nucleus, may also be affected.[161] Thus, the evidence is very suggestive but not conclusive that damage to the medial dorsal thalamic nuclei is necessary for this amnestic syndrome.

Newer Concepts in the Anatomy of Memory

Studies on memory in animals have been difficult, because the verbal memory function of the human cannot be duplicated. However, some strategies, especially the delayed nonmatching-to-sample (DNMS) tests, have been useful.[162,163] In this test, a sample object is shown to the animal. The object is removed from view and later reintroduced, accompanied by a novel object. The food reward lies under the new object. The animal is allowed to discover this, then the objects are removed. The previous object is then reintroduced accompanied by a new novel object under which lies the food reward. The objects are again removed and, after a delay, two more objects are introduced: again, the last "novel" object and a newer object under which the food lies. Thus, the animal has to remember the object from the previous trial and to look under the truly novel object in each trial to get the food.

Using this testing procedure, the effects of lesions on learning can be observed. A more precise production and determination of lesions is possible than occurs with disease in humans. With this paradigm, it has been found that lesions confined to the hippocampi have only a mild effect on DNMS; if there is an additional lesion in the amygdala, the effect on memory is much more marked.[164] Similarly, when the fornices (the main projection pathway from the hippocampus) are lesioned along with the amygdala outflow, the amnesia is profound, while it is mild when either structure is separately lesioned.[165] Similarly, with bilateral lesions confined to the dorsal medial nucleus of the thalamus, the effect on this specific type of memory is mild.[166] Lesions that include both the anterior (including the anterior nucleus of the thalamus to which the mammillothalamic tract projects) and the posterior medial thalamus produce profound amnesia.[166]

As shown in Fig. 1-9, the amygdala projects to the magnocellular part of the medial dorsal nucleus of the thalamus, which also receives an input from the orbital surface of the frontal lobe. The hippocampus projects by way of the fornix to the mammillary body which, in turn, communicates with the anterior thalamic nucleus via the mammillothalamic tract. Further anatomic, studies have shown a link between the hippocampal-forniceal–mammillo-anterior thalamic and the amygdalo–medial dorsal thalamic systems. There are direct connections between the amygdala and the hippocampus and indirect ones throughout the entorhinal cortex.[167] Thus, one should consider there to be two interconnected systems that are responsible for ongoing anterograde memory functions.

Newer yet are observations of the relative importance of the perirhinal-entorhinal cortices and the hippocampi. Zola-Morgan and colleagues produced *transient* disturbances in memory functions in primates with bilateral lesions of the entorhinal cortex in the anterior temporal neocortex, anterior to the hippocampus.[168] They also showed that damage to this region exacerbates memory impairment following lesions to the hippocampal formation.[169] Thus, the anterior temporal region plays a contributory role in learning. By itself, it is not essential for learning or performance.

Neurochemistry of Long-Term Memory

There are a number of facts that argue for an important role of the putative neurotransmitter acetylcholine in memory function: (1) limbic and paralimbic regions receive a richer supply of cholinergic fibers than other cortical regions;[170] (2) scopolamine causes a loss of memory function that resembles the memory loss found in the early stage of demential illnesses;[171] (3) ablations of CH4, the region of the nucleus basalis that provides cholinergic innervation to the amygdala and cerebral cortex, leads to impaired memory function;[172] (4) loss of cholinergic neurons occurs in the nucleus basalis of Meynert in Alzheimer disease[173]; and (5) some memory and cognitive functions improve in a subgroup of patients with Alzheimer disease being treated with tetrahydroaminoacridine, a reversible inhibitor of acetylcholinesterase, the enzyme that degrades acetylcholine.[174] The role of cholinergic pathways in controlling alertness, and its role in nonspecifically altering the hippocampal theta rhythm, led some workers to propose that the cholinergic system acts as a gating mechanism for the retention of memories by the controlling sensory-limbic interactions and alertness.[175]

In Korsakoff syndrome, some workers have found a decrease in noradrenergic activity, reflected in lower than normal concentrations of the noradrenergic metabolite, 3-methoxy-4-hydroxyphenylglycol (MHPG) in the CSF.[176] Further, others have reported decreased numbers of neurons in the locus ceruleus.[177] Thiamine-depleted rats have shown decreased noradrenergic content in various brain regions and increased concentration of 5-hydroxyindoleacetic acid (5-HIAA, the major metabolite of serotonin) in the thalamus and midbrain.[178] Levels of dopamine, its metabolites, and acetylcholine were not abnormal.[179] Patients with Korsakoff syndrome being treated with clonidine, an α_2-noradrenergic agonist, showed significant improvement in a number of memory subtests, as did patients being treated with methysergide, a serotonin receptor antagonist.[180] Whether the effects were due to altered limbic, especially diencephalic, memory functions has yet to be resolved. Arnsten and Goldman-Rakic have argued that the effects are due to reduced attention rather than a fundamental effect on memory function.[181] In any case, it is of great interest that alterations in the monoaminergic systems may play a role in the pathogenesis and potential therapy in this disorder.

Other Memory Systems

Previously Stored Declarative/Semantic Memory Memories laid down prior to hippocampal lesions may be retained; these must be stored in parts of the brain other than the medial temporal regions. Since some patients with diencephalic lesions also retain or can reactivate previous memories, these are not likely represented solely in the diencephalon. Most likely, neocortical sites are used, e.g., the temporal or parietal neocortex.[182,183]

Implicit Memory Implicit memory refers to the effect of a past event on current experience or behavior. The effects are implicit in the actions of the individual. Often, there is "implicit perception," in which the event/emotion/other phenomenon is not consciously detected.[184] Implicit

learning and effect on behavior (memory) can be spared when explicit (declarative) memory is severely affected; there is a legitimate distinction between these two forms of memory.

Implicit memory can modify declarative knowledge and working memory. It can contribute to self-image and thus play a role in emotions expressed when an event triggers a response; behavioral and physiologic consequences follow.[185]

Cognition

Cognition, like consciousness, is difficult to define satisfactorily. Thought is dependent on all the components of consciousness discussed above and includes an awareness of the cognitive activity, as well. There is a synthesizing role in which the prioritized, processed, sensory information, relevant memories, and motivational input are combined on a background of alertness, attention, and concentration to make discriminative, often sequential, decisions that are passed to the motor system for action. Cognition is varied in its brain components, depending on the nature of the operation; for example, the dominant cerebral hemisphere will play a greater role in language or mathematics-related issues, while the nondominant hemisphere will predominate in visuospatial and most musical tasks.[186] The frontal lobes undoubtedly play an executive role in most cognitive activity, in terms of prioritizing and directing these processes.

SOME CLINICAL CONSIDERATIONS

The following clinical cases are examples of common issues regarding the nature of consciousness:

Case 1
A 53-year-old man with a past history of hypertension is brought to the emergency room by ambulance. His wife observes him to collapse while using a rowing machine. His eyes are closed; he has Cheyne-Stokes respirations and shows spontaneous

decerebrate posturing. Similar posturing follows the application of pressure to his nailbeds. His pupils are 6 mm and unreactive to light. Corneal reflexes are absent. Tonic lateral deviation of the ipsilateral eye occurs following the injection of ice water into each ear canal separately with the head elevated at 30°. The left fundus shows a subhyaloid hemorrhage. A CT scan shows hemorrhage into the third ventricle and rostral midbrain. The patient later loses all cranial nerve reflexes and is totally immobile, unresponsive to stimulation. No breathing movements are seen, despite an arterial carbon dioxide concentration (Pa_{CO_2}) of 70 mmHg, after the patient is disconnected from the ventilator while administering oxygen through a tracheal cannula. These findings are consistent when the patient is reviewed 6 h later.

This patient, who suffered an intracranial hemorrhage from a ruptured intracranial aneurysm, was in coma, an unarousable, unresponsive, unconscious state. At no time was there any apparent alertness, awareness, or responsiveness. There was clearly a loss of "crude consciousness" or alertness that is necessary for awareness of self or the environment. Clinically, he showed evidence of rostral brainstem impairment and later progressed to brain death, *coma depassé* (the "state beyond coma"). Brain death is reviewed in greater detail in the next chapter.

Case 2

A 30-year-old man with a history of epilepsy is waiting for an interview. Others observe him to pause, to stare, and then to rise from his chair. He picks up several magazines from the table and walks from person to person in the waiting room, offering each individual a magazine. The observer notes he has a "Medic Alert" bracelet inscribed with the words "Epilepsy" and "Phenytoin." After being assisted to another room, he gradually returns to his normal self. During recovery, he is confused, disoriented, and argumentative. He later recalls nothing of the incident involving the magazines after he recovered.

This patient developed a typical complex partial seizure with a brief postictal acute confusional state.[187] According to the definition of the International League Against Epilepsy, his consciousness was impaired or lost.[187] However, he was not in a coma, but interacted in a somewhat meaningful way with inanimate objects (the magazines) and people in the environment. Mental functioning was clearly impaired, as manifested by grossly inappropriate behavior, the "offering" of magazines. Nonetheless, the behavior likely related to the activation of previous social behavioral patterns. Although the seizure began focally, it probably spread to other components of the limbic system, resulting in total amnesia for events of the episode.

Loss or impairment of consciousness is also an essential component of absence seizures according to the official definition, yet various complex behaviors can occur and memory may be at least partly spared during absence status epilepticus.[187]

Consciousness was still impaired during recovery, or the postictal period, in this patient, in that he had an acute confusional state. This is discussed further in the next chapter.

Case 3

70 year-old right-handed man is left with permanent global aphasia and complete right hemiplegia as a consequence of ischemic infarction in the left middle cerebral artery territory. Very little improvement occurs over the next few months and he requires chronic institutionalization. In the nursing home, he is able to feed himself with his left hand and rings the buzzer when he has to urinate or defecate. When his family comes to visit, he smiles and nods, although inappropriately, to their comments. However, he utters no words and shows no comprehension to commands even requiring nonverbal responses, e.g., "lift your left arm." With the help of an occupational therapist, he learns to paint using his left upper limb. His portrayals of outdoor scenes, taken from memory, are displayed in the hallways of the nursing home.

This patient suffered global or complete aphasia due to infarction of much of the convexity surface of the dominant cerebral hemisphere. Although this patient could not express himself verbally, comprehend verbal material in any format, and may not have been able to think using language symbols, this man was not unconscious. He was alert, clearly interacted, recognized individuals (functioning memory), showed social behaviors and motivation, and could express himself in art.

Patients with surgical division of the corpus callosum cannot describe objects placed in the left hand or flashed tachistoscopically into the left visual field. Gazzaniga argues that, for conscious awareness, the information has to be transmitted to an interpreter in the left (dominant) cerebral hemisphere. This processing is the function of the brain's "language system." Language allows more complete abstraction, which allows for possibly the highest form of symbolic representation used in cognitive processes. Does this mean, then, that aphasic patients, as in case 3, are unconscious? A number of factors argue that they are conscious:[188]

1. Patients maintain place and time orientation.

2. They may later (after recovery) be able to relate what they experienced while aphasic.

3. In Alzheimer disease, a mirror syndrome sometimes occurs: speech may be preserved, but other aspects of cognitive functioning, including aspects of awareness, may be disturbed.

4. In split brain cases, the individual may be able to identify correctly objects placed in the left hand even though he/she cannot describe them.

Thus, although language forms a very important part of mental function, consciousness can be preserved in the absence of this function.

Case 4

A 25-year-old woman develops a severe Guillain-Barré syndrome (an immune-mediated polyneuropathy) that progresses over a week to causing total paralysis of her limbs, cranial nerve–innervated muscles, and respirations. She is dependent on a mechanical ventilator in the intensive care unit. An EEG shows drowsiness and a normal pattern of 10 Hz (alpha) activity in the posterior head that responds or blocks when the eyelids are opened by the technologist. Auditory or somatosensory evoked potential testing does not yield a response.

Over 8 to 12 months, the patient makes a nearly complete recovery. She recalls only small fragments of her stay in the intensive care unit, mainly as frightening, painful, and distressing experiences. She recalls extreme pain in her limbs that was unrelieved, as she could not communicate her needs. She remembers her thoughts about whether she would survive, past events before she became ill, and sleep with nightmares as well as wakeful thoughts. She has only a rough awareness regarding the temporal aspect of her illness.

This patient had severe deprivation of essentially all sensation. The lack of input into the ARAS probably partly accounts for the exaggerated sleepiness noted on the EEG. The reticular formation does, however, function even without such sensory input. The thalamocortical circuits were working normally and dreams, thoughts, memories, and wake and sleep cycles still go on with total sensory deprivation or outward movements.[48] Hallucinations sometimes occur in sensory deprivation.[189] Their explanation is uncertain, but it has been proposed that spontaneous neuronal activity within central sensory systems gives rise to these experiences.

Thus, the patient in case 4 clearly was not unconscious. In addition to her near complete sensory deprivation (she perceived some [spontaneous?] pain and could see with eyes passively held open, and likely would have been able to perceive odors), she was "locked-in" in the sense of being de-efferented because of the extensive disease of the peripheral nervous system. Despite this, she was capable of dreams, memories, and self-awareness.

CONCLUSIONS AND FUTURE DIRECTIONS

A fusion of neurophysiologic, philosophic, and psychologic, concepts may lead to a closer understanding of consciousness. In any case, a "scientific revolution" with a shift of "paradigms" (accepted models) may be necessary before the riddle of consciousness can be completely solved.[190]

Consciousness is multifaceted. Its essential components appear to be alertness and awareness of self and the environment. Full awareness and appropriate behavioral responses involve sensation, perception, memory functions, attention (with links to motivation), and cognition. It probably is not an all-or-none phenomenon. As Crick stated, when the brain is injured in certain ways, consciousness is impaired.[10] This can be in any of the components described.

From a neurologic perspective, one should first consider *alertness* or arousability as a prerequisite for other aspects of consciousness. Alertness depends on the ascending reticular formation which, although multifaceted in itself, plays an activating role for functions of the rostral structures that are involved in much of the processing that goes on without full conscious awareness, as well as for "conscious" behavior. Next, we should consider *awareness*, a function that depends on an infrastructure of attention, allowing focusing of mental activity. Awareness of the outside world (for all but olfaction) requires the parietal cortex for sensory processing and interpretation, after initial reception in the primary sensory areas. For sensory processing to be meaningful, it must be channeled into the limbic system through the temporal lobes, especially the amygdala. Connections with memory stores allow for appreciation of the relevance or importance of contemporary experiences. Motivation, self-awareness, and communications with the motor system relate to widespread integration of various cortical and subcortical regions. The frontal lobes play an essential executive role in directing and maintaining attention and in planning behavior.[138] The left temporal-parietal region plays an important function in converting processed information into symbols in the form of language, allowing for "internal conversation" and conceptual formulation. Language, so important in human functioning, is used in various cognitive processes and communication.

It is possible for clinicians to use this information in sorting out the localization of disorders that impair alertness and the various aspects of the content of consciousness. These components can be affected singly or in various combinations. In summary, it is important to remember that "loss of consciousness" is a meaningless expression, unless the affected elements are identified and described.[191]

REFERENCES

1. Bisiach E: Understanding consciousness: clues from unilateral neglect and related disorders, In Milner AD, Rugg MD (eds): *The Neuropsychology of Consciousness*. London, Academic Press, 1991, pp 113–137.
2. James W: *The Principles of Psychology*. London, Macmillan, 1890.
3. Block N: How can we find the neural correlate of consciousness. *TINS* 19:456, 1996.
4. Wilber K: *The Spectrum of Consciousness*. Wheaton: Theosophical Printing House, 1989.
5. Strehler BL: Where is the self? A neuroanatomical theory of consciousness. *Synapse* 7:44, 1991.
6. Jackson JH: Evolution and dissolution of the nervous system. Croonian Lectures delivered at the Royal College of Physicians, March 1884. *Br Med J* I:591, 1884.
7. Rosenfield I: *The Strange, Familiar and Forgotten: An Anatomy of Consciousness*. New York, Alfred A Knopf, 1992.
8. Humphrey N: *A History of the Mind*. New York, Harper Collins, 1992.
9. Bogen JE: On the neurophysiology of consciousness: part II. Constraining the semantic problem. *Consciousness Cognition* 4:137, 1995.
10. Crick F: *The Astonishing Hypothesis: The Scientific Search for the Soul*. London, Simon and Shuster 1994.
11. Locke J: *Essay Concerning Human Understanding*, vols 1 and 2, revised ed. London, Dutton, 1965.
12. Haldane ES, Ross GRT: *The Philosophical Works of Descartes*. New York, Dover, 1955.

13. Cassano D: Neurology and the soul: from the origins until 1500. *J History Neuroscience* 5:152, 1996.

14. Wolf-Devine C: *Descartes on Seeing*. The History of Philosophy Monograph Series. Carbondale, Southern Illinois University Press, 1993.

15. Hogan J: Can science explain consciousness. *Scientific American* 271:88, 1994.

16. Ayer AJ: *Language Truth and Logic*. London, Victor Gollancz, 1954.

17. Ryle G: *The Concept of Mind*. New York, Barnes and Noble, 1949.

18. Jibu M, Yasue K: *Quantum Brain Mechanics and Consciousness. An Introduction*. John Benjamins, 1995.

19. Moulyn AC: *Mind-Body. A Pluralistic Interpretation of Mind-Body Interaction Under the Guidelines of Time, Space and Movement*. New York, Greenwood Press, 1991.

20. Tinder G: *Tolerance: Toward a New Civility*. Amherst, University of Massachusetts Press, 1976.

21. Strong CA: *The Origin of Consciousness: An Attempt to Conceive the Mind as a Product of Evolution*. London, Macmillan, 1918.

22. Fancher RE: *Psychoanalytic Psychology: The Development of Freud's Thought*. New York, WW Norton, 1973.

23. Sartre JP: *The Transcendence of the Ego: An Existentialist Theory of Consciousness* (translated by William F and Kirkpatrick R.) New York, Noonday Press, 1957.

24. Archard D: *Conscious and the Unconscious*. La Salle, Open Court, 1984, pp 38–54.

25. Ramón y Cajal S: A new concept of the histology of the nervous system, in Rottenberg DA, Hochberg FH (eds): *Neurological Classics in Modern Translation*. New York, Hafner, 1977, pp 7–29.

26. Ramón y Cajal S: *The structure and connexions of neurons. Nobel Lectures: Physiology or Medicine 1901–1921*. Amsterdam, Elsevier, 1967, pp 220–253.

27. Waldeyer W: Über einige Forschungen im Gebiete der Anatomie des Zentralnervensystems. *Dstch med Wschr* 17:1213, 1891.

28. DuBois-Remond E: *Untersuchungen über thierische Elekrictät*. Berlin, Reimer, 1848–1849.

29. Helmholtz H von: On the role of transmission of the nerve impulse, translated in Dennis W (ed): *Readings in the History of Physiology*. New York, Appleton-Century-Croft, 1948, pp 197–198.

30. Bernard C: *Leçons sur les Phénomènes de la Vie Communs aux Animaux et les Végétaux*. Paris, Baillière, 1878–1879.

31. Erlich P: Chemotherapeutics: scientific principles, methods and results. *Lancet* 2:445, 1913.

32. Moruzzi G. Magoun HW: Brain stem reticular formation and activation of the EEG. *Electroenceph Clin Neurphysiol* 1:455, 1949.

33. Munk MHJ, Roelfsema PR, König P, Engel AK, Singer Q: Role of reticular activation in the modulation of intracortical synchronization. *Science* 272:271, 1996.

34. Castro-Alamancos MA, Connors BW: Short-term plasticity of a thalamocortical pathway dynamically modulated by behavioral state. *Science* 272:274, 1996.

35. Jeffreys JGR, Traub RD, Whittington MA: Neuronal networks for induced "40 Hz" rhythms. *TINS* 19:202, 1996.

36. Ruddell AP, Hua J: The recognition potential and conscious awareness. *Electroenceph Clin Neurophysiol* 98:309, 1996.

37. Hebb DO: *Organization of Behavior*. New York, John Wiley and Sons, 1964.

38. Brodal A: *Neurological Anatomy in Relation to Clinical Medicine*. 3rd ed. New York, Oxford University Press, 1981.

39. Nauta WJH, Whitlock DG: Anatomical analysis of the nonspecific thalamic projection system, in Delafresnaye JF (ed): *Brain Mechanisms and Consciousness*. Oxford, Blackwell, 1954, pp 81–104.

40. Scheibel ME, Scheibel AB: Structural organization of nonspecific thalamic nuclei and their projection toward the cortex. *Brain Res* 13:960, 1967.

41. Scheibel ME, Scheibel AB: The organization of the nucleus reticularis thalami. *Brain Res* 1:43, 1966.

42. Newman J: Thalamic contributions to consciousness. *Consciousness and Cognition*. 4:172, 1995.

43. Yingling CD, Skinner JE: Regulation of unit activity in nucleus reticularis thalami by the mesencephalic reticular formation and frontal granular cortex. *Electroenceph Clin Neurophysiol* 39:635, 1975.

44. Morison RS, Dempsey EW: A study of thalamocortical systems. *Am J Physiol* 135:281, 1942.

45. Groenewegen HJ, Berendse HW: The specificity of the "nonspecific" midline and intralaminar thalamic nuclei. *TINS* 17–54, 1994.

46. Penfield W: Consciousness and centrencephalic organization. *Premier Conf. Inter Sci Neurol Bruxelles*, 21–28 juillet, 1957, 2e journée commune, 1957, pp 7–18.

47. Scheibel AB: Anatomical and physiological substrates of arousal: a view from the bridge, in Hobson JA, Brazier MAB (eds): *The Reticular Formation Revisited.* New York, Raven Press, 1980, pp 55–66.

48. Llinás RR, Paré D: Commentary: Of dreaming and wakefullness. *Neuroscience* 44:521, 1991.

49. Yamada T, Kameyama S, Fuchigami Z, et al: Changes of short latency somatosensory evoked potential in sleep. *Electroenceph Clin Neurophysiol* 70:126, 1988.

50. Kinomura S, Larsson J, Gulyás B, Roland PE: Activation by attention of the human reticular formation and thalamic interlaminar nuclei. *Science* 271:512, 1996.

51. Dingledine R, Kelly JS: Brainstem stimulation and the acetylcholine-evoked inhibition for neurons in the feline nucleus reticularis talami. *J Physiol* (London) 271:135, 1977.

52. Brudzynski SM, Eckersdorf M, Golebiewski H: Emotional-aversive nature of the behavioral response induced by carbachol in cats. *J Psychiatr Neurosci* 18:38, 1993.

53. Brudzynski SM, Eckersdorf B, Golebiewski H: Regional specificity of the emotional-aversive response induced by carbachol in the cat brain: a quantitative mapping study. *J Psychiatr Neurosci* 20:119, 1995.

54. Kinai T, Szerb JC: The mesencephalic reticular activating system and cortical acetylcholine output. *Nature* 205:80, 1965.

55. Stewart DJ, MacFabe DF, Vanderwolf CH: Cholinergic activation of electrocorticogram: role of the substantia innominata and the effects of atropine and quinuclidinyl benzylate. *Brain Res* 322:219, 1984.

56. Vanderwolf CH: The role of the cerebral cortex and ascending activating systems in the control of behavior, in Satinoff E, Teitelbaum P (eds): *Handbook of Behavioral Neurobiology,* vol. 6: *Motivation.* New York, Plenum Press, 1983, pp 67–104.

57. Consolo S, Bertorelli R, Forloni GL., Butcher LL: Cholinergic neurons of the pontomesencephalic tegmentum release acetylcholine in the basal nuclear complex of freely moving rats. *Neuroscience* 37:717, 1990.

58. Hayes RL., Pechura CM, Katayama Y, et al: Activation of pontine cholinergic sites implicated in unconsciousness following cerebral concussion in the cat. *Science* 223:301, 1984.

59. Saija A, Hayes RL., Lyeth BG, et al: The effect of concussive head injury on central cholinergic neurons. *Brain Res* 452:303, 1988.

60. Leichnetz GR, Carlton SM, Katayama Y, et al: Afferent and efferent connections of the cholinoceptive medial pontine relicular formation (region of the ventral tegmental nucleus) in the cat. *Brain Res Bull* 22:665, 1989.

61. Foote SL, Bloom FE, Aston-Jones G: Nucleus locus ceruleus: new evidence of anatomical and physiological specificity. *Physiol Res* 63:844, 1983.

62. Ashton-Jones G, Bloom FE: Activity of norepinephrine-containing locus ceruleus neurons in behaving rats anticipates fluctuations in the sleep-waking cycle. *J Neurosci* 1:876, 1981.

63. Spoont MR: Modulatory role of serotonin in neural information processing: implications for human psychopathology. *Psychol Bull* 112:330, 1992.

64. Carskadon MA, Dement WC: Normal human sleep: an overview, in Kryger MH, Roth T, Dement WC (eds): *Principles and Practice of Sleep Medicine.* Philadelphi, Saunders, 1989.

65. Cooper JR, Bloom FR, Roth RH: *The Biochemical Basis of Neuropharmacology.* New York, Oxford University Press, 1991.

66. Eccles JC: *The Neurophysiological Basis of Mind.* Oxford, Clarendon, 1952.

67. Engel J Jr: *Seizures and Epilepsy.* Philadelphia: FA Davis, 1989.

68. Tsumoto T: Excitatory amino acid transmitters and their receptors in neural circuits of the cerebral neocortex. *Neurosci Res* 9:79, 1990.

69. Vanderwolf CH: Near total loss of "learning" and memory as a result of combined cholinergic and serotonergic blockade in the rat. *Behav Brain Res* 23:43, 1987.

70. Feeney DM, Baron J-C: Diaschisis. *Stroke* 17:817, 1986.

71. Ingvar DH, Sourander P: Destruction of the reticular core of the brainstem. A pathoanatomic follow up of a case of cotna of three years duration. *Arch Neurol* 23:1, 1970.

72. Chase TN, Moretti L, Prensky AL: Clinical and electroencephalographic manifestations of vascular lesions of the pons. *Neurology* 18:357, 1968.

73. Kaada BR, Harkmark W, Stokke O: Deep coma associated with desynchronization in EEG. *Electroenceph Clin Neurophysiol* 13:785, 1961.

74. Wilkus RJ, Harvey F, Ojeman LM, Lettich E: Electroencephalogram and sensory evoked

potentials. Findings in an unresponsive patient with pontine infarcts. *Arch Neurol* 24:538, 1971.

75. Plum F, Posner JB: *The Diagnosis of Stupor and Coma*. Philadelphia, FA Davis, 1966.
76. Markand ON: Electroencephalogram in the "locked-in" syndrome. *Electroenceph Clin Neurophysiol* 40:529, 1976.
77. Plum F: Coma and related global disturbances of the human conscious state, in Peters A, Jones EG (eds): *Cerebral Cortex: Normal and Altered States of Function*. New York, Plenum Press, 1991, chap 9, pp 359–425.
78. Brodal A: *Neurological Anatomy in Relation to Clinical Medicine*. New York, Oxford University Press, 1981, pp 444–445.
79. Bremer F: Cerveau isolé et physiol du sommeil. *CR Soc Biol* 118:1235, 1935.
80. Scheibel ME, Scheibel AB: The anatomy of constancy. *Ann NY Acad Sci* 290:421, 1977.
81. Schiller PH, Sandell JH: Interactions between visually and electrically elicited saccades before and after superior colliculus and frontal eye field ablations in the rhesus monkey. *Exp Brain Res* 49:391, 1983.
82. Bushnell MC, Goldberg ME, Robinson DL: Behavioral enhancement visual responses in monkey cerebral cortex. Modulation in posterior parietal cortex related to visual attention. *J Neurophysiol* 46:755, 1981.
83. Mills RP, Swanson PD: Vertical oculomotor apraxia and memory loss. *Ann Neurol* 4:149, 1978.
84. Guberman A, Stuss D: The syndrome of bilateral paramedian thalamic infarction. *Neurology* 33:540, 1983.
85. Gentilini M, De Renzi E, Crisi G: Bilateral paramedian thalamic artery infarcts: Report of eight cases. *J Neurol Neurosurg Psychiatry* 50:900, 1987.
86. Bogousslavsky J, Regli F, Uske A: Thalamic infarcts: clinical syndromes, etiology and prognosis. *Neurology* 38:837, 1988.
87. Castaigne P, Lhermitte F, Buge A, Escourolle R, Hauw JJ, Lyon-Caen O: Paramedian thalamic and midbrain infarcts: Clinical and neuropathological study. *Ann Neurol* 10:127, 1981.
88. Mehler MF: The rostral basilar artery syndrome. *Neurology* 38:9, 1989.
89. Wall M, Slamovits TL, Weisberg LA, Trufant SA: Vertical gaze ophthalmoplegia from infarction in the area of the posterior thalamo-subthalamic paramedian artery. *Stroke* 17:546, 1986.
90. Katz DI, Alexander MP, Mandell AM: Dementia following strokes in the mesencephalon and diencephalon. *Arch Neurol* 44:1127, 1987.
91. Shuster P: Beitrage zur pathologie du thalamus opticus. Part 4. *Arch Psychiatr Nervenkr* 106:201, 1937.
92. Castaigne P, Buge A, Cambier J, Escourolle R, Brunet P, Degos JD: Demence thalamique d'origine vasculaire par ramolissement bilateral, limite au territoire du pedicule retromamillaire. *Rev Neurol* 114:89, 1966.
93. Square LR, Amaral DG, Zola-Morgan S, Kritchevsky M, Press G: Description of brain injury in the amnestic patient NA based on magnetic resonance imaging. *Exp Neurol* 105:23, 1989.
94. Feinberg WM, Rapcsak SZ: "Peduncular hallucinosis" following paramedian thalamic infarction. *Neurology* 39:1535, 1989.
95. Von Monakow C: Diaschisis [1914 article translated by G. Harris], in Prebram KH (ed): *Brain and Behavior I: Mood States and Mind*. Baltimore: Penguin, 1969, pp 27–36.
96. Knott JR, Dogram WR, Chilès WD: Effect of subcortical lesions on cortical electroencephalogram in cats. *Arch Neurol Psychiatry* 73:203, 1985.
97. D'Antona R, Baron JC, Pantano P, et al: Effects of thalamic lesions on cerebral cortex metabolism in humans. *J Cereb Blood Flow and Metab* 5 (suppl 1):S457, 1985.
98. Girault JA, Savaki HE, Desban M, et al: Bilateral cerebral metabolic alterations following lesion of the ventromedial thalamic nucleus: mapping by the ^{14}C-desoxyglucose method in conscious rats. *J Comp Neurol* 231:137, 1985.
99. Feeney DM, Baron J-C: Diaschisis. *Stroke* 17:817, 1986.
100. Serefetinides EA, Hoare RD, Driver MV: Intracarotid sodium amylobarbitone and cerebral dominance for speech and consciousness. *Brain* 88:107, 1965.
101. Albert ML, Silverberg R, Reches A, Berman M: Cerebral dominance for consciousness. *Arch Neurol* 33:453–454, 1976.
102. Salazar AM, Grafman JH, Vance SC, Weingartner H, Dillon JD, Ludlow C: Consciousness and amnesia after penetrating head injury: Neurology and anatomy. *Neurology* 36:178, 1986.
103. Moskovitch M: Information processing and the cerebral hemispheres, in Gazzinga MS (ed): *Handbook of Behavioral Neurobiology*, vol 2: *Neuropsychology*. New York, Plenum Press, 1979, pp 379–446.

104. Posner MI. Attention: the mechanisms of consciousness. *Proc Natl Acad Sci USA* 91:7398, 1994.

105. Posner MI, Raichle ME. *Images of Mind.* New York: Sci Am Library, 1994.

106. Pardo JV, Pardo PJ, Janer KW, Raichle ME: The anterior cingulate cortex mediates processing selection in the Stroop attention-conflict paradigm. *Proc Natl Acad Sci USA* 87:256, 1990.

107. Paus T, Petrides M, Evans AC, Meyer E: Role of the anterior cingulate cortex in the control of oculomotor, manual and speech responses: a positron emission tomographic study. *J Neurophysiol* 70:453, 1993.

108. Eccles JC: *The Physiological Basis of Mind: The Principles of Neurophysiology.* Oxford, Clarendon Press, 1952.

109. Petrides M, Milner B: Deficits on subject-ordered tasks after frontal- and temporal-lobe lesions in man. *Neuropsychologia* 20:249, 1982.

110. Stuss DT, Benson DF: *The Frontal Lobes.* New York, Raven Press, 1986, pp 180–193.

111. Corbetta M, Miezin FM, Shulman GL, Petersen SE: A PET study of visuospatial attention. *J Neurosci* 13:1202, 1993.

112. Watson RT, Heilman KM, Miller BD, King FA: Neglect after mesencephalic reticular formation lesions. *Neurology* 24:294, 1979.

113. Battersby WS, Bender MB, Pollack M, Kahn RL: Unilateral spatial agnosia (inattention) in patients with cerebral lesions. *Brain* 79:68, 1956.

114. Heilman KM, Howell G: Seizure-induced neglect. *J Neurol Neurosurg Psychiatry* 43:1035–1040.

115. Watson RT, Heilman KM: Thalamic neglect. *Neurology* 29:690, 1979.

116. Stuss DT, Benson DF: Neuropsychological studies of the frontal lobes. *Psychol Bull* 95:3, 1984.

117. Milner B: Effects of different brain lesions on card sorting. *Arch Neurol* 9:90, 1963.

118. Wurtz RH, Goldberg ME, Robinson DL: Behavioral modulation of visual response in the monkey: stimulus selection for attention and movement, in Sprague JM, Epstein AN (eds): *Progress in Psychobiology and Physiological Psychology,* vol 9, New York, Academic Press, 1980, pp 43–83.

119. Bouyer JJ, Montaron MF, Rougeul A: Fast fronto-parietal rhythm during combined focused behavior and immobility in cat: cortical and thalamic localizations. *Electroenceph Clin Neurophysiol* 51:244, 1981.

120. Harter MR, Guido W: Attention to patter orientation: negative cortical potentials, reaction time and the selection process. *Electroenceph Clin Neurophysiol* 49:461, 1980.

121. Knight RT, Hilliard SA, Woods DL, Neville HJ: The effects of frontal cortex lesions on event-related potentials during auditory selective attention. *Electroenceph Clin Neurophysiol* 52:571, 1981.

122. Wood CC, Allison T, Goff WR, Williamson PD, Spencer DD: On the neuronal origin of P300 in man, in Kornhuber HH, Deecke L (eds): *Progress in Brain Potential Research,* vol 59, *Motivation, Motor and Sensory Processes of the Brain: Electrical Potentials, Behavior and Clinical Use.* Amsterdam: Elsevier/North Holland, 1980, pp 51–56.

123. Halgren ENK, Squires CL, Wilson J, Rohrbraugh WJ, Babb TL, Crandall PH: Endogenous potentials generated in the human hippocampal formation and amygdala by infrequent events. *Science* (Wash DC) 210:803, 1980.

124. Hillyard SA, Picton TW: Electrophysiology of cognition, in Plum F (ed): *Handbook of Neurophysiology.* Bethesda, American Physiological Society, 1987, chap 13, pp 519–584.

125. Marshall JF, Berrios N, Sawyer S: Neostriatal dopamine and sensory inattention. *J Comp Physiol Psychol* 94:833, 1980.

126. Mason JF, Fibiger HC: Noradrenaline and selective attention. *Life Science* 25:1949, 1979.

127. Hubel DH, Wiesel TN: Receptive fields and functional architecture of monkey striate cortex. *J Physiol* 195:215, 1968.

128. van Essen D, Anderson CH: Information processing strategies and pathways in the primate retina and visual cortex, in Zorbetzer SF, Davis JL, Lau C (eds): *An Introduction to Neural and Electronic Networks.* San Diego, Academic Press, 1990, pp 43–72.

129. Spillmann L, Werner JS: Long-range interactions in visual perception. *TINS* 19:428, 1996.

130. Yukie M, Iwai E: Direct projection form the dorsal lateral geniculate nucleus to the prestrite cortex in macaque monkeys. *J Comp Neurol* 201:81, 1981.

131. Stoerig P: Varieties of vision: from blind responses to conscious recognition. *TINS* 19:401, 1996.

132. Seki S: The visual association cortex. *Curr Opin Neurobiol* 3:155, 1993.

133. Damasio AR, Tranel D: Disorders of higher brain function, in Rosenberg RN (ed): *Comprehensive Neurology.* New York, Raven Press, 1991, chap 19, pp 639–657.

134. Libet B, Pearl DK, Morledge DE, et al: Control of the transition from sensory detection to sensory awareness in man by the duration of a thalamic stimulus. *Brain* 114:1731, 1991.

135. Brown JW: Psychology of time awareness. *Brain Cogn* 14:144, 1990.

136. Gardner H: *The Shattered Mind. The Person After Brain Damage.* New York, Alfred A Knopf, 1975, pp 142–175.

137. Critchley M. *The Parietal Lobes.* New York, Hafner, 1969, pp 236–255.

138. Picton TW, Stuss DT: Neurobiology of conscious experience. *Curr Opin Neurobiol* 4:256–265, 1994.

139. Pöppel E, Schwender D: Temporal mechanisms of consciousness. *Int Anesthesiol Clin* 31:13–25, 1993.

140. Basiach E, Vallar G, Geminiani G: Influence of response modality on perceptual awareness of contralesion visual stimuli. *Brain* 112:1627, 1989.

141. Tegnér R, Levander M: Through a looking glass. A new technique to demonstrate directional hypokinesia in unilateral neglect. *Brain* 114:1943, 1991.

142. Kinsbourne M: Integrated cortical field model of consciousness. *Ciba Found Symp* 174:43–50, 1993.

143. Goldman-Rakic PS: Cellular and circuit basis of working memory in prefrontal cortex in nonhuman primates. *Prog Brain Res* 85:325, 1990.

144. Baars BJ: How does a serial, integrated and very limited stream of consciousness emerge from a nervous system that is mostly unconscious, distributed parallel and of enormous capacity? *Ciba Found Symp* 174:282–290, 1993.

145. Prigatano GP: Anosognosia, delusions, and altered self-awareness after brain injury: an historical perspective. *BRI Quarterly* 4:40, 1988.

146. Mesulam M-M: *Principles of Behavioral Neurology.* Philadelphia, FA Davis, 1985.

147. Wjite J: Autonomic discharge from stimulation of the hypothalamus of man. *Assoc Res Nerv Ment Dis* 20:854, 1940.

148. Salovey P, Mayer JD: Emotional intelligence. *Imagination Cognit Personal* 9:185, 1990.

149. Zola-Morgan S, Squire LR: Memory impairments in monkeys following lesions of the hippocampus. *Behav Neurosci* 100:155, 1986.

150. LeDpux JE: Emotion and the amygdala, in Aggleton JP (ed): *The Amygdala: Neurobiological Aspects of Emotion, Memory and Mental Dysfunction.* New York, Wiley-Liss, 1992, 339–351.

151. Berthier M, Starkstein S, Leiguarda R: Aymbolia for pain: a sensory-limbic disconnection syndrome. *Ann Neurol* 24:41, 1982.

152. Jackendoff R: *Consciousness and the Computational Mind.* Cambridge, Bradford Books, MIT Press, 1988.

153. Sacks O: *The Man who Mistook His Wife for a Hat.* New York, Summit Books, 1985, p 29.

154. Mishkin M, Malamut B, Bachevalier J: Memories and habits: two neural systems, in Lynch G, McGaugh JL, Weinberger NM (eds): *Neurobiology of Learning and Memory.* New York, Guilford Press, 1984.

155. Scoville WB, Milner B: Loss of recent memory after bilateral hippocampal lesions. *J Neurol Neurosurg Psychiatry* 20:11, 1957.

156. Zola-Morgan S, Squire LR, Amaral DG: Human amnesia and the medial temporal region: enduring memory impairment following a bilateral lesion limited to field CA1 of the hippocampus. *J Neurosci* 6:2950, 1986.

157. Victor M, Adams RD, Collins GH: *The Wernicke-Korsakoff Syndrome.* Oxford, Blackwell, 1971.

158. McEntee WJ, Biber MP, Perl DP, Benson DF: Diencephalic amnesia: a reappraisal. *J Neurol Neurosurg Psychiatry* 39:436, 1976.

159. Mills RP, Swanson PD: Vertical motor apraxia and memory loss. *Ann Neurol* 4:427, 1978.

160. Casaigne P, Lhermitte F, Buge A, Escourolle R, Hauw, JJM Lyon-Caen O: Paramedian thalamic and midbrain infarcts: clinical and neuropathological study. *Ann Neurol* 10:127, 1981.

161. Mair WGP, Warrington EK, Weiskrantz L: Memory disorder in Korsakoff's psychosis. A neuropathological and neuropsychological investigation of two cases. *Brain* 102:749, 1979.

162. Aggleton JP, Nicol RM, Huston AE, Fairbairn AF: The performance of amnestic subjects on tests of experimental amnesia in animals. *Neuropsychologica* 26:265, 1988.

163. Squire LR, Zola-Morgan S, Chen KS: Human amnesia and animal models of amnesia: performance of amnesic patients on tests designed for the monkey. *Behav Neurosci* 102:210, 1988.

164. Mishkin M: Memory in monkeys severely impaired by combined, but not by separate removal of amygdala and hippocampus. *Nature* 273:297, 1978.

165. Bachevalier J, Parkinson JK, Mishkin M: Visual recognition in monkeys: effects of separate vs. combined transection of fornix and amygdalofugal pathways. *Exp Brain Res* 57:554, 1985.

166. Aggleton JP, Mishkin M: Memory impairments following restricted medial thalamic lesions in monkeys. *Exp Brain Res* 52:199, 1983.

167. Aggelton JP: A description of the amygdalo-hippo-campal system. *Exp Brain Res* 64:515, 1986.

168. Leonard BW, Amaral DG, Squire LR, Zola-Morgan S: Transient memory impairment in monkeys with bilateral lesions of the entorhinal cortex. *J Neurosci* 15:5637, 1995.

169. Zola-Morgan S, Squire LR, Clower RP, Rempel NL: Damage to the perirhinal cortex exacerbates memory impairment following lesions to the hippo-campal formation. *J Neurosci* 13:251, 1993.

170. Houser CR, Crawford GD, Barber RP, Salvaterra PM, Vaughn JE: Organization and morphological characteristics of cholinergic neurons: an immuno-histochemical study with monoclonal antibody to choline acetyltransferase. *Brain Res* 266:97, 1983.

171. Drachman DA, Leavitt J: Human memory and the cholinergic system—a relationship to aging. *Arch Neurol Psychiatry* 30:113, 1974.

172. Flicker C, Dean RL, Watkins DL, Fisher SK, Bartus RT: Behavioral and neurochemical effects following neurotoxic lesions of a major cholinergic input to the cerebral cortex of the rat. *Pharmacol Biochem Behav* 18:973, 1983.

173. Davies P, Maloney AJF: Selective loss of central cholinergic neurons in Alzheimer's disease. *Lancet* 2:1403, 1976.

174. Alhainen K, Riekkinen P Sr, Helkala E-L, Parta-nen J, Laulumaa V, Reinikainen K, Soininen H, Airaksinen M: The effect of THA on cognitive functions and spectral power EEG in Alzheimer's disease: preliminary results of an open study, in Iabal K, McLachlan DRC, Winblad B, Wisniewski HM (eds): *Alzheimer's Disease: Basic Mechanisms, Diagnosis and Strategies.* Chichester, John Wiley and Sons, 1991, pp 611–619.

175. Mesulam M-M, Mufson EJ, Wainer BH: Three-dimensional representation and cortical projection topography of the nucleus basalis (CH4) in the macaque: concurrent demonstration of choline acetyltransferase and retrograde transport with a stabilized tetramethylbenzidine method for HRP. *Brain Res* 367:301, 1986.

176. McEntee WJ, Mair RG, Langlais PJ: Neurochem-ical pathology in Korsakoff's psychosis: implica-tions for other cognitive disorders. *Neurology* 34:648, 1984.

177. Mayes AR, Meudell PR, Mann D, Pickering A: Location of lesions in Korsakoff's syndrome: neuropsychological and neuropathological data. *Cortex* 24:367, 1988.

178. Mair RG, Anderson CD, Langlais PJ, McEntee WJ: *Brain Res* 360:273, 1985.

179. McEntee WJ, Mair RG: The Korsakoff syndrome: a neurochemical perspective. *TINS* 13:340, 1990.

180. McEntee WJ, Mair RG: Memory enhancement in Korsakoff's psychosis by clonidine: further evi-dence for a noradrenergic deficit. *Ann Neurol* 7:466, 1080.

181. Arnsten AFT, Goldman-Rakic PS: Alpha-2 adre-nergic mechanisms in prefrontal cortex associated with cognitive decline in aged nonhuman primates. *Science* 230:1273, 1985.

182. Penfield W, Perot P: The brain's record of auditory and visual experience. *Brain* 86:595, 1963.

183. Weiskrantz L, Saunders RC: Impairments of visual object transforms in rhesus monkeys. *Brain* 107:1033, 1984.

184. Kihlstrom JF, Barnhardt TR, Tataryn DJ: The psychological unconscious: found, lost and regained. *Am J Psychol* 47:557, 1992.

185. Kihlstrom JF: The psychological unconscious and the self. *Ciba Found Symp* 174:147, 1993.

186. Zimmerman GN, Knott JR: Slow potentials in the brain related to speech processing in normal speak-ers and stutterers. *Electroenceph Clin Neurophysiol* 37:599, 1974.

187. Commission on Classification and Terminology, International League Against Epilepsy: Proposed revisions of clinical and electroencephalographic classification of epileptic seizures. *Epilepsia* 22:480, 1981.

188. Ivanitsky AM: Consciousness: criteria and possible mechanisms. *Int J Psychophysiol* 14:179, 1993.

189. Schultz G, Melzack R: The Charles Bonnet syn-drome: phantom visual images. *Perception* 20:809, 1991.

190. Kuhn TS: *The Structure of Scientific Revolutions,* 2nd ed. International Encyclopedia of Unified Science, University of Chicago Press, 1970.

191. Gloor P: Consciousness as a neurological con-cept in epileptology: a critical review. *Epilepsia* 27(suppl 2):S14, 1986.

Chapter 2

MAJOR SYNDROMES OF IMPAIRED CONSCIOUSNESS

G. Bryan Young

This chapter discusses the major syndromes in which consciousness is impaired: acute confusional state, stupor and coma, akinetic mutism, persistent vegetative state, and brain death.

ACUTE CONFUSIONAL STATE (DELIRIUM)

The following is a report of an illustrative case:

Case report
A 50-year-old man was brought to the emergency room after suffering a 5-min generalized convulsive seizure at home. He had a history of renal failure, managed conservatively with diet. A febrile illness with vomiting developed a week before the admission. His family encouraged him to drink plenty of fluids.

On arrival, he was awake but seemed distractible. He answered questions that a doctor was asking a patient in an adjacent bed. He was disoriented in time, including the month and year, and in the building. He seemed interested in the questions and showed no evidence of aphasia. However, he could not maintain a line of thought and skipped from topic to topic. He could not remember the examining doctor's name, even though he was told several times. He could

repeat up to three digits forwards but no more than two backwards and could not spell "world" backwards. He made writing errors, misspelling common words and leaving articles out of a sentence. On an alternating task, in which he had to cross out a number then a letter in sequential order, he crossed out series of numbers then of letters.

He showed asterixis, or loss of postural tone, when the upper limbs were outstretched, and a postural tremor.

His serum sodium was 112 mmol/L, but his serum creatinine and urea had not changed from the values of 1 month earlier when he was clear mentally.

The diagnosis of acute confusional state due to dilutional hyponatremia was made. He was managed with water restriction. Although his confusional state fluctuated, with periods of relative normality alternating with disorientation and agitation, his behavior and other aspects of the neurologic status returned to normal 3 days later.

Definition and Clinical Features

Lipowski has defined the acute confusional state as "an acute organic mental syndrome featuring global cognitive impairment, attentional abnormalities, a reduced level of consciousness, increased or decreased psychomotor activity, and

39

a disordered wake-sleep cycle."[1] This is compatible with standard concepts of confusion.[2,3] Synonyms include acute brain syndrome, toxic psychosis, clouded state, global cognitive impairment, pseudodementia, and twilight states.[4] Context-related synonyms are: intensive care unit (ICU) psychosis, postoperative encephalopathy, and postsurgery psychiatric syndrome. Lipowski's definition is appropriate to each of these, but some authors use certain terms in a more restricted manner; e.g., Adams, Victor and Ropper, and Plum and Posner use the term "delirium" to refer to a florid state with disorientation, fear, hallucinations, and agitation (often with heightened sympathetic nervous activity).[5,6] It seems reasonable, however, to conceive of a continuum ranging from a mild, subacute beclouded condition (low type) to an agitated, confusional state (raving type).[3,7]

In confusional states, a variable number of cognitive deficits are superimposed on a defect in *attention*. A defect of attention is *consistently present*.[8] Attention comprises alertness and the ability to select and focus upon a given task or stimulus. To elicit clinical evidence of subtly impaired attention, the following are useful: digit span (number of digits repeated), serial 7s (counting down from 100 by continually subtracting 7), spelling "world" backwards, or counting down from 20 to 1 within 10 s with no more than one error.

Patients may show impaired concentration— probably as a component of impaired attention. Because of the difficulty in maintaining attention, patients who are alert are often distractible. The attention shifts to the loudest or most novel stimulus.

Other components of cognition are affected. Perception, thinking, and memory are usually all impaired to variable extents. Perceptual difficulties include difficulty in processing, discriminating, and integrating stimuli with previously stored memories. Hallucinations and delusions may intrude as internally created altered perceptions. Patients may misperceive information. Hallucinations, either auditory, visual, or tactile (usually formication, or a sense of ants crawling on the skin), may accompany agitation, especially in withdrawal or toxic states, but kinesthetic hallucinations are rare. Some delusions are frightening—e.g., mistaking an intravenous line for a snake—and others may be persecutory.

Thinking includes the ability to reason, to grasp the meaning of words and other phenomena, to solve problems, to anticipate, and to plan. Thought processes are often concrete or more profoundly disturbed with disjointed speech. Patients may be unable to shift attention when necessary and to refocus their attention on a more appropriate task; this may underlie perseveration or inappropriate continued activity at a certain task. Patients may even have insight into impersistence, but are unable to make the necessary behavioral change.[9] Insight is usually lost for more complex behaviors, however. Agraphia, dyscalculia, and anomia or dysnomia reflecting impairment of other complex cognitive components are common, but patients are not otherwise aphasic.[10] Speech can be reduced in quantity and prosody (intonation), or patients may talk rapidly and incessantly in a rambling manner, without coherence of thought. The content of speech may belie preoccupation, misperceptions, delusions or hallucinations, and fears. Although patients can be "brought back" to answer questions or obey commands, this is not sustained and speech resumes its confused quality.

Memory includes the registration, storage and retrieval of new material, and the recall of previously stored material. Usually, the recall of previously stored material is better than the registration and later recall of new material. Recent and immediate memory, especially since the onset of the delirium, are typically very poor. Sequencing, or the temporal ordering of events, is also impaired.

Patients are often disoriented in time and place, but never to person. The problems in processing information may underlie disorientation. Visuospatial problems and constructional apraxia are frequent.

The level of alertness often fluctuates between delirium with agitation, and lethargy with clouding of consciousness, quiet perplexity, or mild stupor. Agitation may be associated with apprehension, paranoia, and tremor. Increased sympathetic nervous system activity frequently accompanies the agitated form of delirium, with facial flushing or pallor, dilated pupils, tachycardia, sweating, and a postural-action tremor. Confusion, agitation, and delusions may be more prominent at night (sundowning), leading to poor sleep.

Emotional-behavioral disturbances that accompany agitated delirium include rage, combativeness, irritability, fear and apprehension, or euphoria. Conversely, depression or apathy may be found alternating with these or with the quiet confusional state.

Alterations in motivation, drive, or conation probably derive from a number of the above alterations in mental functioning. A reduction or deficiency of motivation is termed *abulia* or *hypobulia*. Such individuals appear apathetic with reduced emotional response, speech, and ideation. Motor activity may be reduced, with resistance to the physician's attempts to move or motivate the patient. Patients may persist in a posture or activity. The limbs may sustain a posture for prolonged periods (catatonia). Motor inactivity may be accompanied by emotional depression, but motor activity and emotion can be dissociated. Conversely, motor activity may be increased with restlessness that is similar to the hyperactivity-inattention syndrome of children. Akathisia, a state of restlessness with inability to be still, may be found. Heightened emotionality, with euphoria or irritability, sometimes accompanies the increase in motor activity. Some aspects may be combined: restless patients may resist attempts of the examiner to move or motivate the patient in a certain direction.

From the above, motor signs accompanying acute confusion may occur singly or in combination: i.e., psychomotor retardation (decreased motor responsiveness without paralysis or profound decrease in conscious level), hyperactivity, asterixis, multifocal myoclonus, *gegenhalten* (see below), and a postural-action tremor.

In summary, the acute confusional state encompasses a global dysfunction of cortical areas or the thalamocortical system, coupled with inattention, disorientation, and difficulty in sustaining mental tasks. It may blend with or progress to other states of diminished levels of consciousness, e.g., excessive drowsiness or stupor.

Epidemiology and Importance

The estimated prevalence in the United States of delirium in individuals over 55 years of age who are living in the community is between 0.1 and 1.1 percent, based on a 1981 survey.[11] Data from the 1960s indicate that 10 to 15 percent of patients admitted to acute medical and surgical wards are acutely confused.[12] Since patients currently admitted to acute hospitals tend to be sicker than in the past, the current prevalence is likely to be higher. Some diagnostic groups have a high prevalence of confusion: cardiac surgery (32 percent),[13] surgery for hip fracture (45 to 55 percent),[14] and bacteremia (70 percent).[10]

Delirium tremens (DTs), an acute organic psychosis during alcohol withdrawal, currently accounts for 4.5 percent of inpatients in acute care hospitals.[15] Such patients are admitted for: (1) an illness not directly caused by alcohol, but DTs occur within 7 days after admission; or (2) acute or withdrawal symptoms other than DTs with later DTs; or (3) acute DTs.

The elderly are more prone to acute confusion in hospital; 15 percent of such patients are confused upon admission[16] and probably an additional 20 percent develop confusion during their hospitalization.[17] Drug toxicity features prominently among the most common immediately identified, preventable or treatable causes of the acute confusional state in the elderly.[18]

Acute confusion is important to recognize and act upon for the following reasons:

1. An acute confusional state can be a manifestation of a serious, life-threatening but potentially reversible condition.

2. Mortality is higher in patients with acute confusional states than for patients without this syndrome.[19]

3. Delirium precedes greater degrees of impairment of consciousness that are associated with even greater morbidity and mortality. Early detection and management of delirium may lessen morbidity and mortality.

4. There is a risk of complications (e.g., fractures from falls) from the confusional state or

the treatment (e.g., complications of restraints or tranquilizing drugs) for the patient, and attendant medicolegal risks for the physician.

5. The confusional state adds greatly to the medical and nursing burden of care on wards.

6. Understanding the risk factors for the acute confusional state may lead to the development of preventive strategies. One example is the careful assessment of drug combinations.

Pathophysiology of Confusion

Most, if not all, of the components of confusion are interrelated and may arise from one another. To explain the spectrum of the disorder and the relative emphasis of one set of symptoms over another, e.g., hallucinations being extremely prominent, it is likely that the various brain systems (e.g., neurotransmitter systems, arousal and selection-attention mechanisms) are differentially affected by the multitude of causes.[20,21]

Confusion appears to relate to a disturbance in the integrated function of those brain structures that are involved in alertness and attention: the ascending reticular activating system, including the thalamus, the cingulate, prefrontal regions, and parietal cortices. Confusion may result from focal structural insults to these structures, either singly or in combination.[8] There is probably dysfunction in other regions as well, but these integrated regions are likely the most crucial.

Impaired attention constitutes the most significant or fundamental component of the acute confusional state.[14] Attention (discussed in detail in Chap. 1) depends both on alertness (including arousal) and on selective concentration and directivity in which choices are made between competing stimuli.[22] The prefrontal regions play a major role. In delirium, impairment of other mental functions may relate to impaired attention, since without attention these functions cannot operate, analogous to the "crash" of a computer.[22] As a corollary, it is impossible to adequately assess most aspects of cognition, whether or not they are selectively or irreversibly impaired, in the presence of impaired attention.

Principal cognitive functions include perception, memory, and thinking. Perception, as mentioned in the first chapter, involves processing of information and linking with stored memory for a synthesis allowing recognition of what is currently being attended.

Hallucinations have a varied pathogenesis. Visual hallucinations may result from: lesions of the visual pathways; seizures, migraine, or ischemia involving the visual cortex, parietal or temporal lobes; schizophrenia and some other psychoses; hallucinogenic drugs; drug or alcohol withdrawal; certain toxic encephalopathies; and rapid-eye-movement (REM) sleep rebound following REM sleep deprivation.[23] The nature of the hallucination may give some clue as to the pathogenesis and the anatomic site. For example, flashes or photopsias implicate the primary visual cortex on the contralateral side if the hallucination is lateralized. Simple geometric forms (e.g., squares and triangles) implicate the adjacent visual association areas. Complex or formed visual hallucinations suggest an origin from the junction of the temporal and occipital lobes. Seizures, migraine, or sometimes psychoses may be responsible in various circumstances. The stereotypy or similarity of repeated attacks and associated semiology (clinical symptom complex) and context (circumstances under which the confusional state occurs) often allow a precise categorization. The particular features and stereotypy of attacks may lead one to suspect complex partial seizures, e.g., stereotyped attacks of motionless and unresponsive staring followed by lip smacking and swallowing suggest complex partial seizures of mesial temporal origin. The context of the illness often helps in arriving at the diagnosis, e.g., the onset of complex partial seizures in association with an acute febrile illness raises the possibility of herpes simplex encephalitis.

Sometimes hallucinations may arise as "release" phenomena with fixed lesions of sensory pathways or primary cortical areas. Patients with Anton syndrome, who are cortically blind due to infarction of the visual cortex, may describe various scenes they "see" before them, besides denying their blindness. With deprivation of REM sleep, and possibly during drug and alcohol withdrawal or with toxicity from anticholinergic drugs, hallucinations contain features similar to the dream components of REM sleep. These seem inappropriately to intrude during the awake state. Auditory hallucinations, e.g., those in alcoholics, would not be expected from this mechanism, however. The hallucinations of dreams in REM sleep are usually visual, less commonly olfactory or kinesthetic, but almost never purely auditory.[24] Altered function of neurotransmitter pathways probably plays a role. Functional neuroimaging suggests that the primary sensory cortex (specific to the sensory modality) and its surrounding areas are activated during hallucinations.[25]

The mechanism for the interpretation of hallucinations or other perceptions as being real and external (alien) versus a product of the mind is unknown. The interpretation of the phenomena as real and alien may arise because of a breakdown in communication between cortical areas.[26] It has been proposed that the lack of insight into the aberrant interpretation of phenomena in schizophrenia relates simplification or "pruning" of synaptic connections in the neocortex and hippocampi and the establishment of autonomous "parasitic foci" within cortical regions.[26] Such simplified networks may develop simplified, stereotyped responses to incoming information. The parasitic foci may also "insert" information, e.g., messages, that are interpreted, without critical interpretation from other regions, as coming from an outside source. The misinterpretation of endogenous or exogenous information may relate to impaired processing. The altered information and impaired processing might lead to the creation of delusional systems, sometimes paranoid, in which the patient tries to explain perceived phenomena.

Should such aberrant discharges or distortions arise in a more normal nervous system, e.g., as the result of a seizure, the circuitry may interpret these discharges differently; these mismatches would be less likely to be interpreted as arising from a real, outside source. It is also possible that altered neurotransmitter function plays a role in interpretations. For example, the dopaminergic system regulates signal-to-noise discrimination of individual neurons; disturbed dopaminergic

activity may alter the responses of neuronal circuits to various inputs.[27]

Faulty processing and anosognosia for the deficit probably also underlie confabulation, the utterance of statements that are incorrect, yet the patient *believes them to be true*. In confabulation, often associated with profound memory impairment (e.g., Korsakoff syndrome) or sensory processing (e.g., Anton syndrome), the patient is *unaware of the deficit* and mistakenly strings together material that comes to mind.[28]

A disordered wake-sleep cycle is common to many encephalopathies: sleep staging is disrupted, REM sleep is often reduced, and patients have repeated wakenings.

In one of the most common acute confusional states, delirium tremens, disturbed central neurochemistry is undoubtedly important: i.e., relatively increased glutamate (excitotoxic) activity, downregulation of gamma-aminobutyric acid (GABA; inhibitory), decreased $alpha_2$-inhibitory receptors, augmented dopaminergic activity, and deficiency of the cholinergic system and serotonergic systems.[15,29] This accounts for the agitation, impaired attention, distractibility, hyperexcitability, hallucinations, seizures, sleep disturbances, increased sympathetic activity, and parasympathetic insufficiency in DTs. These features, in whole or in part, occur in other acute withdrawal states.

Etiologies and Differential Diagnosis

A wide variety of disorders can cause the clinical picture of acute confusional state (see Table 2-1).

Older age and dementia are major risk factors for the development of the acute confusional state.[30-34] Other commonly associated etiologic factors in hospitalized patients include a history of neurologic disease (e.g., cerebrovascular disease, Parkinson disease), hyponatremia, hypoalbuminemia, systemic infection, operative hypotension, uremia, and fever.[35-37] Drugs that produce delirium (especially in the hospitalized, disabled elderly) include: drugs with muscarinic anticholinergic properties (e.g., tricyclic antidepressants, atropine, scopolamine), narcotic analgesics, sedative-hypnotics (especially triazolam and alprazolam) and

Table 2-1
Some causes of acute confusional state

Systematic illnesses	Withdrawal syndromes
Sepsis (septic encephalopathy)	Alcohol
Acute uremia	Drugs
Hepatic failure	
Cardiac failure	CNS infections
Pulmonary disease (esp. pneumonia and pulmonary embolism)	Meningitis
Electrolyte disturbances	Encephalitis
Hypercalcemia	
Porphyria	Intracranial lesions
Carcinoid syndrome	Head trauma
	Acute lesions (right parietal, bilateral
Endocrinopathies	occipital, or mesial frontal)
Thyroid dysfunction	Subdural hematoma
Parathyroid tumors	
Adrenal dysfunction	Hypertensive encephalopathy
Pituitary dysfunction	
	Miscellaneous
Nutritional deficiencies	Heat stroke
Thiamine (Wernicke's encephalopathy)	Electrocution
Niacin	Sleep deprivation
Vitamin B_{12}	
Folate	Psychiatric disorders
	Mania (esp. in the elderly)
Intoxications	Schizophrenia
Drugs (esp. anticholinergics in the elderly)	Depression—some forms
Alcohols	
Metals	
Industrial agents	
Biocides	

Source: From Cummings JL, *Clinical Neuropsychiatry*. Orlando, Grune & Stratton, 1985, p 71, with permission.

antiparkinsonian agents.[38–42] Among antihypertensive drugs, methyldopa has the worst reputation for its association with acute confusional state in the elderly.[43] Histamine-2 receptor blockers infrequently produce delirium in critically ill patients.[44] Delirium and hallucinations are common toxic effects of street drugs[45] or with toxic doses of standard drugs (see Chap. 16). Nonconvulsive status epilepticus may be the underlying cause for acute confusion in late life, either without an apparent precipitant or in the context of a systemic illness such as hepatic failure or hyponatremia.[46]

    Withdrawal of chronically ingested alcohol, sedative drugs, antidepressant and antipsychotic drugs may be associated with an agitated confusional state.[47] The sudden withdrawal of monoamine oxidase (MAO) inhibitors may precipitate a life-threatening delirium with hypertension or hypotension, severe anxiety, agitation, pressured speech, sleeplessness or drowsiness, hallucinations, cognitive impairment, delusions of persecution, and suicidal tendencies.[48]

    Excess corticosteroids or adrenocorticotropic hormone (ACTH) can produce a characteristic encephalopathy that includes an affective component, commonly depression with crying and mood changes without affective thought content.[49] In medically ill patients, the addition of corticosteroids can cause wildly fluctuating mental changes including mood changes, irritability, poor concentration, or psychosis with hallucinations.

Differential Diagnosis of Toxic Confusional State from Other Disorders

Several features favor toxic-metabolic disorders over structural lesions or destructive damage to the brain: (1) fluctuations in level of consciousness or degree of impairment throughout the day (however, fluctuations are seen in extra-axial lesions such as subdural hematoma); (2) agitation with hallucinations, delusions, and increased sympathetic nervous system activity; (3) lack of cranial nerve abnormalities (however, extraocular palsies are found in Wernicke's encephalopathy and pupillary nonreactivity in overdoses of glutethimide and tricyclics); (4) lack of consistent or persistent focal signs; (5) presence of certain motor phenomena: multifocal myoclonus, asterixis (although lateralized asterixis is seen in some midbrain and parietal lesions), and tremor (see Chap. 3 on clinical evaluation); and (6) certain features of the electroencephalogram (EEG) feature (e.g., bisynchronous rhythmic delta activity or triphasic waves, each against a slow or suppressed background) strongly suggest a metabolic encephalopathy (see Chap. 3).

Although lesions of specific cortical regions can cause confused behavior, there are usually unique characteristics that are peculiar to the affected location. There are also dissociations, so that even large cortical lesions may not be accompanied by confusion. The development of confusion may depend on the acuity and recency, as well as the size, location, and disturbed connectivity of the region, and, occasionally, certain phenomena such as seizures.[50] Lesions of both prefrontal regions can cause lack of judgement, foresight and planning, emotional changes, and perseveration. More localization-specific behaviors include: lack of emotional tone, and impersistence (inability to persist with a task), with nondominant frontal damage; aphasic errors, apraxia, and reduced verbal and gestural fluency (dominant frontal damage); and problems with bimanual tasks, unrepressed (utilization) behavior with usage of perceived objects in the environment, and gait and continence problems (bifrontal damage).

With temporal lobe lesions, amnesia accompanies bitemporal lesions; temporal lobe seizures tend to be stereotyped repetitive behaviors (automatisms) often preceded by visceral (e.g., rising epigastric) sensations, emotional change, especially fear, or dysmemory phenomena (déjà vu or déjà écouté). Often, there are more localization-specific features to indicate a temporal origin, such as aphasic errors or verbal or nonverbal memory deficits, with dominant and nondominant temporal lesions, respectively.

Parietal lesions can be associated with neglect syndromes (either parietal lobe), apraxia (usually the dominant parietal lobe), spatial disorientation, and attentional disorders (the latter two with nondominant parietal lobe dysfunction). Usually, there will be accompanying features, such as language disturbance, features of Gerstmann syndrome (right-left disorientation, finger agnosia, and agraphia and acalculia) lateralized neglect, and somatosensory or visual field deficits, to allow clinical localization that can be confirmed with neuroimaging tests. Parietal or occipital seizures usually are associated with positive visual or somatosensory phenomena. Features tend to be discrete and stereotyped, as opposed to phenomena in acute global confusion.

Table 2-2 shows the differential aspects of delirium, dementia, and depression.

The following features are more typical of toxic-metabolic encephalopathies than demential illnesses (e.g., Alzheimer disease): acute onset and fluctuating course, impaired attention, short duration, reduced awareness and level of consciousness, impaired remote memory, altered perceptions, and disorganized rather than impoverished cognitive function.[23] In contrast, patients with Alzheimer disease show a chronic, persistent loss of intellectual and cognitive function that is ultimately incapacitating for social function. In the early stages of Alzheimer disease, the mental disturbance largely relates to memory dysfunction.

Acute schizophrenia or mania may mimic delirium, but such patients usually do not show the degree of cognitive deficits found in delirium.

Table 2-2
Delirium versus dementia and depression

Feature	Delirium	Dementia	Depression
Onset	Acute or subacute, often "sundowning"	Chronic, insidious	Coincides with life changes, often abrupt
Course	Short, diurnal fluctuations	Long, no diurnal effects, progressive	Variable and uneven
Progression	Abrupt	Slow, even	Variable
Duration	Hours to several weeks	Months to years	Weeks to years
Awareness	Reduced	Clear, aware	Clear
Alertness	Fluctuates	Usually normal	Minimally impaired, distractible
Attention	Impaired	Relatively unaffected	Aspects selectively affected
Orientation	Fluctuates, usually impaired	May be impaired	Aspect selectively impaired
Memory	Immediate and recent, often impaired	Recent worse than remote, both impaired	Intact (themes of hopelessness expressed)
Thinking	Disorganized, fragmented	Perseveration and confabulation, difficulty with abstraction	Intact; delusions and hallucinations only in severe cases
Perception	Often distorted, delusions and hallucinations, problems with reality	No misperceptions	Intact; delusions and hallucinations only in severe cases
Speech	Incoherent, hesitant slow or rapid	Word finding problems, neologisms	Unaffected
Sleep-wake cycle	Always disrupted	Fragmented	Disturbed, often early morning wakening
Psychomotor behavior	Variable, hyperkinetic, hypokinetic, or mixed	Normal, may have apraxia	Variable, psychomotor retardation or agitation
Mental status testing	Distractible from task	Failings, good effort, frustration in early cases	Failings, poor effort, frequent "don't know" answers, gives up
Physical illness or drug toxicity	Either or both present	Often absent, especially in Alzheimer disease	Variable

The delusions and hallucinations of delirium are less systematized than those of functional psychoses; auditory hallucinations are much more common in functional than organic psychoses.[14] The affect may be flattened and not in keeping with thoughts and actions, in contrast to delirium, where they tend to covary. Differentiation can be difficult, however. Although the EEG may help in the differential diagnosis of an agitated confusional state, it is usually impractical because of the patient's agitation, and, furthermore, it may not be sufficiently distinctive in early delirium.

Depression is an affective disorder characterized and dominated by lack of enjoyment of life and a dysphoric mood. Slowing that simulates confusion or dementia only occurs in very severe psychotic depression. Differentiation from a confusional state can be problematic, especially if a serious medical illness coexists.

In delirium, paraphasic errors are not common. If one encounters language-related problems, a specific aphasia, e.g., Wernicke's aphasia, should be suspected. Wernicke's aphasia is commonly mistaken for an acute confusional state. Such patients have fluent speech with paraphasias and striking impairment of repetition, comprehension, and naming. Such patients usually do not have the motor, emotional, and autonomic changes that accompany an agitated delirium.

Laboratory Tests for Causes of the Acute Confusional State

The history, physical and neurologic examinations will likely provide the diagnosis in most cases, but diagnostic procedures are necessary to confirm the clinical suspicions. The following tests are indicated when specific concerns arise, but many of these need to be done when the etiologic possibilities are wide:

1. Lumbar puncture: to exclude meningitis, encephalitis, or subarachnoid hemorrhage.

2. Blood, urine, sputum, and cerebrospinal fluid (CSF) cultures for systemic or central nervous system (CNS) infection. A Venereal Diseases Research Laboratory (VDRL) test on serum and/or CSF for syphilis is probably worth doing, especially when the diagnosis is uncertain.

3. Toxic screen: when there is even a remote possibility, or upon admission through emergency.

4. Metabolic screen for serum concentrations of electrolytes, glucose, urea, calcium, albumin, magnesium, bilirubin, ammonia, aspartate aminotransferase (AST), phosphate, and serum vitamin B_{12} concentration: for most cases.

5. Complete blood count (CBC) and platelet count: for most cases.

6. Blood gases: for most cases.

7. Endocrine studies: thryoid function tests, especially thryoid-stimulating hormone assay, in selected cases, for hypo- or hyperhyroidism.

8. EEG: use to confirm altered cerebral cortical function, to exclude seizure activity (EEG is the only reliable test for nonconvulsive status epilepticus), and to grade the severity of the encephalopathy.[51] Middle- and long-latency evoked potentials, including cognitive evoked electrophysiologic responses (e.g., the "P300" response), can be used in the detection of problems in cortical processing.[52]

9. Neuroimaging [e.g., computed tomography (CT) or magnetic resonance imaging (MRI)]: indicated if there are consistent focal signs or if there is a possibility of an extra-axial lesion such as a subdural hematoma or bilateral intracerebral or extra-axial lesions.

Management

Prevention The acute confusional state in the elderly is often prevented by more appropriate use of medications. Drugs should be used only when necessary, taking renal and hepatic function in mind for the dosage schedule. Whenever possible, polypharmacy should be avoided: an increase from one to four different medications augments ninefold the probability of drug-induced confusion.[53] Unfortunately, our ability to predict the consequences of specific drug combinations is inadequate; therefore, it is best to be both cautious and vigilant. Regular drug utilization reviews are a good idea. It is a good policy to discontinue, if feasible, any drugs that could cause a confusional state, as soon as the altered mental status is recognized.

To prevent drug withdrawal reactions, it is best to taper medications that have been used for some time. Special precautions need to be taken in the discontinuance of MAO inhibitors, clonidine, narcotics, barbiturates and antiepileptic drugs.

Since the debilitated elderly are more susceptible than most other groups, and since sensory and sleep deprivation may play a causative role in

Table 2-3

The standardized Mini-Mental State Examination

Item comment	Maximum correct score	Patient's score	Question / Instruction and
1.	5	( )	What is the: date ____, week day ____, month ____, season ____, year ____?
2.	5	( )	Where are we: country ____, province or state ____, city ____, building ____, floor ____?
3.	3 One point for each correct answer	( )	Name three objects (ball, car, man). Take one second to say and ask the patient to repeat them. Repeat trials until the patient remembers, or a maximum of six trials. Count trial and record: ____ trials.
4.	5 One point for each correct answer	( )	Serial 7s. $100 - 7 = ($ $)$, $93 - 7 = ($ $)$. Alternatively, have the patient spell "world" backwards.
5.	3 Given one point for each answer, regardless of order	( )	What were the three objects you were asked to remember?
6.	9	( )	• Name a watch and a pencil (2 pts) • Repeat "no ifs, ands, or buts" (1 pt) • Follow this command: "Take the paper in your right hand, fold it in half and put it on the floor" (3 pts) • Look at the command "Close your eyes," read the words and do it (1 pt) • Write a complete sentence (1 pt) • Copy the design (intersecting pentagons)
Total score Note level of consciousness: • hypervigilant • alert • drowsy • obtunded • confused	Maximum 30	( )	

Source: From Ref. 60, with permission.

producing confusion in such patients, it is reasonable to control this, as well as possible, with orientation, emotional support, and judicious use of medication.[54] Recent controlled trials that used such strategies revealed only modest benefits, mainly in surgical rather than in medical patients.[55,56]

Investigation and Treatment   Early recognition and prompt investigation and management of the acute confusional state should lessen morbidity and mortality. Mortality for DTs was 10 to 20 percent in the 1960s but has fallen to 1.7 percent with modern management.[57] Nurses initially document 60 to 90 percent of such instances on the wards.[35] An acute onset of altered awareness, disorientation, memory impairment, aggressive behavior, and impaired ability to interact are important indicators.[58] Nurses should be sensitive to the early manifestations of the acute confusional state.[59] Families and close friends are sensitive to changes in mental status; their concerns should be taken seriously. In high-risk patients, it is reasonable to monitor the patient's attention and orientation and/or to perform the Mini-Mental State Examination (see Table 2-3) daily at the bedside.[60] The Confusion Assessment Method (CAM), a standardized test battery for delirium, was developed as a quick and reliable method of detecting the acute confusional state.[61] The diagnosis of delirium is based on four features: (1) acute onset and fluctuating course, (2) inattention, (3) disorganized thinking, and (4) altered level of alertness. The diagnosis of delirium requires both features 1 and 2 as essential factors and either of features 3 or 4. The CAM, administered by nurses, physicians, or trained lay interviewers, was shown to have a positive predictive value of over 90 percent when compared with a psychiatrist's evaluation. The scoring can be completed in less than 5 min. A specific Delirium Symptom Interview has also been developed for diagnostic and monitoring purposes.[62]

Prompt investigation (Table 2-1) and correction of the *underlying illness* are essential. Supportive therapy is also needed: basic fluid and electrolyte balance, and adequate nutrition and vitamin supplementation must be initiated and maintained.

Agitation in the critically ill patient requires nearly continuous nursing care, a well-lit room, a regular routine, constant reorientation and reassurance, but it often requires pharmacologic treatment as well. Haloperidol and short-acting benzodiazepines (e.g., lorazepam) are the safest and most useful drugs;[63] in general, barbiturates should be avoided. Psychoses with hallucinations,

paranoia, etc., may relate to excessive dopaminergic stimulation, and are better treated with parenteral haloperidol than with other drugs that are not as specific and often have anticholinergic or cardiovascular side effects.[64] Carbamazepine, up to 800 mg/day, is sometimes helpful for psychotic features in DTs.[15]

Agitation and fear without psychotic features are best treated with an anxiolytic, such as lorazepam.[65]

Restraints may add to patients' agitation and are best avoided except when absolutely necessary.[66] When used, restraints should be a very temporary measure.

If pain is associated with agitation, narcotics are usually necessary. The brief use of neuromuscular blocking agents in agitated, ventilated patients is sometimes necessary if other measures have failed.[18] However, this should be a last resort because of the attendant risks of complications, as discussed below. Paralyzed patients may still be aware and suffer tremendous psychologic distress unless they are appropriately sedated as well.

Increased sympathetic activity (perspiration, tachycardia, and hypertension) can be treated with clonidine, a centrally acting alpha$_2$ adrenergic agonist. For mild cases, 0.2 mg one to three times a day is sufficient; for more severe cases, up to 2.3 mg/day of oral or intravenous clonidine have been used. If given intravenously, an initial dose of 0.025 mg/h is recommended.[15]

Therapeutic attempts at augmenting serotonergic activity have not been attempted. Although serotonin deficiency probably occurs in alcoholism, excessive serotonin activity, e.g., as induced by large doses of specific serotonin reuptake inhibitors, may cause an agitated delirium—the "serotonin syndrome"[67] (Chap. 16).

Prophylaxis against seizures is controversial. When seizures do occur, phenytoin or barbiturates are often effective. Standard therapy for status epilepticus is sometimes required (Chap. 17).

It is important to be aware of possible complicating conditions, e.g., subdural hematoma, hepatic failure, meningitis, or pneumonia with sepsis in the alcoholic. Hence, the investigations mentioned earlier should be always considered.

Because variables may operate synergistically, potentially contributing factors should be altered, e.g., nonessential drugs should be stopped; infections and metabolic imbalances should be corrected; and vitamins, especially thiamine, should be administered.

STUPOR AND COMA

Stupor and coma are characterized by impairment in the arousal system. In coma, the patient cannot be roused to consciousness, while in stupor, the patient will awaken only briefly and will lapse back into a sleep-like state when the stimulation ceases. The patient must be awake before the other higher mental functions can be assessed clinically. It follows that the assessment of the nervous system of such patients is seriously hampered.

Stupor and coma are precarious states that should be regarded as medical emergencies. Speed in assessment, and supportive and definitive management are of the essence. With the use of all available clinical information and appropriate investigative strategies, a diagnosis and prognosis can often be achieved.

The anatomy and physiology of the arousal system are discussed in Chap. 1, while the clinical features, differential diagnosis, investigation, and management are dealt with in detail in Chap. 3.

Coma is contrasted with other states of impaired responsiveness in Tables 2-4 and 2-5.

AKINETIC MUTISM

Definition and Clinical Features

The syndrome of akinetic mutism was best defined and described in the seminal paper by Cairns and colleagues concerning a 14-year-old girl with an epidermoid cyst of the third ventricle.[68]

"In the fully developed state she lay alert except that her eyes followed the movement of objects or could be diverted by sound. A painful stimulus would produce reflex withdrawal of a limb... but without tears, noise or other sign of pain or displeasure.... [There were] bilateral signs of pyramidal tract involvement, and she was totally incontinent. As one approached her bedside her steady gaze seemed to promise speech but no sound [was produced]. She showed.... "loss of feeling tone, loss of emotional expression, of spontaneous and most of other voluntary movements. She was incapable of originating movements of any kind, with the notable exception that ocular fixation and movement occurred in response to the movement of external objects and to sounds."

Additional descriptive comments concerned distractibility, the presence of wake and sleep cycles, excessive sleep, and arousability from sleep. After the cyst was drained, the patient's behavior transiently returned to normal, during which time she could not recall anything of events during the state of akinetic mutism. Thus, memory mechanisms were impaired during akinetic mutism.

The clinical syndrome is not always manifest in such a complete form. The syndrome may show some fluctuation and, at times, allows for understanding speech and obeying simple commands. Such efforts are, however, ineffective or incomplete. Although there are almost always some signs of pyramidal tract involvement, this can be associated with the extreme progression to decorticate or decerebrate posturing.[68]

Etiology

Akinetic mutism occurs in association with acute hydrocephalus, tumors of the pineal gland or thalamus, hemorrhage into the dorsal medial thalamus, posterior thalamic-rostral midbrain lesions, strokes affecting the anterior limbs of the internal capsules, various lesions of the white matter of the frontal lobes, or destructive lesions of the medial surfaces of the frontal lobes, especially these involving the cingulate gyri.[69-75] In some cases of encephalitis, the main damage is in the posterior hypothalamus. Other diencephalic and limbic structures are also often involved with inflammatory lesions.

Table 2-4
Characteristics of major syndromes

Characteristics	Persistent vegetative state	Coma	Brain death	Locked-in syndrome	Akinetic mutism	Dementia
Self-awareness	Absent	Absent	Absent	Present	Present	Present, but lost gradually or in stages
Sleep-wake cycles	Intact	Absent	Absent	Intact	Intact	Intact
Motor functions	No purposeful movement	No purposeful movement	None, or only spinal-originating	Quadriplegia+ pseudobulbar palsy[a]	Paucity of movement	Variable, limited with progression
Experience of suffering	No	No	No	Yes (if facial/eye movements present)[a]	Questionable: variable avoidance	Yes, but lost in late stages
Respiratory function	Normal	Variable, may be depressed	Absent	Usually normal[a]	Normal	Normal
EEG	Suppressed or slow	Variable, dependent on severity, topography and etiology	Electrocerebral silence	Normal	Nonspecific slowing	Generalized slowing
Cerebral metabolism	Reduced to 50% or more	Reduced by 50% or more (increased if seizures)	Absent	Normal or minimally decreased	Unknown	Variably reduced
Prognosis for neurologic recovery	Depends on cause and duration	Recovery, PVS, or death (usually known by 2 weeks)	No recovery	Recovery unlikely for pontine strokes[a]	Recovery unlikely (depends on cause)	Irreversible (ultimately, depends on cause)

[a] The locked-in syndrome is usually related to a lesion of the basis pontis. If the definition is expanded to include other conditions associated with decreased responsiveness but intact cognition (see text), these variables will be different.
Source: Modified from Ref. 82, with permission.

Table 2-5
Components of consciousness

Characteristics	PVS	Coma	Brain death	Locked-in syndrome	Akinetic mutism	Dementia (e.g. Alzheimer disease)	Psychogenic Unresponsiveness
Wakefulness	+	−	−	+	+	+	+
Attention	−	−	−	+	r	+/r	+
Working memory	−	−	−	+	−	+/r	+
Perception	−	−	−	+	r	r	+
Long-term memory	−	−	−	+	−	r	+
Motivation	−	−	−	+	−	+/r (Late)	Aberrant
Cognition	−	−	−	+	−	r	+/Aberrant
Purposeful motor response	−	−	−	−	−/r	+/r	Aberrant
EEG	Abnormal: suppressed/slow: W&S	Abnormal: wide range (including seizures)	Electrocerebral silence	Normal W&S	Slow (marked); W&S	Slow (usually mild): W&S	Normal; W&S

Key: r = present, but reduced from previous state; W&S = wake and sleep cycles present; + = present; − = absent.

Pathophysiology

The syndrome is usually associated with impairment of thalamic and prefrontal functions, on either the mesial or the orbital-frontal surface. Cairns deduced that the seat of the trouble lay with the diencephalon as decompression of the third-ventricular cyst relieved the symptomatology while drainage of the lateral ventricle did not.[68] Intracranial pressure is not necessarily increased at a time of akinetic mutism.[68]

There are two conceptual mechanisms for akinetic mutism: (1) impaired "activation" of cortical, especially prefrontal, and function from reduced thalamic input; and (2) impaired connectivity of the motor system from frontal damage.[76] However, these mechanisms alone would not explain the associated, profound disturbance in cognitive function that accompanies most cases. It is likely that integrated diencephalic-cortical function is disturbed in these cases. There may be a spectrum, however, in which some cases show predominantly the motor deficit and others have both motor and cognitive problems.

Akinetic mutism is sometimes at least partially reversed by dopaminergic agents, e.g., Sinemet or bromocriptine.[77-80] This implies that there is a functional deficiency of dopaminergic activity—probably in the rostral forebrain (median forebrain bundle).

Differential Diagnosis

The syndrome of akinetic mutism is not difficult to identify when it is fully developed. Because of fluctuations and the presence of milder cases (there may be a spectrum), it is instructive to consider the differential diagnosis of apathetic behavior. The word apathy is derived from *pathos* (Greek for passion); thus, apathy is literally the absence of passion. In psychiatric-neurologic usage, apathy signifies an absence of motivation. Apathy is seen in a number of conditions; it should be assured, however, that motivational lack is the prime problem. For example, patients with depressive illness may appear apathetic, but they are suffering from emotional distress in the form of depression.

Marin proposes the following psychiatric-neurologic classification of apathy[81].

1. General physical, social or environmental factors: e.g., emigration to another cultural region; natural disasters (psychic numbing), loss of hearing or visual ability in the elderly.

2. Neurological disorders: Wernicke-Korsakoff's psychosis. Typical akinetic mutism. Lateralized frontal lesions that produce *abulia*, a hypoactive state short of akinetic mutism (abulic patients register information and have memories, in contrast to patients with akinetic mutism). Basal ganglia disorders, associated with akinesia or lack of movement, are sometimes associated with apathy. (Because of the immobility, however, some may only *appear* to be apathetic.) Blunted emotionality with bitemporal lesions.

3. Psychiatric disorders: psychoses including chronic or catatonic schizophrenia, catatonia and "psychotic depression" with psychomotor retardation.

4. Drug effects: drugs which reduce dopaminergic activity, e.g., phenothiazines, postamphetamine immobility, as with neuroleptic malignant syndrome or extreme parkinsonism.

5. Some medical conditions: chronic renal or hepatic failure, apathetic hyperthyroidism, hyperparathyroidism and pseudohyperparathyroidism.

6. A primary or pure apathetic state as a pervasive abnormality of personality. Apathy as a psychiatric term should refer to a pervasive as opposed to a selective lack of motivation or interest (which often occurs normally). As such, it is part of a personality disorder.

The locked-in syndrome, usually related to a lesion in the basis pontis, also needs to be differentiated from akinetic mutism (Tables 2–4 and 2–5). Such patients are conscious, possess wake and sleep cycles, but have quadriparesis and pseudobulbar palsy, preventing voluntary movements of the jaw, facial, laryngeal, pharyngeal, and tongue muscles. Horizontal gaze is typically lost but voluntary vertical gaze and control of eye opening are intact. Such patients can communicate by eye blinks and vertical eye movements. Thus, they are mute and nearly akinetic but have intact mentation. Management and humane care implications are obvious.

Similarly, pseudobulbar palsy causes limited mutism by interruption of corticobulbar tracts alone.

Laboratory Tests

Usually, the cause will be apparent, either from the patient's history or from neuroimaging. Neuroimaging is usually necessary to exclude structural lesions in the brain, especially the frontal lobes or medial diencephalic region. Functional neuroimaging, e.g., functional MRI positron emission tomography (PET) or single photon emission computed tomography (SPECT) with various agents, may show decreased perfusion of the frontal lobes. The EEG shows diffuse delta waves.

Management

The treatment is dependent on the underlying condition. The decompression of diencephalic structures can relieve the condition, as shown by Cairns' case described above.

Symptomatic treatment with dopamine precursors, such as Sinemet, or agonists, such as bromocriptine, is used for patients who cannot be helped surgically or who remain abulic after surgical decompression, ventricular drainage, or shunting.[78,79] This treatment can be maintained for as long as necessary, but it is sometimes feasible to gradually withdraw such drugs in a few weeks.

PERSISTENT VEGETATIVE STATE

Definition and Conceptual Description

In the persistent vegetative state (PVS), patients have the capacity for wakefulness but not *awareness*. The patient has wake and sleep cycles and can be roused from sleep, but cannot interact with stimuli or carry out any motor act that requires planning or cognitive function. There is no

evidence of cognition or awareness of self or the environment.[82] Reactions to stimuli are simple, automatic, stereotypic, and predictable, rather than goal-directed. Hypothalamic functions and cranial nerve and spinal reflexes are usually, but not necessarily completely, preserved.

In PVS, the *arousal system* is functioning, but the *cognitive* component of consciousness is lacking. Because we cannot know what an unresponsive person is thinking, our clinical conclusions must be inferred. Supportive evidence includes: (1) Behavior occurs in stereotypic responses that are thought to arise at subcortical regions in a reflexive or almost reflexive fashion. (2) The PET studies (see above) show a marked reduction in cerebral metabolism compared with normals and patients with locked-in syndrome. (3) All available pathologic material indicates that PVS is associated with lesions that would have made conscious awareness highly improbable.[82]

When Jennett and Plum coined the term "persistent vegetative state," "persistent" meant that the state was consistently sustained over the period of observation.[83] The term was not meant to imply permanency. To prognosticate that the vegetative state is *permanent* requires time and observation. Despite arguments to the contrary,[84] we argue that ancillary tests are very helpful when appropriately applied (see below).

Epidemiology

The estimated prevalence of PVS in the United States is 10,000 to 25,000 for adults and 4,000 to 10,000 for children.[82]

Etiologies of Persistent Vegetative State

Etiologies of PVS (Table 2-6) can be classified into:

1. Acute brain insults: these are acute brain disorders that lead to a vegetative state following a period of coma lasting days to weeks. During the comatose period, there may be compromise of ventilatory drive, autonomic functions, etc., but these basic functions recover alongside the reappearance of arousal and wake-sleep behavior. The succeeding vegetative state may become *per-*

Table 2-6

Principal causes of the persistent vegetative state for adults and children

Acute insults	Subacute and chronic insults (degenerative, metabolic, and infectious)
Traumatic	*In adults*
Motor vehicle accidents	Alzheimer disease
Gunshot wounds/other direct injury	Multi-infarct dementia
Nonaccidental injury in chidren	Pick disease
Birth injury	Creutzfeldt-Jakob disease
	Parkinson disease
Nontraumatic	Huntington disease
Hypoxic-ischemic encephalopathy	
Cardiorespiratory arrest	*In children*
Perinatal asphyxia	Ganglioside storage disease
Prolonged hypotensive episode	Adrenoleukodystrophy
Near-drowning	Neuronal ceroid lipofuscinosis
Suffocation or strangulation	Organic acidurias
Cerebrovasular injury	Mitochondrial encephalopathy
Cerebral hemorrhage	Gray matter degenerative disorders
Cerebral infarction	
Subarachnoid hemorrrhage	**Developmental malformations**
CNS infection	Anencephaly
Bacterial meningitis	Hydranencephaly
Viral meningoencephalitis	[a] Lissencephaly
Brain abscess	[a] Holoprosencephaly
CNS tumor	[a] Encephalocele
CNS toxins or poisoning	[a] Schizencephaly
	[a] Congenital hydrocephalus
	[a] Severe microcephaly

[a] For some severe cases only.

Source: From Ref. 82, with permission.

manent or the patient may have various degrees of cognitive recovery. The most common acute causes of the vegetative state in both children and adults are head trauma and hypoxic-ischemic encephalopathy.[82] Certain encephalitides, e.g., St. Louis, Eastern and Western equine, and Japanese B, may also produce a coma followed by a vegetative state; this is related to diffuse cerebral cortical damage.[85]

2. Subacute and chronic disorders: these include various degenerative, metabolic, and infectious conditions. These include progressive or cumulative brain diseases, progressing through cognitive and multifocal deficits to dementia to loss of all cognitive function, but with preservation of basic arousal and wake-sleep cycles.[82,86] From an epidemiologic perspective, the most common condition is Alzheimer disease. Other relentlessly progressive disorders, such as Creutzfeldt-Jakob disease, subacute sclerosing panencephalitis, and metabolic storage diseases of infancy, e.g., Tay-Sachs disease, can produce terminal PVS.

3. Developmental malformations: these are conditions that develop during embryogenesis and in which the cerebral structures (in which cognition

would take place) never develop into functioning anatomic structures. Thus, these patients do not have the *potential* for cognition, based on our knowledge of the nervous system. Even before cognitive function would develop in the normal neonate, it should be possible to identify those extreme cases of brain maldevelopment where the patients could never achieve self- and environmental awareness.

Anatomic Basis of Persistent Vegetative State

There are three basic topographic patterns of neuropathology in patients who have died of PVS that was persistent to death.

1. Predominantly Neocortical The most common finding in PVS patients who suffered severe anoxic-ischemic insult is diffuse laminar cortical necrosis.[87–92] This involves the larger cell layers—3, 5, and 6 especially—but the necrosis can involve all layers. In addition, there is almost invariable involvement of the hippocampus (especially the CA1 and CA4–6 regions) and variable involvement of subcortical gray matter structures and the cerebellar Purkinje cells. A markedly suppressed or "flat" EEG is commonly found.[93]

2. Predominantly Thalamic An alternative pattern has recently been proposed following a very careful study of the brain of Karen Ann Quinlan.[94] Karen Ann Quinlan suffered a cardiopulmonary arrest at age 21 years. She survived for nearly a decade in a persistent vegetative state, in which she showed wake and sleep cycles, and spontaneous eye opening as well as eye opening to auditory stimuli. She showed simple withdrawal-type responses to stimuli, more than spinal reflex movements, but not goal-directed, purposeful actions.

At postmortem, the thalamus was shown to be severely affected, especially in the paramedian and lateral regions of the central and posterior portions. (It is of special interest that the "nonspecific" and reticular thalamic nuclei were severely

ravaged, given their proposed function in arousal.) The forniceal system and mammillary bodies were badly damaged. The cerebral cortex was especially affected in the parasagittal watershed zones posteriorly and in the occipital lobes. However, other cortical regions were relatively spared. Thus, her PVS appears to have been due largely to diencephalic disease.

The postmortem study gives reasonable evidence that: (1) the thalamus plays an important role in cognitive function; and (2) extrathalamic mechanisms may cause alerting and "activation" of the cerebral cortex as an alternative pathway to the traditional ascending reticular activating system (ARAS).

3. Diffuse Axonal Injury and Subcortical White Matter Damage Diffuse axonal injury results from acute trauma in which shearing decelerating-accelerating and rotational forces tear white matter axons. This effectively isolates the cortex from subcortical structures.[95] There may be associated brainstem injury, but this is not an essential or consistent feature.[82]

Leukoencephalopathies following anoxic insults or carbon monoxide poisoning (often appearing a week or two after apparent recovery), necrotizing hemorrhagic leukoencephalopathy, or necrotizing leukoencephalopathies from methotrexate-radiation damage (Chap. 7) could produce PVS.

Clinical Features

Criteria for the diagnosis of PVS have been established by the Multi-Task Force on PVS[82]:

1. No evidence of awareness of self or environment and an inability to interact with others.

2. No evidence of sustained, reproducible, purposeful, or voluntary behavioral responses to visual, auditory, tactile, or noxious stimuli.

3. No evidence of language comprehension or expression.

4. Intermittent wakefulness manifested by the presence of wake-sleep cycles.

5. Sufficiently preserved hypothalamic and brainstem autonomic functions to permit survival with medical and nursing care.

6. Bladder and bowel incontinence.

7. Variably preserved cranial-nerve reflexes (pupillary, oculocephalic, corneal, vestibulo-ocular, and gag) and spinal reflexes.

The patient in PVS is not immobile, but he/she moves the eyes, limbs, and trunk in meaningless ways. There is no goal-directed behavior and the patient does not visually track or show a behavioral, emotional, or avoidance response to the image projected on the retina. Primitive orienting reflexes, such as turning the head and eyes towards the source of a sound or tactile stimulus, may be present.

As a corollary, when patients do visually track or show more than reflexive or instinctive behavior on testing and retesting, they are no longer in PVS.

Recovery from PVS occurs in some patients. Usually, the first feature is the return of visual tracking, followed by primitive behaviors, then the obeying of commands and, next, spontaneous purposeful activity. Speech, cognitive function, and motor abilities have been fully or nearly fully recovered in a small number of patients. Significant improvement is very unlikely in a child or adult who has been in PVS for more than 12 months.[82] Some very exceptional cases occur, where recovery of reactivity occurs after more than a year in PVS.[96] Laboratory assessment of cerebral function (see above) should allow more reliable predictors than clinical features alone. Better guidelines are needed.

Differential Diagnosis

The main conditions to be differentiated are conditions of reduced responsiveness. These and their principal differentiating features are given in broad outline in Tables 2-4 and 2-5. It should be noted that decreased responsiveness does not necessarily imply decreased consciousness or cognitive function. Patients may have psychogenic unresponsiveness (e.g., from malingering, psychosis, or conversion reaction) or may be locked-in (either from the classic basis pontis lesion or peripheral de-efferentation, e.g., severe Guillain-Barré syndrome, myopathy, or neuromuscular transmission defect).

The recognition of PVS on clinical grounds alone, especially in patients with severe motor deficits, can be very difficult. This applies especially to patients with severe motor disabilities. Andrews et al reported a careful assessment of 40 patients admitted to a rehabilitation unit with the clinical diagnosis of PVS several months to years after the initial insult.[97] Occupational therapists worked with these patients daily for 2 weeks and sought to obtain consistent button push responses to questions, with the patient using either a limb or the head and neck. Seventeen (43 percent) of the patients were able to respond, indicating misdiagnosis of PVS.

Management

Management decisions are dependent on the accurate diagnosis of PVS (see criteria for diagnosis above) and then determination of prognosis. The value of adherence to valid guidelines in arriving at a diagnosis in PVS was emphasized in a recent survey at London's Royal Hospital for Neuro-disability. Seventeen of 40 patients deemed to be in PVS were, in fact, aware.[97] A similar American study showed inaccurate diagnosis in 18 of 49 (37 percent) patients thought to be in PVS.[98]

With developmental abnormalities, e.g., hydranencephaly, and the chronic progressive degenerative, subacute, and chronic infectious disorders discussed above, there is no hope of meaningful recovery when PVS is reached. Establishing the prognosis in the acute brain disorder category is the most difficult, as the outcome is often not as clear in the early phase of the illness. Consulting the literature for guidance is problematic because: (1) most studies are retrospective, and therefore biased; (2) outcome measures in some studies in some patients are often not clearly defined, e.g., "poor outcome" refers to PVS as well as patients with various degrees of disability who are not vegetative; and (3) the perceived prognosis affects the quality of care, i.e., the care is less vigorous in

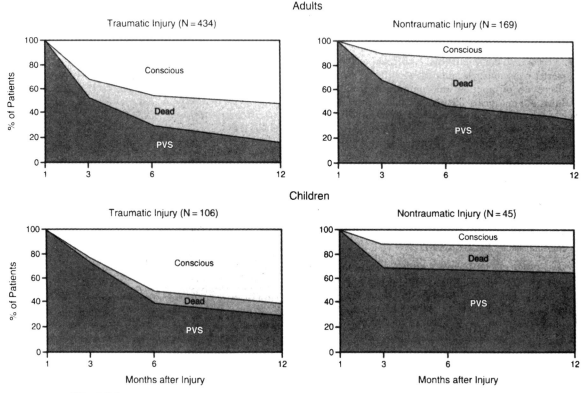

Figure 2-1

Outcome for patients in PVS after traumatic and nontraumatic insults. Discussion is given in the text. (From Multi-Society Task Force on PVS,[101] with permission.)

patients who are perceived to have a poor outcome.[99,100]

Establishing the Prognosis Clinically

Figure 2-1 shows the outcome in patients with PVS after traumatic and nontraumatic injuries.[101] With trauma in either adults or children, recovery of consciousness after 6 months is unusual, but it does occasionally occur.[102] In contrast, recovery of consciousness after nontraumatic PVS is uncommon (15 percent of adults and 13 percent of children) and rare after 3 months in both adults and children. This led the American Academy of Neurology to issue the following diagnostic standards for a permanent vegetative state[103]:

1. PVS is usually permanent if it persists for 12 months following *traumatic* injury in adults and children. Special attention to signs of awareness should be devoted to children during the first year after traumatic injury.

2. PVS can be judged to be permanent for *nontraumatic* injury in adults and children after 3 months.

3. The chance for recovery after these periods is exceedingly low, and recovery is almost always to a severe disability.

A Role for Investigative/Confirmatory Tests

Electroencephalogram   These have shown varied results as they are heavily dependent on the anatomic site of maximum damage. Since the EEG records only cerebral cortical synaptic activity, it is most helpful in those cases in which the cortex is primarily affected. Thus, in severe anoxic-ischemic insult, the EEG shows suppression of various degrees. Complete suppression in such cases is associated with a *permanent* vegetative state, if the patient survives for several weeks or more.

With white matter and thalamic lesions, EEG rhythms are better preserved. These show various degrees of slowing and reactivity, as well as differences between wakefulness and sleep.[94,104,105]

Evoked Potential Studies Somatosensory evoked potentials (EPs) are useful in the early assessment of the probability of death or PVS following all three anatomic types of insult.[106] They are most reliable in the coma after anoxic-ischemic insult, where bilateral absence of the N20 potential after median nerve stimulation (in the presence of intact earlier potentials, e.g., N14) is reliably predictive that PVS is permanent.[107-109] They are also of considerable value in the post-trauma patient (see Chap. 6).

Neuroimaging Standard neuroimaging is of value in PVS. Patients with PVS are more likely to have abnormal CT or MRI scans than those who recover.[110,111] Predictive guidelines for PVS based on degrees of structural change have not been developed, but cases of large bihemispheric near-total destruction, such as in cases of hydranencephaly or complete bilateral middle cerebral artery territory infarctions, would be predictive of PVS.

Functional Neuroimaging The tests that have potential value in prognosis include PET and blood flow studies. Positron emission tomography studies of regional cerebral oxygen and glucose metabolism show widespread reduced metabolism in the cerebral cortex of PVS patients by at least 40 percent that of normal or of patients with locked-in syndrome.[112,113] It is not yet certain whether this consistently reflects irreversible damage (e.g., in cases of multiple infarcts, could recovering multiple "penumbra" show improvement?) and to what extent this represents the metabolism of neuronal versus nonneuronal cells.

Cerebral blood flow (CBF) studies show variable patterns shortly after coma-producing insult.[114,115] However, after the PVS is established, there is a reduction in CBF. The use of HMPAO-SPECT (hexamethylpropylaminoxime–single photon emission computed tomography) shows similar results in at least one preliminary study.[116]

Withdrawal of Care

Management issues hinge on an accurate diagnosis (see above) and prognosis. After this is established, the management of the "whole person" needs to include both science and considerations of the individual case.[117] Usually, if the PVS is a permanent one, most individuals would not wish to be medically supported to prolong such a low quality of existence. The issue of deciding on the level of care is discussed in Chap. 24 on "Ethics."

BRAIN DEATH

Definition

Death is defined as the irreversible end of life. All cultures recognize this as death, even though most have the idea of a spiritual afterlife. These concepts do not appear to conflict with each other.[118] Unlike the definition of other medical disorders, death is entrusted to the law rather than to medicine. In other words, the law has the ultimate authority to declare a person dead. Prior to the concept of brain death, death was identified as irreversible cessation of heartbeat and respirations. This definition still applies, but, with the advent of intensive care units and ventilators, another form of death, that of the brain, became recognized as being equivalent to death.

Death of the brain without cessation of the heartbeat required assisted ventilation and intensive medical care. With ventilatory support, it is possible to maintain the heartbeat of even those with massive, irreversible structural brain damage who could never awaken or breathe on their own. Cessation of heartbeat without recovery of consciousness inevitably follows in days or weeks, even with continued support. Such individuals have no recognizable brain function (including respiration) and are unable even to maintain their own internal milieu: they develop diabetes insipidus, poikilothermia, and require pressor support for blood pressure. In 1959, the term *coma depassé* (the state beyond coma) was coined by French neurologists to describe the state of such individuals.[119] This concept was slow to be accepted in other countries until the published conclusions of the 1968 "A definition of irreversible coma: report of the Ad Hoc Committee of the Harvard Medical School to examine the definition of brain death".[120] Subsequently, there has been a general acceptance that death of the brain is a necessary and sufficient condition for death of the individual. As argued by Korein, brain death is not "a new way of being dead" or a totally new idea, but it represents the essential nugget of human death.[121] Even the old criteria of cessation of heartbeat and respirations were not valid if patients were successfully resuscitated. However, if the heart had stopped and the brain was nonviable, this was death. Thus, brain death allowed the medical profession and society to consider and refine the definition of death.[118]

The matter of declaring brain death has enormous implications for legal purposes, notably the transplantation of organs. Clearly, for brain death declaration and subsequent organ transplantation, it is essential that the individuals are truly dead; the issue is not at all equivalent to predicting a poor outcome, persistent vegetative state, or severe disability.[122]

Criteria for Brain Death

The brain death criteria of the Harvard Committee of 1968[120] are given in Table 2-7. This document is of great historical importance as: (1) it gave official recognition to brain death; and (2), it served as a model for other efforts at developing criteria for determining brain death in a reliable and timely manner. The official recognition of brain death by society allowed for the removal of vital organs for transplantation purposes, as often such organs were viable even though the brain was not. Subsequent refinements of brain death criteria were

Table 2-7
"Harvard criteria" for brain death (1968)

1. Unreceptivity and unresponsivity—no response even to intensely painful stimuli.
2. No movement or spontaneous respiration for 3 min off respirator.
3. No reflexes: fixed, dilated, and unresponsive pupil; no ocular movements with head turning and irrigation of the ears with ice water, no blinking; no postural activity; no corneal or pharyngeal reflexes; no swallowing, yawning, or vocalization; no biceps, triceps, pronator, quadriceps, or gastrocnemius reflexes, and no plantar response.
4. Flat EEG for at least 10 min of technically adequate recording is of great confirmatory value; no reactivity to noise or pinch.
5. All of the above tests repeated in 24 h with no change.
6. No evidence of hypothermia or CNS depressants.

Source: Ref. 120.

made in the United States in 1981 (Table 2-8).[123] These have recently been revised in the United Kingdom; the essentials are contained in Table 2-9.[124] Criteria have also been officially revised by the American Academy of Neurology; the main points are listed in Table 2-10.[125] These are all clinical guidelines that can only be validly applied when (1) there is an acute CNS catastrophe that is capable of causing brain death; (2) conditions that might prevent valid application of clinical criteria (severe electrolyte, acid-base or endocrine disturbance, or shock with systolic blood pressure less than 90 mmHg) have been excluded; (3) drug intoxication or poisoning are absent: and (4) the core body temperature is at least 32.2°C.

Clinical Evaluation

Before considering whether brain death has occurred, the diagnosis should be known and the condition should be one that is capable of causing neuronal death. Such conditions include trauma, intracranial hemorrhage, or severe brain swelling. Determination of irreversibility is dependent on the cause, completeness of the dysfunction, the passage of time (to demonstrate consistency), and

Table 2-8
Guidelines for brain death proposed by medical consultants on the diagnosis of death to the President's Commission for the Study of the Ethical Problems in Medicine and Biomedical and Behavioral Research (1981)

An individual with irreversible cessation of all functions of the entire brain including the brainstem is dead.

1. Cessation is recognized when evaluation discloses findings of (a) and (b):

    a. Cerebral functions are absent. There must be cerebral unresponsivity and unreceptivity.

    b. Brainstem functions are absent. These include pupillary light, corneal, oculocephalic, oculovestibular, oropharyngeal, and respiratory reflexes. Apnea is tested with a nasal cannula delivering oxygen and demonstrating failure of respiratory effort with Pa_{CO_2} greater than 60 mmHg. Spinal cord reflexes may persist after death. True decerebrate and decorticate posturing or seizures are inconsistent with the diagnosis of death.

2. Irreversibility is recognized when evaluation discloses findings of (a) and (b) and (c):

    a. The cause of the coma is established and is sufficient to account for the loss of brain functions.

    b. The possibility of the recovery of any brain function is excluded.

    c. The cessation of all brain functions persists for an appropriate period of observation or trial of therapy ... confirmation of clinical findings by EEG is desirable when objective documentation is needed to substantiate the clinical findings ... complete cessation to the normothermic adult brain for more than 10 min is incompatible with the survival of brain tissue ... absent cerebral blood flow, in conjunction with the clinical determination of cessation of all brain functions for at least 6 h, is diagnostic of death ....

Complicating conditions:

A. Drug and metabolic intoxication
Drug intoxication is the most serious problem in the determination of death.... In cases where there is any likelihood of sedative presence, toxicology screening for all likely drugs is required. If exogenous intoxication is found, death may not be declared until the intoxicant is metabolized or intracranial circulation is tested and found to have ceased ... before irreversible cessation of brain functions can be determined, metabolic abnormalities should be considered and, if possible, corrected.

B. Hypothermia
Criteria for reliable recognition of death are not available in the presence of hypothermia (below 32.2°C core temperature).

C. Children: The brains of infants and young children have increased resistance to damage and may recover substantial functions even after exhibiting unresponsiveness on neurologic examination for longer periods than do adults. Physicians should be particularly cautious in applying neurologic criteria to determine death in children younger than 5 years.

D. Shock: Physicians should also be particularly cautious in applying neurologic criteria to determine death in patients in shock because the reduction in cerebral circulation renders clinical examination and laboratory tests unreliable.

Source: Ref. 123.

confirmation by retesting. With anatomic disruption of the brainstem, e.g., by hemorrhage or trauma, the intervals between assessments can be just a few hours apart. With generalized anoxic-ischemic encephalopathy from cardiac arrest, or with fat or air embolism, it may take longer, e.g., 24 h or more, to establish a confident prognosis. Ancillary tests, e.g., those of cerebral perfusion, can be used to make earlier diagnoses of brain death or a more timely prognostic evaluation.

The presence of potentially reversible causes of coma (especially sedatives or hypothermia), neuromuscular blocking agents, severe neuropathy, or drugs with anticholinergic effects preclude application of the clinical criteria alone.

Table 2-9
U.K. criteria for the diagnosis of brainstem death (Working Group convened by the Royal College of Surgeons, 1995)
(This incorporates and updates the previous U.K. code for brain [stem] death of 1976)[186]

Definition of death
Death is defined as "the irreversible loss of the capacity for consciousness, combined with the irreversible loss of the capacity to breathe." The irreversible cessation of brainstem function (brainstem death), whether induced by intracranial events or the result of extracranial phenomena such as anoxia, will produce the same clinical state. Therefore, brainstem death is equivalent to death of the individual. It is suggested that the more correct term "brainstem death" should henceforth replace the term "brain death" used in previous papers produced by the Conference of Colleges and the Department of Health.

The diagnosis of brainstem death
The clinical criteria for the diagnosis of brainstem death identified by the Conference of Colleges during the period 1976–1981 have been confirmed by all published series and have been adequately validated. The following issues are incorporated into the discussion in the text: (a) a beating heart in brainstem death, (b) endocrinologic and metabolic abnormalities (recognizes that some endocrinologic abnormalities arise as a result of brain death rather than as a cause, e.g., diabetes insipidus, electrolyte and fluid balance abnormalities, hypothermia), (c) limb and trunk movements, (d) investigations, (e) children, (f) the persistent vegetative state (differentiation from brain death), (g) peripheral nervous syndromes of critical care.

Conditions under which the diagnosis of brainstem death should be considered
1.   There should be no doubt that the patient's condition is due to irremediable brain damage of known etiology (discussed in text).

2.   The patient is deeply comatose:

   (a) There should be no suspicion that this state is due to depressant drugs (discussed in text).
   (b) Primary hypothermia as a cause of coma must have been excluded.
   (c) Potentially reversible metabolic and endocrine disturbances must have been excluded as a likely cause of coma. It is recognized that metabolic and endocrine disturbances are a likely accompaniment of brainstem death but these are the effect rather than the cause of that condition and do not preclude the diagnosis of brainstem death.

3.   The patient is being maintained on the ventilator because spontaneous respiration has become inadequate or ceased altogether (discussed in text). It is essential that these conditions be satisfied before the diagnosis of brain death is considered or further investigated.

Source: From Ref. 124, with permission.

This applies whether such factors are present in isolation or in association with potentially lethal etiologies.

After it is established that the patient's condition is due to irreversible brain damage of known etiology, three necessary clinical components of brain death are: unresponsiveness, absence of brainstem reflexes, and apnea. These will be discussed in turn:

1.   Unresponsiveness   There should be no motor response of the limbs or grimacing to nailbed and supraorbital pressure. Because of the possibility of a neuropathy or spinal cord lesion, applying a stimulus to a somatosensory branch of a cranial nerve is essential. The supraorbital branch of the ophthalmic division of the cranial nerve is the most practical one to test: one applies pressure with a finger against the medial supraorbital region. For peripheral stimulation, vigorous compression of the patient's nailbed by a pen is adequate.

No spontaneous movements arising from the brain (e.g., dystonic, decerebrate, or decorticate posturing or seizures) should be present. It is notable that movements of spinal cord origin may

Table 2-10

Practice parameters for determining brain death in adults (Report of the Quality Standards Subcommittee of the American Academy of Neurology [1995])

The following captures the essential aspects of the previous American guidelines "Proposed by Medical Consultants on the Diagnosis of Death to the President's Commission for the Study of the Ethical Problems in Medicine and Biomedical and Behavioral Problems" of 1982. Some aspects are clarified and updated.

I. Diagnostic criteria for the clinical diagnosis of brain death.

    A. Prerequisites. Brain death is the absence of clinical brain function when proximate cause is known and demonstrably irreversible.

        1. Clinical or neuroimaging evidence of an acute CNS catastrophe that is compatible with the clinical diagnosis of brain death.

        2. Exclusion of complicating medical conditions that may confound clinical assessment (no severe electrolyte, acid-base, or endocrine disturbance).

        3. No drug intoxication or poisoning.

        4. Core temperature $\geq 32°C$ (90°F).

    B. The three cardinal findings in brain death are coma or unresponsiveness, absence of brainstem reflexes, and apnea.

        1. Coma or unresponsiveness—no cerebral motor response to pain in all extremities (nailbed and supraorbital pressure).

        b. Ocular movement:

            (i) No oculocephalic reflex (testing only when no fracture or instability of the cervical spine is apparent).

            (ii) No deviation of the eye to irrigation of each ear with 50 mL of cold water (allow 1 min after injection and at least 5 min between sides).

        c. Facial sensation and facial motor response:

            (i) No corneal response to touch with a throat swab.

            (ii) No jaw reflex.

            (iii) No grimacing to deep pressure on nailbed, supraorbital ridge, or temporomandibular joint pain.

        d. Pharyngeal and tracheal reflexes:

            (i) No response after stimulation of the posterior pharynx with a tongue blade.

            (ii) No cough response to bronchial suctioning.

        3. Apnea. Testing procedure as follows:

        a. Prerequisites:

            (i) Core temperature $>36.5°C$ or 97°F.

            (ii) Systolic blood pressure ≥ 90 mmHg.

            (iii) Euvolemia. *Option:* positive fluid balance in the previous 6 h.

            (iv) Normal P_{CO_2}. *Option:* $P_{CO_2} > 40$ mmHg.

            (v) Normal P_{O_2}. *Option:* preoxygenation to obtain arterial $P_{O_2} > 200$ mmHg.

        b. Connect a pulse oximeter and disconnect the ventilator.

        c. Deliver 100% O_2, 6 L/min, into the trachea. *Option:* place a cannula at the level of the carina.

        d. Look closely for respiratory movements (abdominal or chest excursions that produce adequate tidal volumes).

        e. Measure arterial P_{O_2}, P_{CO_2}, and pH after approximately 8 min and reconnect the ventilator.

        f. If respiratory movements are absent and arterial P_{CO_2} is ≥ 60 mmHg (*Option:* 20 mmHg increase in P_{CO_2} over a baseline normal P_{CO_2}), the apnea test is said to be positive (i.e., it supports the diagnosis of brain death).

(Continued overleaf)

Table 2-10 *Continued*

g. If respiratory movements are observed, the apnea test is negative (i.e., it does not support the clinical diagnosis of brain death) and the test should be repeated.

h. Connect the ventilator if, during testing, the systolic pressure becomes <90 mmHg or the pulse oximeter indicates significant oxygen desaturation and cardiac arrythmias are present; immediately draw an arterial blood sample and analyze arterial blood gases. If P_{CO_2} is >60 mmHg or the P_{CO_2} rise is >20 mmHg, the apnea test is said to be positive (i.e., it supports the diagnosis of brain death); if P_{CO_2} is <60 mmHg or P_{CO_2} is <20 mmHg over baseline P_{CO_2}, the result is indeterminate, and an additional confirmatory test can be considered.

Other recommendations, including pitfalls, clinical observations compatible with the diagnosis of brain death, and optional confirmatory tests, are discussed in the text and in the original document.

occur during hypoxia or hypotension (e.g., Lazarus' sign).[126] There may be neck and hip flexion, arching of the back, or short excursion breathing movements. Testing motor responsiveness is not valid if there is neuromuscular paralysis from a severe neuropathy or neuromuscular blockade.[127] If neuromuscular blocking agents have been administered, it should be demonstrated, by eliciting deep tendon reflexes or by the use of a peripheral nerve stimulator, that the block is no longer operative.[128]

2. Absence of Brainstem Reflexes See Fig. 2-2.

Pupils A bright light is shone in each pupil independently, examining for direct and consensual (opposite) pupillary constriction. The pupils could be midposition or dilated but should not react to light.[129] Round, oval, or irregular-shaped pupils are all compatible with brain death.

Atropine inadvertently dropped on the cornea, overdoses of drugs with antimuscarinic

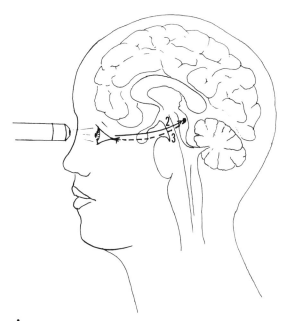

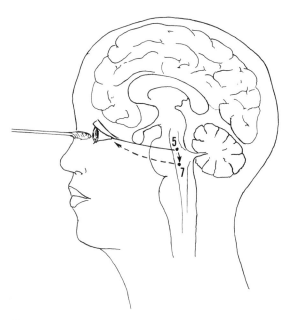

A   **B**

blocking properties, or traumatic mydriasis may cause pupillary nonreactivity. In conventional doses, intravenous atropine does not affect the pupillary response.[130] A report of fixed, dilated pupils after extremely high doses of intravenous dopamine has not been confirmed.[131] This author's

group has observed fixed pupils in the context of *both* shock *and* high doses of dopamine, however.

Ocular Movements   In brain death, ocular movements are absent along with the oculocephalic (head turning) and oculovestibular (caloric)

Figure 2-2

The four main brainstem reflexes to be tested as part of the assessment for brain death. A. Pupillary reflexes are tested by shining a bright light alternatively in each eye, while looking for a direct and consensual constriction of the pupil. 2= optic nerve and 3= oculomotor nerve and nucleus. B. The corneal reflex is tested by touching each cornea with a cotton swab while looking for contraction of the orbicularis oculi and/or upward deviation of the eyes (Bell's phenomenon). 5= trigeminal nerve, serving corneal sensation and 7= facial nerve, supplying orbicularis oculi. C. The oculovestibular reflex is tested by irrigating the ear canal with up to 150 cm³ of ice water with the head at 30° up from horizontal. Any eye movement is looked for. In the unconscious patient with intact brainstem and afferent connections from the ear and efferent connections to the extraocular muscles, the eyes tonically deviate to the side of irrigation. No grimacing should be noted with the application of painful stimulation. As part of this test, the painful stimulation should be applied in cranial nerve (usually the fifth) territory. 3= oculomotor nerve on one side, 6= contralateral abducens nerve and nucleus, 8= vestibular nerve; mlf= medial longitudinal fasciculus. D. The pharyngeal reflexes are tested by stimulating the larynx and trachea by the passage of a suction catheter into the back of the throat and down the nasogastric tube. 9= glossopharyngeal nerve (afferent limb of reflex), 10= vagus nerve (efferent limb of reflex). *The asterisk represents the outflow of the vagus to the pharyngeal muscles and palatal elevators. (Patients may also cough, reflecting a fixed action reflex driven by a central program.) (Redrawn from Pallis,[187] with permission.)

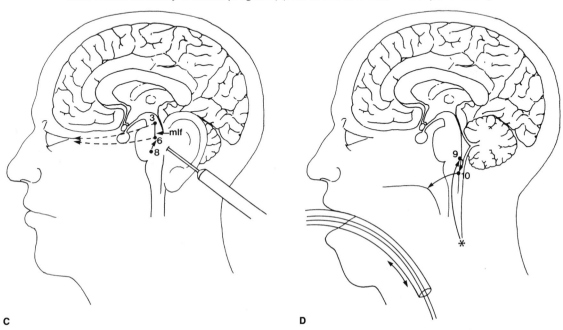

C   D

testing. Caloric testing is a more potent stimulus; it should always be used if the oculocephalic reflex is absent. A syringe is used to inject $50 \, cm^3$ of ice water into the canal. In the unconscious patient with an intact brainstem, both eyes tonically deviate to the irrigated side. One minute of observation should be allowed after each injection which should be at least 5 min apart.

Drugs that may abolish the caloric response include high doses of sedatives, aminoglycosides, most antiepileptic drugs, tricyclic antidepressants, anticholinergic drugs, and certain chemotherapeutic agents.[132] Closed head injury, facial trauma, lid edema, or chemosis of the conjunctiva can preclude assessment of eye movements. Basal skull fractures involving the petrous bone (often with Battle's sign or hemotypanum) may abolish the caloric response on the same side. The canals should be cleared of clotted blood and cerumen and the oculovestibular reflex testing should be repeated after visual inspection reveals the ear canals to be clear.

Facial Sensation and Movements Corneal reflexes are usually tested with a cotton swab. Facial movements can be assessed by applying pressure to the supraorbital ridge or over the condyles near the temporomandibular joint. Severe facial trauma can limit validity of the interpretation.

Pharyngeal and Tracheal Reflexes The gag response is tested by touching the posterior pharynx with a tongue depressor. This is often difficult in the orally intubated patient, in whom the cough reflex can be demonstrated by tracheal suctioning or tracheal tug.

3. Apnea Testing Two problems occurred with the Harvard (1968) recommendations[120] re apnea testing in brain death determination: (a) desaturation of arterial oxygen during the period of disconnection from the ventilator; and (b) insufficient partial pressure of carbon dioxide in arterial blood (Pa_{CO_2}) to stimulate respirations. The first problem was effectively prevented in most patients by preoxygenating with 100% oxygen for 10 min

before apnea testing and then administering 100% oxygen, through a tracheal cannula or cannula inserted to the level of the carina, at 6 to 8 L/min during disconnection from the ventilator. Respiratory movements are looked for during the time that the ventilator is stopped. The second problem is somewhat more difficult as the optimal Pa_{CO_2} concentration for stimulation of the medullary respiratory center has not been established.[133] In most cases, however, a rise of Pa_{CO_2} to greater than 60 mmHg, generally accepted as a sufficient stimulus, is met by ensuring that the Pa_{CO_2} is 40 ± 5 nmHg before disconnection, that the temperature is $> 36.5°C$, and by allowing at least 8 min of disconnection. In most cases, this is sufficient to allow the Pa_{CO_2} to rise above 60 mmHg.[133] This should obviate the need to administer 5% carbon dioxide, a procedure that can lead to severe hypercarbia and respiratory acidosis.[134] In all but patients with chronic chest disease and insensitivity to Pa_{CO_2}, this should serve as a powerful stimulus to the medullary respiratory centers for respiration.

Because apnea testing constitutes a stress and may cause intracranial pressure (ICP) to rise, it should only be done if there is a strong suspicion of brain death and cranial nerve areflexia. Euvolemia, preferably a positive fluid balance, and a stable, normal blood pressure are recommended prerequisites before the apnea test is performed.

Respiration or spontaneous ventilation is defined as abdominal or chest movements that produce adequate tidal volumes. If present, respiration is present in the early phases of testing. Some respiratory-like movements, despite brain death, arise as spinal cord phenomena. These may occur at the end of testing if oxygenation is marginal or with continued use of continuous positive airway pressure. Such movements (shoulder elevation and adduction, back arching, and intercostal expansion) do not produce a tidal volume; this can be confirmed by spirometry.

During apnea testing, if the systolic blood pressure falls to less than 90 mmHg, the pulse oximeter shows marked desaturation, or cardiac arrhythmias occur, one should immediately draw a blood gas sample and reconnect the ventilator. Testing is considered valid if there is apnea during the test and the Pa_{CO_2} rises to greater than 60 mmHg, unless other exclusions apply.

Exclusions and Caveats

It must be emphasized that the clinical criteria occasionally cannot be adequately applied for the determination of brain death. Severe facial trauma may preclude assessment of cranial nerve reflexes. Hypothermia, shock, or toxic levels of various drugs (e.g., sedatives such as barbiturates, carbamazepine, and tricyclics) may produce reversible unresponsiveness and depression of cranial nerves or spontaneous respirations. Overdoses of drugs with antimuscarinic properties may produce unreactive pupils. In these events, the clinical criteria are not valid and ancillary tests are necessary. Benzodiazepines are very cumulative. It is essential that the drug history be carefully reviewed. The possibility of drug intoxication being the cause of, or contributing to, the patient's clinical state precludes the clinical diagnosis of brain death.

Peripheral neurologic syndromes can invalidate the application of clinical criteria, e.g., the assessment of any movements, including apnea testing, or reflexes. These include neuromuscular transmission defects (including the use of neuromuscular blocking agents), polyneuropathies (including Guillain-Barré syndrome, critical illness polyneuropathy, and porphyria), severe myopathies, or anterior horn cell disorders.[135]

Advances in Concepts of Brain Death Since the 1968 Guidelines

Important conceptual advances include:

1. Acceptance of brain death as death even with preservation of spinal cord reflexes.

2. Recognition that brainstem death is the essential and necessary component of brain death.

3. Improved apnea testing (discussed above).

4. Appropriate use of ancillary tests.

5. Consideration of neonates and young infants.

Along with this, it is necessary to have established practice parameters. For example, a recent survey of methods of apnea testing in brain death showed considerable variation among neurologists in their technique and duration of observation.[136] A major problem is that there are very few well-designed clinical studies to validate the criteria for brain death.[133,137]

These concepts will be discussed in turn. Apnea testing has already been discussed above.

1. A Dead Brain and an Alive Spinal Cord Not long after the publication of the Harvard criteria, a number of single and collaborative studies pointed out that the spinal reflexes could be preserved in cases that otherwise met the criteria for brain death, with appropriate confirmation that the brain was nonviable.[138–142] These reflexes included movements of the trunk and limbs usually related to segmental spinal activity. It then became accepted that brain death could occur in the presence of intact spinal reflexes.

2. Brainstem Death Three years after the publication of the Harvard criteria, Mohandas and Chou from Minnesota published their study showing that most cases of brain death could be reliably diagnosed using clinical criteria alone.[143] The EEG was thus not mandatory. Furthermore, they noted that irreversible damage to the brainstem was "the point of no return." They also introduced the idea of etiologic preconditions, i.e., that the etiology had to be something capable of causing irreversible structural damage or necrosis of tissue. This report had considerable influence in the United Kingdom, where thinking on the topic was led by Christopher Pallis. He conceived of "brainstem death" as being the essence of brain death. In other words, if the brainstem is dead, all the conditions of the Harvard and other criteria are met. It is then irrelevant to ensure that all the intracranial neurons are dead. His ideas formed the basis for the U.K. set of criteria for brain death (see Table 2-7). This has subsequently been accepted in Canada.[144] In the United States, the current guidelines are those of the President's Commission for the Study of Ethical Problems in

Medicine and Biomedical and Behavioral Research, published in 1981 (Table 2-8).[123] There is still widespread opinion in the United States that death of the entire brain must be ascertained and that "brainstem death" is inadequate.[145] Arguments against relying on Pallis' set of criteria for brainstem death include the consideration of potentially reversible conditions, such as severe Guillain-Barré syndrome, similar to our case 4 in Chap. 1, the Miller Fisher variant of Guillain-Barré syndrome (mistakenly termed brainstem encephalitis), and a single case report of a four-ventricular hemorrhage in a premature infant.[146-148] None of these cases, however, would have been accepted if the British criteria were properly applied. The etiology would have precluded the first two; concerns about prematures, neonates, and young infants should have created extra caution with the last case (see below). Philosophically, it is of great comfort to the attending physician to feel that the "whole brain" is dead. However, this is most often an unobtainable goal when one considers the difficulties in excluding some neuronal activity in deep cerebral structures. The relevance of such surviving neurons above a dead brainstem is unclear; it seems analogous to persisting neuronal activity in the spinal cord, which is also a CNS structure.

3. Improved Ancillary Testing

Angiography Angiography is regarded as a final determinant in the diagnosis of brain death: the finding of "blocked intracranial circulation."[149] Its chief use is in cases where clinical criteria cannot be applied: i.e., unsuitability for cranial nerve (e.g., enucleation of one or both eyes, swollen face, or petrous fracture) or apnea testing (e.g., severe acute or chronic pulmonary disease). Angiography creates technical problems: namely, moving an unstable patient to the angiography suite and assuring that the patient is not hypotensive during the injection. This would be even more problematic for premature neonates (see below). Systemic hypotension may prevent the angiographic dye reaching the intracranial compartment, unless the dye is injected under pressure

with the catheter filling the lumen of the vessel. Injection into the wall (usually deep to the intima) will also prevent dye from reaching the intracranial compartment. Vertebral as well as carotid injections are necessary to ensure that the intracranial circulation is arrested.

Radioisotope Nuclide Scanning Conventional scanning with technetium 99m-labeled agents is convenient and can be done at the bedside in the intensive care unit with adequate monitoring and support.[150] A major drawback is that such scanning does not adequately assess the posterior fossa circulation.[151] After all, if brainstem death is the essential element that must be proven, perfusion of the brainstem should be the essential part of the assessment. Brain flow studies by themselves are thus generally not regarded as sufficient evidence of brain death, but they are of considerable ancillary value.[152]

Perfusion imaging with ^{99m}Tc-hexamethyl-propylamineoxime (^{99m}HMPAO) constitutes an advance: the result is independent of the adequacy of the bolus injection; there are no problems with venous sinus activity; posterior fossa circulation (at least to the cerebellum) can be assessed.[153-156] The test can be performed at the bedside with two planar views; the CT technique is not needed.[157] See Fig. 2-3.

Nuclear Magnetic Resonance (NMR) There are distinctive nuclear magnetic resonance imaging (MRI) features of brain death (Fig. 2-4)[158]:

1. Loss of the subarachnoid spaces.

2. Slow flow in the intracavernous and cervical internal carotid arteries.

3. Loss of flow void in the small and large intracranial arteries and the major intracranial venous sinuses.

4. Relative loss of normal gray-white differentiation on T1-weighted images but preservation of gray-white differentiation on T2-weighted images, producing a "supernormal" appearance.

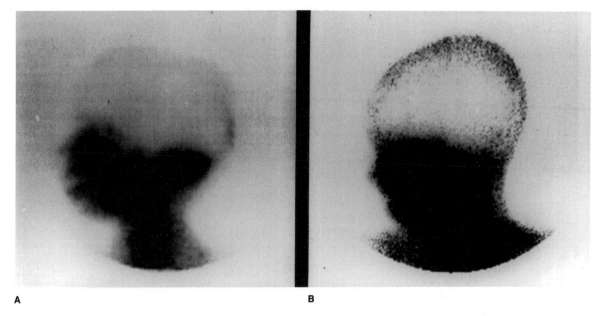

A   B

Figure 2-3
^{99m}Tc-Hexamethylpropylamineoxime brainscan performed at the bedside. A. This scan was taken when brainstem reflexes were partially preserved; there is uptake in the cerebellum. B. This scan, taken 4 h later when brainstem reflexes were absent, shows no perfusion of posterior fossa structures.

Magnetic resonance angiography and MRI may play an important future role; this needs further study and confirmation. Nonparamagnetic ventilator equipment must be used; transportation to the scanner and the time involved may be problematic. Functional MRI has not been examined; NMR spectroscopy may also play a future role.

Transcranial Doppler Transcranial Doppler flow studies can give supportive evidence of absent flow through middle cerebral and basilar arteries.[159] The latter technique is difficult, however, and one needs to be certain that one has insonated a vessel or feeding vessel before one can be certain that there is no flow. Patterns compatible with greatly increased ICP include: (1) absent diastolic or reverberating flow, indicating flow only through systole or retrograde diastolic flow; and (2) small systolic peaks in early systole with absent or reversed flow, indicating very high

vascular resistance (see Fig. 2-5).[160] The pattern of brief systolic forward flow appears to be specific for brain death in several series.[126,161,162] Lack of transcranial Doppler signals is necessary, but this finding is not confirmatory of brain death as 10 percent of patients do not have temporal insonation windows. An exception might be in patients who had previously documented transcranial Doppler signals. The sensitivity and specificity of transcranial Dopplers in brain death are 91.3 and 100 percent, respectively.[163]

Transcranial Doppler velocities can be markedly affected by significant changes in Pa_{CO_2}, hematocrit, and cardiac output.[163] The techniques require considerable practice, patience, and skill. Because of such marked operator-dependence, it is not universally recommended.

Other Tests of Brain Blood Flow These include nitrous oxide flow studies,[164] tests of pulsatile midline echo on ultrasound,[165] and arteriovenous

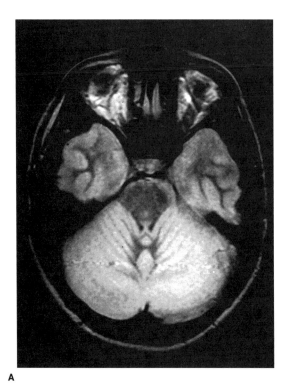

A

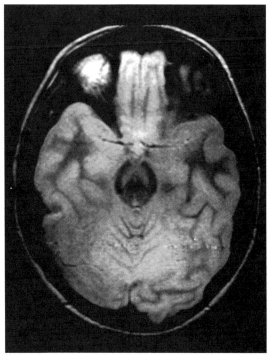

B

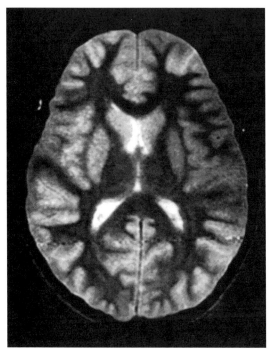

C

Figure 2-4

Typical MRI findings in brain death. The patient was a 16-year-old girl who suffered hypoxic-ischemic brain damage. She met the criteria for brain death shortly after these images were taken. A. This shows loss of subarachnoid spaces, loss of anatomic definition with the brainstem, and no flow void in the basilar artery. B. This shows flow void in the proximal middle cerebral artery which correlates with the transcranial Doppler study in Fig. 2-5. The more distal middle cerebral artery does not show flow void, nor did other arteries or venous sinuses. C. This shows the "supernormal appearance" of the brain with very distinct cortical–white matter definition, thought to be due to increased cellular and interstitial edema and the absence of brain pulsations. Also note the absence of subarachnoid space.

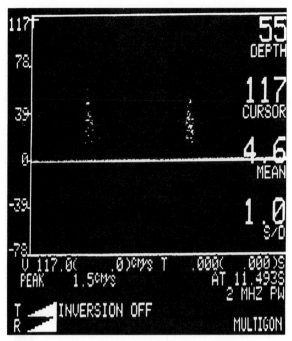

Figure 2-5

Transcranial Doppler studies of a middle cerebral artery from the same patient as in Fig. 2-4. There is a systolic peak only and no diastolic component.

oxygen difference. Nitrous oxide brain flow studies can provide useful prognostic information, but have not been tested adequately in very low flow states. Hyperoxia of jugular venous blood is characteristic of brain death.[166] None of these tests, however, have achieved general acceptance as stand-alone criteria or replacements for clinical criteria when the latter cannot be applied.

Electroencephalogram Pallis maintains that the EEG is irrelevant in the diagnosis of brain death. If patients meet all the clinical criteria, no patient of over 1000 surveyed has survived or recovered consciousness despite being ventilated until asystole.[167] Many of these patients did not have isoelectric EEGs. Conversely, when the EEG shows no electrical activity over $2\,\mu V$, some patients may survive, especially with drug intoxication, hypothermia, or immediately following

circulatory arrest.[93] The EEG may be some confirmatory value in some circumstances, but in the author's opinion, this is very limited. However, the EEG has historically been a part of the diagnostic protocol in the United States. Since electrical cortical activity indicates some function of cerebral cortical neurons, it is difficult for many physicians to conceptually declare brain death when such potentials are present, even though it makes no difference to outcome.

Evoked Potentials Brainstem auditory and somatosensory evoked potentials are relatively insensitive to barbiturate and other drug effects.[168,169] Their absence is an indication of very serious disruption of the intrinsic brain function, providing the potentials that precede them indicate that the signal has reached up to the CNS. However, they sample only a small component of brain function in restricted sensory pathways. Furthermore they can be technically difficult in the hostile electrical environment of the ICU; it is more difficult to standardize the quality than many other diagnostic tests.

4. Neonates and Very Young Children
Early guidelines for the determination of brain death raised cautions about their application to infants and children under 5 years of age, because their brains had "increased resistance to damage" and a greater likelihood of recovery compared with adults.[170] Some early studies suggested that application of "adult criteria" to children, even those under 3 years of age, was appropriate.[171,172] Anecdotal reports of newborns who had no evidence of brainstem or EEG activity, but who survived, added greatly to the doubt about applying standard criteria.[173,174] More recently, the British have concluded that brainstem death criteria can be applied to infants of more than 2 months postterm.[124,175]

Evoked responses hold some promise; they have been used in infants to predict with some accuracy an outcome no better than PVS.[176] However, they have not been adequately tested in brain death. Sensory evoked responses can be used to assess sensory pathways and way stations for auditory and somatosensory pathways, but are specific to those anatomic locations.

Angiography to demonstrate absence of intracranial flow in the carotid and vertebrobasilar systems is the gold standard, but the procedure is difficult, time and labor-intensive, risky, and invasive, especially in the neonate and more so in the premature infant.

Problems with other ancillary tests have been recognized. Cranial sector scanning using the anterior fontanelle can examine for the absence of pulsations in the anterior and middle cerebral arteries, but the brainstem circulation is not examined. Thus, some neonates may show facial movements or may survive with intact respirations despite absent flow on cranial ultrasound.[177] Similar issues are found with nuclear medical scanning.[178] Although such infants are severely disabled, they are not brain dead. Some of the issues can be resolved by waiting a suitable period of time, and then reapplying clinical criteria.[179]

In the United States, a Special Task Force published guidelines for the determination of brain death in children.[180] These were similar to previous "adult criteria" except that times of observations were specified for different ages: (1) For infants of 7 days to 2 months and gestational age of more than 38 weeks, two examinations and EEGs separated by 48 h are recommended. (2) For infants of 2 months to 1 year, two examinations and EEGs separated by 24 h are recommended. A repeat exam is not necessary if a concomitant cerebral radionuclide angiographic study demonstrates no filling of the cerebral arteries. (3) For infants over 1 year, an observation period of at least 12 h is recommended. The observation period can be shortened if the EEG shows electrocerebral silence or if cerebral radionuclide angiographic study demonstrates no filling of the cerebral arteries.

Soon after this, however, a number of articles raised concern. The cause of coma in the neonate may be antenatal and not as clearly obvious as with adult cases.[181] Hypotension is often difficult to exclude or properly define in the newborn.[181] The results of ancillary tests may not be definitive.[181] Sufficient numbers had not been tested to allow a high probability of certainty; especially if there is no available proof a priori of brain death.[122] The validity of the EEG as a test for brain death was questioned, as nearly 20 percent of clinically brain dead patients had residual EEG activity, a finding noted also in children.[181,182] The rationale for the times suggested by the task force was questioned because supportive, scientifically validated evidence was lacking.[183] There were additional concerns. Toxic screens for children are not all inclusive; some ingested but commonly available drugs may not be assayed.[184] Some metabolic disorders in neonates may not be detected in hospital laboratories. Premature and even full-term neonates may not be very responsive normally, raising the validity of testing reactivity.

On the positive side, brainstem function can be adequately assessed in neonates over 48 weeks gestational age. Thus, if we use brainstem death as the benchmark, the clinical evaluation is likely valid in neonates, providing the other provisions of the task force are met. The EEG seems insufficient and unnecessary, but it may provide some support; some neonatologists and pediatric neurologists use a "flat" EEG as a screen for apnea testing.

CONCLUSIONS

Ethical issues surrounding the management of cases that do not quite meet "whole brain" or brainstem death criteria are discussed in Chap. 24.

For clinicians, it is vital to follow established guidelines in the diagnosis of brain death and to *document* the essential steps in arriving at the diagnosis. Brain death should never be diagnosed hurriedly in the emergency room. There should be an appropriate period of observation and the clinical examination should be repeated, mainly for confirmatory purposes. The diagnosis of brain death should be clearly separated from the decisions and exigency for organ transplantation.

The explicit legal recognition that brain death is death varies among different countries, as do the guidelines for making the diagnosis of brain death.[185] Some countries have no legal statutes but allow a medical recognition of brain death. In Japan and Israel, there is not a social acceptance or full recognition of brain death. All countries use the clinical criteria, but some require ancillary tests—brain flow studies, electroencephalography, or brainstem evoked responses—as options or in various combinations. One must be aware of the national regulations and guidelines as well as those of the institution in which such decisions are made.

REFERENCES

1. Lipowski ZJ: *Delirium. Acute Confusional States.* New York, Oxford University Press, 1990.
2. Adams RD, Victor M, Ropper AH: *Principles of Neurology*, 6th ed. New York, McGraw-Hill, 1997, p 405.
3. Watt DF: Delirium and DSMI-IV. *J Neuropsychiatry* 5:459, 1993.
4. Lipowski ZJ: Update on delirium. *Psychiatr Clin N Am* 15:335, 1992.
5. Adams RD, Victor M, Ropper AH: *Principles of Neurology*, 6th ed. New York, McGraw-Hill, 1997, p 406.
6. Plum F, Posner JB: *Diagnosis of Stupor and Coma.* Philadelphi: FA Davis, 1980, pp 4–5.
7. Yeaw EM, Abbate JH: Identification of confusion among the elderly in an acute care setting. *Clin Nurse Specialist* 7:192, 1993.
8. Mesulam M-M: Attention, confusional states and neglect, in Mesulam M-M (ed): *Principles of Behavior in Neurology*. Philadelphia, FA Davis, 1986, pp 125–168.
9. Suss DT, Benson DF: *The Frontal Lobes.* New York, Raven Press, 1986, pp 98–103.
10. Young GB, Bolton CF, Austin TW, et al: The encephalopathy associated with septic illness. *Clin Invest Med* 13:297, 1990.
11. Folstein MF, Bassett SS, Romanski AJ, Nestadt G: The epidemiology of delirium in the community: The Eastern Baltimore Mental Health Survey. *Int Psychogeriatr* 3:169, 1991.
12. Engel GL: Delirium: In Friedman AM, Kaplan HS (eds): *Comprehensive Textbook of Psychiatry*. Baltimore, Williams and Wilkins, 1967, p 711.
13. Smith LW, Dimsdale JE: Postcardiotomy delirium: Conclusions after 25 years. *J Psychiatry*. 146:452, 1989.
14. Berggren D, Gustafson Y, Erickson B, et al: Postoperative confusion after anesthesia in elderly patients with femoral neck fractures. *Anesth Analg* 66:497, 1987.
15. Schuchardt V, Bourke DL: Alcoholic delirium and other withdrawal syndromes, in Hacke W (ed): *NeuroCritical Care*. Berlin, Springer Verlag, 1994, p 846.
16. Francis J, Martin D, Kapoor WN: Delirium in hospitalized elderly. *JAMA* 263:1097, 1990.
17. Liptzin B, Levkoff SE, Cleary PD, et al: An empirical study of diagnostic criteria for delirium. *Am J Psychiatry* 148:454, 1991.
18. Larson EB, Reifler BV, Sumi S, et al: Diagnostic evaluation of 200 elderly outpatients with suspected dementia. *J Gerontol* 40:536, 1986.
19. van Hemert AM, van der Mast RC, Hengeveld MW, Vorstenbosch M: Excess mortality in general hospital patients seen in psychiatric patients with delirium: 5 year follow-up of 519 patients seen in psychiatric consultation. *J Psychosom Res* 38:339, 1994.
20. Ross CA: CNS arousal systems: possible role in delirium, *Int Psychogeriatr* 3:353, 1991.
21. Gibson GE, Blass JP, Huang HM, Freeman GB: The cellular basis of delirium and its relevance to age-related disorders including Alzheimer's disease. *Int Psychogeriatr* 3:373, 1991.
22. Watts DF: Delirium and DSM-IV. *J Neuropsychiatry* 5:459, 1993.
23. Komel HW: Visual illusions and hallucinations. *Baillières Clin Neurol* 2:243, 1993.
24. Symons D: The stuff that dreams aren't made of: why wake and sleep-state sensory experiences differ. *Cognition* 47:181, 1993.
25. Erkwoh R, Ebel H, Kachel F, et al: 18FDG-PET and electroencephalographic findings in a patient suffering from musical hallucinations. *Nuklearmedizin* 32:159, 1993.
26. Hoffman RE, McGlashan TH: Parallel distributed processing and the emergence of schizophrenic symptoms. *Schizophr Bull* 19:119, 1993.
27. Cohen JD, Servan-Schreiver D: A theory of dopamine function and its role in cognitive deficits in schizophrenia. *Schizophr Bull* 19:85, 1993.
28. Fisher CM: Neurologic fragments. *Neurology* 39:127, 1989.
29. Miller NS: Pharamacotherapy in alcoholism. *J Addictive Dis* 14:23, 1995.
30. Erkinjunti T, Wikstrom J, Palo J, et al: Dementia among medical inpatients: evaluation of 2000

consecutive admissions. *Arch Intern Med* 146:1923, 1986.

31. Thomas RI, Cameron DJ, Fahs MC: A propsective study of delirium and prolonged hospital stay. *Arch Gen Psychiatry*. 45:937, 1988.

32. Gustafson Y, Berggren D, Brannstrom B, et al: Acute confusional states in elderly patients treated for femoral neck fracture. *J Am Geriatr Soc* 36:525, 1988.

33. Rockwood K: Acute confusion in elderly medical patients. *J Am Geriatr* 37:150, 1989.

34. Schor JD, Levkoff SE. Lipsitz LA, et al: Risk factors for delirium in hospitalized elderly. *JAMA* 267:827, 1992.

35. Francis J: Delirium in older patients. *J Am Geriatr Soc* 40:829, 1992.

36. Hill CD, Risby E, Morgan N: Cognitive deficits in delirium: assessment over time. *Psychopharmcol Bull* 28:401, 1992.

37. Verslegers W, De Deyn PP, Saerens J, Martin P, et al: Slow progressive bilateral posterior cerebral artery infarction presenting as agitated delirium, complicated with Anton's syndrome. *Eur Neurol* 31:216, 1991.

38. Tollefson GD, Montague-Clouse, J, Lancaster SP: The relationship of serum anticholinergic activity to mental status performance in an elderly nursing home population. *J Neuropsychiatry Clin Neurosci* 3:314, 1991.

39. Kaiko RF, Foley KM, Grabinki PY, et al: Central nervous system excitatory effects of meperidine in cancer patients. *Ann Neurol* 13:180, 1983.

40. Rothschild AJ: Disinhibition, amnestic reactions, and other adverse reactions secondary to triazolam: a review of the literature. *J Clin Psychiatry* 53(suppl):69, 1992.

41. Cummings JL: Behavioral complications of drug treatment of Parkinson's disease. *J Am Gertiatr Soc* 39:708, 1991.

42. Tune LE, Bylsma FW: Benzodiazepine-induced and anticholinergic-induced delirium in the elderly. *Int Psychogeriatr* 3:397, 1991.

43. Croog SH, Levine S, Testa MA, et al: The effects of antihypertensive therapy on the quality of life. *N Eng J Med* 314:1657, 1986.

44. Cantu TG, Korek JS: Central nervous system reactions to histamine-2 receptor blockers. *Ann Intern Med* 114:1027, 1991.

45. Mirchandani HG, Rorke LB, Sekula-Perlman A, Hood IC: Cocaine-induced agitated delirium, forceful struggle and minor head injury. A further definition of sudden death during restraint. *Am J Forensic Med Pathol* 15:95, 1994.

46. Primavera A, Giberti L, Scotto P, Cocito L: Non-convulsive status epilepticus as a cause of confusion in later life: a report of 5 cases. *Neuropsychobiology* 30:148, 1994.

47. Dilsaver SC: Withdrawal phenomena associated with antidepressant and antipsychotic agents. *Drug Saf* 10:103, 1994.

48. Dilsaver SC: Withdrawal phenomena associated with antidepressant and antipsychotic agents. *Drug Saf* 10:103, 1994.

49. Starkman MN, Schteingart DE: Neuropsychiatric manifestations of patients with Cushing's syndrome. *Arch Intern Med* 141:215, 1981.

50. Damasio A: The frontal lobes, in Heilman KM, Valenstein EV (eds): *Clinical Neuropsychology*. New York, Oxford University Press, 1979, pp 360–472.

51. Brenner RP, Utility of EEG in delirium: past views and current practice. *Int Psychogeriatr* 3:211, 1991.

52. Sutton S, Braren M, Zubin J, John ER: Evoked potential correlates of stimulus uncertainty. *Science* 150:1187, 1965.

53. Larson EB, Kukull WA, Buchner D, Reifler BV: Adverse drug reactions associated with global cognitive impairment in elderly persons. *Ann Intern Med* 107:169, 1987.

54. Rabins PV: Psychosocial and management aspects of delirium. *Int Psychogeratr* 3:319, 1991.

55. Cole MG, Primeau FJ, Bailey RF, et al: Systematic intervention for elderly patients with delirium: a randomized trial. *Can Med Assoc J* 151:965, 1994.

56. Cole MG, Primeau F, Clusher J: Effectiveness to prevent delirium in hospitalized patients: a systematic review. *Can Med Assoc J* 155:1263, 1996.

57. Pfitzer F, Schuchardt V, Heitmann R: The treatment of severe alcoholic delirium. *Nervenzart* 59:229, 1988.

58. Rasmussen BH, Creason NS: Nurses' perception of the phenomenon of confusion in elderly hospitalized inpatients. *Vard Nord Utveckl Forsk* 11:5, 1991.

59. Inaba-Roland KE, Maricle RA: Assessing delirium in the acute care setting. *Heart Lung* 21:48, 1992.

60. Folstein MF, Folstein SE, McHugh PR: "Mini-Mental State," A practical guide for grading the cognitive state of patients for the clinician. *J Psychiatr Res* 12:189, 1975.

61. Inouye SK, Can Dyck CH, Alessi CA, et al: Clarifying confusion: the Confusion Assessment

Method. A new method for the detection of delirium. *Ann Intern Med* 113:941, 1990.

62. Levkoff S, Liptzin B, Cleary P, Reilly CH, Evans D: Review of research instrumentats and techniques used to detect delirium. *Int Psychogeriatr* 3:253, 1991.

63. Fish DN: Treatment of delirium in the critically ill patient. *Clin Pharm* 10:456, 1991.

64. Stiefel F, Holland J: Delirium in cancer patients. *Int Psychogeriatr* 3:333, 1991.

65. Earnest MP, Parker WD Jr: Metabolic encephalopathies and coma from medical causes, in Grotta JC (ed): *Management of the Acutely Ill Neurological Patient*. New York, Churchill Livingstone, 1993, chap 1, pp 1–15.

66. Brungardt GS: Patient restraints: new guidelines for a less restrictive approach. *Geriatrics* 49:43, 47, 1994.

67. Tueth MJ: Emergencies caused by side effects of psychiatric medications. *Am J Emerg Med* 12:212, 1994.

68. Cairns H, Oldfield RC, Pennybacker JB, Whitteridge D: Akinetic mutism with an epidermoid cyst of the 3rd ventricle. *Brain* 64:273, 1941.

69. Fesenmeier JT, Kuzniecky R, Garcia JH: Akinetic mutism caused by bilateral anterior cerebral tuberculous obliterative arteritis. *Neurology* 40:1005, 1990.

70. Cairns H: Disturbances of consciousness with lesions of the brain-stem and diencephalon. *Brain* 75:8, 1952.

71. Park-Matsumoto YC, Ogawa K, Tazawa T, et al: Mutism developing after thalamo-capsular lesions by neuro-Behcet disease. *Acta Neurol Scand* 91:297, 1995.

72. Gugliotta MA, Silvestri R, De Domenico P, et al: Spontaneous bilateeral anterior cerebral artery occlusion resulting in akinetic mutism. A case report. *Acta Neurol* 11:252, 1989.

73. Ishii N, Nishihara Y, Imamura T: Why do frontal lobe symptoms predominate in vascular dementia with lacunes? *Neurology* 36:340, 1986.

74. Gütling E, Landis, T, Kleihues P: Akinetic mutism in bilateral necrotizing leucoencephalopathy after radiation and chemotherapy: electrophysiological and autopsy findings. *J Neurol* 239:125, 1992.

75. Yamamori C, Ishino H, Inagaki T, et al: Neuro-Behcet disease with demyelination and gliosis of the frontal white matter. *Clin Neuropathol* 13:208, 1994.

76. Ackermann H, Ziegler W: Akinetic mutism—a review of the literature. *Forschr Neurol Psychiatr* 63:59, 1995.

77. Milhaud D, Berrardin G, Roger PM. Traitment d'un état de mutisme akinetique par la bromocriptine. *Presse Medicale* (Paris) 22:688, 1993.

78. Anderson B: Relief of akinetic mutism from obstructive hydrocephalus using bromocriptine and ephedrine. *J Neurosurg* 76:152, 1992.

79. Barret K: Treating organic abulia with bromocriptine and lisuride: four case studies. *J Neurol Neurosurg Psychiatry* 54:718, 1991.

80. Echiverri HC, Tatum WO, Merens TA, Coker SB: Akinetic mutism: pharmacologic probe of the dopaminergic mesencephalofrontal activating system. *Pediatr Neurol* 4:228, 1988.

81. Marin RS: Differential diagnosis and classification of apathy. *Am J Psychiatry* 147:22, 1990.

82. Multi-Society Task Force on PVS: Medical aspects of the persistent vegetative state. *N Eng J Med* 330:1499, 1994.

83. Jennett B, Plum F: Persistent vegetative state after brain damage: a syndrome in search of a name. *Lancer* 1:734, 1972.

84. Jennett B, Dyer C: Persistent vegetative state and the right to die: the United States and Britain. *BMJ* 302:1256, 1991.

85. Barrett R, Merritt HH, Wolf A: Depression of consciousness as a result of cerebral lesions. in Ket SS, Evarts EV, Williams HL (eds): Sleep and altered states of consciousness. *Res Publ Ass Nerv Ment Dis*. New York, Raven Press, vol. XLV:241–276, 1967.

86. Walshe TM, Leonard C: Persistent vegetative state: extension of the syndrome to include chronic disorders. *Arch Neurol* 42:1045, 1985.

87. Brierley JB, Graham DI, Adams JH, Simpson JA: Neocortical death after cardiac arrest: a clinical neurophysiological, and neuropathological report of two cases. *Lancet* 2:560, 1971.

88. Dougherty JH Jr, Rawlinson DG, Levy DE, Plum F: Hypoxic-ischemic brain injury and the vegetative state: clinical and neuropathological correlations. *Neurology* 3:31, 1981.

89. Ingvar DH, Brun A, Johansson L, Samuelsson SM: Survival after several cerebral anoxia with destruction of the cerebral cortex; the apallic syndrome. *Ann NY Acad Sci* 315:184, 1978.

90. French JD. Brain lesion associated with prolonged unconsciousness. *Arch Neurol Psychiatry* 68:727, 1952.

91. Korein J, Maccario M: On the diagnosis of cerebral death: a prospective study on 55 patients to define

irreversible coma. *Clin Electroencephalogr* 2:178, 1971.

92. Brierley JB, Miller AA: Fatal brain damage after dental anaesthesia: its nature, etiology, and prevention. *Lancet* 2:869, 1966.

93. Pollack MA, Kellaway, P: Cortical death with preservation of brainstem function: Correlations of clinical, electrophysiologic and CT scan findings in 3 infants and 2 adults with prolonged survival. *Trans Am Neurol Ass* 103:36, 1978.

94. Kinney HC, Korein J, Panigraphy A, Dikkes P, Goode R: Neuropathological findings in the brain of Karen Ann Quinlan. *N Eng J Med* 330:1469, 1994.

95. Jennett B: Vegetative state: causes, management, ethical dilemmas. *Curr Anaesth Crit Care* 2:57, 1991.

96. Braakman R, Jennet WB, Minderhoud JM: Prognosis of the posttraumatic persistent vegetative state. *Acta Neurochir* (Wien) 95:49, 1988.

97. Andrews K, Murphy L, Munday R, Littlewood: Misdiagnosis of the vegetative state: retrospective study in a rehabilitation unit. *BMJ* 313:13, 1996.

98. Childs NL, Mercer WN, Childs HW; Accuracy in the diagnosis of persistent vegetative state. *Neurology* 43:1465, 1993.

99. Shewmon DA, DeGiorgio CM: Early prognosis in anoxic coma. *Neurol Clin* 7: 823, 1989.

100. Murray LS, Teasdale GM, Murray GD, et al: Does prediction of outcome alter patient management? *Lancet* 341:1487, 1993.

101. Multi-Society Task Force on PVS: Medical aspects of the persistent vegetive state (second of two parts). *N Eng J Med* 330:1572, 1996.

102. Childs NL, Mercer WN: Brief report: late improvement in consciousness after post-traumatic vegetative state. *N Eng J Med* 334:24, 1996.

103. Report of the Quality Standards Subcommittee of the American Academy of Neurology: Practice parameters: assessment and management of patients in the persistent vegetative state. *Neurology* 45:1015, 1995.

104. Hansotia PL: Persistent vegetative state: review and report of electrodiagnostic studies in eight cases. *Arch Neurol* 42:1048, 1985.

105. Danze F, Brule JF, Haddad K: Chronic vegetative state after severe head injury: clinical study; electrophysiological investigations and CT scans in 15 cases. *Neurosurg Rev* 12(suppl 1):477, 1989.

106. Geurit JM: Evoked potentials: a safe brain death confirmatory tool? *Eur J Med* 1:233, 1992.

107. Zegers de Beryl D, Brunko E: Prediction of chronic vegetative state with somatosensory evoked potentials. *Neurology* 36:134, 1986.

108. Brunko E, Zegers de Beyl D: Prognostic value of early cortical somatosensory evoked potentials after resuscitation from cardiac arrest. *Electroenceph Clin Neurophysiol* 66:15, 1987.

109. Rothstein TL, Thomas EM, Sumi SM: Predicting outcome in hypoxic-ischemic coma. A prospective clinical and electrophysiologic study. *Electroenceph Clin Neurophysiol* 79:101, 1991.

110. Levin HS, Saydjari C, Eisenberg HM, et al; Vegetative state after closed head injury: a Traumatic Coma Data Bank Report. *Arch Neurol* 48:580, 1991.

111. Mutoh K, Nakagawa Y, Hojo H: CT appearance of children in a persistent vegetative state. *Brain Dev* 9:605, 1987.

112. Shalit, MN, Beller AJ, Feinsod M: Clinical equivalents of cerebral oxygen consumption in man. *Neurology* 22:155, 1972.

113. Levy DE, Sidtis JJ, Rottenberg DA, et al: Differences in cerebral blood flow and glucose utilization in vegetative versus locked-in patients. *Ann Neurol* 22:673, 1987.

114. Jaggi, JL, Obrist WD, Gennarelli TA, Langfitt TW: Relationship of early cerebral blood flow and metabolism to outcome in severe head injury. *J Neurosurg* 72:176, 1990.

115. Muizelaar JP, Marmarou A, DeSalles AAF, et al: Cerebral blood flow and metabolism in severely head-injured children: part I, relationship with GCS score, outcome, ICP and PVI. *J Neurosurg* 71:63, 1989.

116. Oder W, Goldenberg G, Podreka I, Deeke L: HMPAO-SPECT in persistent vegetative state after head injury: prognostic predictor of the likelihood of recovery? *Intensive Care Med* 17:149, 1991.

117. Cassell EJ: Clinical incoherence about persons: the problem of the persistent vegetative state. *Ann Intern Med* 125:146, 1996.

118. Lamb D: *Death, Brain Death and Ethics.* Albany, SUNY Press, 1985.

119. Mollaret, P, Goulon M: "Le coma dépassé." *Revue Neurologique* 101:3, 1959.

120. Beecher HK: A definition of irreversible coma: report of the Ad Hoc Committee of the Harvard Medical School to examine the definition of brain death. *JAMA* 205:85, 1968.

121. Korein J: The problem of the brain death. *Ann NY Acad Sci* 315:19, 1978.

122. Shewmon DA: Commentary on guidelines for the determination of brain death in children. *Ann Neurol* 24:798, 1988.

123. President's Commission for the Study of Ethical Problems in Medicine and Biomedical and Behavioral Research: Defining death: medical, legal and ethical issues in the determination of death. US Government Printing Office, 1981.

124. Working group convened by the Royal College of Physicians and endorsed by the Conference of Medical Royal Colleges and their Facilities in the United Kingdom. *J Royal College of Physicians of London* 29:381, 1995.

125. Report of the Quality Standards Subcommittee of the American Academy of Neurology: Practice parameters for determining brain death in adults (summary statement). *Neurology* 45:1012, 1995.

126. Ropper AH: Unusual spontaneous movements in brain-dead patients. *Neurology* 34:1089, 1984.

127. Segredo V, Caldwell JE, Matthay MA, et al: Persistent paralysis in critically ill patients after long-term administration of vecuronium. *N Eng J Med* 327:524m, 1992.

128. Partridge BL, Abrams JH, Bazemore C, Rubin R: Prolonged neuromuscular blockade after long-term infusion of vecuronium bromide in the intensive care unit. *Crit Care Med* 18:1177, 1990.

129. Black P McL: Brain death (first of two parts). *N Eng J Med* 299:388, 1978.

130. Goetting MG, Contreras E: Systematic atropine administration during cardiac arrest does not cause fixed and dilated pupils. *Ann Emerg Med* 20:55, 1991.

131. Ong GL, Bruning HA: Dilated fixed pupils due to high doses of dopamine hydrochloride. *Crit Care Med* 9:658, 1981.

132. Snavely SR, Hodges GR: The neurotoxicity of antibacterial agents. *Ann Intern Med* 101:92, 1984.

133. Wijdicks EFM: Determining brain death in adults. *Neurology* 45:1003, 1995.

134. Ivanow SD, Nunn JF: Methods of elevation of P_{CO_2} for restoration of spontaneous breathing after artificial ventilation of anaesthetized patients. *Br J Anaesth* 41:28, 1969.

135. Bolton CF, Gilbert JJ, Hahn AF, et al: Polyneuropathy in critically ill patients. *J Neurol Neurosurg Psychiatry* 47:1223, 1984.

136. Earnest MP, Beresford HR, McIntyre HB: Testing for apnea in suspected brain death: methods used by 129 clinicians. *Neurology* 36:542, 1986.

137. Report of the Quality Standards Subcommittee of the American Academy of Neurology. *Neurology* 45:1012, 1995.

138. Becker DP, Robert CM, Nelson JR, et al: An evaluation of the definition of cerebral death. *Neurology* 20:459, 1970.

139. Invgar DH, Widén L, Hjäendöd: Sammanfattning av ett symposium *Läkartidningen* 69:3804, 1972.

140. Jørgensen EO: EEG without detectable cortical activity and cranial nerve areflexia as parameters of brain death *Electroenceph Clin Neurophysiol* 36:70, 1974.

141. Ivan LP: Spinal reflexes in cerebral death. *Neurology* 23:650, 1973.

142. Editorial: An appraisal of the criteria of cerebral death: a summary statement: a collaborative study. *JAMA* 237:982, 1976.

143. Mohandas A, Chou SN: Brain death—a clinical and pathological study. *J Neurosurg* 35:211, 1971.

144. CMA Position Statement: Guidelines for the diagnosis of brain death. *Can Med Assoc J* 136:355, 1987.

145. Byrne PA, Nilges RG: The brain stem in brain death: a critical review. *Issues Law Med* 9:3, 1993.

146. Amer SN, Al Din: Coma and brain stem areflexia in brain stem encephalitis (Fisher's syndrome). *Br Med J* 291:535, 1985.

147. Drury I, Westmoreland BF, Sharbrough FW: Fulminant demyelinating polyradiculopathy resembling brain death. *Electroenceph Clin Neurophysiol* 67:42, 1987.

148. Pasternak JF, Volpe JJ: Full recovery from prolonged brainstem failure following intraventricular hemorrhage. *J Pediatr* 95:1046, 1979.

149. Heiskanen O: Cerebral circulatory arrest caused by acute increase in intracranial pressure. *Acta Neurol Scand* 40(suppl 7):7, 1964.

150. Kung HF: New technetium-99m-labeled brain perfusion imaging agents. *Semin Nucl Med* 20:150, 1990.

151. Kricheff II, Pinto RS, George AE, Braunstein P, Korein J: Angiographic findings in brain death. *Ann NY Acad Sci* 315:168, 1978.

152. Black P McL: Conceptual and practical issues in the declaration of brain death by brain criteria. *Neurosurg Clin N Am* 2:493, 1991.

153. George MS: Establishing brain death: the potential role of nuclear medicine in the search for a reliable confirmatory test. *Eur J Nucl Med* 18:75, 1991.

154. Yatim A, Mercatello A, Coronel B, et al. ^{99m}Tc-HMPAO cerebral scintigraphy in the diagnosis of brain death. *Transplant Proc* 23:2491, 1991.

155. Laurin NR, Driedger AA, Hurwitz GA, et al: Cerebral perfusion imaging with technetium-99m HMPAO in brain death and severe central nervous system injury. *J Nucl Med* 30:1627, 1989.

156. Roine RO, Launes J, Lindroth L, Nikkinen P: ^{99m}Tc-hexamethylpropylamineoxime scans to confirm brain death (Letter). *Lancet* 2:1223, 1986.

157. Masdeu JC: Brain single-photon emission computed tomography (Special Review). *Neurology* 44:1970, 1994.

158. Lee DH, Nathanson JA, Fox AJ, Pelz DM, Lownie SP: Magnetic resonance imaging of brain death. *Can Assoc Radiol J* 46:174, 1995.

159. Ropper AH, Kehne SM, Weschler L: Transcranial Doppler in brain death. *Neurology* 37:1733, 1987.

160. Ropper AH, Kehne SM, Weschler L: Transcranial Doppler in brain death. *Neurology* 37:1733, 1987.

161. Shiogai T, Sato E, Tokitsu M, et al: Transcranial Doppler monitoring in severe brain damage: relationships between intracranial hemodynamics, brain dysfunction and outcome. *Neurol Res* 12:205, 1990.

162. Feri M, Raly L, Felici M, Vanni D, Capria V: transcranial Doppler and brain death diagnosis. *Crit Care Med* 22:1120, 1994.

163. Petty GW, Mohr JP, Pedley TA, et al: The role of transcranial Doppler in confirming brain death: sensitivity, specificity and suggestions for performance and interpretation. *Neurology* 40:300, 1990.

164. Overgaard J, Tweed WA: rCBF in impeding brain death. *Acta Neurochir* 31:167, 1975.

165. Uematsu S, Smith TD, Walker AE: Pulsatile cerebral echo in diagnosis of brain death. *J Neurosurg* 48:866, 1978.

166. Minami T, Ogawa M, Sugimoto T, et al: Hyperoxia of internal jugular venous blood in brain death. *J Neurosurg* 39:442, 1973.

167. Pallis C: Prognostic value of brain lesion. *Lancet* I: 379, 1981.

168. Star A: Brainstem auditory evoked responses in brain death. *Brain* 99:543, 1976.

169. Goldie WO, Chiappa KH, Young RR, et al: Brainstem auditory and short-latency somatosensory evoked responses in brain death. *Neurology* 31:248, 1989.

170. Guidelines for the determination of death: Report of the medical consultants on the diagnosis of death to the President's Commission for the study of ethical problems in medicine and biomedical and behavioral Research. *Neurology* 32:395, 1982.

171. Rowland TW, Donnelly JH, Jackson AH, Jamroz SB: Brain death in the pediatric intensive care unit. *Am J Dis Child* 137:547, 1983.

172. Moshe SL, Alvarez LA: Diagnosis of brain death in children. *J Clin Neurophysiol* 32:239, 1982.

173. Okamoto K, Sugimoto T: Return of spontaneous respiration in an infant who fulfilled current criteria to determine brain death. *Pediatrics* 96:518, 1995.

174. Ashwal S, Schneider S: Failure of electroencephalography to diagnose brain death in comatose children. *Ann Neurol* 6:512, 1979.

175. British Paediatric Association: *Diagnosis of brain stem death in infants and children. Report of a working party*. London, BPA, 1991.

176. De Meirleir L, Taylor MJ: Prognostic utility of SEPs in comatose children. *Pediatr Neurol* 3:78, 1987.

177. Furgiuele TL, Frank M, Riegle C, Wirth F, Earley LC: Prediction of cerebral death by cranial sector scan. *Crit Care Med* 12:1, 1984.

178. Ashwal S, Smith AJK, Torres F, Loken M, Chou SN: Radionuclide bolus angiograpphy: a technique for verification of brain death in infants and children. *J Pediatr* 91:722, 1977.

179. Coulter DL: Neurologic uncertainty in newborn intensive care. *N Eng J Med* 316:840, 1986.

180. Report of Special Task Force: Guidelines for the determination of brain death in children. *Pediatrics* 80:298, 1987.

181. Volpe JJ: Brain death determination in the newborn. *Pediatrics* 80:293, 1987.

182. Grigg MM, Kelly MA, Celesia GG, et al: Electroencephalographic activity after brain death. *Arch Neurol* 44:948, 1987.

183. Freeman JM, Ferry PC: New brain death criteria in children: further confusion. *Pediatrics* 81:301, 1988.

184. Kohrman MH, Brain death in neonates. *Seminars in Neurology* 13:116, 1993.

185. Pallis C, Harley DH: *ABC of Brainstem Death*, 2nd ed. London, BMJ Publishing Group, 1996, pp 40–44.

186. Editorial: Criteria for the diagnosis of brain death of the Conference of the Royal Colleges and Faculties of the United Kingdom. *Br Med J* 2:1187, 1976.

187. Pallis C: *ABC of Brainstem Death*. London, BMJ Publications, 1983, p 15.

Chapter 3

INITIAL ASSESSMENT AND MANAGEMENT OF THE PATIENT WITH IMPAIRED ALERTNESS

G. Bryan Young

Impairment of consciousness demands immediate investigation, simultaneous support, and definitive treatment. In the following discussion, coma will be emphasized, as it is the most urgent and challenging category of impaired consciousness. However, lesser degrees of obtundation, e.g., the acute confusional state (see Chap. 2), are also of urgent importance: morbidity and mortality are reduced if the patient does not become comatose. Many cases present to the emergency room; other patients deteriorate in hospital beds. These context-dependent presentations are discussed in consolidated form in Part 6.

CLINICAL APPROACH

Figure 3-1 shows an algorithm for approaching a patient with impaired responsiveness. The clinical assessment of the patient's condition is fundamental for diagnosis and management. One must first establish that the patient is in a coma rather than a state of psychogenic unresponsiveness or paralysis with preserved alertness. The neurologic examination should assess the depth of impairment of arousability and more specific deficits. The general examination is useful for additional etiologic clues and management.

Next, one establishes the anatomic localization of the lesion causing coma: is it due to a single supratentorial lesion, an infratentorial lesion, or a multifocal or diffuse process?

Supportive and specific management steps are conducted simultaneously with further clinical and laboratory diagnostic procedures that define the etiology. Thus, the assistance of nurses and fellow physicians is necessary.

History

The history can be of considerable help in giving direction to diagnostic pursuits. It is often possible to deduce that the coma is an expected result of a progressive illness, a complication of a pre-existing condition, or a totally unexpected event. The circumstances in which the patient is found can give clues, e.g., the patient who suddenly collapses on the street versus the patient found alone with medication bottles nearby. It is important to speak to those who found the patient in a state of collapse, anyone who saw the individual take ill, or friends and relatives who know the patient well. Also, checking the patient's wallet or purse, clothing and person may provide clues (e.g., a "Medic Alert" bracelet or necklace may disclose diagnoses, drugs in use, and allergies). Suitable questions

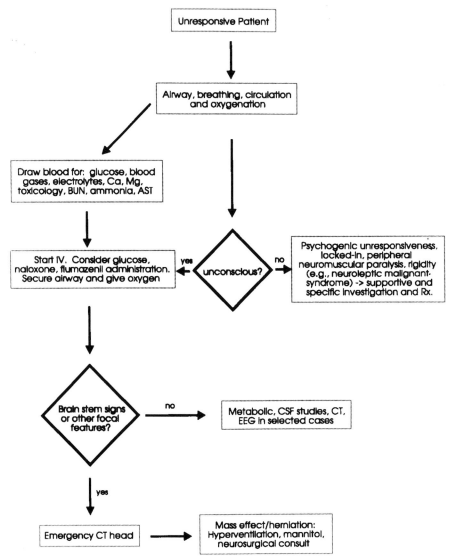

Figure 3-1

Algorithm for coma assessment and management. AST= glutamic-oxaloacetic transaminase; BUN= blood urea nitrogen; IV= intravenous solution; Rx= treatment.

(which should be appropriately paraphrased) for witnesses are:

1. Was the loss of consciousness gradual and progressive or abrupt; did the level of consciousness fluctuate, stay the same, or worsen? This often gives valuable diagnostic clues. For example, a sudden onset suggests trauma, a vascular cause, or seizures. Fluctuation suggests metabolic disorders, seizures, intoxications, or, sometimes, an extra-axial lesion (e.g., a subdural hematoma) or fluctuations in intracranial pressure (ICP). Progressive worsening suggests accumulating pathology or increasing metabolic or toxic derangement, e.g., a

CNS infection, an increasing destructive or compressive lesion, or progressive organ failure.

2. Did focal signs such as a hemiparesis or altered speech precede the loss of consciousness? This suggests a structural lesion.

3. What chronic conditions has the patient suffered (e.g., epilepsy; diabetes; cancer; hypertension; disorders of immunodeficiency; autoimmune diseases; psychiatric, cardiac, vascular, pulmonary, hepatic, or renal problems)? What were the reasons for previous hospitalizations?

4. What drugs does the patient take regularly and what drugs has he/she taken recently (both prescription and nonprescription, including street drugs)? Is there a history of alcoholism?

5. Were there previous lapses of consciousness or transient neurologic symptoms (e.g., transient speech problems, lateralized weakness, visual disturbances)?

6. Has he/she been ill lately (e.g., fever or headache) or has there been a noted change in behavior or mental functioning? Have there been any falls or accidents, especially with injury to the head?

7. What is the detailed eyewitness account of today's illness? Did the patient collapse; if so, did the patient fall limply (to suggest a faint) or like a tree (to suggest a seizure)? Was there a convulsion; if so, how did it start? Did anyone feel for a pulse (absent, fast, slow, or regular, irregular)?

Historical clues favoring one or more structural lesions include: a history of progressive focal deficit (e.g., language impairment, lateralized weakness), trauma, alcoholism, cancer, bleeding disorder or anticoagulant therapy, recent sinusitis, or sudden collapse.

Clues from the General Examination

The general physical examination can often provide important clues. Signs of traumatic brain injury include lacerations or bruising about the scalp or face. Findings suggestive of a basal skull fracture: (1) There may be unilateral or bilateral periorbital ecchymosis (raccoon eyes) with fractures of the orbital roof (floor of the anterior cranial fossa): blood tracks through the loose orbital connective tissue until it is stopped by the attachment of the orbital periosteum at the margins of the orbit (see Fig. 6-6)—unlike the ordinary "black eye" in which blood tracks into the facial tissues. (2) There may be bruising confined to the skin over the mastoid (Battle's sign) from a fracture of the petrous temporal bone; again, the blood is confined, as there is no subgaleal space into which it can diffuse. (3) Blood may be visible behind the ear drum (hemotypanum). (4) Fractures of the cranial vault may bleed beneath the galea aponeurotica, the latter being separate from the underling periosteum. This allows for a swollen, boggy area of scalp overlying the fracture. (5) There may be bruising on other parts of the body. Linear bruises often result from assault with a club or stick.

A bitten tongue or lacerations of the buccal mucosa imply a recent convulsive seizure.

Vital signs provide important diagnostic clues and prompt management endeavors. Fever suggests an infection that may have directly (e.g., meningitis or encephalitis) or indirectly (e.g., sepsis, or endocarditis with septic emboli) involved the nervous system, or sometimes salicylate poisoning, heat prostration, a recent seizure, or brainstem stroke (see Table 12-1). Hypothermia raises the possibility of hypothyroidism, environmental exposure, barbiturate or alcohol intoxication, Wernicke's encephalopathy, or profound circulatory failure. Severe hypertension due to hypertensive encephalopathy is almost invariably associated with papilledema (Fig. 3-2). Otherwise, hypertension with coma is *secondary* to the intracranial process. A widened pulse pressure and slow pulse (the Cushing response) suggest raised intracranial pressure. Severe hypotension, hopefully promptly treated, suggests inadequate global brain perfusion. Possibilities include volume depletion (e.g., bleeding, excessive diuresis, or adrenal failure), low-output cardiac failure, vasodilatation (as in sepsis), or autonomic failure.

Features of the skin, nails, and mucous membranes may also assist with the diagnosis. There may be jaundice or other stigmata of liver disease in patients experiencing hepatic coma. An extreme

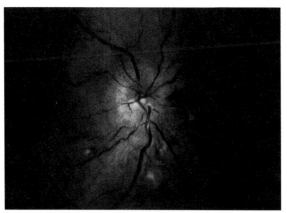

Figure 3-2
Papilledema in association with malignant hypertension. In addition to disk swelling and retinal hemorrhages, there is marked arteriolar narrowing and white retinal infarcts. Hemorrhages are often farther from the disk than in the papilledema of raised ICP.

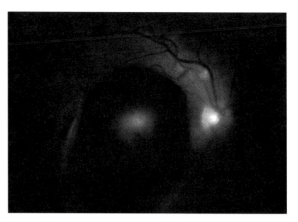

Figure 3-3
Subhyaloid hemorrhage. A large hemorrhage in the vitreous chamber is present in this patient with a ruptured intracranial berry aneurysm arising from the internal carotid artery. Such hemorrhages occur in about one-quarter of patients with ruptured berry aneurysms.[64]

ruddy color may imply carbon monoxide poisoning. Petechiae raise the possibility of meningococcemia, thrombotic thrombocytopenic purpura, disseminated intravascular coagulation, bacterial endocarditis, or Rocky Mountain spotted fever. Bullous lesions of the skin are found in barbiturate intoxication. Needle marks of the drug addict may point to drug intoxication. Hyperpigmentation of the skin and mucous membranes suggests Addison disease. The skin is sweaty in shock and hypoglycemia but is usually dry in diabetic coma. The facies of myxedema coma include periorbital puffiness, large tongue, and pale, cool, doughy, skin. Pituitary insufficiency is associated with a sallow appearance.

The breath may suggest alcohol intoxication (but this is related to the type of alcoholic beverage—ethyl alcohol or vodka is odorless), hepatic failure (fetor hepaticus, a fishy odor), uremia (uremic fetor, a uriniferous odor), ketosis (a sweet, fruity odor), oral or pulmonary infection (severe halitosis), or cyanide poisoning (an almond smell).

The optic fundi should be carefully examined. A subhyaloid hemorrhage indicates a ruptured berry aneurysm until otherwise disproven (see Fig. 3-3).[1] Bilateral papilledema (Fig. 3-4) usually

Figure 3-4
This shows florid papilledema due to raised ICP, with a swollen, elevated optic disk with indistinct margins. There are some small retinal hemorrhages near the disk. Papilledema is caused by an obstruction to the axoplasmic flow from retinal ganglion cells as they course through the optic nerve. The sign is reliable for sustained elevation of ICP. Some patients with raised ICP, however, do not have papilledema.

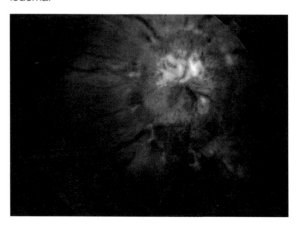

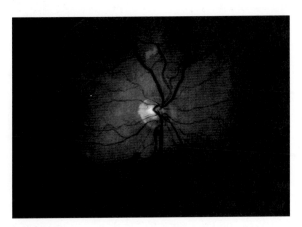

Figure 3-5
A "Roth spot" or white-centered hemorrhage. These are commonly associated with bacterial endocarditis (as in this patient), but may be seen in a number of other infectious (e.g., sepsis with emboli, candidiasis, and AIDS), hematologic (e.g., leukemia and multiple myeloma), and vascular disorders (e.g., vasculitis including systemic lupus erythematosis, and diabetic retinopathy) in which a capillary leak of plasma proteins or leukocytes may occur.

indicates raised intracranial pressure, but malignant hypertension is occasionally responsible (Fig. 3-2). Roth spots, pale areas (leukocytes or fibrin) surrounded by hemorrhages in the retina, indicate vascular leakage, as seen in emboli from bacterial endocarditis or various vascular and hematological conditions (see Fig. 3-5).

Cardiac murmurs raise the possibility of cerebral embolism; if occurring with fever, bacterial endocarditis should be considered.

Abdominal examination may reveal signs of liver disease (ascites, portal hypertension) or signs of a ruptured viscus and sepsis. Polycystic kidneys raise the possibility of subarachnoid hemorrhage.

Meningismus is suggestive of meningeal irritation, e.g., from infection or subarachnoid blood. This can be demonstrated by resistance to forward neck flexion relative to other passive neck movements and by Kernig's sign in which the resistance of flexion of the hip is tested when the knee is extended. With Brudzinski's sign for meningeal irritation, there is flexion of the contralateral thigh when one hip is flexed. The presence of resistance to neck flexion when Kernig's and Brudzinski's signs are negative suggests a cerebellar pressure cone. Resistance to all neck movements, including rotation, suggests a problem in the cervical spine or paratonic rigidity (see below). In drowsiness or stupor, resistance to passive neck movements seems to be a protective response. In deep coma, the resistance encountered in these tests for meningeal irritation is lost; one cannot exclude a central nervous system (CNS) infection or intracranial hemorrhage.

Principal Aspects of the Neurologic Examination

1. Level of Consciousness   The degree of obtundation is best described in terms of the patient's spontaneous activity and responsivity to stimulation. For example, it is much more useful and specific to know that the patient opened their eyes and looked about only when their nailbeds were squeezed than to have stated that the patient was in "moderate coma."

One should note behavior when the patient is undisturbed. Arousability is then assessed by stimulating the patient by speaking in their ear, and by applying pressure to above the medial portion of the supraorbital ridge as well as to the nailbeds.[2] Patients in coma will not rouse, but may push against the stimulating hand or posture. In a stupor, the patient will open their eyes and verbalize, but will then lapse back into unconsciousness. The specific behavioral response should be charted, with the behavior and specific description of responsiveness, so that the level of consciousness is trended over time.

Standardized documentation of the severity and course of neurologic illness in the patient record is invaluable for patient care: for *confused patients*, the standardized Mini-Mental State Examination (Table 2-3) is suitable, while "coma scales" (see Tables 3-3 to 3-6) are useful over a wide range of obtundation, with emphasis on stupor and coma.[3] Better standardization should improve intra- and interinstitutional communication.

2. Cranial Nerves It is usually possible to assess at least components of functions related to cranial nerves II through X. Metabolic and toxic causes of coma tend to spare the pupillary light reflex (involving cranial nerves II and III), while single structural lesions impair these functions when coma is present. The oculovestibular reflexes (involving cranial nerves III, IV, VI, and VIII) are more sensitive to metabolic and toxic causes of coma, but their integrity is good evidence that the brainstem is intact. These statements have some caveats (discussed below), but serve as a practical clinical guide.

Direct and consensual pupillary light reflexes are easily assessed, as shown in Fig. 3-6. The eyes usually need to be passively held open; then the light in shone in both eyes alternatively, looking for constriction of the ipsilateral and contralateral pupils. With complete, one-sided optic nerve damage, neither pupil will react when light is shone in the affected eye. When light is shone into the spared eye, however, both pupils constrict.

Pupils are normally 3 to 7 mm in diameter, symmetrical, and constrict to 2 to 6 mm with light stimulation directly (eye stimulated) and consensually (opposite eye stimulated). Twenty percent of persons have unequal pupils by less than 1 mm (anisocoria), but the difference remains the same with different degrees of illumination. The major criterion for normality is reactivity to light.[49] The presence of a normal pupillary light reflex indicates that its afferent and efferent limbs are intact, including the rostral brainstem. An early manifestation of a herniation syndrome (see Chap. 4) is the decline in pupillary reactivity, usually on the side of a mass. The pupils may be affected symmetrically by metabolic/toxic factors. Patients

Figure 3-6
A. *This shows a patient with normal-sized pupils.* B. *This shows the direct (same side) and consensual (contralateral) pupillary constriction when a bright light is shone into the left eye. This is a normal pupillary light reflex.*

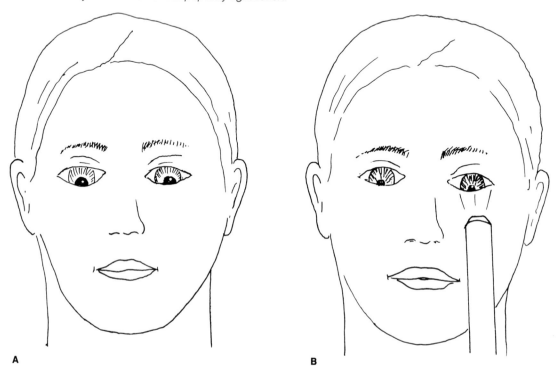

A   B

Table 3-1

Etiologies of third cranial nerve palsy

Site	Example	Site	Example
Nuclear	Infarction	Intra-axial, nonnuclear	Infarct, hemorrhage, inflammation, compression, late herniation
Subarachnoid space	Aneurysm (typically posterior communicating), meningitis (neoplastic or infectious), herniation, trauma	Cavernous sinus and superior orbital fissure	Carvernous sinus thrombosis (bland or septic), aneurysm, tumor (including pituitary apoplexy), herpes zoster, cardotid-cavernous fistula
Orbit	Trauma	Uncertain	Migraine, postviral or post-immunization

Source: Constructed from text in Nadeau SE, Trobe D: Pupil sparing in oculomotor palsy: a review. *Ann Neurol* 13:193, 1983.

with chronic lung disease or chronic hypoxemia may have large, sluggishly reactive pupils. Systemic opiates, organophosphates, or miotic eye drops may produce small pupils.

With a unilateral oculomotor nerve palsy, the ipsilateral pupil is typically dilated and unreactive; the eye is turned laterally and there is complete or nearly complete ipsilateral ptosis. Further, with oculovestibular or oculocephalic testing, the eye will not move medially or vertically. In coma, a third nerve palsy with pupillary involvement implies a structural, rather than a metabolic-toxic, cause for coma. The causes of third nerve palsies, based on anatomic sites, are given in Table 3-1.

Oculomotor nerve palsy must be differentiated from traumatic or drug-induced mydriasis as well as from mechanical problems with eye movement (e.g., blowout orbital fracture) or neuromuscular transmission failure (caused by muscle relaxants or myasthenia).

Extraocular movements (Figs. 3-7 to 3-10) are examined to provide diagnostic information. The structures involved in conjugate eye movements lie in the brainstem tegmentum; structures that compromise the brainstem reticular formation would be expected to alter conjugate eye movements. Comatose patients generally do not make quick or saccadic eye movements unless they are driven by epileptic nystagmus or opsoclonus. Epileptic nystagmus refers to jerky conjugate eye movements due to cerebral cortical discharges,

often in the occipital lobe.[4] Otherwise, quick conjugate movements of the eyes imply that the patient is not unconscious, as in psychogenic unresponsiveness and in the locked-in syndrome. In the latter, a lesion in the basis pontis causes quadriplegia, pseudobulbar palsy, and a paralysis of abducens function. The patient has vertical saccades, as these are related to the pretectal area and the third nerve complex, which are intact.

Conditions that spare the centers for horizontal gaze and the medial longitudinal fasciculi that allow for conjugate, eye movements (Figs. 3-7 and 3-8) are usually of a metabolic rather than a structural nature. These can be assessed by watching for spontaneous conjugate eye movements or by stimulating eye movements using the vestibulo-ocular reflex (Figs. 3-9 and 3-10). With the oculocephalic (doll's eyes) maneuver, the head is rapidly rotated in horizontal and vertical planes to test ocular movements that occur in the same plane. The eyes move conjugately in the direction opposite to that of head movement if the internuclear pathways of the brainstem are spared (Fig. 3-9). This test can be used if one is certain that there is no cervical spine instability. With the oculovestibular test (caloric testing), the head is elevated at 30° from the horizontal. The ear canal is irrigated with water that is at least 10°C cooler than body temperature. In the unconscious patient, the eyes conjugately move tonically towards the irrigated ear. (The eyes move conjugately to the opposite side if

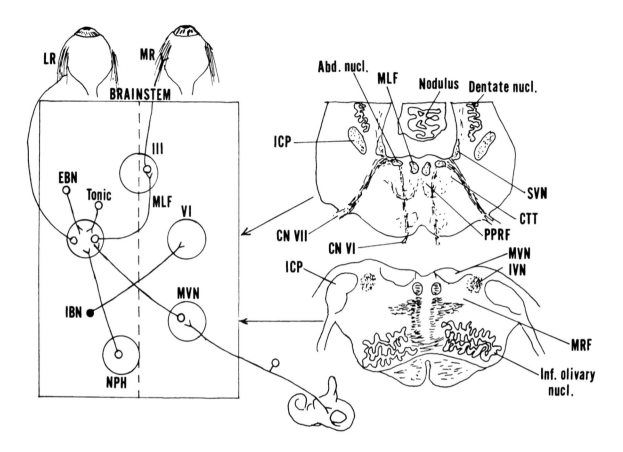

Figure 3-7

Anatomic pathways for horizontal eye movements. The horizontal semicircular canal connects with the medial vestibular nucleus (MVN) that synapses with neurons in the contralateral nerve VI nucleus. The abducens nucleus (Abd. nucl.) has neurons that innervate the ipsilateral lateral rectus (LR) and internuclear neurons that project into the contralateral medial longitudinal fasciculus (MLF) to synapse onto neurons in the oculomotor (III) nucleus that supplies the medial rectus (MR) on that side. This allows the eyes to move conjugately to the left, in a tonic manner, when warm water is injected into the right ear with the head elevated at 30° from the horizontal. There are excitatory and inhibitory burst neurons (EBN and IBN, respectively) that allow for saccades (rapid eye movements) in conscious patients. The IBN neurons also cause the antagonist eye muscles to relax during eye movements.

The anatomic sections on the right correspond to the levels of the brainstem shown in the diagram on the left (as indicated by the arrows). Abbreviations: CN VI = abducens nerve VI (facial nerve); CN VII = cranial nerve VII (facial nerve); CTT = central tegmental tract; Dentate nucl. = dentate nucleus; ICP = inferior cerebellar peduncle; MRF = medullary reticular formation; NPH = nucleus prepositus hypoglossi (a center for integrated eye movement information); PPRF = paramedian pontine reticular formation (a center for eye position information); SVN = superior vestibular nucleus; IVN = inferior vestibular nucleus.

(Redrawn from Leigh and Zee[65] and Carpenter and Sutin,[66] with permission.)

Figure 3-8

Vestibular-ocular reflexes involved in vertical eye movements. In A, afferents from the anterior semicircular canals (AC) synapse in the superior vestibular nucleus (SV) and their excitatory influences are relayed by the brachium conjunctivum (BC, superior cerebellar peduncle) to the oculomotor subnuclei that drive the ipsilateral superior rectus (SR) and the contralateral inferior oblique (IO) muscles.

In B, afferents from the posterior semicircular canals (PC) synapse in the medial vestibular nucleus and their axons and their excitatory signals are then transmitted via the contralateral medial longitudinal fasciculus (MLF) to the trochlear (IV nerve) nucleus controlling the superior oblique (SO) muscle (note the nerve itself crosses over outside the brainstem to innervate the opposite muscle) and the oculomotor subnucleus that controls the inferior rectus (IR).

C and D represent inhibitory pathways from the anterior and posterior semicircular canals, respectively.

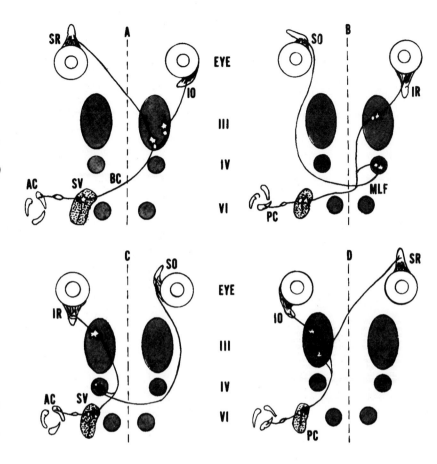

water at > 44°C is used.) The oculovestibular test is performed in place of the oculocephalic test when moving the neck is contraindicated, especially when there is even a possibility of a cervical spine injury or if the neck is too stiff to move. Caloric testing with ice water is a more potent test of brainstem function than the oculocephalic maneuver. Before declaring the oculovestibular reflexes absent, caloric testing must be performed with at least 50 mL of ice water. Vertical gaze can be elicited by the near simultaneous application of cold water in both ear canals, producing tonic downward deviation of both eyes, or by warm water injection bilaterally, causing tonic upward deviation in the unconscious patient (Fig. 3-9).

The testing of *vertical* eye movements, with either oculocephalic or oculovestibular maneuvers, should not be omitted. Structural lesions, such as infarctions restricted to the thalamus or rostral midbrain, may closely resemble metabolic coma if the problem with vertical eye movements is not appreciated.[5,6]

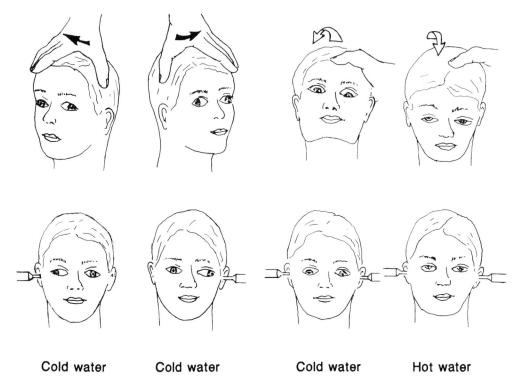

Cold water   Cold water   Cold water   Hot water

Figure 3-9
Ocular movements in an unconscious patient with an intact brainstem. The top row of figures represent oculocephalic (doll's head) maneuvers that cause conjugate eye movements in the angular direction opposite the direction of passive head movement. The bottom row shows ocular responses to caloric stimulation. With cold water irrigation of the head at 30° elevation from the horizontal, the eyes deviate tonically toward the ear irrigated. When cold water is injected simultaneously into both ear canals, the eyes deviate tonically downwards; the reverse occurs with simultaneous warm water irrigation.

If the patient is conscious, as in psychogenic unresponsiveness, nystagmus occurs with the fast phase away from the irrigated ear. If these tests give the above-mentioned results, brainstem function is likely intact; the pathogenesis of coma is more likely to be a diffuse or multifocal process.

Deviation of the eyes to one side indicates an imbalance in the activity of the lateral gaze center. Seizures involving either the frontal or the parietal occipital gaze centers may drive the eyes to the contralateral side. Dysfunction of these centers may lead to the eyes being driven to the side of the lesion by the intact, tonically active contralateral gaze center. It should be possible to overcome such supratentorial influences by stimulating the oculovestibular reflex with caloric testing. Thus, the patient with a supratentorial gaze preference "looks away" from the hemiplegic side, but the eyes can be made to turn towards that side using the vestibulo-ocular reflex. With infratentorial lesions, if one lateral gaze center is not functioning, the eyes will be driven to the affected side by the intact contralateral side. In this situation, the eyes cannot be moved using caloric testing.

Lesions of the medial longitudinal fasciculus (MLF) prevent the yoking of eye movements, so that the globes become dysconjugate. There may be a skew deviation, with one eye above the other in

Figure 3-10
A and B. *The effects of ice water irrigation in an unconscious patient with a brainstem lesion interrupting the medial longitudinal fasciculus. There is abduction of the eye ipsilateral to the irrigated ear, but the other eye fails to adduct. Note the pupillary inequality.*

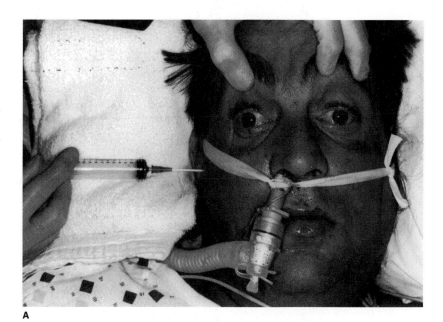

A

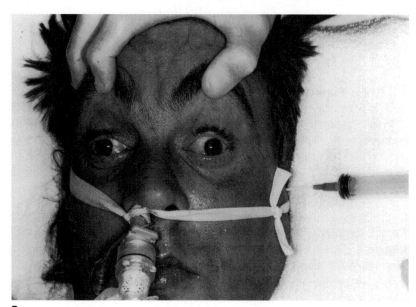

B

the horizontal plane (see Fig. 3-8). An example of internuclear ophthalmoplegia due to bilateral MLF lesions is shown in Fig. 3-10.

The corneal reflex is elicited by touching the cornea with a cotton-tipped swab or tissue. Through connections in the brainstem, this stimu-

lates the dorsal part of both seventh-nerve nuclei, causing the eyes to close, and the third nerve complex and fourth nerve, causing the eyes to roll up (Bell's phenomenon).

Nystagmus retractorius and convergence nystagmus are due to diffuse excitation of the oculomotor complex, causing the eyes to retract or converge with simultaneous contraction of all the third nerve-innervated muscles. This is usually due to dysfunction (structural or functional) at the pretectal and midbrain tegmentum.

Ocular bobbing is a rapid conjugate movement of the eyes downwards, followed by a slow return to the horizontal plane. It is a sign of a lesion, most often ischemia from a basilar occlusion, in the caudal pons.[7] It is not specific for this condition, and has been described in compressive posterior fossa lesions, brainstem encephalitis, and, rarely, in metabolic encephalopathy.[8–10] Inverse bobbing (ocular dipping) is a slow downward deviation with a rapid upward return. Ocular dipping is common in anoxic encephalopathy. Reverse bobbing is a rapid upward deviation with a slow downward return. All these movements indicate pontine dysfunction.

Palatal and pharyngeal reflexes, like ocular bobbing, are anatomically located caudal to centers involved in alertness, but they are worthwhile assessing to determine the extent of dysfunction (Chap. 2).

3. Motor Function The presence and type of spontaneous activity and the response to stimulation are valuable in determining the level of consciousness. The exact description of the patient's spontaneous movements and response to pain, including the nature of the stimuli and the sites of application, are valuable for initial assessment and trending purposes. Adequate somatosensory and auditory stimuli must be applied before concluding that there is no response.

Observed Motor Activity Yawning, sneezing, crossing the legs in a natural posture, or normal shifts of posture indicate less severe impairment of consciousness. Swallowing and hiccups imply that the lower brainstem is intact, but these are among the last motor responses to disappear in brainstem dysfunction. Hiccups may correspond to an irritative process in the medullary reticular formation.

Spontaneous movements include seizures or myoclonus and some tremors. Some spontaneous movements at rest—e.g., some "extrapyramidal movements" such as dystonia, chorea, athetosis, or ballismus—require an alert state. The appearance of some abnormal movements may also require the active support of a limb against gravity, as with tremor and asterixis.

Restlessness, athetosis, ballistic movements, tremor, rhythmic myoclonus, or heterogenous movements may be seen with acute mass lesions.

In some instances, the patient is "locked-in", i.e., conscious but unable to move because of motor paralysis (see earlier and Chap. 2).

TREMOR, ASTERIXIS, AND MULTIFOCAL MYOCLONUS Tremor is a rhythmic oscillation of a body part. Tremor associated with impaired consciousness is mainly a "postural-action" tremor—absent at rest, but noted with the upper limbs outstretched, or with active displacement of the limb through space, e.g., touching a target with the index finger. The tremor typically involves the upper limbs, but may include the head and neck (not the jaw or tongue separately), and, when extreme, may affect the lower limbs. It is usually coarse at about 10 Hz. Tremor is commonly associated with an acute confusional state related to a metabolic or toxic etiology. Common associations are uremia, hepatic failure, alcohol or drug withdrawal, and carbon dioxide narcosis.

Asterixis is a sudden loss of postural tone, so that the body must be actively supported against gravity for it to be seen. Most commonly, asterixis is detected by having the patient hold the upper limbs extended in front of the body, with the wrists dorsiflexed and the fingers extended at the metacarpophalangeal and interphalangeal joints. There is initially a lateral or rotatory tremor-like movement of the fingers, followed by a coarse loss of tone, so that a flexion-type movement occurs. The original posture is quickly regained, and the cycle may be repeated. If both upper limbs are involved, the "flapping" is usually asynchronous. Asterixis may involve any appendicular or axial group of muscles. There may even be a total body asterixis, causing a "drop attack" in which the patient may fall limply to the floor without further impairment of consciousness. Asterixis is due to abnormal function of the motor component of the brainstem reticular formation that is responsible for maintenance and adjustments of postural tone. Asterixis is almost invariably symptomatic of a metabolic or toxic disorder, but unilateral asterixis has been described with midbrain and contralateral parietal lesions.

Multifocal myoclonus is the scattered asynchronous active twitching of various muscle groups on both sides of the body. In contrast to asterixis, the movements are due to "active" neurally driven muscle twitching rather than a relaxation of tone. Patients vary from mild to severe encephalopathy. When symptomatic of metabolic or toxic disorders, the severity is usually more advanced than with tremor or asterixis. Also, in multifocal myoclonus, in contrast to tremor and asterixis, the body part does not need to be actively moved or maintained against posture (except in action myoclonus) and the patient may be in coma.

MOTOR RESPONSES AND POSTURES   See Fig. 3-11. Hemiplegia is characterized by the absence of upper and lower limb movements on one side of the body, either observed spontaneously or following the application of noxious stimuli. This implies dysfunction of the upper motor neuron system, especially the descending system from the frontal regions, the posterior limb of the internal capsule, the cerebral peduncle, the basis pontis of the midbrain and pons, respectively, or the medulla (usually more than the pyramid). A flexion response of the upper limb usually indicates an incomplete cerebral lesion contralateral to the posturing. Extension implies a deeper cerebral or brainstem lesion.

Flexion, extension, and adduction as gross motor responses should be regarded as reflex responses indicating deep bicerebral or brainstem dysfunction affecting the motor system. No response could reflect marked dysfunction in either the central (especially the lower medulla) or peripheral nervous systems, or indicate psychogenic unresponsiveness. These abnormal motor responses may be dissociated from impairment of the arousal system.[1] The motor systems are

spatially separate from the ascending reticular activating system (ARAS).

Bilateral upper limb flexion responses, usually accompanied by extension and plantar flexion of the lower limbs, are usually referred to as decorticate posturing. This may relate to the "released" influences of subcortical pathways such as the rubrospinal pathways.

"Decerebrate posturing" (Fig. 3-11F) consists principally of extension of the upper limbs at the elbows and extension of the lower limbs at the hips and knees. In the full decerebrate response there is opisthotonus, trismus of the jaws, internal rotation of the upper limbs at the shoulders, fisting, and plantar flexion. Decerebrate posturing, usually a sign of more advanced motor system dysfunction than is decorticate posturing, is found principally in: deep bilateral cerebral hemispheric lesions, the late stages of rostral-caudal syndrome (see Chap. 4), bilateral structural lesions of or compressing the brainstem (midbrain and upper pons), and profound metabolic disturbances, e.g., advanced hepatic coma, severe hypoglycemia, anoxia, or drug intoxication.[11]

Bouts of decerebrate or decorticate posturing (Fig. 3-11E and F) are often mistaken for seizures. This phenomenon is common following rebleeding from ruptured berry aneurysms.

Occasionally, patients will have decerebrate posturing on one side and decorticate posturing on the other. If this is consistent, it is usually the more extensive cerebral lesion (or a single lesion with marked mass effect) that is on the side contralateral to the decerebrate posturing.[2]

Extension of the upper limbs and flexion at the hips and knees, or no movement of the lower limbs, usually indicates a lesion at the pontine tegmentum or below, usually related to basilar artery occlusion (Plum and Posner[2]; Ropper, A.H., personal communication, 1996).

Abduction of the arm at the shoulder or the lower limb at the hip is usually a purposeful response and indicates that the corticospinal system on that side is intact and that the person is only mildly obtunded (Fig. 3-11D). Symmetrical grimacing is a favorable sign, but drawing down of the corners of the mouth represents a lower

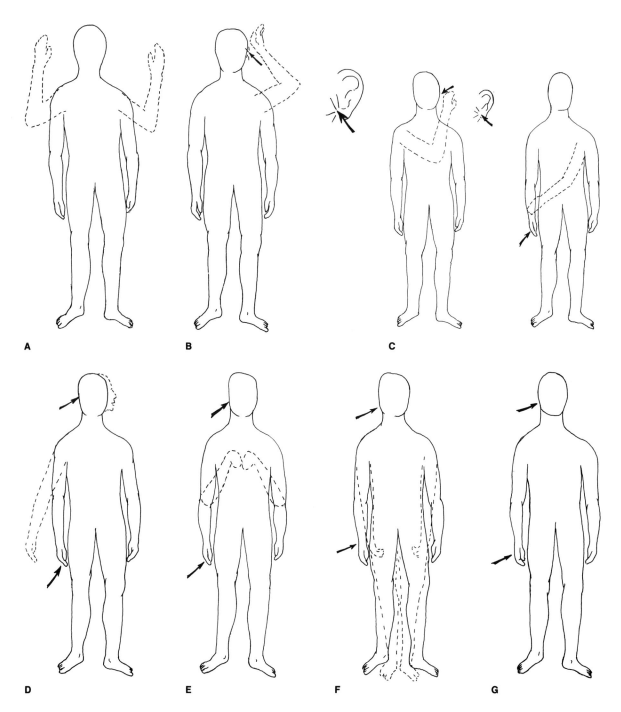

Figure 3-11

A. *Normal motor reactivity. The patient was asked to raise his arms.* B. *A patient with only mild obtundation wards off a painful stimulus to the ear.* C. *A patient who does not respond to commands and who cannot ward off pain can still localize a painful stimulus* brainstem phenomenon and is not necessarily favorable.[1]

Forced grasping is a "release sign," in which the fingers flex, usually curling about or "grasping" the examiner's fingers as they stroke the patient's palm. Forced grasping affects the hand that is contralateral to a large frontal lesion. The main brain region involved is the supplementary motor region on the side contralateral to the grasp reflex.[12]

Trismus or biting-down, either spontaneously or on something placed in the mouth, implies the dysfunction is above the midpons. Deviation of the head and/or eyes to one side is, in general, a lateralizing sign of a supratentorial or infratentorial lesion.

Turning towards a noxious stimulus is always a reflex response, while turning to the opposite side, away from the stimulus, may be purposeful.[13]

With seizures, turning movements or clonic activity usually indicate that the focus lies in the opposite cerebral hemisphere.

Patients with psychogenic unresponsiveness will actively close the eyes by vigorous contraction of the orbicularis oculi. A "purposeful" motor response is one that avoids the noxious stimulus or attempts to push it away.

Convulsive or myoclonic status epilepticus is readily recognized. Nonconvulsive status epilepticus is characterized by impaired consciousness without such motor activity. It should be considered in the following situations: (1) when the patient has a prolonged "postictal state" following a recognized seizure; (2) during prolonged recovery from a neurologic insult, such as trauma, or an anoxic-ischemic event, such as a cardiac arrest or a hypotensive event; (3) during prolonged recovery from an intracranial neurosurgical procedure; (4) when the patient is unconsciousness with myoclonus of the facial (palpebral, periorbital, facial) or jaw muscles; and (5) when there is abrupt, unexplained loss of consciousness with intact brainstem function.[14]

The differential diagnosis includes tremors. Tremulous extensor movements of the lower limbs may follow acute lesions of the corticospinal tracts with basilar artery occlusion. These can, at times, resemble seizures. The author's group has also seen limb tremors in comatose patients in association with hypoxemia and hypotension. Multifocal myoclonus, usually in association with a metabolic encephalopathy, does not usually indicate a cortical seizure, but probably reflects discharges in the reticular formation.[15]

4. Respiration Decreased level of consciousness is often accompanied by both upper and lower airway dysfunction (see Fig. 3-12). In upper airway obstruction, there is a loss of strength and tone in the oropharynx, and the tongue of the supine patient falls backward. Pieces of food, vomitus, or thick saliva may cause further obstruction. With complete obstruction, the examiner's hand over the mouth and throat will not feel any movement of air and breathing will be silent. Partial obstruction causes noisy breathing that becomes a high-pitched stridor if the airway is severely narrowed. Upper airway obstruction leads to indrawing of the supraclavicular fossa and descent of the larynx and trachea (tracheal tug) due to the increased negative intrathoracic pressure. There

---

Figure 3-11 (Continued).
by moving the hand across the midline. (The arrows in this and other figures indicate the site(s) of painful somatosensory stimulation.) D. This patient, more severely affected than the one in part C, makes a withdrawal abducting movement of the arm or a contraversive head movement. E. With progressive worsening, the patient assumes a bilateral decorticate response; a slow mechanical upper limb flexion posture is adopted. F. The next most abnormal response is a stereotyped extensor posturing. The arms are extended and internally rotated at the sides. The feet are plantar flexed and the head is extended backwards. G. In the final stages of brainstem failure, there is no response or posturing to painful somatic stimulation.

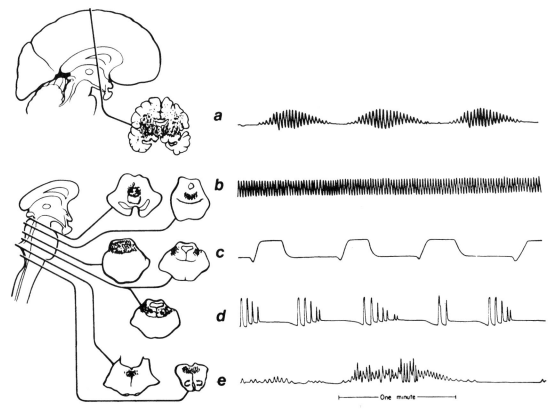

Figure 3-12

Respirations: respiratory patterns associated with lesions/dysfunction at various levels of the neuraxis. (a) Long-cycle Cheyne-Stokes respirations with bilateral cerebral hemispheric lesions. (b) Central neurogenic hyperventilation (originally attributed to midbrain lesions), now mainly found with neurogenic pulmonary edema. (c) Apneustic breathing with inspiratory and expiratory cramping. (d) and (e) Cluster and ataxic breathing, respectively, with caudal pontine or medullary lesions. (From Plum F, Posner JB: The Diagnosis of Stupor and Coma, *3rd ed. Philadelphia, FA Davis, 1980, p 34, with permission.)*

is often a rocking (alternating) motion of the chest and abdomen: with attempted inspiration, the abdomen moves out with descent of the diaphagm coincident with a retraction of the chest wall. Immediate blood gas analysis reveals a marked reduction of Pa_{O_2} and increase in Pa_{CO_2}. This emergent situation requires prompt suctioning of the oropharynx and anterosuperior traction on the mandible to open the oropharynx. With an oropharyngeal airway to keep the tongue from obstructing air flow, the upper airway can usually be kept open for some time with oxygen delivered by mask. For longer-term maintenance of the upper airway and greater protection against aspiration, an endotracheal tube is necessary.

Once upper airway patency is secured, observing the pattern of respiration, coupled with blood gas determination, can give clues as to the site and cause of the ventilatory problem. Problems with ventilatory insufficiency (vital capacity <12 mL/kg, or rising Pa_{CO_2}) may appear in association with the upper airway obstruction or may manifest later. This requires ventilatory support.

Cheyne-Stokes respiration is a common abnormality, indicating bicerebral dysfunction or reduced cardiac output. It is a sign of only mild neurologic dysfunction and implies that the patient is *not* in imminent danger. The stage of maximal impairment is during the apneic phase of Cheyne-Stokes breathing, when responsiveness diminishes, the eyes close, the pupils constrict, and spontaneous movement ceases.[1]

So called "short-cycle Cheyne-Stokes respiration" consists of three or four rapid deep breaths while the waxing and waning phases each consist of one breath. This has a much more sinister prognosis and is usually associated with intracranial hemorrhage. A variant of this is "Biot's breathing" in which the respirations are very irregular and associated with incomplete lower brainstem failure.

Apneustic breathing is characterized by deep breathing, with pausing in both inspiration and expiration.

Kussmal breathing is a regular, deep respiration usually related to a metabolic acidosis. "Central neurogenic hyperventilation" is regular deep respiration associated with a respiratory alkalosis; it is related to brainstem lesions not uncommonly associated with pulmonary edema.[16]

Weakness of the muscles of respiration from dysfunction of anterior horn cells, the phrenic nerve, or the neuromuscular junction or muscle may be caused by a variety of neuromuscular disorders. Such patients have rapid, shallow breathing with blood gases showing a progressive rise in Pa_{CO_2}. With predominant diaphragmatic weakness, paradoxical respiration will be present: in inspiration, the abdomen moves inwards or remains immobile instead of moving outwards. If the weakness is primarily in the chest wall muscles, the opposite paradoxical movement will be present: there will be a retraction of the chest wall, but the abdomen moves out appropriately with descent of the diaphragm.

Unfortunately, these clinical signs may be absent if the patient has already undergone endotracheal intubation and is on a ventilator before neurologic assessment is performed. Thus, we find that electrophysiologic studies are of great value in localizing a nervous system cause for ventilatory insufficiency (see below).

Summary of Clinical Neurologic Examination

Synthesizing the information from the exam, some localizing deductions can be made:

1. Signs of a *solitary supratentorial lesion* include contralateral hemiparesis with eye deviation to the side opposite the paretic limbs and contralateral focal motor (e.g., "jacksonian") seizures. With further progression, signs of a third nerve palsy appear ipsilateral to the lesion: i.e., pupillary dilatation with loss of light reflex, then paresis of adduction so that the affected eye is abducted to the temporal side of the midline, accompanied by ptosis.

2. Signs of *infratentorial lesions* include cranial nerve palsies, dysconjugate eye movements (such as an internuclear ophthalmoplegia), ocular bobbing (caudal pons localization), retractory or convergence nystagmus (rostral midbrain tegmental lesion), quadriparesis before loss of consciousness, and loss of oculovestibular response with hemi- or quadriparesis. A gaze palsy causing the eyes to face the hemiparetic side usually indicates a caudal pontine lesion, affecting the brainstem paramedian lateral gaze center and the corticospinal fibers before they cross in the caudal medulla.[17] Such gaze palsies cannot be overcome by oculocephalic or oculovestibular testing if the brainstem paramedian pontine reticular formation is compromised or if the vestibular input is disconnected from this gaze center, e.g., in Wernicke's encephalopathy.

The earliest features and sequence of deficits provide useful clinical data. For example, in cerebellar hemorrhage or infarction, the patient is alert, usually not paretic in the limbs, but has headache, vertigo, and severe lateralized or midline ataxia. Then, a lateral rectus palsy and extensor plantar response occur, followed by impairment of consciousness and a lateral gaze palsy, with the eyes deviated away from a lower motor seventh nerve palsy. This may be followed by further brainstem signs, pupillary abnormalities, and bilateral corticospinal tract signs. Since surgical decompressive treatment can be life-saving, if performed before severe brainstem compromise has occurred, it is important to recognize, investigate, and treat such cases early.

An acute presentation of intrinsic brainstem signs, e.g., bilateral long-tract motor signs, with cranial nerve palsies such as deafness and eye movement disorders, in an adult raises the possibility of an acute or impending basilar artery occlusion. There may be an earlier history of transient brainstem ischemia. Intravenous or intra-arterial thrombolysis is sometimes feasible if the patient presents within 3 h and has a normal computed tomography (CT) scan (see Chap. 14).

3. *Multifocal supratentorial lesions* or *metabolic or toxic encephalopathies* typically spare the pupils and oculovestibular reflexes, which are almost invariably affected by the time a single supra- or infratentorial mass lesion causes coma. Morphine and heroin produce small pupils that should still react. Massive overdoses of barbiturates, and hypothermia or profound metabolic disorders, such as extreme, prolonged hypoglycemia, may cause the pupillary reflexes to be lost in a reversible fashion (sometimes to the point of mimicking brain death). Wernicke's encephalopathy can cause gaze paresis, single extraocular movement paresis (especially abductor weakness), or internuclear ophthalmoplegia as well as loss of oculovestibular reflexes and impaired consciousness *without compromising the pupillary reflexes*.

Subhyaloid hemorrhages indicate a ruptured berry aneurysm until proven otherwise.

Acute obstructive hydrocephalus is usually associated with headaches, mental changes (inattention and distractibility, then reduced alertness), abnormal gait, and poor bladder control. Upward gaze may be impaired if there is pressure on the rostral midbrain. There is no paralysis of movements in the early stages.

Multifocal myoclonus or abundant twitching usually indicates a metabolic encephalopathy or a nonconvulsive seizure. Isolated facial twitching is often an indication of nonconvulsive seizures.

If the patient has signs of brainstem dysfunction, including loss of pupillary reflexes and absent caloric responses, it is often impossible, when the patient is first seen to determine from the neurologic examination alone whether the problem began in the posterior fossa or if the patient has experienced advanced rostral-caudal deterioration from a supratentorial mass lesion. Occasionally profound, diffuse toxic or metabolic processes may also compromise brainstem function. Emergency neuroimaging is necessary to exclude a structural lesion and, if one is present, to clarify the site, cause, and reversibility.

INVESTIGATION

Tests are guided by the clinical categorization of the problem (see Fig. 3-1).

The respiratory pattern and simple arterial or capillary blood gas determination reduces the number of possibilities. *Hyperventilation with a metabolic acidosis pattern* (pH < 7.30; Pa_{CO_2} < 30 mmHg; HCO_3 < 15 mmol/L can result from renal failure, lactic acidosis, diabetic ketoacidosis and salicylate, methanol, or ethylene glycol poisoning. *Hyperventilation with respiratory alkalosis* (pH > 7.45; Pa_{CO_2} < 30 mmHg; HCO_3 > 15 mmol/L) is associated with hepatic failure, early sepsis, early salicylate intoxication, cardiopulmonary disease (e.g., pulmonary embolism or pneumonia), or psychogenic unresponsiveness. *Hypoventilation with respiratory acidosis* (pH < 7.35; Pa_{CO_2} > 55 mmHg; HCO_3 > 15 mmol/L) may be the end result of medullary failure from structural or toxic depression, hypothyroidism, or coma-producing severe respiratory failure itself.

With ventilatory failure, the central nervous system can now be tested by the technique of transcranial magnetic stimulation, with recording from the diaphragm using surface electrodes, and by somatosensory evoked potential studies from the contralateral parietal cortex.[18,19] The peripheral nervous system can be tested with phrenic nerve conduction studies. Repetitive phrenic nerve stimulation, in trains of 3 Hz or more, can be used to detect a neuromuscular transmission disorder.[20] Needle electromyography of the diaphragm also gives important information on central and peripheral causes of neuromuscular respiratory insufficiency.[21]

Multifocal or diffuse problems without focal signs are likely to be due to metabolic, septic, or toxic causes, or problems reflected by abnormal cerebrospinal fluid (CSF) (i.e., infections or hemorrhage). Occasionally, bicerebral damage from trauma or stokes may mimic this picture.

For diffuse or multifocal problems, the following screening tests are indicated: complete blood count, serum glucose, electrolytes, urea, creatinine, calcium, magnesium, hepatic function tests (especially serum bilirubin and ammonia), urinalysis, arterial blood gases, and a serum and urinary screen for drugs. Blood cultures should be carried out in systemic and CNS infections (e.g., sepsis or bacterial endocarditis). Serum ammonia and other liver function tests help to confirm hepatic encephalopathy. Thyroid or adrenal function tests may also be necessary. For coagulation problems, a blood smear, disseminated intravascular coagulation (DIC) screen, antiphospholipid antibody test, platelet count, and antithrombin III determination are needed. Carboxyhemoglobin determination should be carried out when carbon monoxide intoxication is suspected.

The investigation and management of patients suspected of *toxin exposure* is given in Chap. 16. Some clues that one may be dealing with a toxin include:

1. Hypoventilation with intact brainstem reflexes, no primary neuromuscular dysfunction, and a normal chest examination.

2. Hyperventilation with metabolic acidosis without uremia, ketosis, or lactate excess.

3. Intact brainstem function with a negative CT scan of the cerebral hemispheres.

4. Miotic, reactive pupils (opiates).

5. General examination clues: stigmata of drug or alcohol abuse (e.g., needle marks, signs of hepatic dysfunction), or cherry-red skin and mucous membranes (carbon monoxide poisoning).

6. History of depression, previous suicide attempts or gestures, drug or alcohol abuse, or use of any medication.

A *lumbar puncture* may confirm meningitis, encephalitis, or a subarachnoid hemorrhage if the CT scan is normal. The main contraindications are evidence of an intracranial lesion of significant size, a coagulopathy, or an infection in the tissues overlying the lumbar spine (Chap. 11).

For suspected multifocal *structural brain lesions*, e.g., from trauma, metastases, or multiple embolic strokes, prompt neuroimaging is important.

Neurophysiological Tests for Coma

Electroencephalography   Electroencephalography (EEG) comprises standard, 30-min recordings as well as serial recordings, continuous EEG monitoring, quantitative EEG, and evoked potentials. These will be discussed in turn. It is important to understand the nature of the information given by each of these tests, along with the individual strengths and limitations of these procedures. Electrophysiologic investigations are tests of *function*. They have only approximate localizing value and rarely have diagnostic specificity. They can, however, be helpful in broadly classifying various conditions associated with unresponsiveness.

The standard/routine EEG records electrical activity arising in the cerebral cortex underlying the scalp electrodes. The recorded waveforms arise from summated synaptic activity arising from the larger neurons lying in the deeper layers. The synchronized synaptic activity, in turn, reflects intrinsic cortical rhythms and those due to interaction with the thalamus. Thus, the EEG allows a dynamic examination of cortical-thalamic *function*. This can be especially useful in patients with impaired consciousness, especially those who in coma or who are paralyzed and in intensive care units (ICUs). Such patients may be clinically similar, yet the EEG will show a wide range of types

Table 3-2

Electroencephalogram classification

Category	Subcategory
I. Delta/theta >5% of record (not theta coma)	A. Reactivity B. No reactivity
II. Triphasic waves	
III. Burst-suppression	A. With epileptiform activity B. Without epileptiform activity
IV. Alpha/theta/spindle coma (unreactive)	
V. Epileptiform activity (not in burst-suppression pattern)	A. Generalized B. Focal or multifocal
VI. Suppression	A. $< 20 \,\mu V$ but $> 10 \,\mu V$ B. $\leq 10 \,\mu V$

Guidelines:

1. Burst-suppression pattern should have generalized flattening at standard sensitivity for ≥ 1 s at least every 20 s.
2. Suppression: for this category, voltage criteria should be met for the entire record: there should be no reactivity.
3. When more than one category applies, select the most critical:
   - Suppression is the most serious category.
   - Burst-suppression is more important than the category of triphasic waves, which is more significant than dysrhythmia or delta.
   - Alpha pattern coma is more important than focal spikes, triphasic waves, dysrhythmia, or delta categories.

Source: Reproduced from Young GB, McLachlan RS, Kreeft JH, Demelo JD: An EEG classification for coma. *Can J Neurol Sci*, in press.

and severity of dysfunction reflecting different processes with various degrees of reversibility.

Guidelines and standards for EEGs and related neurophysiologic tests on comatose patients have been developed recently by a special committee of the International Federation of Clinical Neurophysiology.[22] This author and coworkers have developed a classification system that accommodates all possible categories.[23] This is given in Table 3-2, and representative EEGs from patients with impaired consciousness are shown in Fig. 3-13.

The EEG has been used for the following:

1. To verify and classify the brain dysfunction. The EEG is always abnormal in comatose patients, but is normal in patients with psychogenic coma. In a normal EEG, during wakefulness in a relaxed state with the eyes closed, the predominant rhythm is posteriorly situated, symmetrical, and is in the "alpha" range, between 8 and 13 Hz. Typically, such activity is blocked by eye opening. Drowsiness or nervous tension may also diminish alpha activity. Since the EEG in psychogenic unresponsiveness may be of low voltage or may show faster frequencies, it is important to test for EEG reactivity, including the response to passive eye opening, before it is concluded that the EEG indicates psychogenic unresponsiveness. In delirium, an agitated confusional state, the EEG may be of low voltage and "desynchronize," but may not show much slowing. A normal alpha rhythm, responsive to eye opening, may also be found in the "locked-in" syndrome (see Chap. 2).

The type of abnormality can reflect the depth and severity of the underlying dysfunction or it may give diagnostic clues. The EEGs are usually standard, discontinuous, single or serial recordings.

This author's group has developed an EEG classification system with high interrater agreement (Table 3-2).[24] This was modified from an earlier

Figure 3-13

EEG illustrations.

A. A burst of slow frequency waves is evidence of reactivity to the sound of a clap near the ear (arrow) in this patient with a toxic encephalopathy. The patient survived.

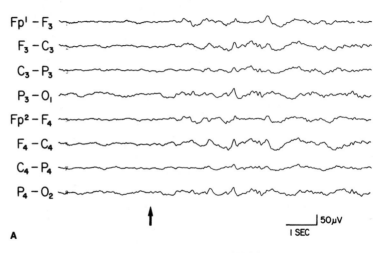

B. Delta, a rhythm of 4 Hz or less, is the predominant frequency in this patient with renal failure and sepsis (Category I, Table 3-2). Faster frequencies are reduced in the right side (bottom four channels) due to a previous cerebral infarction. The patient recovered.

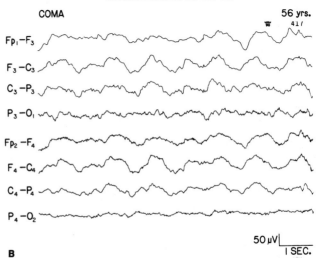

RENAL FAILURE AND SEPSIS

COMA   56 yrs.

C. Triphasic waves (Category II, Table 3-2) are present in this patient with septic encephalopathy. The patient later died of multiorgan failure.

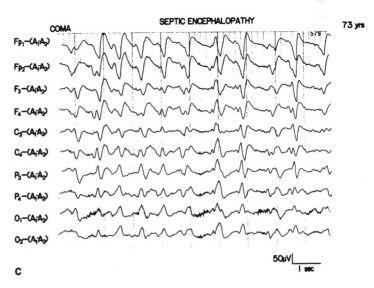

SEPTIC ENCEPHALOPATHY   73 yrs

COMA

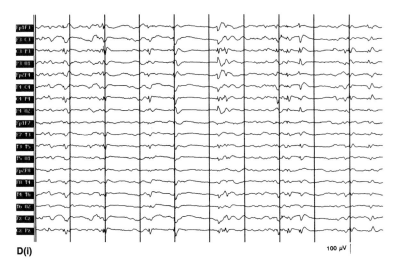

D(i)

100 µV

Figure 3-13 *(Continued)* D. *A burst-suppression pattern consists of generalized bursts containing various frequencies (i) with or (ii) without epileptiform activity (Categories IIIA and IIIB, respectively, Table 3-2).*

BURST-SUPPRESSION

COMA   74 yrs

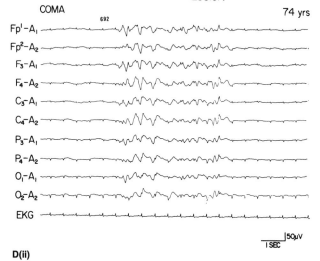

D(ii)

50µV

I SEC

ALPHA-THETA COMA

COMA   50 yrs

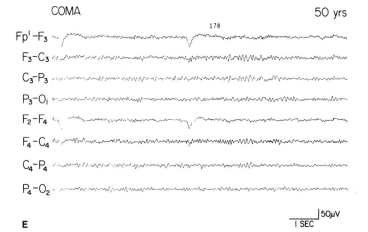

E

50µV

I SEC

E. *An alpha pattern coma (Category IV, Table 3-2) consists of frequencies between 5 and 13 Hz with widespread distribution and no reactivity, as seen in this patient with anoxic-ischemic encephalopathy from cardiac arrest. He died without recovery of consciousness.*

Figure 3-13 *(Continued)*
F(i). This 47-year-old man suffered a cardiac arrest 4 days before the recording. Generalized epileptiform discharges (Category VA, Table 3-2) are present against a suppressed background. The patient was in deep coma with only a flexor response to noxious stimuli. He had generalized myoclonus when not on muscle relaxants. He died shortly afterwards without recovery of consciousness.

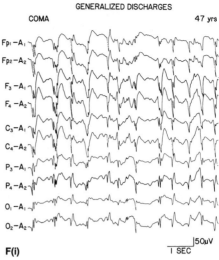

GENERALIZED DISCHARGES
COMA   47 yrs

F(i)   50μV
                        1 SEC

F(ii). This 44-year-old man had seizures associated with nystagmoid horizontal eye movements while in coma after open heart surgery. A seizure consisting of augmenting epileptiform discharges (Category VB, Table 3-2) begins in the right occipital region (last channel) and spreads to the left posterior head (fourth channel). The patient ultimately made a complete recovery.

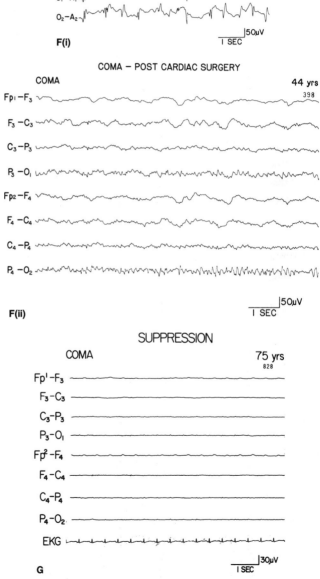

COMA – POST CARDIAC SURGERY
COMA   44 yrs
                                         398

F(ii)   50μV
                        1 SEC

SUPPRESSION
COMA   75 yrs
                                         828

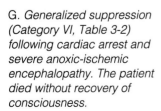

G. Generalized suppression (Category VI, Table 3-2) following cardiac arrest and severe anoxic-ischemic encephalopathy. The patient died without recovery of consciousness.

G   30μV
                        1 SEC

classification system by Synek[25] and is arranged roughly in order of severity of the abnormality and underlying brain dysfunction. Using this system and the contained guidelines, it is possible to classify nearly all EEGs without ambiguity.

The EEG is the most specific and sensitive test for detecting seizures or interictal epileptiform activity. An urgent EEG is indicated when there is a previous history of seizures, bitten tongue, tonic eye deviation (especially with nystagmoid eye movements), or twitching about the face or limbs. This applies especially if movements are lateralized or bilaterally synchronous, or no there is other explanation for the comatose state.[26] The EEG is especially useful in the detection of nonconvulsive seizures or cerebral seizure activity in the paralyzed, ventilated patient. The treatment of status epilepticus is greatly facilitated by EEG monitoring during injections, as discussed in Chap. 17.

Some patterns are highly suggestive of, but not diagnostic of, metabolic encephalopathies: i.e., generalized triphasic waves or intermittent rhythmic delta activity on a slow, suppressed background. These can be seen in some advanced degenerative or systemic inflammatory response syndromes.

2 To evaluate the depth of coma. The degree of slowing for many metabolic and toxic encephalopathies follows the anesthetic model. These are listed in detail, along with the caveats, in Chap. 13.

Many patients in the ICU are treated with opiates or benzodiazepines. Clearance of these drugs is slowed by hepatic and/or renal failure. These and other drugs with similar actions can significantly alter rhythmicity, voltage, and reactivity. The interpreter of EEGs must be aware of drugs taken recently by the patient. In some cases, one should consider the intravenous administration of flumazenil or naloxone to block benzodiazepine or opiate receptors, respectively.

3. To monitor the course or trends. Trending is facilitated by continuous recording with quantification of rhythms and voltage, as allowed by compressed spectral arrays. This can be helpful in examining for potentially reversible developments such as vasospasm, reduced cerebral perfusion, or increased mass effect. The effects of treatments can also be gauged.

4. Prognosis. Prediction of clinical outcome is closely linked to etiology. Because many EEG patterns are nonspecific, it is vital to know the etiology before an estimate of disease severity or reversibility is attempted. Drugs, hypothermia (temperature $< 32.2°C$), and many metabolic disorders may cause reversible slowing, burst-suppression, or suppression patterns. On the other hand, cardiac arrest may produce neuronal death, and such patterns may be predictive of a poor prognosis. Apart from finding complete suppression, it is unlikely that a single EEG recording is reliably predictive of a poor or hopeless outcome. This author and coworkers have found serial EEGs to be useful in the prediction of generalized anoxic-ischemic encephalopathy. Alpha, theta, or alpha-theta pattern coma is common after cardiac arrest. About 20 percent of such patients regain conscious awareness.[27] A prognositically useful pattern usually develops by day 5: those who survive develop continuous rhythms and regain electrographic reactivity to stimulation, while those who fail to recover develop a burst-suppression pattern without reactivity.[27]

Continuous Electroencephalography Continuous EEG (CEEG) recording is now feasible with the availability of digital EEG displays at the bedside, storage on electronic media such as optical disks, quantified methods, and computerized sampling and recognition programs. Some early studies have shown potential value in detecting nonconvulsive seizures and other patterns of diagnostic and prognostic value in comatose ICU patients.[28,29] This is a promising technology, but evidence-based indications are yet to be developed.

A minimum of eight channels is necessary to provide for adequate bilateral coverage of the cerebrum. Because technologists and electroencephalographers cannot be continuously present, nurses may be taught to interpret basic patterns.[28] This can be facilitated by automation for trending, and automated spike and seizure detection with alarms. However, in general, nurses perform seizure detection as well or better than automated systems. The trending capabilities of quantitative EEG are of considerable help in continuous monitoring. There should be a ready means of communication of the nurses' observations along with transmission of the signal to the electroencephalographer for interpretation and feedback. It is the feedback with action and subsequent monitoring for further effect that constitutes an effective CEEG monitoring *system*.[28-30]

Continuous EEG could be used for trending the severity of cerebral dysfunction, determining if seizures are occurring, surveying for regional abnormalities, and noting the effects of therapy, including sedative drugs. The latter, especially benzodiazepines and opiates, can confound evaluations of encephalopathy, adequate perfusion, and other general assessments, just as sedation hampers the clinical evaluation. The usefulness of CEEG in the management of status epilepticus is discussed in Chap. 17. Further work needs to be carried out on determining the indications for such monitoring, where the monitoring makes a difference in patients' outcomes and management.

Evoked Responses Evoked responses are produced by repetitive sensory stimulation, performed in a standardized format. The EEG electrodes are attached to the scalp using standardized landmarks.[22] The stimulation is repeated many times; with computer averaging, the potentials that occur regularly in a time-locked fashion relative to the stimulus are summated and are able to be viewed. Evoked responses are usually performed in discrete or separate sessions by the technologist, who brings the equipment to the bedside for each evaluation. The technology for automatically performing continuous or frequent evoked responses and trending results has been developed.[31] This would allow for quantitative monitoring of sensory pathways. The indications and application of this emerging technology for management and outcome issues require assessment.

Somatosensory evoked responses, usually performed with median nerve stimulation, produce a series of waves, including a negative brainstem peak at 14 ms after the stimulus. The response from the primary sensory area, S1, occurs at about 20 ms.

Brainstem auditory evoked responses are produced by introducing clicks at about 60 dB above presumed hearing threshold.

The main value of the evoked responses is in helping to establish a prognosis. They are only worthwhile in cases of coma where the etiology is a condition capable of causing neuronal death. Loss of early or some middle and later components is usually associated with a poor outcome, but the persistence of normal responses does not assure a good recovery, because such responses are so robust.[22]

Evoked responses can be useful in the evaluation of sensory pathways; the early (short-latency) components are relatively resistant to metabolic, toxic substances, drugs, and even hypothermia down to less than 27°C.[32] This makes these factors of value in assessing the integrity of sensory pathways, including primary somatosensory cortical areas, in the presence of such factors. Differentiation between cortical and subcortical, especially brainstem, lesions is achieved. As a proviso, the peripheral receptors and nerves, and spinal and central subcortical regions must be intact before one can assess the thalamocortical component. The use of somatosensory and auditory evoked responses are especially useful in providing prognostic information.

Note that evoked potentials (EPs) are not useful in examining the depth of coma or in looking for epileptiform activity. They have not been adequately evaluated in neonates and very young infants.

Neuroimaging

The advent of CT greatly facilitated the evaluation of patients with suspect structural intracranial lesions or hemorrhage. Scanning of the head by CT allows diagnostic, prognostic, and management decisions to be made quickly. This has been shown in a comparative study matching clinically similar groups of head-injured patients before and after CT scanning was available.[33] Neuroimaging, especially repeated CT scanning, allowed earlier and more definitive recognition of operable lesions than did cerebral angiography. This would be expected, given CT's significantly superior imaging of soft tissues and ventricles.

Neuroimaging should not, however, be carried out indiscriminately before adequate evaluation and stabilization of the patient. It should not be allowed to delay more specific management, e.g., the treatment of seizures or suspected bacterial meningitis.

The CT scans show changes that correlate with raised intracranial pressure.[34] In children with nontraumatic coma, the obliteration of CSF spaces (sulci, fissures, chiasmatic and ambient or quadrigeminal cisterns) and narrowing of ventricular dimensions is consistently associated with markedly raised ICP.[34] In patients with white matter or basal ganglionic lesions detected on CT scanning, there was not a consistent relationship between some loss of CSF spaces and raised ICP. Also, some of the patients in this series, who had initially normal CT scans, developed raised ICP and reduced cerebral perfusion. Thus, CT scanning is not always a reliable guide to ICU management in such children with nontraumatic coma.

Magnetic resonance imaging (MRI) is superior to CT in showing early tissue signal changes in a number of conditions, such as herpes simplex encephalitis, infarction, and brainstem lesions. In the assessment of white matter, e.g., with ischemic or traumatic lesions, MRI is superior to CT and functional neuroimaging.[35] Magnetic resonance angiography (MRA) allows the assessment of flow as well as a low-resolution "angiogram." However, MRI and MRA are more difficult to perform on the ICU patient, especially in the presence of assisted ventilation or multimodal monitoring. In addition, these procedures are contraindicated in patients with electronic pacemakers, epidural pacing, or ferromagnetic aneurysmal clips. Standard cerebral angiography is now used mainly for the identification of the sites of intracranial aneurysms and the nature of arterial lesions (e.g., dissection), after the nature of the disease process is determined.

Anatomic and functional neuroimaging are sometimes used for the confirmation of brain death (see Chap. 2). Neuroimaging test results in specific disease states are discussed in later chapters.

Other

A number of other investigative techniques, such as transcranial Doppler, jugular venous oxygen determination, cerebral blood flow determinations, and ICP measurements, are helpful, in specific cases, for monitoring and prognostic purposes in patients in the ICU rather than in the initial assessment of patients with impaired consciousness. The roles of these tests are briefly reviewed here; specific applications are addressed in more detail in the relevant chapters.

Transcranial Doppler Transcranial Doppler (TCD) ultrasonography provides a noninvasive method of examining the intracranial circulation, at least for the basal intracranial arteries.[36] Transcranial Doppler ultrasonography uses the Doppler principle that relates the blood velocity to the shift in frequency of sound waves in the ultrasonic frequency range, as illustrated in Figs. 3-14 and 3-15. There are several "acoustical windows" through which various intracranial arteries can be examined with the Doppler probe (Fig. 3-16).

The change in velocity is inversely related to the cross-sectional area of the insonated vessel, but the relationship is linear only over a restricted portion of the diameter-flow curves (Fig. 3-15).

Doppler studies have been useful in looking for vasospasm (increased blood velocity) in patients with subarachnoid hemorrhages. With raised ICPs, vessels become constricted and blood velocity increases. However, this is a comparatively late finding with raised ICP; often, the course is set or damage is done when ultrasonography becomes positive in this situation. Transcranial Doppler testing has a potential role in brain death determination (see Chap. 2). In head injury, TCD can reveal a number of important changes: increased velocities in hyperemia or vasospasm, vascular occlusion, and findings of carotid-cavernous fistula, among

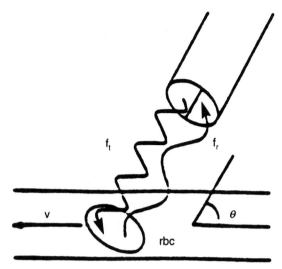

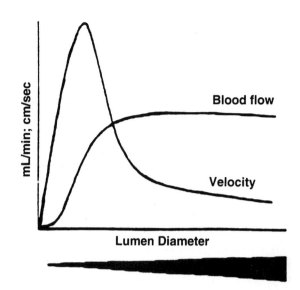

Figure 3-14

The Doppler principle. The velocity of blood is proportional to the Doppler shift and the cosine of the angle between the sound beam and the flow axis. $\Delta f = Z f_t V \cos \theta / c$, where f_t = transmitted frequency; V = velocity of blood; c = velocity of sound; Δf = Doppler shift; θ = angle between the sound beam and flow axis. f_r = rebound frequency; rbc = red blood cell.

Figure 3-15

The relationship of the flow velocity and vessel lumen diameter. Note that with narrow lumen diameters, the velocity is increased at a time when flow is decreasing. With very narrow vessels, both flow and velocity are greatly diminished. (Adapted from Spencer and Reid,[67] with permission.)

others.[36] There are potential roles for TCD in assessing autoregulation of cerebral blood flow.

Functional neuroimaging may prove superior to MRI in the assessment of cortical and subcortical gray matter disease.[35] Single photon emission computed tomography (SPECT) uses radioactively labeled compounds that pass into the brain parenchyma from the capillaries. The "trapped" compound then releases photons that can be imaged with rotating gamma cameras to create image slices similar to CT images. The amount of radioactive material in each unit volume of brain is roughly proportional to regional blood flow. Thus, SPECT is a test of regional blood flow, which is linked to metabolism.

The resolution of SPECT is superior to nuclear scans obtained without multiple detectors and computed image capacity.[37] Images can be superimposed on MRIs or CTs to allow a better correlation of functional defects with anatomic structures.[38] There is a potential role for SPECT in investigating relative deficiencies in regional

Figure 3-16

Skull acoustical windows used in the "freehand" transcranial Doppler technique. (From Newell and Asalid,[68] with permission.)

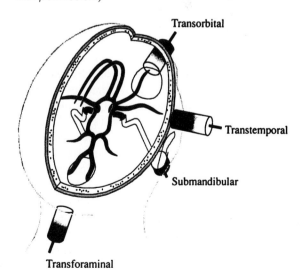

blood flow with ischemia (including acute ischemic stroke and vasospasm following subarachnoid hemorrhage), and increased activity with seizures, and it has been used to determine brain death.[39,40] There may be a role in examining altered blood flow or metabolic activity in herpes simplex encephalitis, encephalopathies [including the dementia in acquired immunodeficiency syndrome (AIDS)], and prognosis in cases of persistent vegetative state.[41] These all require further study. The application of radiolabeled ligands for specific receptors (e.g., acetylcholine, benzodiazepine, and dopamine) may expand the usefulness of SPECT beyond its current role as a test of blood flow and, indirectly, of metabolism.[42–44] The cost-effectiveness and availability are obvious advantages over functional MRI and positron emission tomography (PET).

Intracranial Pressure Monitoring Intracranial pressure is normally less than 10 mmHg when measured at the level of the foramen magnum in a supine patient.[45] The intracranial volume is fixed in older children and adults. the brain and its interstitial spaces constitute about 80 percent of the intracranial volume; CSF and blood each constitute about 10 percent. An increase in the volume of one of these components must be accompanied by a decease in one or more of the others to prevent a rise in ICP. Such accommodation depends on the time course of the increased volume. Once this compensating mechanism is exhausted, the ICP rises as shown in Fig. 3-17.

Increased ICP in itself is not harmful to the brain unless it leads to tissue ischemia by compromising cerebral blood flow, usually at pressures of >50 mmHg. The (global) cerebral perfusion pressure (CPP) is the gradient allowing for perfusion of the brain; it is equivalent to the mean arterial blood pressure minus the intracranial pressure. Normally, CPP is 70 to 100 mmHg. This allows for adequate perfusion of the brain as determined by metabolic needs. "Autoregulation" refers to the brain's ability to maintain a constant brain blood flow over a wide range of perfusion pressures. This is illustrated in Fig. 3-18, which also shows the

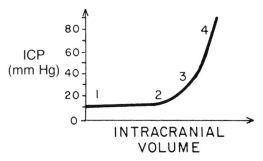

Figure 3-17

The relationship of ICP and intracranial volume, when extra volume is added abruptly. (From Shapiro HM: Intracranial hypertension: therapeutic and anesthetic considerations. Anesthesiology *43:447, 1975, with permission.)*

effects that the concentrations of oxygen and carbon dioxide in the arterial blood have on the the cerebral blood flow, When CPP falls below 60 mmHg, e.g., due to raised ICP, the brain perfusion is threatened and is pressure passive, i.e., there is no autoregulation and the brain becomes ischemic with further drops in pressure.

Measurements of global ICP and CPP have limited value. They are crude replacements for measures of regional blood flow and metabolism. Local tissue changes with altered perfusion, mass

Figure 3-18

The relationship of Pa_{O_2} and Pa_{CO_2} on CBF in normal brain. CBF=cerebral blood flow; BP= blood pressure. (From Shapiro HM: Intracranial hypertension: therapeutic and anesthetic considerations. Anesthesiology *43:447, 1975, with permission.)*

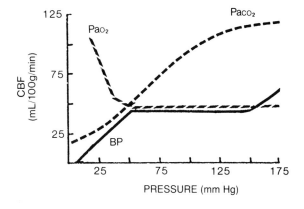

effects, herniations, and displacements often occur without significant changes in ICP or CPP until the effects become great. Nonetheless, ICP and CPP do provide a method of monitoring general aspects of the intracranial compartment and, when coupled with clinical judgment, measurements of blood pressure, blood gases, and jugular venous oxygen determination, they can be helpful.

The indications for ICP monitoring have not been firmly established, nor has a standardized approach or a set of guidelines been developed. However, patients who suffer from acute or sub-acute illnesses with increased volume of a component of the intracranial compartment, especially the brain, are commonly monitored. Head trauma, intracranial hemorrhage of any type, some tumors with brain swelling, and certain cases of encephalitis or ischemic stroke edema seem to be especially suitable. Uses are discussed in the chapters regarding those specific topics.

Methods of ICP monitoring include: fluid-coupled systems (e.g., intraventricular catheter, subarachnoid bolt) and nonfluid coupled systems (e.g., the intraparenchymal Casimo monitor or the Ladd epidural monitor). The advantages of the intraventricular monitor include the ability to withdraw CSF for both the relief of ICP and the sampling of CSF. The risks include intracranial infection. The Ladd epidural monitor does not give as accurate readings but allows for trending and is less invasive.

A more complete discussion of the use of ICP monitoring is found in standard textbooks about neurocritical care, such as those edited by Ropper and by Hacke.[46,47]

Jugular Oxygen Measurement Cerebral blood flow is normally tightly linked to the metabolic needs of the brain. The measurement of the oxygen concentration of venous blood leaving the brain provides an estimation of the relationship of cerebral blood flow to metabolism.

Normal jugular venous oxygen saturation is 50 to 75 percent.[48] Less than 50 percent indicates brain ischemia, while more than 75 percent indicates hyperemia relative to cerebral needs. Jugular venous oxygen concentration, when coupled with information about mean arterial blood pressure and ICP, allows for rational therapeutic measures to ensure cerebral perfusion. The usefulness in management strategies is illustrated in the algorithm shown in Fig. 3-19.

Jugular venous oxygen measurement is usually performed with a catheter inserted into the internal jugular vein and advanced to the jugular bulb, so that blood from the brain is sampled before it is mixed with that in the vessels draining into the internal jugular vein farther down in the neck.

MANAGEMENT

General Measures

Before the neurologic assessment of the comatose patient is undertaken, the "ABCs" (airway, breathing, and circulation) needs must be met. The clinical assessment should reveal the degree of obtundation, and the degree to which the patient can support his/her ventilation and airway, and maintain blood pressure, tissue perfusion, and temperature. Arterial blood gases are a useful guide. Ventilatory failure is present when Pa_{CO_2} values are elevated or fail to fall below 40 mmHg during hypoxemia. The institution of mechanical ventilation is indicated in the face of hypoventilation, obstruction of the upper airway, or if there is significant risk of aspiration. In general, if the coma is not likely to reverse quickly, endotracheal intubation and assisted ventilation should be undertaken. The physician should look for signs of upper airway obstruction and apnea with indrawing or stertorous breathing. If the patient is deeply comatose, it is often necessary to have an endotracheal tube inserted. The goals are to secure an adequate airway, to prevent aspiration, to permit adequate oxygenation and ventilation, and to facilitate further management, e.g., the use of hyperventilation for raised ICP, if necessary. Assisted ventilation with enhanced oxygen concentration may be required to provide adequate oxygenation so that the Pa_{O_2} is at least 90 to 105 mmHg.[49] Adequate protection/stabilization of the cervical spine, e.g., with a firm collar, should be provided if there is any

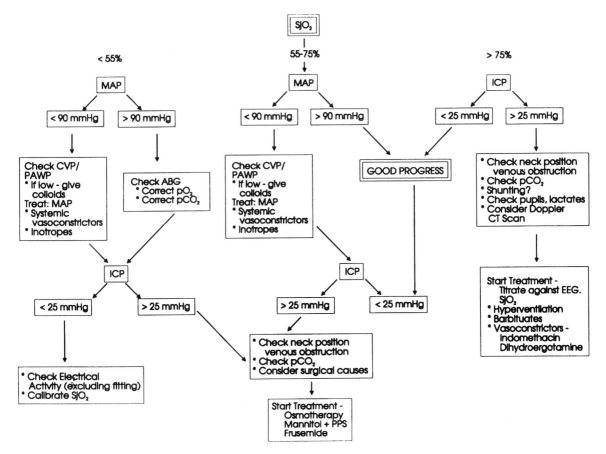

Figure 3-19

Algorithm for investigation and management using jugular venous oxygen measurement and other parameters. Abbreviations: ABG= arterial blood gases; CT= computed tomography of brain; CVP= central venous pressure; ICP= intracranial pressure; MAP= mean arterial blood pressure; PAWP= pulmonary arterial wedge pressure; pCO₂= arterial partial pressure of carbon dioxide; pO₂= arterial partial pressure of oxygen; SjO₂= jugular venous oxygen value. (Adapted from Souter MJ, Andrews PJD: A review of jugular venous oximetry. Intensive Care World *13:32, 1996.)*

history of trauma or if the cause of coma is unknown, especially when using endotracheal intubation. The technique of rapid sequence intubation, in which a neuromuscular blocking agent is administered with a potent sedative, is especially useful for head-injured patients.[50]

Pulse and blood pressure are assessed promptly, and intravenous access should be obtained immediately. Blood and urine should be taken for analysis at the time. If the patient is hypotensive or shows evidence of poor tissue perfusion (i.e., severe vasoconstriction, elevated serum lactate), the cause should be remedied as quickly as possible. Emergency volume replacement or the use of inotropic or vasoconstrictive agents may be necessary to maintain a cerebral perfusion with a mean arterial blood pressure of greater than 80 mmHg. Episodes of hypotension usually indicate an extracerebral cause of coma, but advanced brainstem failure may produce hypotension.[51]

Hypertension should not be treated immediately unless it is life-threatening, i.e., malignant hypertension, usually associated with mean arterial pressures of greater than 120 mmHg. Hypertension in association with raised ICP is sometimes helpful is assuring adequate cerebral perfusion. A cardiac monitor should be available allowing recognition and treatment of serious arrythmias.

Hypoglycemia is a common, correctable cause of impaired consciousness. The serum glucose concentration should be meaured immediately in the emergency room. An intravenous bolus of glucose as 50 mL of 50% solution should be given promptly if there is strong suspicion of hypoglycemia or if a spot test shows low serum glucose. Thiamine should be coadministered if there is a possibility of vitamin deficiency.

Epileptic seizures should be treated promptly to prevent additional brain damage and to lessen morbidity and mortality. Specific management is discussed in Chap. 17.[52] The effectiveness of treatment is best assessed by serial or continuous EEG if the patient fails to recover consciousness quickly.

It is wise to protect the patient from vitamin deficiency, before glucose is administered, by administering thiamine (50 mg intramuscularly). This is also a life-saving, specific therapy for Wernicke's encephalopathy. Naloxone or flumazenil can reverse the sedative effects of opiates and benzodiazepines, respectively (see Chap. 16).

As part of management, prophylactic eye care should be administered by taping the eyes shut in the comatose patient or by using ophthalmic ointment in the less obtunded patient if one or both eyes are open from facial nerve palsy.

Prioritization

It is important to organize and prioritize management steps. Too often, comatose patients with metabolic problems or meningitis are sent to the CT suite as an initial step. This wastes valuable time and jeopardizes patient safety and care. Ideally, the essential investigations and management can go hand-in-hand with initiation of treatment in the emergency room.

Monitoring

To monitor is derived from the Latin word *monere*, meaning "to warn." Implicit in this derivation is communication of findings to a physician or decision-maker who acts upon them. Thus, monitoring is a *system of management* rather than a piece of equipment. Monitoring includes the monitoring technique or device, the warning or feedback to a physician, the treatment strategy, and the further monitoring for effectiveness of treatment.

The monitoring of various physiologic variables in a long-term, continuous or semicontinuous fashion has, until recent times, been on a clinical basis, with serial neurologic examinations and charting by nurses and house staff. This is limited in the unconscious patient. The cerebral hemispheres are largely inaccessible in coma; findings of brainstem compromise are often late events. Recent technologic advances have extended observations to more direct and quantitative measures of important, clinically inaccessible variables in the unconscious patient. There is some evidence that the inclusion of these measures in a monitoring system will lead to improved outcomes, at least in selected patient populations. This needs further study.

COMA SCALES

Scoring systems were developed for the quantification and standardization of the severity of acute illnesses and for the prediction of outcome.[53] Motivations for their development included the need for reliable, standardized data for resource allocation, and quality assurance and improvement initiatives. Such "clinimetrics" rest on pragmatic, clinical observational data that can be treated in a scientific fashion to develop scoring systems that can be validated and tested for clinical relevance.[54] Coma scales serve the following purposes: (1) standardization of the level of consciousness for clinical research (e.g., inclusion in a series and allowing comparison of studies); (2) monitoring of the course of an illness; (3) allowing prognostic estimations; and (4) allowing management decisions to be made from information from points 2 and 3.

The ideal coma scale should have (1) good validity; (2) ordinal arrangement of the degree of severity; (3) linearity (there should be an equal weighting to individual units of score); (4) correlation with outcome; (5) ease of use (brevity, simplicity, unambiguity, and practicality); and (6) little redundancy.[55]

Specific Scales

Glasgow Coma Scale The Glasgow Coma Scale (GCS) (Table 3-3) is almost universally used in emergency rooms and ICUs and is by far the most common coma scale cited in the neurosurgical literature.[56,57] However, it has not been used consistently in different hospitals and the later versions of the GCS have not been adequately tested for reliability.[58,59] The GCS was designed for the initial assessment of patients with head injury. Problems with the use of the GCS arise when patients are intubated, and cannot respond verbally, or if the eyes are swollen shut, preventing verbal response from the patient and ocular assessment, respectively.[60] A theoretical disadvantage is the three-dimensional assessment: the total score is

Table 3-3
Glasgow Coma Scale

Item	Factor	Score
Best motor response	Obeys	6
	Localizes	5
	Withdraws (flexion)	4
	Abnormal flexion	3
	Extensor response	2
	Nil	1
Verbal response	Oriented	5
	Confused conversation	4
	Inappropriate words	3
	Incomprehensible sounds	2
	Nil	1
Eye opening	Spontaneous	4
	To speech	3
	To pain	2
	Nil	1

Source: From Ref. 56, with permission.

Table 3-4
Innsbruck Coma Scale

Neurological assessment	Score
Turning towards stimuli	3
Better-than-extension movements	2
Extension movements	1
None	0
Reactive to pain	
Defensive movements	3
Better-than-extension movements	2
Extension movements	1
None	0
Body posture	
Normal	3
Better-than-extension movements	2
Extension movements	1
Flaccid	0
Eye opening	
Spontaneous	3
To acoustic stimuli	2
To painful stimuli	1
None	0
Pupil size	
Normal	3
Narrow	2
Dilated	1
Completely dilated	0
Pupil response to light	
Sufficient	3
Reduced	2
Minimum	1
None	0
Position and movements of eyeballs	
Fixing of eyes	3
Sway of eyeballs	2
Divergent	1
Divergent fixed	0
Oral automatisms	
Spontaneous	2
To external stimuli	1
None	0

Source: From Ref. 61, with permission.

obtained by adding the values for three motor activities—eye opening, best motor response, and best verbal response. These are assumed to be independent variables, but they are not. Because they covary, their addition may not be valid. Furthermore, to achieve a score of 6 to 12, there are more than 10 simple combinations of variables, each with very different clinical profiles. It seems unlikely that all patients with specific scores between 6 and 10 will be equivalent in disease severity. Further, there is little difference in outcome over several different score values, e.g., between 10 and 15. The GCS is often insufficiently sensitive for the detection of changes in the level of consciousness of patients following head injury or those with masses and the risk of herniation when they are in lighter stages of impaired consciousness. Further, in the application of the GCS to patients who have been in the ICU for an extended period of time, eye opening does not equal conscious awareness, as patients with persistent vegetative state may show this and patients with seizures may show spontaneous eye opening.

Having said this, the GCS has been the standard scoring assessment around the world for 20 years. It seems unlikely that it will be easily replaced, even by potentially superior scoring systems.

Innsbruck Coma Scale The Innsbruck Coma Scale (ICS) was also developed for assessment of victims of trauma.[61] The total score is analogous to that the GCS in having a number of separate assessments that are scored separately but are added for an aggregate score (see Table 3-4). The same theoretic disadvantages for the GCS can be applied to the ICS, but the score can be more readily applied to intubated patients. An anomaly is that the score rates dilated, fixed pupils of greater severity (lower score) than midposition nonreactive pupils.[62] Thus, a patient with brain death (where midposition pupils are the general rule) would achieve a better score than one who is not brain dead. The maximum score is 23, but since oral automatisms also occur in the vegetative state, the maximum score for late assessments probably should be 21. The ICS was shown to be highly predictive of nonsurvival by 21 days if an aggregate score of 0 or 1 is achieved at the first neurologic examination after admission.

Edinburgh-2 Coma Scale The Edinburgh-2 Coma Scale (E2CS) is shown in Table 3-5. The best response is the one that is used in tabulating the score which is inversely related to conscious level. The E2CS has some advantages in that it does not add covarying factors. It is a single-line scoring system. The E2CS shows excellent corre-

Table 3-5

Edinburgh-2 Coma Scale

Stimulation (maximum)	Response (best)	Score
Two sets of questions:	Answers correctly to both	0
Month?	Answers correctly to either	1
Age?	Incorrect for both	2
Two sets of commands:		
1. Close and open hand	Obeys correctly to both	3
2. Close and open eyes	Obeys correctly to either	4
	Neither correct	5
Strong pain	Localizing	6
	Flexion	7
	Extension	8
	No response	9

Source: From Ref. 63, with permission.

lation with the GCS and the Glasgow Outcome Score for mortality and morbidity: the levels are arranged in the appropriate order.[63] Because the E2CS scale is ordinal, the intervals are not linearly related to percentage mortality or morbidity. For values from 1 to 3, the morbidity rate rises rapidly, but mortality is less than 30 percent until the E2CS value of 5, and then it rises in a nonlinear fashion to reach 100 percent with an E2CS score of 10.

A disadvantage is that the E2CS makes the assumption that obeying of commands is preserved when oral responses are lost or inaccurate. The test procedure cannot be applied to intubated patients who may have been able to give an oral response.

Reaction Level Scale The Reaction Level Scale (RLS 85) (Table 3-6), developed in Sweden in 1985, is an eight-grade single-line ordinal scale for the assessment of patients in

Table 3-6
Reaction Level Scale (RLS 85)

Score	Clinical descriptor	Qualifying factors
1. Normal	Alert. No delay in response	Alert. Not drowsy, oriented. Intubated patient: no delay in reaction
2. Mildly drowsy or confused	Drowsy or confused. Responsiveness to light stimulation	Drowsy: drowsy or shows delay in reaction Confused: wrong answer to: What is your name? Where are you? What year and month is it?
3. Very drowsy or confused. Response to strong simulation	Strong stimulation: loud verbal or painful stimulation	Mental responsiveness: arousable. Performs at least one of the following: obeys commands (incl. nonverbal response—e.g., "Lift up your arms," orienting eye movements, wards off painful stimulus
4. Unconscious: localizes but does not ward off pain	Unconscious: no mental response. Cannot perform any activity defined under mental responsiveness	Localizes: with retromandibular pain, patient moves one hand above chin level; with pain to nailbeds, the other arm crosses the midline
5. Unconscious: withdraws	Withdrawing movement: with retromandibular pressure, patient turns head away.	With nailbed pressure, patient makes withdrawal movement with abduction at shoulder
6. Unconscious: stereotypic flexion movement	Stereotypic movement: with retromandibular or nailbed pressure, the patient slowly assumes decorticate posture	The movement is "mechanical" and clearly different from the withdrawal response described above
7. Unconscious: stereotypic extension movements	Stereotyped extension movement: with retromandibular or nailbed pressure, the patient extends the limbs	If there is a mixture of extension and flexion, the flexion (best response) is recorded
8. Unconscious: no response	With retromandibular or nailbed pressure, there is no response of limbs or face	

Source: From Ref. 13, with permission.

the ICU.[57] It has advantages over the GCS in that in can be applied to patients who are intubated or whose eyes have swollen shut. There is no addition of covarying values. Although the numeric values are not necessarily separated by steps of equal value, the order appears to be valid. The test compares favorably with the GCS and outcome is inversely related to the achieved score. It has also shown good inter-rater reliability. Further, any change in the RLS 85 is related to a significant change in patient status, and it is superior to the GCS in this respect.

The scale cannot be applied to cases where the patient is clinically or pharmacologically paralyzed yet alert (e.g., polyneuropathy, spinal cord lesion, locked-in syndrome, use of neuromuscular blocking agents) or those with psychogenic unresponsiveness. These are usually not difficult to identify and exclude. Then, the scale should be applicable to almost all patients with impaired consciousness in the Neuro-ICU.

REFERENCES

1. Fisher CM: The neurological examination of the comatose patient. *Acta Neurol Scand* 45 (Suppl 36):4, 1969.
2. Plum F, Posner JB: The *Diagnosis of Stupor and Coma*, 3rd ed. Philadelphia. FA Davis, 1980, pp 53–54.
3. Folstein ME, Folstein SE, McHugh PR: "Mini-mental state": a practical method for grading the cognitive state of patients for the clinician. *J Psychiatr Res* 12:189, 1975.
4. White JC: Epileptic nystagmus. *Epilepsia* 12:157, 1971.
5. Castaigne P, Lhermitte F, Buge A, et al: Paramedian midbrain and thalamic infarcts: clinical and neuropathological study. *Ann Neurol* 10:127, 1981.
6. Schuaib A, Farah S: Stroke involving the midbrain and thalamus and causing "nonfocal" coma. *South Med J* 85:49, 1992.
7. Fisher CM: Ocular bobbing. *Arch Neurol* 11:543, 1964.
8. Finelli PF, McEntee WJ: Ocular bobbing with extraaxial hematomas of posterior fossa. *J Neurol Neurosurg Psychiatry* 40:386, 1977.
9. Rudick R, Staram R, Eskin TA: Ocular bobbing in encephalitis. *J Neurol Neurosurg Psychiatry* 44:441, 1981.
10. Braems M, Dehaene I: Ocular bobbing: clinical significance. *Clin Neurol Neurosurg Psychiatry* 78:99, 1975.
11. Plum F, Posner JB: *The Diagnosis of Stupor and Coma* 3rd ed. Philadelphia: FA Davis, 1980.
12. Penfield W, Welch K: The supplementary motor area of the cerebral cortex. A clinical and experimental study. *Arch Neurol Psychiatry* 66:289, 1951.
13. Starmark J-E, Stålhammar D, Holmgren E: The reaction level scale (RLS 85). *Acta Neurochir* 91:12, 1988.
14. Young GB, Jordan KG, Doig GS. An assessment of nonconvulsive seizures in the intensive care unit using continuous EEG monitoring: an investigation of variables associated with mortality. *Neurology* 47:83-89, 1996.
15. Zuckermann EC, Glaser GH: Urea-induced myoclonic seizures: all experimental study of the site of action and mechanism. *Arch Neurol* 27:14, 1972.
16. Gottlieb D, Michowitz SD, Steiner I, Wald U: Central neurogenic hyperventilation in a patient with medulloblastoma. *Eur Neurol* 27:51, 1987.
17. Fisher CM: Some neuro-ophthalmological observations. *J Neurol Neurosurg Psychiatry* 30:383–392, 1967.
18. Zifko U, Remtulla H, Power K, Harker L, Bolton CF: Transcortical and cervical magnetic stimulation with recording of the diaphragm. *Muscle Nerve* 19:614, 1996.
19. Zifko U, Slomka PJ, Reid RH, et al: The cortical representation of somatosensory evoked potentials from the phrenic nerve. *J Neurol Sci* 139:197, 1996.
20. Nicolle MW, Stewart DJ, Remtulla H, et al: Lambert-Eaton myasthenic syndrome presenting with severe respiratory failure. *Muscle Nerve* 19:1328, 1996.
21. Bolton CF: AAEM minimonograph #40: Clinical neurophysiology of the respiratory system. *Muscle Nerve* 16:809, 1993.
22. Chatrian G-E, Bergamasco B, Bricolo A, Frost JD Jr, Prior PE: IFCN recommended standards for electrophysiologic monitoring and other unresponsive states. Report of an IFCN committee. *Electroenceph Clin Neurophysiol* 99:103, 1996.
23. Young GB, McLachlan RS, Kreeft JH, DeMelo JD: The electroencephalogram in coma. *Can J Neurol Sci*, in press.

24. Young GB, McLachlan RS, Kreeft JH, DeMelo JD: An EEG classification for coma. *Can J Neurol Sci*, in press.

25. Synek VM: Prognostically important EEG coma patterns in diffuse anoxic and traumatic encephalopathies in adults. *J Clin Neurophysiol* 5:161, 1988.

26. Jordan KG: Continuos EEG and evoked potential monitoring in the neuroscience intensive care unit. *J Clin Neurophysiol* l0:445-475, 1993.

27. Young GB, Blume WT, Campbell VM, et al: Alpha, theta and alpha-theta coma: a clinical outcome study using serial recordings. *Electroenceph Clin Neurophysiol* 91:93, 1994.

28. Jordan KG: Continuous EEG and evoked potential monitoring in the neuroscience intensive care unit. *J Clin Neurophysiol* 10:445, 1993.

29. Nuwer MR: Electroencephalograms and evoked potentials. Monitoring cerebral function in the neurosurgery intensive care unit. *Intensive Care Med* 13:249, 1994.

30. Jordan KG: Neurophysiologic monitoring in the neuroscience intensive care unit, in Jordan K (ed): *Neurologic Critical Care. Neurologic Clinics*. Philadelphia, Saunders, 13:579–626, 1995.

31. Miskiel E, Ozdamar O: Computer modeling of auditory brainstem responses. *Comput Biol Med* 17:185, 197.

32. Mauguière F, Garcia-Larrea L, Murray NMF, Rogers T: Evoked potential diagnostic strategies. EPs in coma, in Binnie CD, Cooper R, Fowler CJ, Mauguiére F, Prior PF, Osselton JW, (eds): *Clinical Neurophysiology. EMG, Nerve Conduction and Evoked Potentials*, part 3: *Evoked Potentials*. Oxford, Butterworth-Heineman, 1995, pp 494–502.

33. Turazzi S, Bricolo A, Pasut ML, Formenton A: Changes produced by CT scanning in the outlook of severe head injury. *Acta Neurochir* 85:87, 1987.

34. Tasker RC, Matthew DJ, Kendall B: Computed tomography in the assessment of raised intracranial pressure in non-traumatic coma. *Neuropediatrics* 21:91, 1990.

35. Oder W, Podreka I, Spatt J, Goldenberg G: Cerebral function following catastrophic brain injury: relevance of single photon emission computed tomography and positron emission tomography, in Levin HS, Benton AL, Muizelaar JP, Eisenberg HM (eds): *Catastrophic Brain Injury*. New York, Oxford University Press, 1996, pp 51–78.

36. Newell DW, Aaslid R: Transcranial Doppler: clinical and experimental uses. *Cerebrovasc Brain Metab Rev* 4:122, 1992.

37. Masdeu JC, Brass LM, Holman L, Kushner MJ: Brain single-photon emission computed tomography. *Neurology* 44:1970, 1994.

38. Holman BL, Zimmerman RE, Johnson KA, et al: Computer-assisted superimposition of magnetic resonance and high-resolution technetium-99m HMPAO and thallium-201 SPECT images of the brain. *J Nucl Med* 32:1478, 1991.

39. De Roo M, Mortelmans L, Devos P, et al: Clinical experience with Tc-99m HM-PAO high resolution SPECT of the brain in patients with cerebrovascular accidents. *Eur J Nucl Med* 15:9, 1989.

40. Laurin NR, Driedger AA, Hurwitz GA, et al: Cerebral perfusion imaging with technetium-99m HM-PAO in brain death and severe central nervous system injury. *J Nucl Med* 30:1627, 1989.

41. Masdeu JC, Brass LM, Holman BL, Kushner MJ: Brain single-photon emission computed tomography. *Neurology* 44:1970, 1994.

42. Eckelman WC, Reba RC, Rzeszotarski EJ, et al: External imaging of cerebral muscarinic acetylcholine receptors. *Science* 233:291, 1984.

43. Schubiger PA, Hasler PH, Wohlfahrt B, et al: Evaluation of a multicenter study with Iomazenil—a benzodiazepine receptor ligand. *Nucl Med Commun* 12:569, 1991.

44. Kung HF: Radiopharmaceuticals for CNS receptor imaging with SPECT. *Int J Rad Appl Instrum* 17:85, 1990.

45. Beks JWF: Increased intracranial pressure. *Clin Neurol Neurosurg* 79:245, 1976.

46. Ropper AH, ed: *Neurological and Neurosurgical Intensive Care*, 3rd ed. New York, Raven Press, 1993.

47. Hacke W, ed: *NeuroCritical Care*. Berlin, Springer Verlag, 1994.

48. Souter MJ, Andrews PJD: A review of jugular venous oximetry. *Intensive Care World* 13:32, 1996.

49. Ivan L, Bruce D: *Coma: Pathophysiology, Diagnosis and Management*. Springfield, Charles C Thomas, 1982.

50. Walls RM: Advances in trauma: airway management. *Emerg Clin North Am* 11:53, 1993.

51. Finklestein S, Ropper A: The diagnosis of coma: its pittfalls and limitations. *Heart Lung* 8:1059, 1979.

52. Working Group on Status Epilepticus: Treatment of convulsive status epilepticus: recommendations of the Epilepsy Foundation of America's Working Group on Status Epilepticus. *JAMA* 270:854–859, 1993.

53. Wisner DH: History and current status of scoring systems for critical care. *Arch Surg* 127:352, 1992.

54. Feinstein AR, Horowitz RI: Choosing cases and controls: the clinical epidemiology of "clinical investigation." *J Clin Invest* 81:1, 1988.

55. Price DJ: Factors restricting the use of coma scales. *Acta Neurochir* suppl 36:106, 1986.

56. Teasdale G, Jennett B: Assessment of coma and impaired consciousness: a practical scale. *Lancet* 2:81, 1974.

57. Starmark J-E, Holmgren E, Stålhammar D: Current reporting of responsiveness in acute cerebral disorders. *J Neurosurg* 69:692, 1988.

58. Marion DW: The Glasgow Coma Scale score: contemporary application. *Intensive Care World* 11:101, 1994.

59. Knaus WA: Measuring the Glasgow Coma Scale in the intensive care unit: potentials and pitfalls. *Intensive Care World* 11:102, 1994.

60. Starmark J-E, Holmgren E, Stålhammar D: Current reporting of responsiveness in acute cerebral disorders. *J Neurosurg* 69:692, 1988.

61. Benzer A, Mitterschiffthaler G, Marosi M, et al: Prediction of non-survival after trauma: Innsbruck Coma Scale. *Lancet* 338:977, 1991.

62. De'Clari F: Innsbruck coma scale. *Lancet* 338:1537, 1991.

63. Sugiura K, Fukuya R, Kunimoto K, et al: Significance of different levels of the Edinburgh 2 Coma Scale calculated from the outcome of neurosurgical patients. *Neurosurgery* 31:1023, 1992.

64. Garfinkle AM, Danys IR, Nicolle DA, et al: Terson's syndrome: a reversible cause of blindness following subarachnoid hemorrhage. *J Neurosurg* 76:1992.

65. Leigh RJ, Zee DS: *The Neurology of Eye Movements.* Philadelphia, FA Davis, 1983.

66. Carpenter MB, Sutin J: *Human Neuroanatomy,* 8th ed. Baltimore, Williams and Wilkins, 1983.

67. Spencer MP, Reid JM: Quantification of carotid stenosis with continuous wave Doppler ultrasound. *Stroke* 10:326, 1979.

68. Newell DW, Aaslid R: Transcranial Doppler: clinical and experimental uses. *Cerebrovasc Brain Metab Revs* 4:125, 1992.

Part 2

IMPAIRED CONSCIOUSNESS AND PHYSICAL AND STRUCTURAL INSULTS

Chapter 4

TRANSTENTORIAL HERNIATION

Allan H. Ropper

One of the basic tenets of clinical neurology has been that a mass inside the cranium can cause coma. It is also widely accepted that the mass need not necessarily destroy the crucial areas at the upper reticular formation that sustain arousal, but that secondary compression of these regions, largely through displacement of tissue at a distance from the mass, have the same effect. Coma can therefore be thought of as a false localizing sign of a supratentorial mass. Over the years, this concept has been expanded further and subdivided into several discrete anatomic configurations that describe the manner in which the upper brainstem is compressed by dramatic displacements of brain tissue through apertures of the dural folds separating the main compartments of the brain. Moreover, groups of clinical signs have been explicitly assigned to each type of brainstem compression. Indeed, one of the major advances in clinical neurology in this century has been the delineation of these coma syndromes. It has become customary to refer to the anatomic configurations and their corresponding syndromes with a unitary term, "herniations."

This chapter reviews the classic herniation syndromes, but it is also meant to offer an alternative or revised view of the precise anatomic relationships between a supratentorial mass and the upper brainstem in cases of coma—a view that is gleaned from imaging studies rather than from pathologic specimens, as in the past. The fundamental premise in this discussion remains that the relatively fixed volume of the cranial cavity, bounded as it is by the skull, forces a mass to compress adjacent tissue, and eventually to cause coma by deforming crucial neurons and their connections at the upper end of the reticular formation. In question is the precise mechanism of this compression and whether herniation per se is the cause. There are other herniations than the ones outlined in this chapter (e.g., transfalcial) but they are not addressed in detail because they have less relevance to coma.

HISTORY OF HERNIATION

Although transtentorial herniation from an intracranial mass has been discussed in the literature for approximately seventy-five years, most observations have been of pathologic material only. "Herniation," a term used by pathologists, was coined by Meyer in 1920[1] from his investigation of post-mortem material in cases of brain tumor. He described in detail the displacement of the medial temporal lobe over the free edge of the tentorium and into the space between the tentorium and the lateral edge of the midbrain. Jefferson[2] and, later, Van Gehuchten[3] confirmed these findings and were the first to systematically correlate compression of the upper brainstem with clinical signs, although few of their clinical observations would be accepted as valid today. In all this work, there was an essential implication that the herniated medial temporal lobe compressed the midbrain at the tentorial opening and caused clinical signs (although not necessarily coma), but it is interesting that these observations preceded the seminal work by Moruzzi and Magoun[4] that established the role of the reticular activating system in maintaining alertness.

This entire subject was comprehensively, but somewhat disjointedly, reported as a group of "dislocational syndromes" by Burdenko's group from Moscow in a 1972 monograph.[5] The seminal work on the subject, however, appeared in a paper by McNealy and Plum,[6] and in a book that followed, now in its third edition, by Plum and Posner.[7] It was a breakthrough in that it collected and codified the clinical signs that had been previously reported as a result of a large supratentorial mass, organizing them into syndromes and implicitly associating them with the pathologic configurations of uncal and central herniation. It is notable that the original paper ends with a comment indicating the authors' desire not to emphasize a direct relationship between the postmortem appearance of the brain and the like-named clinical syndromes, but the detail and lucid organization of the "herniation syndromes" has left a notion among all physicians that transtentorial herniation causes relatively stereotyped constellations of signs.

What made these herniation syndromes so compelling at the time, and has led to their durability in clinical jargon, was the observation by Plum and colleagues that a series of signs leading to coma progressed in a predictable manner from those that correspond to damage in the upper midbrain, thence to the pons, and, finally, to respiratory and cardiovascular collapse and death when the medullary stage is reached. It was stated by the original authors that the orderly progression is due to sequential brainstem ischemia at each level. The ease that is allowed, by using these constructs, of teaching medical students and residents the signs related to a mass and to coma, and their utility in showing the anatomic organization of the brainstem tegmentum, has established the herniation concept during the early stages of medical education and thereby

fortified it as a tenet of medicine for generations of medical students.

HERNIATION SYNDROMES

It is useful to begin with an explication of the main herniation syndromes as they are traditionally taught. The central syndrome has been felt to be more common than the uncal type, and both may occur together, in which case the features are combined but the progression of signs that are attributable to each portion of the brainstem still proceeds in an orderly fashion from top to bottom. These descriptions are taken from the previously mentioned text, *The Diagnosis of Stupor and Coma.*[7]

Uncal Herniation

This syndrome is anchored by early pupillary enlargement on the side of the mass, presumably from the medially displaced anterior portion of the temporal lobe, namely the uncal gyrus, coming into contact with the third nerve which is situated just inside the anterior margin of the tentorial dura. As the temporal lobe tissue is displaced further, the upper midbrain is compressed from the side and drowsiness or stupor ensue, but wakefulness depends on the extent to which the diencephalon above is compressed. The pupil may, at first, be sluggishly reactive or there may be only minimal anisocoria (early third nerve stage). Once the pupil fully enlarges, generally 6 mm or larger in diameter, there is also supposed to be external ophthalmoplegia and signs of brainstem dysfunction may appear rapidly (late third nerve stage). As more of the upper brainstem is displaced, coma soon occurs and there may be compression of the opposite cerebral peduncle leading to hemiparesis ipsilateral to the mass (the Kenrohan notch phenomenon). The signs then progress caudally, presumably from progressive ischemia, and indications of pontine damage appear (upper pontine stage), manifest as loss of elicitable eye movements and corneal responses, and decerebrate rigidity. Finally, the medulla is compressed, and aberrant respiratory rhythms are followed by respiratory arrest. Along the way, the pupil opposite to the mass also becomes enlarged or attains a midposition size (5 mm), and eventually both pupils become midsized. The essential feature of the uncal syndrome, early third nerve compression by the uncus, was first described explicitly by Macewen,[8] although the sign itself had been noted 25 years earlier, in 1867, by Hutchinson.[9]

Central Syndrome

In this constellation, the earliest signs are referable to compression of the uppermost reticular activating system in the dorsal thalamus. This is manifest as confusion, drowsiness, and, later, stupor (diencephalic stage). The pupils tend to be initially small (2 to 3 mm) and this perhaps distinguishes the two syndromes most clearly. Periodic breathing or similar abnormalities are common. There may be roving conjugate eye movements or the eyes may be still and move passively by head turning (the ill-named "doll's eyes," or oculocephalic maneuver). If there is a contralateral hemiplegia from the mass itself, it tends to worsen, and corticospinal signs appear on the other side (i.e., both sides). This stage is marked by bilateral Babinski signs, and, later, by decorticate posturing. As midbrain compression occurs, the pupils enlarge and become light unresponsive, irregular or asymmetric, and near midposition (midbrain–upper pons stage). The eye movements then become progressively more difficult to elicit and the globes are dysconjugate, all of which are signs of severe pontine dysfunction. At the lower pontine stage, these signs are consolidated; breathing abnormalities supervene, the limbs become flaccid, the pupils remain in midposition and fixed, and eye movements are unobtainable. The final stage is marked by irregularities in blood pressure and breathing, and, finally, by cardiovascular collapse.

Cerebellar Herniations

The two types, upward transtentorial and downward foramen magnum "pressure cone," are perhaps the least well-defined clinical herniation syndromes, and the primary effects of the initiating lesion are difficult to separate from the secondary effects of compression. Certain characteristics of upward transtentorial cerebellar hernation are commonto most descriptions. Compression of the pretectal area has been thought to occur early and to produce failure of upgaze or conjugate downward deviation of the globes.[10] The pontine component of compression, more common than tectal in this author's experience, produces gaze paresis followed by loss of all eye movements, miotic pupils, and fairly symmetric decerebrate posturing. The corneal responses may be lost early. Respiration is initially normal or slowed, but degenerates into irregular sighing or periodic breathing.

The cerebellar pressure cone with impaction of the medulla at the foramen magnum is quite dramatic at the autopsy table and has therefore been assumed to be related to sudden apnea and death. This mechanism is often invoked when deterioration follows lumbar puncture.

HERNIATIONS AS CLINICAL AND RADIOLOGIC PHENOMENA

From a clinical perspective, not all experience has been entirely concordant with these well-defined herniation syndromes. In part, this is because a hybrid uncal-central syndrome is so frequent, but also because pressure throughout the posterior fossa is likely to be elevated quickly once a supratentorial mass has exhausted the buffering effects of cerebrospinal fluid (CSF) translocation and changes in blood volume. This often leads to sudden ischemia of the brainstem and complete loss of all brainstem function almost simultaneously. For the same reasons, the sequence of signs with posterior fossa masses is even less predictable. It does seem valid, however, that in cases of supratentorial mass, pontine or medullary signs rarely precede medullary or thalamic signs. As an example of the inconsistency of the syndrome when a relatively uniform supratentorial mass is considered, in 12 consecutive stroke cases with massive hemispheral swelling, progressive drowsiness was almost always the first sign of the expanding mass, soon followed by minor pupillary asymmetry or by periodic breathing, but in only one case by small pupils corresponding to the early diencephalic stage of the central syndrome.[11] Four of the 12 cases developed a homolateral Babinski sign or posturing at various times. The sequence of progression from the early pupillary asymmetry varied greatly, sometimes with both pupils enlarging virtually simultaneously. None followed the patterns as traditionally set forth, except, again, that eye movements referable to the pons were generally not disrupted before the pupils and consciousness were affected.

If transtentorial herniation is defined as entrapment of medial temporal lobe tissue in the lateral perimesencephalic space due to downward pressure, or descent of central diencephalic tissue below the plane of the tentorium, then herniation can be accepted as distorting the upper midbrain reticular system sufficiently to cause coma and pupillary changes. There is also general acceptance of a number of secondary pathologic changes from transtentorial herniation, particularly occlusion of the first branches of the circle of Willis as they pass over the tentorial edge, as well as brainstem hemorrhages and ischemic lesions adjacent to herniated tissue (Table 4-1). Ventricular enlargement is quite common with a unilateral mass and has been attributed to "entrapment" of a lateral ventricle —a sort of internal herniation. Closer inspection in

Table 4-1
Changes caused by herniations and horizontal shifts

Clinical
Abulia, stupor, coma
Pupillary enlargement
Eye movement abnormalities
Ipsilateral hemiparesis (Kernohan notch phenomenon)
Respiratory alterations

Vascular
Posterior cerebral artery entrapment (occipital
  infarctions)
Anterior cerebral artery entrapment (frontal infarctions)
Secondary brainstem hemorrhages

Cerebrospinal fluid spaces
Compression of upper brainstem cisterns
Unilateral or bilateral enlargement of lateral ventricles

many cases shows this to be simply the result of compression of the third ventricle juxtaposed upon compression of the ipsilateral lateral ventricle; viz., a bilateral dilatation of the lateral ventricles cannot manifest itself. Several other secondary phenomena, however, have been attributed uncritically to herniation, such as pupillary enlargement or entrapment of the opposite ventricular horn where the anatomic changes and their effects on tissue at a distance are not as evident.

AN ALTERNATIVE VIEW OF HERNIATION

Whatever the cause and effect relationship between herniations and the clinical signs associated with them, a problem has been created by utilizing the pathoanatomy that is seen well after the clinical signs have ensued. The precise configuration at the moment stupor or coma commence, or at the time the ipsilateral pupil enlarges, cannot be gleaned from pathology specimens since the shift and distortion created by a mass invariably progress beyond the stage at which clinical signs were created. Downward transtentorial shift, an extreme pathologic entity, may have been adopted uncritically as a plausible clinical paradigm, in part because it is so obvious and its secondary features, such as brainstem hemorrhage, are evident in the removed brain, whereas the effects of horizontal shift are not appreciated once the hemispheres have been sectioned from the upper brainstem. The opportunity to view the proximate anatomic changes as a patient becomes stuporous or comatose is the great advantage presented by computed tomography (CT) and magnetic resonance imaging (MRI). A review of both the literature and of MRI scans suggests that downward transtentorial herniation is not required for diminished consciousness or for unilateral pupillary enlargement.

If downward displacement of brain tissue through the tentorial aperture does not cause coma, how else does a mass alter the configuration of crucial structures at a distance? An alternative is that horizontal displacement away from a mass is a more consistent and important early distortion than vertical movement. There must, of course, be both horizontal and vertical shift away from a mass, as allowed by the main dural restrictions and by the pliability of the ventricular system. In what follows, "coma" will be used as a shorthand for the entire range of diminished consciousness. These comments express a view previously offered by C. M. Fisher,[12] and by Hasenjäger and Spatz in 1937.[13]

With regard to supratentorial masses, the effects of medial temporal lobe herniation should be considered separately from those of central herniation, although the two often occur, together. The former is reflected radiologically by obliteration of the lower perimesencephalic cistern on the side of the mass between the dural edge and the adjacent low midbrain; the latter is reflected radiologically by vertical descent of midline structures such as the pineal or the iter of the cerebral aqueduct (its upper entry point). There are four main points against herniation or downward movement as the cause of coma, the first two applying mainly to medial temporal herniation and the latter two to central herniation. (1) The upper brainstem cistern is usually open, if not enlarged, on the side of a mass when viewed on CT and MRI scans, and in many patients there is no herniation into this space in autopsy material inspected in situ and obtained soon after the onset of coma. (2) Rapid clinical improvement from herniation syndromes with mannitol or hyperventilation treatment is unlikely to be the result of disimpaction and upward movement of herniated tissue that is trapped between the edge of the dura and the lateral midbrain. (3) The degree of horizontal shift of midline structures, generally greater in magnitude than vertical displacement, correlates well with the level of consciousness, while there is no such relationship between the degree of vertical shift and the clinical state. (4) Extreme and relatively acute downward displacement of the upper brainstem occurs in low-pressure CSF syndromes without a change in alertness. These are detailed below.

Medial Temporal Lobe Herniation

The earliest change resulting from a large supratentorial mass is enlargement, not compression, of

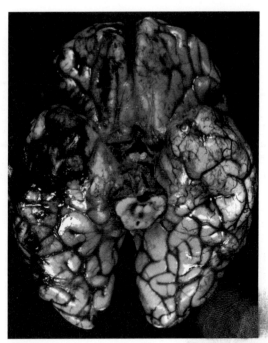

Figure 4-1

Underside of brain in case of traumatic contusion of the right hemisphere and brain swelling. The upper brainstem is pushed downward and shows compressive-hemorrhagic lesions. The right perimesencephalic space (reader's left), however, is enlarged rather than being closed by herniation of the medial temporal (parahippocampal) gyrus. Compression of the contralateral peduncle is evident.

the cistern on the side of the mass, while the cistern opposite the mass is simultaneously compressed (Figs. 4-1 and 4-2). This configuration occurs as patients become drowsy and then stuporous, and probably persists in early coma, suggesting that medial temporal herniation into the cistern does not occur at this stage. In contrast to the prevailing concept that herniation into the tentorial notch causes midbrain distortion from direct sideways pressure, the configuration of the cisterns indicates that horizontal translation of central brain tissue above the tentorial plane is the predominant early shift from a unilateral supratentorial mass. Appreciating this pivotal point requires a visual comprehension of the relations between the medial temporal lobe, the tentorial reflection (edge), and

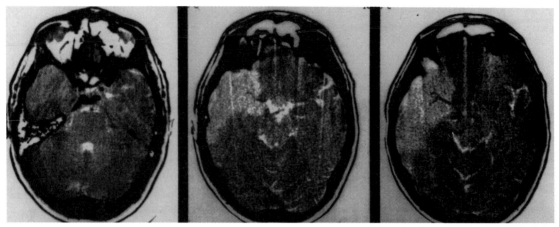

Figure 4-2
Axial CT scans in a patient with a large right middle cerebral artery territory infarction and brain swelling. The ambient and perimesencephalic cisterns on the side of the infarction are widened, without herniation at a time when the patient was progressing from stupor to coma.

the lateral border of the midbrain. Although the relationships between these structures vary between individuals, the tentorial edge is located several millimeters below the midbrain-pontine sulcus in most specimens.[14] As a mass drives brain tissue towards the tentorial opening, the horizontal displacement compresses the entire midbrain well above the plane of the tentorium. As the shift continues, the medial temporal lobe is pushed laterally into the upper recesses of the lateral mesencephalic cistern (the space of Bichat), without the necessity of tissue descending into the tentorial notch. The medial temporal lobe could, if displaced along a more caudal vector, compress the midbrain below the tentorial plane, but the parahippocampal gyrus must first fill the cisterns above the tentorial plane and, in doing so, should still push the midbrain horizontally at a level above that plane.

Taking these observations further, it may be appropriate to question if any compression of the midbrain, even in the cisterns above the tentorial plane, is necessary for diminished consciousness. Coronal MRI scans in drowsy and in some stuporous patients demonstrate that the cisterns surrounding the upper brainstem initially remain open while the lower diencephalon is bowed away

from the mass (Fig. 4-3). Because this convex distortion continues above the tentorial plane as a mass enlarges, it is difficult to separate the effects of midbrain compression from those of extreme horizontal diencephalic compression in causing coma. Moreover, there must be (and is, on MRI scans) some degree of downward displacement of tissue as the mass fills the space of Bichat and brain is crammed towards the tentorial opening. This entire polemic may therefore be semantic since the upper midbrain region is certainly compressed by tissue displacement of some kind; at issue is the observation that *temporal lobe herniation per se seems to be a late phenomenon that is probably not responsible for the initial stages of reduced consciousness.* By the time coma occurs, horizontal shift, filling of cisterns above the tentorium (the sign usually highlighted in CT studies of mass effect), and true herniation below the tentorial opening are all evident.

Central Downward Herniation

Downward descent of the thalamus, subthalamic region, and upper midbrain below the tentorial plane is associated with large masses and is seen in pathologic specimens taken from patients in

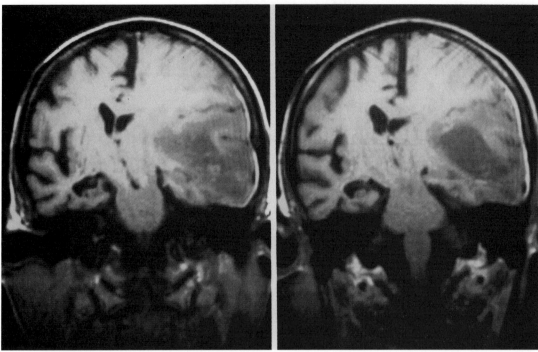

Figure 4-3

Coronal MRI images in a patient with putaminal hemorrhage showing the characteristic bowing of the deep brain structures away from the mass and obligate canting of the upper brainstem. There may be a small knuckle of medial temporal lobe herniation, but the brainstem distortion is occurring above the level of the tentorial plane.

deep coma with fixed pupils—typically advanced cases in which death (and pathologic examination) occurs hours or days after the onset of coma. Extreme central herniation is said to "buckle" the brainstem at the upper pons.[15] Vertical shift occurs mostly with bilateral supratentorial masses or those located high in the cranium near the vertex. The main issues of contention are the extent to which downward movement is related to the level of consciousness, and the relative amounts of vertical compared with horizontal shift. Feldmann et al,[16] and Reich and colleagues[17] have convincingly demonstrated that downward displacement of the upper brainstem may result from a mass during life. But, in the majority of patients, they found no concordance between the level of consciousness and the degree of downward displacement, in part explained by the subacute nature of

the lesions in their series. Although vertical displacement of the pontomesencephalic junction from Twining's line (Feldman's method), or of the iter (inlet of the aqueduct) from a line that approximates the incisural plane (Reich's method), lessened with treatment for raised intracranial pressure, patients nonetheless remained awake with up to 11 mm of downward displacement. In Feldman's patients, mainly with brain tumors, maximal downward displacement, calculated as a normalized ratio, represented, at most, 4 mm of downward shift. Neither study was able to compare the absolute amount of horizontal and vertical shifts because midsagittal MRI images were used. Feldman encountered instances of almost pure vertical or horizontal shift, although most patients had both. In an MRI series,[18] using coronal scans to judge vertical shift (a method that is inferior to

Reich's), horizontal displacement of the upper brainstem was consistently greater than vertical shift.

Finally, a condemning point against downward herniation is made by the observation of almost pure downward displacement in patients with acute low spinal fluid pressure syndromes. Panullo and Reich's group have shown that these patients have 9 to 11 mm of downshift of the upper aqueduct without any reduction in consciousness.[19] There is, however, a difference between this passive downward dragging of the brainstem, due to pressure gradients, and the situation in which a mass pushes tissue ahead of it and downward through the tentorial opening.

Central downward shift therefore occurs during life, but its effect upon consciousness, or at least its obligate role, must be questioned since coma occurs without central herniation and its presence is not always associated with an alteration in alertness. It cannot be determined whether a small amount of vertical shift creates more physiologic damage in the midbrain than do lesser degrees of horizontal shift.

Horizontal Shift

The anatomy of secondary tissue shifts has been summarized above, but the clinical correlates need amplification. This author and others have found a fairly consistent and graduated relationship between the absolute horizontal displacement of supratentorial midline structures and the level of consciousness in patients with *acute* unilateral masses.[20,21] Most patients remain awake with up to 3 to 4 mm of pineal shift, become drowsy with 3 to 6 mm, stuporous with 6 to 9 mm, and comatose with greater than 9 mm (all true dimensions), or slightly less if the lesion evolves abruptly. There is less correspondence between shift of the septum pellucidum and the level of consciousness, as much as 10 mm of displacement being tolerated acutely with only drowsiness resulting. The unqualified use, in the literature, of the term "midline shift," without clarifying the structure chosen for measurement, is a major deficiency. The perimesencephalic cisterns of patients with more than

about 9 mm of pineal shift, most of whom are comatose, are invariably obliterated on both sides above and at the level of the tentorium.[22,23]

If the predominant displacement is horizontal in most cases of unilateral mass effect, then a Kernohan notch phenomenon might be expected fairly consistently as drowsiness progresses to coma. I have found a newly aquired Babinski sign, or posturing, homolateral to the mass in approximately two-thirds of patients just as they become stuporous, but the precise frequency of this sign has not been studied. When coma occurs without Kernohan's hemiplegia, the reticular formation is presumably compressed above the level of the cerebral peduncle, since either frank herniation or medial temporal impaction into the space of Bichat should depend on squeezing of the midbrain against the opposite dural edge. The shape of the tentorial opening and the arrangement of the midbrain cisterns may explain some of the variability in the appearance of this sign.

Bilateral symmetrically balanced masses may cause coma, either by pressing downward and shifting the upper brainstem or by a "pincer-like" compression of the upper brainstem, the latter being the more frequently observed radiologic configuration (Fig. 4-4). In the latter case, each mass acts as a barrier to the horizontal shift caused by the other, playing the role of the fixed tentorial edge that deforms the brainstem in horizontal shift from a unilateral mass.

Practical Use of Horizontal Shift Measurements

In making use of the concept of horizontal displacement, several factors need to be considered. First, some patients with deep hematomas have a tongue of clot that extends directly into the diencephalic-mesencephalic junction, thus destroying the upper reticular system directly.[24] This was the case in a recent report which suggested that downward herniation was the proximate cause of clinical deterioration.[25] There is in these circumstances no direct relationship between shift of any kind and the level of consciousness. Second, the location of the mass, in addition to its size and rapidity,

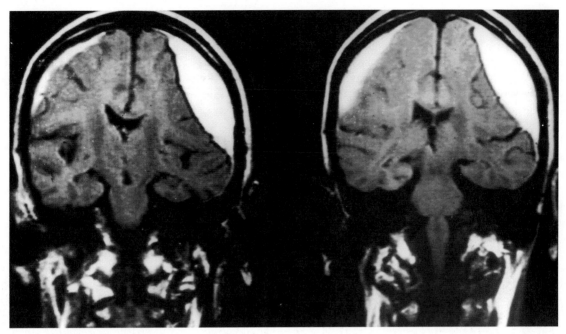

Figure 4-4
Coronal MRI images in a patient with bilateral chronic subdural hematomas and drowsiness. The central structures are compressed in a pincer-like fashion and there is slight horizontal displacement of the brain away from the larger clot, but there is no evident herniation or downward movement.

determines the amount of horizontal shift and consequently the level of consciousness; a large mass in the frontal or occipital lobe, no matter how striking on CT, may cause little in the way of change in consciousness and this will be reflected by minor shift. Third, masses that enlarge over days move the expected brackets upward by 1 to 2 mm and, conversely, slowly enlarging masses may cause pineal and septal shifts of over 10 mm without alteration in alertness. The appearance of a large shift that is disproportionate to the level of consciousness generally indicates chronicity.

The following method can be used to make a quick assessment of the horizontal shift in true dimensions from a CT scan. Measure the distance from the inner table of the skull to the center of the pineal calcification from both sides; take the difference and halve it (thus measuring midline shift in minified CT dimensions), and then multiply by 2.7 (the approximate minification factor on CT

radiographic film arrayed as 3 × 4 CT images). A more accurate conversion factor from CT films to true dimension can be found by dividing the 50-mm graticule at the edge of most scans by its measured length, using a ruler. Of course, a CT console cursor can also be used for computerized measurements of midline shift.

Flaws in the Horizontal Shift Approach

An apparent limitation of the horizontal shift view is its inability to explain acute clinical deterioration in patients with a mass after lumbar puncture. This should be due to purely downward displacement of central hemispheral or lower posterior fossa structures. When no mass is present, as in the post-lumbar puncture low-pressure syndrome noted previously, vertical displacement seems to do little harm. An important element, however, is the tendency for patients in whom deterioration occurs to have balanced masses, such as subdural hematomas, meningitis, or obstructive hydrocephalus, or to have a large posterior fossa mass. In most instances, where careful clinical description is available, the syndrome includes a component of cerebellar tonsillar herniation with abrupt apnea. Nonetheless, downward movement does occur after lumbar puncture, as Panullo and coworkers have shown,[19] leading to exaggeration of existing cerebellar tonsillar impaction. Any increase in temporal lobe shift at the tentorium also increases posterior fossa pressure, thereby also increasing tonsillar herniation. Neither the vertical nor horizontal thesis addresses sixth nerve paresis with raised intracranial pressure, but downward shift better accounts for bilateral sixth nerve signs since horizontal shift would make one nerve taut and the other slack.

PUPILLARY ENLARGEMENT

Here, again, the maxim has been that the third nerve is compressed by uncal herniation, or perhaps by the downward displaced posterior cerebellar artery. Numerous pathologic specimens support these mechanisms, particularly the work of Sunderland[26,27] and Reid and Cone,[28] but there are clearly examples in which neither mechanism pertains and the third nerve is instead stretched over the clivus as the midbrain is displaced laterally.[29,30] The medial uncus comes into contact with the third nerve in many normal specimens, and there are numerous cases of pupillary enlargement in which there is no uncal herniation, so this mechanism has probably been overrated as a unifying explanation. It seems likely that the third nerve dysfunction in cases of an advancing mass may have several configurations, depending on the shape of the tentorial opening and the relationship of the edge of the tentorium to the third nerve in a given patient.

The situation with enlargement of the opposite pupil, after the one on the side of the mass has already been affected, is far more complex and has so far eluded explanation.[31] The idea that the opposite temporal lobe also herniates seems very unlikely since the corresponding perimesencephalic cistern is closed off. The initial enlargement of a pupil opposite a mass is just as puzzling. This author's thinking has been that a central (midbrain) mechanism of third nerve nuclear or fascicular compression may play a role.

CEREBELLAR HERNIATION

Fisher[32] alluded to several cases of fatal cerebellar hematoma in which no downward cerebellar pressure cone was found (some even had lumbar punctures), and to others in which a cone was present but there were no referable symptoms. Beyond this, there is little evidence to attach upward or downward shift of the cerebellum to any particular signs, and it has been taken for granted that progressive deterioration by way of brainstem failure is somehow connected to the pathologic change. In most cases, the signs that accompany progressive enlargement of a brainstem mass, or with cerebellar edema, can be explained as easily by direct compression of the brainstem going forward or laterally. Indeed, in one such case studied with MRI and autopsy, the ventral medulla was pushed anteriorly against the lower clivus, creating pyramidal signs.[33]

SUMMARY

Large supratentorial masses create both horizontal and vertical displacements of central brain structures adjacent to the tentorial aperture. The role of transtentorial herniation seen at autopsy, whether central or medial temporal, is not well established as the proximate cause of coma or of pupillary enlargement; CT and MRI scans suggest that herniation may arise after the events leading to the compression of crucial upper midbrain structures. Horizontal shift from an acute lesion correlates better with the level of consciousness and this leads to several practical ways of understanding the radiologic correlates of coma and following its clinical course. As Plum and his colleagues have pointed out, these issues should not eclipse the importance of upper brainstem dysfunction, whether rostral-caudal, lateral, or due to impaction of the temporal lobes with little displacement, as a sign of imminent danger.[34]

The signs related to secondary effects of a mass in the cranium follow several general patterns, but are not stereotyped in detail. After reduced alertness, pupillary changes of several types are excellent indicators of progressive displacement of brain tissue in the neighborhood of the tentorium. Moreover, the mechanism of coma and of the cardinal sign of pupillary enlargement on the side of a mass is still in dispute, although historical dictum attaches them all to herniations.

REFERENCES

1. Meyer A: Herniation of the brain. *Arch Neurol Psychiat* 4:387–400, 1920.
2. Jefferson G: The tentorial pressure cone. *Arch Neurol Psychiat* 40:857–876, 1938.
3. van Gehuchten MP: Le méchanisme de la mont dans certain cas de tumeurs cérébrale. *Rev Neurol* 65:702–728, 1936.
4. Moruzzi G, Magoun HW: Brain stem reticular formation and activation of the EEG. *Electroenceph Clin Neurophysiol* 1:455, 1949.
5. Blinkov SM, Smirnov NA: Brain Displacements and Deformations, translated by Onischenko GT, Lindsley DB (translation ed). New York, Plenum Press, 1971.
6. McNealy DE, Plum F: Brainstem dysfunction with supratentorial mass lesions. *Arch Neurol* 7:10-32, 1962.
7. Plum F, Posner JB: *The Diagnosis of Stupor and Coma*. Philadelphia, FA Davis, 1966.
8. Macewen W: *Pyogenic Infective Diseases of the Brain and Spinal Cord*. Glasgow, Maclehose and Sons, 1893.
9. Hutchinson J: Four lectures on compression of the brain. *Clin Lec Rep Lond Hosp* 4:10–55, 1867.
10. Cuneo RA, Caronna JJ, Pitts L, et al: Syndrome of upward cerebellar herniation. *Arch Neurol* 36:618–623, 1979.
11. Ropper AH, Shafran B: Brain edema after stroke. *Arch Neurol* 41:26–29, 1984.
12. Fisher CM: Acute brain herniation: a revised concept. *Semin Neurol* 4:417–421, 1984.
13. Hasenjäger T, Spatz H: Über örtliche Veränderungern der Konfiguration des Gehirns beim Hindruck. *Arch Psychiat Nevenkr* 107:193–222, 1937.
14. Ono M, Ono M, Rhoton AJ Jr, et al: Microsurgical anatomy of the region of the tentorial incisura. *J Neurosurg* 60:365–399, 1984.
15. Howell DA: Upper brainstem compression and foraminal impaction with intracranial space-occupying lesions and brain swelling. *Brain* 82:525-550, 1959.
16. Feldmann E, Gandy SE, Becker R, et al: MRI demonstrates descending transtentorial herniation. *Neurology* 38:697–701, 1988.
17. Reich JB, Sierra J, Camp W, Zanzonico P, Deck MD, Plum F: Magnetic resonance imaging measurement and clinical changes accompanying transtentorial and foramen magnum brain herniation. *Ann Neurol* 33:159–170, 1993.
18. Ropper AH: A preliminary MRI study of the geometry of brain displacement and level of consciousness with acute intracranial masses. *Neurology* 39:622–627, l989.
19. Panullo SC, Reich JB, Krol G, Deck MDF, Posner JB: MRI changes in intracranial hypotension. *Neurology* 43:919–926, 1993.
20. Ropper AH: Lateral displacement of the brain and level of consciousness in patients with an acute hemispheral mass. *New Eng J Med* 314:953–958, 1986.
21. Ross DA, Olsen, Ross AM, et al: Brain shift, level of consciousness, and restoration of consciousness in patients with acute intracranial hematomas. *J Neurosurg* 71:498–502, 1989.
22. van Dongen KJ, Braakman R, Gelpke GJ: The prognostic value of computerized tomography in comatose head injured patients. *J Neurosurg* 59:951–957, 1983.
23. Toutant SM, Klauber MR, Marshall LF, et al: Absence or compressed cisterns on first CT scan: ominous predictors of outcome in severe head injury. *J Neurosurg* 61:691–694, 1984.
24. Ropper AH, Gress DR: CT and clinical features of large cerebral hemorrhages. *Cerebrovasc Dis* 1:38–42, 1991.
25. Wijdicks EFM, Miller GF: MR imaging of downward herniation of the diencephalon. *Neurology* 48:1456–1459, 1997.
26. Sunderland S: The tentorial notch and complications produced by herniations of the brain through that aperture. *Br J Surg* 45:422–438, 1958.
27. Sunderland S: Mechanism responsible for changes in the pupil unaccompanied by disturbance of

extra-ocular muscle function. *Br J Ophthalmol* 36:638–644, 1952.

28. Reid WL, Cone WV: Mechanism of fixed dilation of the pupil. *JAMA* 112;2030–2034, 1939.

29. Ropper AH, Cole D, Louis DL: Clinicopathologic correlation in a case of pupillary dilation from cerebral hemorrhage. *Arch Neurol* 48:1166–1169, 1991.

30. Fischer-Brügge E: Das "Klivukantensyndrom." *Acta Neurochir* (Wien) 2:36–68, 1951.

31. Ropper AH: The opposite pupil in herniation. *Neurology* 40:1707–1710, 1990.

32. Fisher CM: The neurological examination of the comatose patient. *Acta Neurol Scand* 45(suppl 36): 1–56, 1969.

33. Kanis K, Ropper AH, Adelman L: Homolateral hemiparesis as an early sign of cerebellar mass effect. *Neurology* 44:2194–2197, 1994.

34. Plum F, Deck M, Reich J: Reply to letter re: Magnetic resonance imaging measurements and clinical changes accompanying transtentorial and foramen magnum brain herniation. *Ann Neurol* 34:748–749, 1992.

Chapter 5

INTRACRANIAL HEMORRHAGE

Eelco F. M. Wijdicks

Acute impairment of consciousness or rapid progression in coma, within minutes, often bespeaks intracranial hemorrhage. In most compiled stroke registries, coma or stupor is prominent in patients with parenchymal hemorrhages. Obviously, these series have been skewed toward patients who have received medical attention and, therefore, do not include a considerable proportion of patients with large supratentorial hemorrhages or destructive pontine lesions, or patients suffering sudden death due to aneurysmal subarachnoid hemorrhage.

Transient loss of consciousness, impaired consciousness at presentation, or gradual deepening of coma have many potential explanations in patients with intracranial hemorrhages. It is important not only to identify the anatomic location of an intracranial hemorrhage, but also to be familiar with secondary deterioration in a previously alert patient. This chapter reviews these clinical courses.

CLINICAL FEATURES OF INTRACRANIAL HEMATOMA

Intracranial hematoma produces distinct clinical profiles that should lead to the diagnosis in most patients. Impaired consciousness is common for disease reasons. Coma or impaired consciousness in patients with intracranial hemorrhage can be studied by anatomic location and compartment. Worsening clinical conditions in an alert patient

has many possible explanations, and the causes are different for each type of hemorrhage. The causes of coma and possible reasons for worsening of the degree of coma are summarized in Table 5-1.

Subarachnoid Hemorrhage

Most subarachnoid hemorrhages are caused by rupture of an aneurysm in the circle of Willis. Blood floods the basal cisterns, and about one-half of the patients have a brief loss of consciousness. Neurologic examination of patients with aneurysmal subarachnoid hemorrhage may indicate the location of the aneurysm. The presence of retinal hemorrhages generally indicates that the hemorrhage is extensive. Retinal hemorrhage is explained largely by transmission of the intracranial pressure surge wave. (The presence of subhyaloid hemorrhages, however, is not predictive of outcome and merely confirms subarachnoid hemorrhage under arterial pressure.) (See Fig. 3-3.)

Persistent coma and significant impairment of consciousness is uncommon with aneurysmal subarachnoid hemorrhage. Most of the patients admitted to an intensive care unit are alert, cooperative, and able to comprehend complex tasks. An acute confusional state is rare, and, when it is present, it may point to rapid filling of the interhemispheric fissure with blood that may extend into the parenchyma of the frontal lobe producing a frontal lobe hematoma. Cranial nerve deficits are seldom observed, but, when they are, they localize

Table 5-1

Causes of coma and impaired level of conciousness in patients with intracranial hematoma

Anatomic location	Case	
	Initial coma	Worsening coma
Subarachnoid hemorrhage	• Massive intraventricular hemorrhage and acute hydrocepalus • Early seizures • Raised ICP and global ischemia	• Acute hydrocepalus • Cardiac arrhythmia • Iatrogenic sedation • Several electrolyte or acid-base abnormality • Seizures • Rebleeding • Delayed cerebral ischemia • Temporal lobe hematoma
Supratentorial parenchymal hemorrhage or subdural or epidural hematoma	• Diencephalic destruction • Massive subfalcial horizontal shift with midbrain distortion	• Trapping of ventricles from occlusion of foramen of Monro • Perihematoma edema • Enlargement of clot • Rebleeding
Cerebellum or pontine hemorrhage	• Destruction of ARAS • Secondary shearing hemorrhage in in brainstem (Duret's lesion)	• Acute hydrocephalus

Abbreviations: ICP = intracranial pressure; ARAS = ascending reticular activating system.

the aneurysm. A third nerve palsy usually indicates direct compression or bleeding into the nerve by a recently ruptured posterior communicating artery aneurysm. Pupillary reflexes may be spared. Other abnormalities of extraocular eye movements, especially sixth nerve palsy, indicate a ruptured basilar artery aneurysm.

Nuchal rigidity is an important clinical finding. Although this sign is not present immediately after aneurysmal rupture, or may be absent in comatose patients with pathologic withdrawal or extensor motor responses, it can be demonstrated by failure to flex the neck in neutral position and to retroflex when both shoulders are lifted.

The physiologic changes underlying sudden unresponsiveness during arterial rupture are complicated and not fully understood. Even though about the same amount of blood is seen on computed tomography (CT) scans, some patients awaken fully and others remain in a coma, with extensor responses. The reason for this difference in response is unclear. A sharp increase in intracranial pressure occurs at the time of aneurysmal rupture. This has recently been confirmed by transcranial Doppler (TCD) measurements. These data became available when patients reruptured during TCD studies. Rebleeding resulted in a pattern of absent diastolic or reverberating flow or small systolic peaks, reminiscent of patterns in brain death.[1] This brief period of absent effective cerebral blood flow is a global ischemic insult; therefore, failure of patients to awaken after a subarachnoid hemorrhage may be due to global ischemic encephalopathy. However, this biologic mechanism does not account for sudden death after subarachnoid aneurysmal hemorrhage. In a series of 13 patients who did not reach medical attention after subarachnoid hemorrhage because they died, massive intraventricular hemorrhage and pulmonary edema was very frequently found at autopsy.[2] Marked dilatation of the fourth ventricle may contribute to coma in these patients. In a study of terminal intracranial hemorrhages, hemorrhagic dilatation of the fourth ventricle was associated with multiple pressure-associated medullopontine infarcts.[3]

Another possible cause of initial coma after subarachnoid hemorrhage is distortion of the brainstem caused by a large temporal lobe hematoma, usually associated with rupture of a middle cerebral artery aneurysm. In a significant proportion of these patients, the presentation is coma or a rapidly deteriorating level of consciousness due to direct compression of the brainstem or shift of the midbrain.[4] In contrast, bilateral or unilateral frontal hematoma caused by rupture of an aneurysm of the anterior cerebral artery is usually associated with acute confusional state and akinetic mutism and seldom causes coma.

Brainstem function may become lost in moribund patients with subarachnoid hemorrhage, and the clinical criteria for brain death are met several hours after presentation. Many patients have only corneal reflexes, trigger the ventilator, and have yet pharmacologically unsupported blood pressure. This gradual deterioration of the patient's condition to brain death after the initial rupture of an aneurysm is not well understood, but the development of edema, probably associated with the initial global ischemic event, has been documented on CT (Fig. 5-1).

Normal or near-normal findings, such as sedimentation of blood in the fissures or ventricles, on the initial CT scan or xanthochromic cerebrospinal fluid (CSF) as the only laboratory confirmation of subarachnoid hemorrhage should point immediately to a systemic factor in patients presenting in a coma due to subarachnoid hemorrhage. Systemic causes of coma in cases of subarachnoid hemorrhage are seizures, severe hyponatremia, and metabolic alkalosis caused by severe dehydration associated with vomiting. The use of cocaine, a substance typically associated with subarachnoid hemorrhage, must be considered as a cause of coma in the appropriate setting. Subarachnoid hemorrhage may be the first presentation of granulomatous vasculitis.[5] In these patients, multiple territories of cerebral infarction, not initially visualized on CT, may impair the level of consciousness.

Worsening coma in patients with recent aneurysmal subarachnoid hemorrhage has several causes. Gradual decrease in the level of consciousness on the day of the ictus, or on the next day, indicates acute hydrocephalus. Most patients with hydrocephalus are able to perform simple tests (e.g., showing fingers or making a fist) with adequate prodding, but, when left alone, they drift into a sleep-like state. Pinpoint pupils are seen only in patients with considerable enlargement of the ventricles, and, then, vertical eye movements often become sluggish.[6] Repeat CT demonstrates enlargement of the ventricles, which subsequently decreases (often to a volume smaller than baseline) after ventriculostomy (Fig. 5-2).

Worsening coma on the day of admission may also be caused by enlargement of a temporal lobe hematoma. The condition of patients with a temporal lobe hematoma tends to deteriorate fairly rapidly because of rerupture (the hematoma may indicate that the hemorrhage represents rebleeding) or edema developing around the clot.

An unusual but well-documented cause of sudden deterioration is an acute cardiac arrhythmia, with a marked decrease in blood pressure and loss of consciousness. Life-threatening cardiac arrhythmias include brief ventricular tachycardia, asystole, and torsades de pointes.[7] Seizures may cause a decrease in the level of consciousness and are observed mostly at the time of the initial rupture or during rebleeding.

Iatrogenic causes of coma associated with subarachnoid hemorrhage must be excluded. Repeated doses of morphine for pain control or benzodiazepines for agitation can occasionally be implicated but the effect can be reversed with antidotes such as naloxone or flumazenil.

Cerebral vasospasm (more accurately termed "delayed cerebral ischemia") may cause worsening coma in subarachnoid hemorrhage, especially if it is observed 3 days or more after the most recent rupture.

In many of these patients, the level of consciousness had already been fluctuating, and they had lost their ability to concentrate on a simple task. The clinical features of delayed cerebral ischemia are recognized mainly by progressive

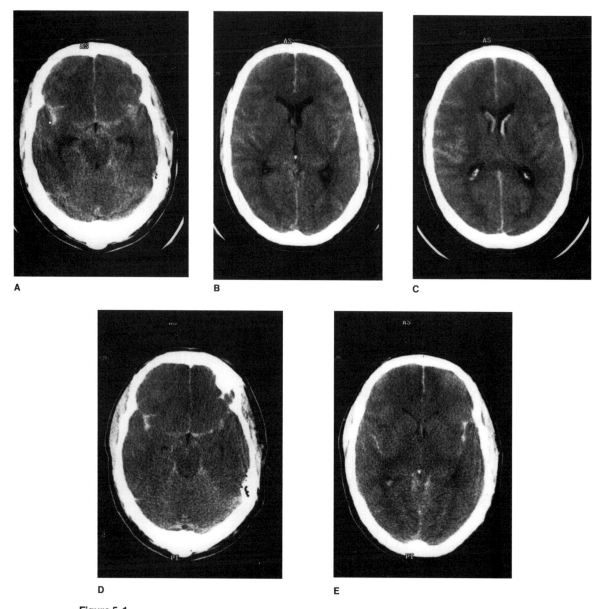

Figure 5-1
Development of massive hypodensity and loss of gray-white matter differentiation in a patient with low-grade subarachnoid hemorrhage, indicating a major global ischemic event.

sleepiness, aphasia or sudden mutism, or hemiparesis. Transcranial Doppler ultrasonographic examination may be helpful if the results of earlier studies were equivocal or if a marked increase (more than 50 cm/s in the middle cerebral artery segment) in velocities is seen. Repeat CT is seldom helpful, because it rarely demonstrates new hypodensities. Cerebral angiography is often indicated to confirm cerebral vasospasm and to provide opportunity for intervention, such as infusion of

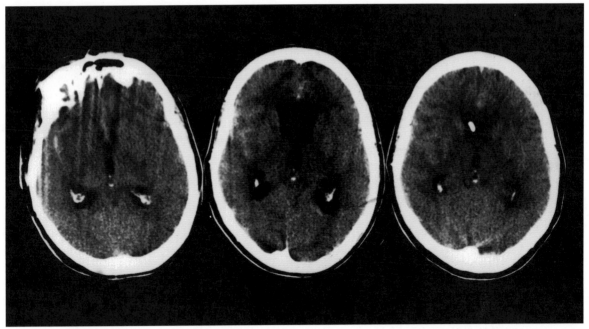

Figure 5-2
Progression of acute hydrocephalus in subarachnoid hemorrhage, followed by success-ful drainage of CSF and clinical improvement.

intra-arterial papaverine or angioplasty when cere-bral vasospasm is localized in a single segment of the middle cerebral artery.

With subarachnoid hemorrhage, a patient's condition may deteriorate because of rebleeding at any time after the initial rupture. The factors that make a patient susceptible to rebleeding have not been identified, but those who survive an episode of rebleeding are at high risk for a second episode.

The first 24 h are the time with the highest prevalence of rebleeding, and the risk of rebleeding during the following weeks is 20 percent.[8] Rebleed-ing is readily recognized by apnea and the loss of virtually all brainstem reflexes. New, fresh blood in the basal cisterns, but, more often, in the ventricles, is often seen on CT. A less common presentation of rebleeding is sudden worsening of headache with-out loss of consciousness. Emergency endotracheal intubation and total mechanical ventilation are often indicated, and patients may remain in coma for several hours, with sluggish brainstem reflexes.

Few patients recover to a previous clinical state, and, then, surgical intervention is the only way to prevent a fatal second episode of rebleeding.

In summary, the principal factors that are likely to contribute to the immediate development of coma from subarachnoid hemorrhage are a major surge in intracranial pressure with secondary global ischemic damage, temporal lobe hematoma, or, less likely, a systemic cause. Worsening coma in previously alert patients may indicate the develop-ment of acute hydrocephalus, delayed cerebral ischemia, seizures, or severe metabolic derange-ment.

Spontaneous Supratentorial Parenchymal Hemorrhage

Patients with a sizable supratentorial hemorrhage are rarely alert. The initial volume of parenchymal hemorrhage generally corresponds to the level of consciousness. Large-volume (>60 mL) clots may disconnect the diencephalon from the ascending

Table 5-2
Major distinguishing clinical features of supratentorial parenchymal hemorrhages

Location	Features
Putamen	• Nonfluent or global aphasia (fluent aphasia if hemorrhage spreads to temporal lobe) • Conjugate deviation of eyes • Hemiparesis (severity depends on spread of hemorrhage to internal capsule) • Hyperreflexia • Hemisensory findings (may be prominent neglect)
Caudate	• Restlessness, amnesia, abulia • Neck stiffness • Hemiparesis (only with extension of hemorrhage to internal capsule)
Thalamus	• Aphasia (paraphasic errors, fluent but retained repetition) • Pinpoint pupils: vertical gaze paresis (upward > downward) • Significant sensory deficit • Very mild hemiparesis
Lobar	• Headache (common); seizures (1/3 of patients) • Wernicke's aphasia, quadrant hemianopsia (temporal) • Hemiparesis, hemisensory syndrome (parietal) • Homonymous hemianopia (occipital)

reticular activating system or produce bihemispheric dysfunction because of a mass effect and shift. Coma should be expected in patients in whom the CT scan shows a large horizontal shift of the pineal gland (8 mm or more) or in a patient with a diencephalic hematoma (ventral thalamus and hypothalamus). At times, these patients have hydrocephalus, but coma is seldom due to hydrocephalus alone. Small localized occipital or deep-seated hemorrhages in the internal capsule or basal ganglia produce only hemiplegia or a visual field deficit but not an impaired level of consciousness.

Patients with lobar, putaminal, thalamic, or caudate hemorrhage may be distinguished clinically (Table 5-2), although in one large study from the Stroke Data Bank, many clinical features, such as seizures, deficit on awakening, vomiting, or decreased level of consciousness and coma, were similar.[9]

Seizures are uncommon at onset in patients with lobar hematoma; at most, the rate may approach 20 percent. A flurry of seizures with associated prolonged postural episodes are an uncommon cause of impaired consciousness in patients with intracranial hemorrhage.

Crack cocaine, alcohol abuse, or amphetamine-related substances may be implicated as a cause of impaired consciousness in any adult with intracranial hematoma,[10] certainly when the hemorrhage is comparatively small. Fever indicates possible bacterial endocarditis, although an early increase in body temperature with relative bradycardia more commonly indicates absorption of blood rather than an ongoing infectious process. Transesophageal echocardiography is an essential study in these patients.

Worsening coma in parenchymal hematoma has not been studied extensively, but recent studies with sequential CT scans, made at brief intervals, demonstrated a significant (twofold to threefold) increase in hematoma volume in the first 12 h after the hemorrhage, nearly always accompanied by further clinical deterioration.[11] Rarely, sudden dramatic worsening may occur and result in death.[12] Massive enlargement of the hematoma with extension into the ventricular system has been described (Fig. 5-3).[12]

According to one retrospective study, formation of edema around the clot is sufficient to explain a 2-point or greater deterioration on the

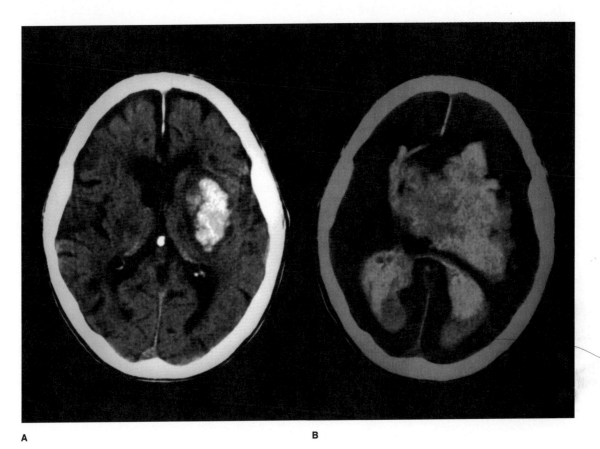

A   B

Figure 5-3
A. *Initial putaminal hemorrhage.* B. *Massive rebleeding with fatal sudden deterioration in putaminal hemorrhage. (From Wijdicks and Fulgham,[12] with permission.)*

Glasgow Coma (sum) Scale, but this study most likely underestimated the contribution of the extension of the hematoma or overestimated clinical deterioration.[13] Trapping of the ipsilateral ventricle with pronounced enlargement at the hematoma site is often seen in patients with thalamic hemorrhages that border the foramen of Monro, and may produce secondary progressive 5 drowsiness (Fig. 5-4). Patients with temporal lobe hematoma are especially at risk for further deterioration clinically, and the hematoma should be evacuated surgically, even if deterioration is subtle.[14,15]

Worsening of coma should also be expected in patients who have an underlying coagulopathy or whose hemorrhage was due to thrombolytic agents.[16] Enlargement of the volume of the hematoma is likely.

Intraventricular, Subdural, and Epidural Hemorrhage

The presentation of the rare entity of intraventricular hemorrhages is striking and often similar to that of aneurysmal subarachnoid hemorrhage. Many patients rapidly become comatose, with most demonstrating extensor motor responses. As with subarachnoid hemorrhage, headache and vomiting may precede the coma, because of the massive bleeding. Neurologic findings are nonlocalizing, and many brainstem reflexes may be muted or lost. Vertical oculocephalic reflexes are

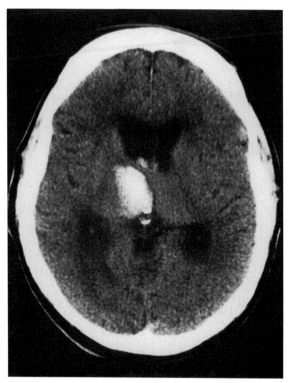

Figure 5-4
Thalamic hemorrhage, with trapping of right ventricle, causing progressive drowsiness.

often lost, and papilledema may occur because of rapid enlargement of the ventricular system under significant pressure. Preretinal hemorrhages are often observed.

Coma is present at the onset, but in about 25 percent of the patients, ventricular hemorrhage is less severe and presents as an acute confusional state.[17] In those who are less affected initially, worsening coma often can be attributed to the development of hydrocephalus. In patients presenting in coma and who have a massive ventricular hemorrhage, ventriculostomy is frequently unsuccessful because of permanent destruction of periventricular tissue, particularly in the midbrain and pons.

Acute subdural hematomas are typically caused by trauma, and they commonly produce impairment of consciousness.[18] The presence of a horizontal shift on CT scans is an important guide for estimating the level of consciousness, because additional hemorrhagic contusions may not be visible on initial CT studies. Coma with only a minimal shift of the pineal gland should point to the presence of additional traumatic brain injury not visualized on the CT at admission. Brain shift, however, does not predict outcome after surgical decompression. Andrews and colleagues showed that pineal shift was poor in predicting outcome in a large proportion of patients with extracranial hematomas.[14] These authors made the important observation that visibility of the ambient cisterns may have better prognostic value. Obliteration of the contralateral ambient cistern may indicate that the shift in the cerebral hemisphere and brainstem is equal. Obliteration of the ipsilateral ambient cistern may indicate a shift of the hemisphere without a proportional shift in the brainstem, resulting in greater distortion and kinking of the brainstem.

According to traditional teaching, patients with a subdural hematoma may have a lucid, virtually asymptomatic interval. In more than two-thirds of the patients, impairment of consciousness is rapid or present from the beginning. However, in some patients with traumatic subdural hematoma, described as "talk and deteriorate," the rapidity of impairment of consciousness and the deepening of the level of coma are characteristic.

Epidural hematomas may evolve so rapidly that patients die of brainstem compression within several hours. Often, the pupil ipsilateral to the compression enlarges and becomes sluggish or unresponsive to bright light. This is soon followed by a similar change in the opposite pupil. Asymmetry in motor response is common. However, asymmetry of motor response and a fixed dilated pupil may both be falsely localizing signs.

Surgical evacuation of the hematoma, preferably after CT has confirmed its presence, may result in awakening, but two-thirds of the patients with an epidural hematoma and a score of 3 on the Glasgow Coma Scale remain in a vegetative state. Bilateral pupillary dilatation associated with acute subdural hematoma does not imply a devastating surgical outcome. Nonreactivity of the pupils bilaterally for at least 3 h increases the probability of severe disability, vegetative state, or death, although a good outcome or moderate disability is possible.[19] Acute subdural or epidural hematoma of the posterior fossa is almost always caused by trauma to the torcula herophili.[20] In these cases, early intervention is successful, with a mortality rate of 20 percent or less.

Hemorrhages in the Cerebellum and Brainstem

Neurologists have a heavy responsibility for recognizing a hemorrhage in the cerebellum, because if it is missed, the patient's condition rapidly deteriorates. A large clot in the cerebellum puts pressure on the contents of the posterior fossa. Impingement of the clot on the brainstem causes impairment of consciousness, loss of brainstem reflexes, and cardiac arrhythmias, particularly episodic sinus bradycardia. Sudden vertigo (with inability to maintain balance), vomiting with any change in position, and severe overwhelming headache are key features. Midline cerebellar hemorrhages are notorious for causing rapid onset of coma, which can be expected when the hemorrhages abut or extend into the pons. Development of a more profound degree of coma can be expected in a large proportion of patients and often within the first 8 h after onset of hemorrhage.[21]

Deterioration in the level of consciousness is difficult to predict in patients with cerebellar hematoma. However, CT findings of obliteration of the fourth ventricle, effacement of the ambient cistern, indentation of the brainstem, and loss of the typical diamond shape of the supracerebellar cisterns are indications of a possible unstable compensation that should urge surgical evacuation of the hematoma if the patient is still alert or drowsy (Fig. 5-5).

Worsening coma can be gradual or acute. Apnea and acute loss of most brainstem reflexes have been noted repeatedly, but the anatomic substrate is not known. Although survival is possible, the disability is significant. Currently, this clinical course is uncommon, partly because, with improved resolution of CT, early brainstem compromise can be demonstrated. More

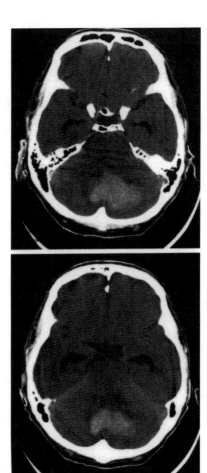

Figure 5-5
Cerebellar hematoma with upward herniation.

commonly, there is gradual deterioration due to obstructive hydrocephalus, resulting in vertical gaze palsy, inability to protect the airway, and apnea (if untreated). Ventriculostomy is usually combined with posterior fossa craniotomy to relieve pressure on the brainstem and especially to decrease the chance of upward herniation caused by CSF drainage.

Primary brainstem hemorrhages are usually located in the pons. Midbrain hemorrhages are often extensions of a large thalamic hemorrhage or typical Duret-type hemorrhages caused by tissue distortion. Midbrain hemorrhages vary in size, and small hemorrhages produce disturbances in extraocular eye movements (internuclear ophthalmoplegia or complete ophthalmoplegia) and hemiparesis. A typical Parinaud syndrome (upward gaze palsy) may be observed if the superior colliculus is affected. The level of consciousness may be affected, but usually only drowsiness occurs. Some patients have visual hallucinations, often of vivid landscapes (peduncular hallucinations).

Statistically, pontine hemorrhages are more common than midbrain or medullary hemorrhages, although they represent only a small percentage of all intracranial hemorrhages. Many pontine hemorrhages cause drowsiness or, more often, frank coma because of destruction of midline structures. Consciousness is spared in patients with small hemorrhages and predominantly segmental localization.

Fairly characteristic findings associated with pontine hemorrhage include sudden coma, early spontaneous extensor responses, and irregular, ineffective breathing. Brief shivering or tonic movements may occur and are often interpreted as seizures by clinical novices. Frequently, small pupils bilaterally are early clinical indicators when observed in patients with sudden collapse and extensor posturing. The pupils often are 2 to 3 mm wide and reactive to light; rarely are they "pinpoint." Horizontal doll's eyes are absent. Ocular bobbing is seen regularly and may inadvertently suggest spontaneous vertical movements, as in locked-in syndrome. (The distinction between ocular bobbing and voluntary vertical eye movements can be difficult to make, and electroencephalography (EEG) may demonstrate a typical alpha coma instead of an essentially normal EEG, as in patients with locked-in syndrome.) Acute hydrocephalus caused by compression of the aqueduct may be indicated on initial CT scan, but this is seldom the cause of worsening coma. In this author's experience, ventriculostomy has not resulted in patients awakening.

Patients with large pontine hemorrhages may have autonomic signs, including significant increases in systolic blood pressure, profuse sweating, and hyperthermia up to 40°C.

LABORATORY INVESTIGATIONS

The most crucial diagnostic test in confirming the presence of intracerebral hemorrhage is CT. The CT localizes the anatomic lesion, often explains the reason for coma in a particular patient, may explain secondary deterioration (e.g., by demonstrating enlargement of the hemorrhage), and, occasionally, may suggest an underlying structural lesion (e.g., tumor, arteriovenous malformation, or aneurysm). The site of the hemorrhage should determine what laboratory tests are performed.

Subarachnoid Hemorrhage

Most subarachnoid hemorrhages are associated with a ruptured aneurysm. The CT demonstration of diffuse layers of blood in the basal cisterns and fissures suggests an aneurysmal source (Fig. 5-6A). Intraparenchymal extension of the hemorrhage strongly predicts location of the aneurysm (frontal lobe, anterior cerebral artery; lateral temporal lobe, middle cerebral artery; basal temporal lobe, carotid artery). Blood in the cortical sulci or localized in the perimesencephalic or pontine cisterns only should point to a different cause than aneurysmal rupture. Blood in the perimesencephalic cistern (so-called "perimesencephalic nonaneurysmal hemorrhage") has been identified as a variant of subarachnoid hemorrhage[22] (Fig. 5-6B). It is distinguished by the lack of impaired consciousness and absence of secondary neurologic deterioration. Cerebral angiography is indicated in these patients to exclude an aneurysm in the posterior circulation, but, in the appropriate clinical setting, the findings will be negative. Impaired consciousness can be expected in perimesencephalic subarachnoid hemorrhage only when acute hydrocephalus (due to CSF block at the tentorial outlet) occurs; the patient's condition may improve remarkably after the block is circumvented by ventriculostomy.

Blood found only in the cortical sulci points to trauma, and impaired consciousness may indicate extensive head injury. In these patients, follow-up CT may demonstrate the evolution of hemorrhagic contusions or demonstrate shear lesions at the white-gray matter junction.

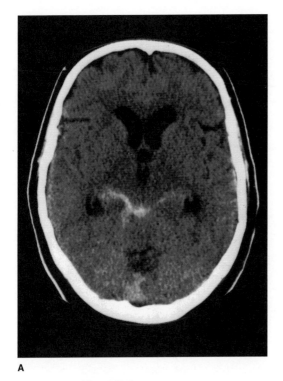

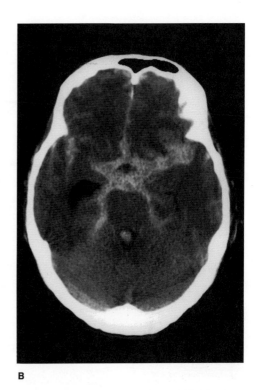

Figure 5-6

A. *Aneurysmal subarachnoid hemorrhage.* B. *Perimesencephalic hemorrhage.*

Impaired consciousness and blood localized only in the cortical sulci also may indicate isolated central nervous system (CNS) vasculitis or cerebral venous thrombosis, conditions that should become clear after magnetic resonance imaging (MRI), or MR angiography, or cerebral angiography is performed.

Blood diffusely located in the subarachnoid space, certainly when large amounts of blood fill the suprasellar cisterns, is compatible with a marked decrease in the level of consciousness, but, as mentioned above, acute hydrocephalus may contribute.

In addition to CT and cerebral angiography, ultrasonography and single photon emission computed tomography (SPECT) may be valuable if a fluctuating level of consciousness is not readily explained. Delayed cerebral ischemia may cause a decrease in alertness, and a marked increase in velocities on TCD ultrasonography may support the diagnosis of global ischemia. Scanning by SPECT is useful especially if TCD ultrasonography findings were abnormal on admission and do not show any further worsening. Global hypoperfusion may be demonstrated but may be compensated by increased oxygen extraction.

Putaminal and Lobar Hematomas

Ganglionic hemorrhage is clearly delineated with CT, which may also indicate intraventricular extension of the hemorrhage and acute hydrocephalus. Significant enlargement of the fourth ventricle is a poor prognostic sign (Fig. 5-7). Massive ganglionic hemorrhages can cause coma because of extention into the diencephalon[23] or because of massive horizontal and vertical shifts (Fig. 5-8). However, herniation seen on CT may not necessarily explain the clinical course, and the deepening coma may be caused by horizontal displacement of the midbrain alone. The MRI scans can be helpful in

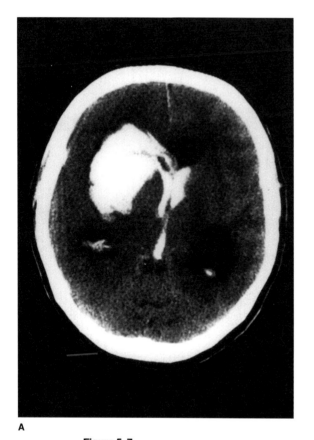

A

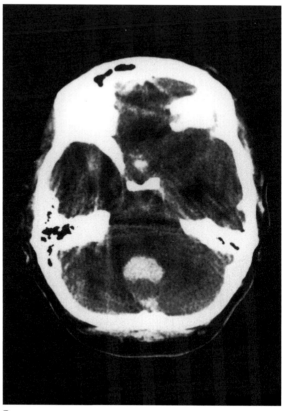

B

Figure 5-7

Massive intraventricular hemorrhage associated with putaminal hemorrhage.

demonstrating the extent of the hemorrhage. Thalamic hemorrhages may extend into the mesencephalon and cause unilateral pupillodilatation, without producing a noticeable change in the level of consciousness (Fig. 5-9).

The evaluation of lobar hematoma is more complex. Most patients with suspected lobar hematoma should undergo cerebral angiography without delay. Cerebral angiography is able to demonstrate an underlying arteriovenous malformation or middle cerebral artery aneurysm, with a reasonable yield of 30 to 40 percent.[24] Whether angiography should be performed on the day of admission depends on the patient's level of consciousness, the shift seen on CT, and, possibly, localization in the temporal lobe. If a temporal lobe hematoma is sufficiently large, it often causes

rapid neurologic deterioration. Usually, surgery is followed immediately with evacuation of the clot and resection of the arteriovenous malformation or clipping of the aneurysm. In small lobar hemorrhages, MRI and MR angiography may be performed to exclude hemorrhage inside a tumor, to diagnose cerebral venous thrombosis, or to demonstrate findings compatible with a venous angioma or an arteriovenous malformation that may go unnoticed on cerebral angiography.

There are many causes of lobar hematomas, and long-standing hypertension should not be accepted automatically as the probable trigger. In elderly patients, cerebral amyloid angiopathy is a common cause, and MRI occasionally shows evidence of small earlier hemorrhages and extensive white matter disease. In young patients with lobar

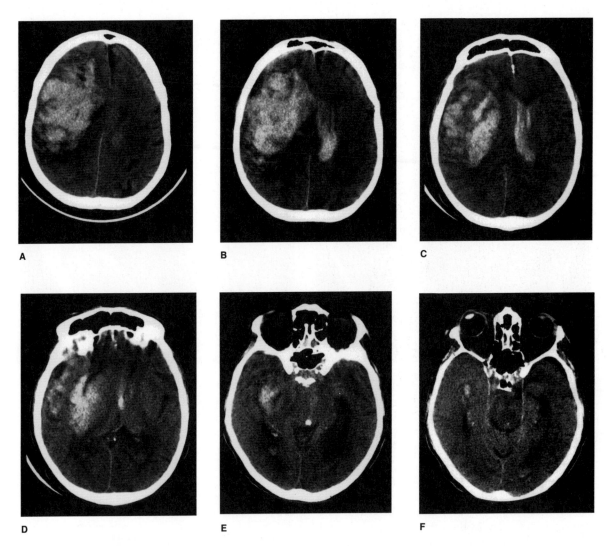

Figure 5-8

Massive lobar intracerebral hematoma. The CT shows characteristic marked edema, horizontal shift (note displacement of third ventricle, filled with blood, and widening of ipsilateral cisterns), and vertical shift (note significant displacement of pineal gland, and possible early hypodensity in the pons due to ischemia caused by tearing of the penetrating arteries).

hematoma, drug abuse should be considered if cerebral angiography does not disclose an underlying vascular malformation or when CT findings do not explain the level of consciousness (e.g., a small hematoma with no shift). A marked surge in hypertension may damage a small penetrating artery; this mechanism is thought to cause intracranial hemorrhages associated with cocaine, amphetamines, and phenylpropanolamine. Fever and lobar intracerebral hematoma in a drug user immediately point to the possibility of a ruptured mycotic aneurysm due to bacterial endocarditis.

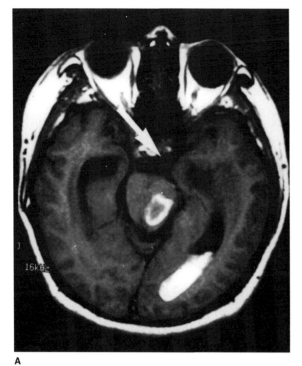 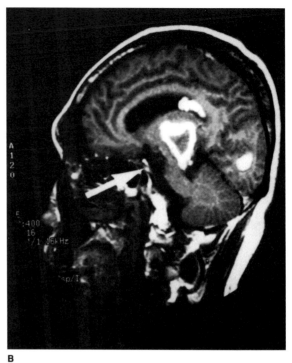

A   B

Figure 5-9

A. *An MRI from a patient with a thalamic hemorrhage with extension into the mesencephalon.* B. *Corresponding MRI (T2-weighted image) showing acute hemorrhage with vertical and horizontal shift of upper brainstem but no uncal herniation.*

Lobar hematomas may be caused by a hematologic-oncologic disorder and, indeed, may be the first manifestation of such disease. A reasonable approach to further evaluation in cases of spontaneous lobar hematoma with negative angiographic findings is outlined in Table 5-3. Typically, intracranial hemorrhages associated with hypertension and localized in the territories of perforating arteries (e.g., in the putamen, thalamus, pons, and cerebellum) do not need extensive laboratory evaluation other than additional MRI and comprehensive evaluation to determine the cause of hypertension if it is of recent onset.

MANAGEMENT AND OUTCOME

The location and size of the intraparenchymal hematoma, the shift of intracranial contents, the

Table 5-3

Evaluation of spontaneous lobar hematoma with negative findings on cerebral angiography[a]

- Transesophageal echocardiography
- IgM rheumatoid factor, antinuclear antibodies specific for double-standard DNA; anticytoplasmatic antineutrophil antibody
- Blood smear
- Coagulation profile (von Willebrand, factor III and IX deficiency)
- Toxicology screen (urine, blood, gastric fluid, gas chromatography with mass spectrometry, and thin-layer chromatography)

[a] Often, arteriovenous malformations, venous angiomas, or aneurysms can be demonstrated only after repeat cerebral angiography.

Table 5-4

Consistently reported poor prognostic signs in intracranial hemorrhage

Location	Variable
Subarachnoid space	• Score ≤ 8 on Glasgow Coma Scale or World Federation of Neurologic Surgeons IV, V • Rebleeding, delayed cerebral ischemia • Intraventricular hemorrhage
Putamen	• Intraventricular extension • Volume >40 mL • Pineal shift >3 mm
Thalamus	• Diameter >3 cm on CT scan (volumetric measurements not available)
Lobar	• Volume >40 mL • Intraventricular extension • Hypertension
Pons	• Midline location (as opposed to segmental location) • Coma at onset
Cerebellum	• Diameter >3 cm • Complete obliteration of cultures on CT

See also Refs. 26–37.

presence of ongoing coagulopathy, the patient's age, and, certainly, coma with clear signs of brainstem dysfunction are factors that determine whether surgical evacuation of the blood is successful. In many medical centers, the presence of alertness or drowsiness in patients with intracranial hematoma discourages neurosurgeons to perform a craniotomy. Only when the level of consciousness is impaired or significantly worsens is surgical evacuation of the clot considered. However, the condition of patients with temporal lobe hematoma and evidence of compression of the lateral ventricles almost always deteriorates because of swelling, despite conservative measures, and early evacuation of the blood should be considered.

Surgical management is rarely a primary measure in the treatment of deep-seated putaminal or thalamic hemorrhages. In some medical centers, early evacuation is considered, but the outcome is dismal for patients with progression to coma. Survival is often at the expense of significant disability, even 1 year after the evacuation was performed.[25]

The predictors of outcome for each localization are shown in Table 5-4. However, coma, certainly at presentation, overrides many other factors in outcome, including the volume of the hematoma. Coma has often been characterized as a score of 8 or less on the Glasgow Coma Scale, but a hematoma volume of 50 mL, ventricular extension of the hematoma, and a 3-mm or more shift of the pineal gland are poor prognosticating features and many patients will not survive. Abnormal pupils, extensor responses, and abnormal eye movements with oculocephalic responses are closely associated with catastrophic bleeding and, thus, indicate a poor chance for survival. In general, neurologic deterioration is a poor prognostic sign in any type of intracranial hematoma. Only hemorrhage into the caudate nucleus is invariably associated with good outcome despite a large volume and intraventricular extension.

REFERENCES

1. Hassler W, Steinmetz H, Gawlowski T: Transcranial Doppler sonography in raised intracranial pressure and in intracranial circulatory arrest. *J Neurosurg* 68:745–751,1988.
2. Schievink W, Wijdicks EFM, Parisi JE, Piepgras DG, Whisnant JP: Sudden death from aneurysmal

subarachnoid hemorrhage. *Neurology* 45:871–874, 1995.

3. Shapiro SA, Campbell RL, Scully T: Hemorrhagic dilation of the fourth ventricle: an ominous predictor. *J Neurosurg* 80:805-809, 1994.

4. Pasqualin A, Bazzan A, Cavazzani P, Scienza R, Licata C, Da Pian R: Intracranial hematomas following aneurysmal rupture: experience with 309 cases. *Surg Neurol* 25:6–17, 1986.

5. Ozawa T, Sasaki O, Sorimachi T, et al: Primary angiitis of the central nervous system: report of two cases and review of the literature. *Neurosurgery* 36:173–179, 1995.

6. Hasan D, Vermeulen M, Wijdicks EFM, Hijdra A, van Gijn J: Management problems in acute hydrocephalus after subarachnoid hemorrhage. *Stroke* 20:747-753, 1989.

7. Andreoli A, di Pasquale G, Pinelli G, Grazi P, Tognetti F, Testa C: Subarachnoid hemorrhage: frequency and severity of cardiac arrhythmias: a survey of 70 cases studied in the acute phase. *Stroke* 18:558–564, 1987.

8. Hijdra A, Vermeulen M, van Gijn J, van Crevel H: Rerupture of intracranial aneurysms: a clinicoanatomical study. *J Neurosurg* 67:29-33, 1987.

9. Massaro AR, Sacco RL, Mohr JP, Foulkes MA, Tatemichi TK, Price TR, Hier DB, Wolf PA: Clinical discriminators of lobar and deep hemorrhages: the Stroke Data Bank. *Neurology* 41:1881–1885, 1991.

10. Brust ICM: Stroke and substance abuse, in *Stroke: Pathophysiology, Diagnosis, and Management.* Barne HJM, Mohr JP, Stein BM, et al (eds): New York, Churchill Livingston, 1986, 903 pp.

11. Chen ST, Chen SD, Hsu CY, Hogan EL: Progression of hypertensive intracerebral hemorrhage. *Neurology* 39:1509–1514, 1989.

12. Wijdicks EFM, Fulgham JR: Acute fatal deterioration in putaminal hemorrhage. *Stroke* 26:1953–1955, 1995.

13. Mayer SA, Sacco RL, Shi T: Neurologic deterioration in noncomatose intracerebral hemorrhage. *Neurology* 44:1379–1384, 1994.

14. Andrews BT, Chiles BW III, Olsen WL, Pitts LH: The effect of intracerebral hematoma location on the risk of brain stem compression and on clinical outcome. *J Neurosurg* 69:518-522,1988.

15. Maiuri F, Corriero G, Passarelli F, Cirillo S, Astarita G: CT indications for surgery and evaluation of prognosis in patients with spontaneous intracerebral haematomas. *Br J Neurosurg* 4:155–160, 1990.

16. Wijdicks EFM, Jack CR: Intracerebral hemorrhage after fibrinolytic therapy for acute myocardial infarction. *Stroke* 24:554–557, 1994,

17. Roos YBWEM, Hasan D, Vermeulen M: Outcome in patients with large intraventricular haemorrhage: a volumetric study. *J Neurol Neurosurg Psychiatry* 58:622–624, 1995.

18. McLaurin RL, Tutor FT: Acute subdural hematoma. Review of ninety cases. *J Neurosurg* 18:61–67, 1961.

19. Haselberger K, Pucher R, Auer LM: Prognosis after acute subdural or epidural haemorrhage. *Acta Neurochir* 90:111–116, 1988.

20. Cervoni L, Rocchi G, Salvati M, Celli P, Maleci A: Extradural haematoma of posterior cranial fossa. *J Neurosurg Sci* 37:47–51, 1993,

21. Dunne JW, Chakera T, Kermode S: Cerebellar hemorrhage—diagnosis and treatment: a study of 75 consecutive cases. *QJ Med* 64:739–754, 1987.

22. Rinkel GJE, Wijdicks EFM, Vermeulen M, Hasan D, Brouwens PJAM, Van Gijn J: The clinical course of perimesencephalic nonaneurysmal subarachnoid hemorrhage. *Ann Neurol* 29:463–468, 1991.

23. Ropper AH, Gress DR: Computerized tomography and clinical features of large cerebral hemorrhages. *Cerebrovasc Dis* 1:38–42, 1991.

24. Toffol GI, Biller T, Adams HP, et al: The predictive value of arteriography in nontraumatic intracerebral hemorrhage. *Stroke* 17:881, 1986.

25. Juvula S, Heiskanen O, Poranen A, et al: The treatment of spontaneous intracerebral hemorrhage: a prospective randomized trial of surgical and conservative treatment. *J Neurosurg* 70:755–758, 1989.

26. Lisk DR, Pasteur W, Rhoades H, Putnam RD, Grotta JC: Early presentation of hemispheric intracerebral hemorrhage: prediction of outcome and guidelines for treatment allocation. *Neurology* 44:133–139, 1994.

27. Longstreth WT: Prediction of outcomes after intracerebral hemorrhage. *Stroke* 24:1761, 1993.

28. Daverat P, Castel JP, Dartigues JF, et al: Death and functional outcome after spontaneous intracerebral hemorrhage: a prospective study of 166 cases using multivariate analysis. *Stroke* 22:1–6, 1991.

29. Dixon AA, Holness RO, Howes WJ, et al: Spontaneous intracerebral hemorrhage: an analysis of factors affecting prognosis. *Can J Neurol Sci* 12:267–271, 1985.

30. Franke CL, van Swieten JC, Algra A, van Gijn J: Prognostic factors in patients with intracerebral

haematoma. *J Neurol Neurosurg Psychiatry* 55:653–657, 1992.

31. Broderick JP, Brott TG: Prediction of outcomes after intracerebral hemorrhage. *Stroke* 24:1761, 1993.

32. Broderick JP, Brott TG, Duldner JE, Tomsick T, Huster G: Volume of intracerebral hemorrhage: a powerful and easy-to-use predictor of 30-day mortality. *Stroke* 24:987–993, 1993.

33. Cerillo A, Villano M, Vizioli L, Narciso N, Tedeschi E, Bucchiero A, Quaglietta P, Cirillo S, La Tessa G: Intracerebral haemorrhage: criteria for prognosis on the grounds of clinical and CT data. *J Neurosurg Sci* 34:123–135, 1990.

34. Tuhrim S, Dambrosia JM, Price TR, et al: Intra-cerebral hemorrhage: external validation and extension of a model for prediction of 30-day survival. *Ann Neurol* 29:658–663, 1991.

35. Tuhrim S, Dambrosia JM, Price TR, et al: Prediction of intracerebral hemorrhage survival. *Ann Neurol* 24:258–263, 1988.

36. Portenoy RK, Lipton RB, Berger AR, et al: Intra-cerebral hemorrhage: a model for the prediction of outcome. *J Neurol Neurosurg Psychiatry* 50:976–979, 1987.

37. Young WB, Lee KP, Pessin MP, et al: Prognostic significance of ventricular blood in supratentorial hemorrhage: a volumetric study. *Neurology* 40:616–619, 1990.

Chapter 6
HEAD INJURY

R. Moulton

EPIDEMIOLOGY

Traumatic brain injury is an extremely common cause of impaired consciousness. Estimates of incidence in the United States vary from 200 to 400 per 100,000 population.[1] Like other forms of traumatic injury, traumatic brain injury has its highest incidence in the second and third decades (usually as a result of vehicular trauma) and declines in later decades. Unlike some other forms of traumatic injury, there remains a considerable incidence in middle and old age, primarily due to injury by falling (Fig. 6-1). Typically, the male/female incidence varies between 2:1 and 3:1.[1] Because of the high incidence of persistent disability in survivors of moderate and severe head injury, and the young age at which many of these disabilities are incurred, traumatic brain injury carries extremely high direct and indirect economic costs, and constitutes a major public health problem. The lifetime direct and indirect costs of hospitalized and fatal head injuries occurring in the year 1985 in the United States have been estimated at 129 billion dollars.[2] Many, if not most, of these injuries are preventable and a number of prevention initiatives have arisen over the last few years, ranging from more general measures (e.g., changes in drinking-and-driving legislation) to the introduction of specific programs to prevent neurologic injury that are targeted at the adolescent population.* Examples of successful prevention strategies include bicycle and motorcycle rider helmet use and legislative initiatives in this regard.[3,4]

Although in virtually all studies, vehicular trauma is the commonest cause of injury (accounting for 27 to 60 percent of all injuries),[1,5] injury etiology typically varies according to the geographic area studied. Falls and injury resulting from interpersonal violence typically occur more often in urban areas.[6] Economic and social factors influence the type of injuries seen from one center to another and this, in turn, may play a considerable role in the variation in outcome from injury between centers.[7]

Alcohol intoxication is an extremely common factor in traumatic brain injury. In the author's own center, the incidence of obvious clinical signs of intoxication varies from 26 percent of patients involved in vehicular trauma to 41 percent of patients who have fallen to over 50 percent of patients who have been assaulted (Fig. 6-2). These figures are typical of those found in the literature.[8] Impairment of judgment and/or coordination caused by alcohol are frequently important factors in causing the injury, and the subsequent examination of patients may be confounded by the sedating effects of alcohol. Patients with evolving intracranial mass lesions occasionally deteriorate while under medical observation, because the earliest changes in their level of consciousness are mistakenly attributed to alcohol intoxication. The effect of alcohol on the injured human brain remains unclear and may vary with the dose, although animal studies indicate a

---

* Think First Foundation, Park Ridge, Ill.

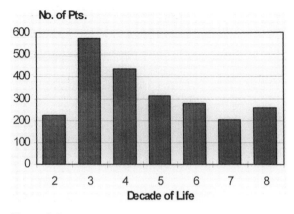

No. of Pts.

Figure 6-1

Patient age distribution by decade at an adult neuro-surgical unit at St. Michael's Hospital, Toronto, Canada. Like other forms of traumatic injury, there is a peak incidence in the second decade. Unlike some other forms of injury, there is a significant "tail" to the distribution in middle and old age. Falls account for the majority of injuries in the latter age group.

deleterious effect of alcohol on injured brain and spinal cord tissue.[9] In the clinical setting, recovery from brain injury may be complicated by the effects of alcohol withdrawal (i.e, delirium, seizures). A history of chronic alcohol usage or an admission

Figure 6-2

Incidence of alcohol intoxication by etiology. The bars are normalized to 100 percent. Mcycle = motorcycle; MVA = vehicle occupant; Ped = pedestrian; Other includes unwitnessed falls and assaults, recreational, industrial, and sporting injuries.

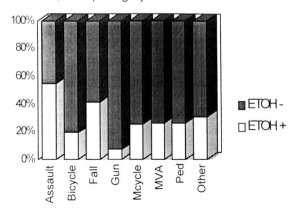

alcohol level ≥ 50 mg% (10.9 mmol/L) has been shown to predispose patients to recurrent intracranial hematomas. This may be due to alcohol-induced hemostatic abnormalities.[10]

Normally, the diagnosis of traumatic brain injury is not difficult, provided a history of injury is available from the patient (in cases of mild injury) or from witnesses (if the patient remains unconscious at the time of assessment). Diagnostic difficulties most commonly arise when a patient is found unconscious and brought to hospital without witnesses to the causative event. A less common source of diagnostic error occurs when a non-traumatic catastrophic neurologic event (usually cerebrovascular) causes a patient to fall or lose control of the vehicle. Neurologic deficits, including impairment of consciousness, may then be falsely attributed to traumatic injury rather than to the inciting event.

CLASSIFICATION

Injury Type (Blunt versus Penetrating)

Injury may first be classified into blunt and penetrating types. In penetrating injury, the skull and meninges are violated and the underlying brain tissue is directly disrupted by the object causing the injury and/or indriven bone and contaminants from the scalp. In missile injuries, the neurologic sequelae of the injury, including disturbance of consciousness, depend on the kinetic energy of the penetrating missile[11] and the site of injury. Stab wounds or low-velocity missile wounds to the hemispheres may produce little or no disturbance in consciousness, and occasionally no focal neurology if a "silent" area of the brain (e.g., single frontal lobe) is involved. High-velocity missile wounds from military assault weapons unleash a large amount of energy to brain remote from the missile tract, typically produce profound coma, and are commonly fatal.[12] All penetrating wounds to the brain expose the patient to the risks of secondary intracranial bleeding and central nervous system infection. These may, in turn, cause delayed deterioration in consciousness.

Blunt head injury is the most common form of civilian head injury. Injury may be confined to the face and skull or may involve the brain as well. To the neurologist or neurosurgeon, the greatest significance of facial, scalp, and skull injuries is that they signify that an impact to the head has occurred and that accompanying brain injury is a real possibility. Evidence of scalp bruising, laceration, facial or skull fracture is extremely useful in sorting out the etiology of unwitnessed coma.

Injury Severity, Level of Consciousness, and Posttraumatic Amnesia

The severity of blunt injury to the brain is primarily judged on the depth and duration of alterations in consciousness. Anatomic injury features (skull fracture, intracranial hematoma, etc.) are of secondary importance. The most common measurement of injury severity used in traumatic brain injury is the Glasgow Coma Scale (GCS).[13] It has received almost universal acceptance based on ease of use, precise characterization of disturbed consciousness, and low rates of interobserver variability. The scale was initially introduced as a 14-point scale based on the observation and documentation of patient responses in three categories of behaviour: eye opening, verbal response, and motor response. The original 14-point scale was subsequently revised to a 15-point scale with the differentiation between normal (withdrawal) and abnormal flexor (flexor posturing) responses. Clinical studies of the GCS at admission to hospital and following resuscitation of systemic physiologic perturbations (e.g. shock, hypoxia) have shown the GCS to be an excellent predictor of patient outcome, more valuable than imaging studies or intracranial pressure (ICP) measurement, and approximately equivalent in prognostic accuracy to multiple modality evoked potentials.[14]

Other coma scores have been proposed since the introduction of the GCS, but none has supplanted it (see discussion of coma scales in Chap. 3). Some of these scores incorporate information about brainstem function. While it is important to examine for and record evidence of brainstem dysfunction in severe injuries, abnormalities therein are not a measure of level of consciousness per se but indicate the anatomic localization of lesions, and their inclusion in a severity scoring system, while potentially strengthening the prognostic value, has the disadvantage of mixing lesion localization with level of consciousness information, thereby lessening the clinical descriptive value. A frequently used scoring system in the multiple trauma literature is the Abbreviated Injury Scale (AIS)[15] for head injury (and other body regions). This is designed as an anatomic injury scoring system. The weakness of a purely anatomic approach to scoring in brain injury has forced inclusion of some data concerning the depth and duration of unconsciousness in patients without intracranial hematomas to improve the predictive value of the score. It still suffers the weakness of scoring patients with acute intracranial hematomas based only on the size of the clot, regardless of the level of consciousness, so that the accuracy of the AIS in predicting outcome from head injury suffers as a result. The gold standard of severity scoring in neurosurgical units remains the Glasgow Coma Scale. Injuries resulting in an admission Glasgow Coma Score of 8 or less are considered *severe*, scores of 9 to 12 are *moderate* injuries, and scores of 13 and above are *mild* injuries.

An older method of classification of injury severity involves the length of posttraumatic amnesia (PTA).[16] Injuries producing less than 1 h of posttraumatic amnesia are considered *mild*, 1-24 h *serious*, and greater than 24 h *severe*. It is important to note that this classification is not intended to correspond to the classification based on the admission GCS, although the terms are similar. This method of injury classification suffers from the disadvantage of being entirely retrospective. One can only determine the length of PTA once the patient has regained consciousness and can describe when they recovered the ability to form new memories. The information is obviously completely subjective, and typically is of little or no use in the initial acute clinical management of patients. The Galveston Orientation and Amnesia Test (GOAT) is a means of attempting to define the end of posttraumatic amnesia prospectively.[17]

However, actual recovery from amnesia and recovery according to the GOAT may not always correspond.[18] The duration of PTA continues to be of value in predicting late cognitive disability.

PATHOLOGY AND PATHOPHYSIOLOGY

Injury Mechanics

At its most fundamental level, blunt brain injury involves the transfer of kinetic energy to the brain by means of inertial forces (acceleration or deceleration). The injury may involve contact of an object with the head (impact injury), or may take place without any contact (impulse injury).[19] Angular (i.e., through an arc) acceleration/deceleration is tolerated much less than translational (straight line) acceleration/deceleration, and, in the experimental situation, rotational forces are required to produce unconsciousness and the diffuse parenchymal changes associated with more severe grades of unconsciousness.[20,21] Pure translational forces, however, may produce intracerebral hematomas in the experimental situation.[20] Typical acceleration/deceleration injury is associated with injury duration of 200 m or less. Impact injury superimposes the sequelae of skull contact (skull fracturing and its complications) on any brain injury produced by the inertial forces. Complications of skull fracture include cranial nerve palsies, epidural hemorrhage, and infection of the cerebrospinal fluid (CSF) and/or brain parenchyma (brain abscess) if the scalp and meninges are breached.

Skull fractures may involve the vault or base and may be closed or open (compound). A fracture is considered to be depressed if the outer table of one of the fragments lies below the inner table of the adjacent skull. Depressed fragments may lacerate the underlying meninges and brain, and, in the latter circumstance, are often associated with parenchymal hemorrhage of varying size.

Fractures of the skull base typically involve the anterior or middle fossae floors, or, much less commonly, the clivus. If the paranasal sinuses or the mastoid air cells are involved with the fracture and the meninges are breached at the fracture site, there may be leakage of CSF through the nose or ears (i.e., rhinorrhea, otorrhea) and the patient is at risk for early or delayed meningitis if the leak either does not seal itself or is not repaired operatively. The usual organism in infection acquired outside hospital is the pneumococcus. Nosocomial infections may involve *Staphylococcus aureus* or possibly gram-negative organisms. Fractures of the petrous bone may disrupt either the middle ear ossicles or the cochlear apparatus. In the latter circumstance, the hearing loss is permanent. Facial nerve palsy may also occur with petrous bone fractures, often on a delayed basis. Lower cranial nerve palsies may rarely occur with fractures in the region of the jugular foramen.

Epidural hemorrhage may occur from tears in meningeal arteries or veins or from the dural sinuses. The most frequent culprit is a tear in the middle meningeal artery resulting from fracturing of the temporal bone, and causing a middle fossa hemorrhage. Epidural hemorrhage from venous sinuses usually occurs at the vertex (sagittal sinus) or in the posterior fossa (transverse sinus). Enlarging hematomas produce compression and shift of the underlying brain, and, depending on the rate and amount of hemorrhage, may rapidly become fatal. Smaller hemorrhages beneath fractures [diagnosed frequently since the advent of computed tomography (CT) scanning] may be clinically insignificant.

Contusion   Contusion of the brain underneath the site of skull impact is called *coup* contusion. Contusion of brain tissue at a site opposite the site of skull impact is referred to as *contre-coup*. Cavitation of brain tissue has been invoked to explain *contre-coup* injury. Abrupt acceleration of the head moves the skull away from the brain opposite the site of the blow due to the inertia of the brain within the skull. Negative pressure of sufficient magnitude to produce cavitation in the brain tissue may be seen at the site opposite the site of a blow to the head.[22] Both *coup* and *contre-coup* contusions are usually confined to the inferior surface of the frontal lobes and the anterior and inferior surfaces of the temporal lobes. The skull at these locations contains sharp and/or irregular projections and a much simpler theory holds that these projections lacerate the brain surface with movement of the brain over the irregular surface of the skull, thus explaining the frontal and temporal preponderance of contusional injury.[22] Laceration of the brain surface may produce continued hemorrhage into the brain substance with the development of a confluent intracerebral hematoma, or may result in bleeding into the subdural space (acute subdural hematoma). The latter may also be produced by tearing of bridging veins, or, much more rarely, from tears of arterial twigs passing between the dura and cortex.[23] Tearing of bridging veins has been shown to be related to the strain rate (i.e., the rate of acceleration/deceleration) produced by the injury.[24]

Diffuse Axonal Injury Most significant in the production of traumatic brain injury is the effect of acceleration/deceleration on the brain parenchyma. The forces involved include compressive, tensile, and shear forces.[19] It is the latter force that is felt to result in the greatest disruption of brain tissue. Shear injury predominates in white matter fiber tracts, and individual axons within these tracts may be disrupted. Studies by Holbourn, and later Strich and others, led to the postulate that shear injury produces immediate physical separation of axons, with immediate loss of function.[25,26] Histopathologic studies were most commonly performed in patients who lived for days or weeks following injury, and these showed axon retraction balls (the retracted ends of a severed axon) throughout the white matter in the affected individuals. More recently, using serial histologic studies in an animal model of head injury, Povlishock has shown that axon changes that ultimately culminate in separation of the axon evolve over hours in initially intact axons.[27] Mechanistic explanations have subsequently invoked cytoskeletal failure.[28] The latter may be due to entry of ionic calcium into the axoplasm.[29] These same evolutionary changes in axon integrity, first demonstrated in animals, have now been shown to occur in humans.[28,29] The potential therapeutic implications of this are considerable, as the clinical treatment of patients with diffuse axonal injury has long been predicated on the somewhat nihilistic view that diffuse axonal injury is not amenable to treatment, based on the assumption of immediate physical disruption of axons. While there are now cautious grounds for optimism in his area, development of efficacious clinical treatment strategies has not yet resulted from this altered view of axonal injury. Development of appropriate therapeutic strategies will likely have to await the elucidation of the precise mechanism(s) of cytoskeletal failure.

Primary Injury

From a clinical standpoint, brain injury is best thought of as occurring in two phases. Primary injury is that injury which is produced at the moment of impact and consists of brain contusion/laceration and diffuse axonal injury. Laceration and contusion of the brain surface may uncommonly take place without loss of consciousness. Alteration of consciousness is the clinical hallmark of diffuse axonal injury. Loss of consciousness may be produced by lesions affecting the rostral brainstem reticular activating system or by diffuse dysfunction of both cerebral hemispheres. The experimental studies of Ommaya and Gennarrelli have shown that the histologic changes associated with inertial injury and loss of consciousness are centrifugally distributed, i.e., they are always greater in the periphery of the hemispheres than in the brainstem or deep portion of the hemispheres.[20] Human studies have confirmed the predominance of hemispheric damage and shown that brainstem neuronal disruption occurs with only the most severe injuries.[26] Isolated blunt brainstem injury is an extremely rare occurrence and is usually associated with fracture of the basisphenoid or basiocciput.

The biochemical events associated with blunt brain injury and loss of consciousness include a sudden increase in extracellular potassium- and calcium-dependent release of excitotoxic amino acids, particularly glutamate.[30] The latter results in a positive feedback loop involving further increases in extracellular potassium beyond physiologic levels, and consequent depression of neuronal activity. Potassium efflux is accompanied by an increase in intracellular glycolysis and consequent increases in intracellular lactate. Increased glycolysis has been demonstrated in both animals and humans by positron tomography (PET) studies.[31] Intracellular calcium also increases. The putative role of Ca^{2+} entry into neurons in human head injury served as the basis of two trials of a calcium channel blocker following human head injury. Both trials were prospective randomized trials of nimodipine and neither showed a beneficial effect on outcome from head injury.[32]

Considerable attention has also been focused on the potential role of glutamate excitotoxicity in head injury. In human head injury, glutamate levels have been found to be elevated above normal control levels early after injury, and this elevation may persist for several days.[33] Further evidence for a putative role of excitotoxicity in human head injury is provided in an autopsy study by Ross et al,[34] describing selective neuronal loss in the thalamic reticular nucleus, thought to be due to sustained excitation of this nucleus by cortico-thalamic projections. It is possible that excitotoxins are passively released from damaged cells, that there is a failure of reuptake mechanisms by neurons or astroglia, or that there is pathologically increased release from neurons in response to secondary ischemia. Clinical trials of glutamate antagonists are now beginning in head injury. It remains to reconcile the putative role of glutamate excitotoxicity in brain injury with the fact that diffuse axonal injury, the major histologic feature of blunt brain injury, occurs in the white matter of the brain where there are no glutamate receptors.

Conversion of arachidonic acid to prostaglandins/leukotrienes culminates in the generation of free radicals of oxygen in experimental models of head injury. Free radicals may damage both cerebral parenchyma and the cerebral microvasculature.[35] Animal experiments have shown some benefit in treatment of head injury with free radical scavenging compounds, and the beneficial effects of methyprednisone in human spinal cord injury are thought to result from the inhibition of lipid peroxidation and the resulting generation of free radicals of oxygen.[36] Unfortunately, the success of glucocorticoids in ameliorating the effects of spinal cord injury has not been duplicated for human head injury. Superoxide dismutase (SOD) is a free radical scavenger. Phase II trials of this agent have shown a trend toward improved clinical outcome in patients with severe head injury and a positive effect on raised ICP following head injury.[37] The latter may be due to a protective effect on the cerebral vascular bed.

Secondary Insults to the Injured Brain

Secondary insults[38] are those injury phenomena that evolve subsequent to the initial impact injury. The occurrence and seriousness of these are often only partially dependent on the severity of the primary impact injury, although, as a general rule, the incidence and severity of secondary insults tends to increase with increasing severity of primary impact injury. The importance of secondary insults is that they are often preventable, most often treatable, and are a significant source of increased morbidity and mortality following head injury.

Intracranial Hemorrhage Traumatic intracranial hemorrhage may occur into the brain parenchyma, the subdural space, or between the outer layer of the dura and the skull (extra/epidural). The mechanism of hematoma formation is discussed above. In the author's own patient population, the overall incidence of operable traumatic intracranial hemorrhages is approximately 26 percent. The incidence rises to 50 percent in patients admitted to hospital in coma. A breakdown of the relative incidence is shown in Fig. 6-3. Acute subdural hemorrhage is the most common; isolated extradural hemorrhage is the least common. Factors that predispose one to the risk of traumatic intracranial hemorrhage include increasing injury severity (lower GCS score), increasing age of the patient, and the presence of a skull fracture.[39,40] Patients from motor vehicle accidents are less prone to develop intracranial hematoma than are victims of assault or car-pedestrian collisions.[24,39]

Hematomas exert both local and distant effects on the injured brain. In the case of contusions/intracerebral hematomas, there is obvious

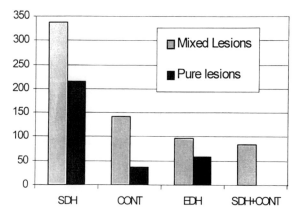

Figure 6-3

Incidence of operable intracranial hematomas in 2310 consecutive admissions to an adult neurosurgical unit. The total number of patients with operable hematoma(s) was 509. SDH= acute subdural hematoma; CONT= contusion/intracerebral hematoma; EDH= isolated extradural hematoma.

disruption of brain parenchyma at the hematoma site. Local damage from surface hematomas may occur due to local ischemia from the pressure of the clot on the surface vessels, ischemia from release of vasoactive substances from the clot in the case of subdural hematomas, or possibly from simple mechanical distortion of the underlying brain. In animal models of acute subdural hematomas, parenchymal ischemia and increased concentrations of glutamate are found under the clot.[41] In the clinical situation, one may occasionally see CT evidence of infarction in the subjacent brain following evacuation of an acute subdural hematoma.

The remote effects of intracranial hematomas occur as the result of raised ICP and brain herniation. These are more fully discussed in the following section.

Raised Intracranial Pressure The volume of the skull is constant and is made up of the brain parenchyma, with its intra- and extracellular spaces, the volume of blood circulating within and around the brain, and the volume of the CSF spaces, intraventricular and subarachnoid. Increments in volume of any of these components, or volume increase occurring as the result of

intracranial bleeding, must be accompanied by reduction in one of the other components or the pressure inside the skull will rise. Compliance is the change in volume per unit change in pressure. This relationship is an exponential one, but can be made linear by plotting log pressure versus volume, the slope of which is the pressure-volume index.[42] The inverse of the compliance is the elastance of the intracranial contents. Typically, changes in volume resulting from brain swelling or traumatic hematomas are compensated for by decrements in the volume of blood circulating through the brain or by displacement of CSF out of the cranium. During the initial period of compensation, there is little or no change in ICP, i.e., compliance is high. Once this capacity for volume compensation is lost, small increments or decrements in volume may produce large pressure fluctuations (Fig. 6-4). These relationships form the basis of treatment of ICP following head injury.

Raised pressure is felt to exert its harmful effects by brain herniation (see Chap. 4) or by lowering the cerebral perfusion pressure, i.e., the difference between cerebral arterial and venous

Figure 6-4

The pressure-volume curve. The volume of the skull is constant—the sum of the various compartments listed in the equation. When CSF and blood can no longer be displaced out of the cranium to compensate for volume increments, the pressure rises sharply with additional small increments in volume.

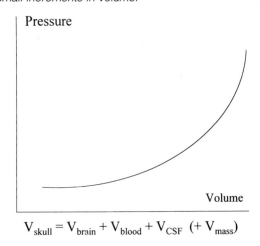

$$V_{skull} = V_{brain} + V_{blood} + V_{CSF} \ (+ \ V_{mass})$$

pressures. The latter pressure is identical to ICP, so that the difference can be measured clinically by subtracting mean ICP from the mean arterial blood pressure. At a cerebral perfusion pressure of about 70 mmHg, there may be an autoregulatory break, i.e., the cerebral blood flow becomes dependent on cerebral perfusion pressure (CPP) (Fig. 3-18).[43] Ideally, therefore, CPP should be maintained at 70 mmHg or greater. In a stable patient, this is normally not difficult. The greatest problems arise in patients who are hypotensive as the result of accompanying systemic injuries. The CPP is also typically reduced below critical levels in the terminal phase of uncontrollable ICP when the ICP may exceed the mean arterial blood pressure with consequent cessation of cerebral blood flow. This phenomenon is the basis for the use of cerebral angiography as an ancillary test in the determination of brain death.

Brain herniation occurs when pressure differentials develop between different compartments within the cranium, or between the cranial and spinal subarachnoid space. These are most often the result of localized masses, and less often the result of diffuse or localized brain swelling without a mass lesion. Dural partitions separate the two hemispheres (falx cerebri) and separate the anterior and middle cranial fossae from the posterior fossa (tentorium cerebelli). Herniation may occur through these dural partitions (subfalcine, transtentorial) or through the foramen magnum (tonsillar/transforaminal). Subfalcine herniation is not associated with any recognizable clinical signs. Transtentorial herniation is a critical clinical event in brain injury. Its occurrence is heralded by the development of ipsilateral pupillary dilatation, loss of pupillary reaction to light, and extra-ocular palsy. This has been attributed to pressure of the herniating uncus on the oculomotor nerve (however, see Chap. 4). Normally, the dilated pupil is associated with a contralateral hemiparesis or hemiplegia as a result of local effects of the mass on the ipsilateral hemisphere. However, the pressure of the mass can sometimes produce impingement of the contralateral cerebral peduncle on the adjacent contralateral edge of the tentorium (Kernohan's notch), resulting in paralysis that is ipsilateral to

the mass and dilated pupil. The ipsilateral posterior cerebral artery may become distorted and ipsilateral occipital lobe infarction can occur. With continued herniation, the midbrain becomes compressed from side to side and the entire brainstem may become displaced downward. Perforating branches of the basilar artery become stretched and may tear, producing hemorrhages within the substance of the midbrain or pons (Duret hemorrhages). Typically, signs of brainstem dysfunction are present (bilateral absence of pupillary reaction, loss of oculocephalic and oculovestibular responses). At this stage, the patient's condition becomes irretrievable and the outcome is usually death or permanent total disability. For this reason, the development of signs of early transtentorial herniation constitutes a surgical emergency. Rapid removal of mass effect early in the above sequence of events may allow for substantial recovery. This is particularly true in the case of isolated extradural hemorrhages that are associated with little or no primary impact injury.

Herniation of the cerebellar tonsils through the foramen magnum produces abrupt loss of brainstem function (apnea, loss of gag and corneal responses, vasomotor collapse). It is normally the penultimate event in cases of uncontrollable ICP and often occurs at some time subsequent to the development of transtentorial herniation in traumatic brain injury. This sequence of events occurs in head injury because of the preponderance of both diffuse brain injury and traumatic intracranial hematomas in the supratentorial compartments. Isolated hematomas in the posterior fossa are quite unusual, and only in this circumstance might one see development of tonsillar herniation without prior tentorial herniation.

Hypoxia / Ischemia   Ischemia and/or hypoxia occur when there is inadequate blood flow to the brain to meet metabolic requirements, or there is inadequate oxygenation of the blood flowing to the brain. Post-mortem studies of patients dying from traumatic brain injury show a very high incidence of ischemic change in neurons, even when one eliminates patients dying of uncontrolled ICP.[44] Until recently, these autopsy findings were difficult to reconcile with studies of cerebral blood flow in patients following head injury. The pioneering work of Obrist showed an extremely low incidence of ischemic levels of blood flow in measurements conducted in the early days following head injury.[45] Most often, flows were found to be normal for metabolic requirements, elevated for metabolic levels, but within normal limits for awake patients (relative hyperemia), or elevated for even normal awake patients (absolute hyperemia). More recent studies by Bouma and Muizelaar[46] have shown that if one studies patients early enough after injury (within 12 h), there is a significant incidence (33 percent) of ischemic levels of blood flow. This incidence rises the earlier one is able to study the patients. In almost all patients who survive the first day or two of injury, the flows tend to return to normal or hyperemic levels after the first 24 to 36 h.[46] The tendency for blood flows to increase to normal levels is shown in Fig. 6-5, derived from a group of patients with severe head injury who were monitored in the author's intensive care unit.

Clinically obvious causes of ischemia or hypoxia are usually systemic. By far the most common cause of hypoxia and ischemia early after brain injury is the failure to adequately manage the airway and resuscitate patients from shock due to accompanying injuries. Early uncontrolled posttraumatic seizures may result in a situation in which even normal levels of blood flow and oxygenation are inadequate to meet the heightened metabolic requirements of the brain. In this circumstance, one must control the seizures in addition to carrying out the appropriate supportive systemic measures.

Loss of consciousness due to brain injury normally produces reduction of respiratory drive and depression or loss of reflexes that control and protect the upper airway. The tongue may partially or completely obstruct the airway. The patient loses control of swallowing and gag reflexes and there is suppression of cough reflexes. Frequently, patients regurgitate gastric contents into the pharynx and these are aspirated into the trachea. There is loss of sensitivity to rising levels of CO_2 and there is often inadequate ventilation in response to elevated CO_2 levels. All of these conspire to produce increased partial pressure of CO_2 in the blood and decreased oxygen content. The former causes cerebral vasodilatation, increased cerebral blood volume, and raised ICP. The latter results in direct damage to brain tissue by depletion of brain energy stores. Occasionally, one may see centrally driven hyperventilation, Cheyne-Stokes respiration, or other abnormal breathing patterns. The localizing significance of these patterns of respiration is dubious, and they are often the harbinger of impending respiratory arrest. This is particularly true in the case of ataxic respiration. There is no role for continued observation of respiratory disturbances in the acute management of comatose head-injured patients. All comatose patients require endotracheal intubation with a cuffed endotracheal tube to protect the airway, and almost all will require mechanical ventilation to ensure adequate oxygenation and to avoid hypercarbia.

Hypotension is not the result of brain injury unless the injury is so severe that the vasomotor centers in the medulla oblongata have become compromised. This is normally seen only in established or impending brain death. In virtually all other circumstances, hypotension is the result of

Figure 6-5
Cerebral blood flow (CBF) measurements at 12-h intervals postinjury in a series of 52 patients with severe head injuries. The units of measurement (ordinate) are mL per 100 g brain tissue per min.

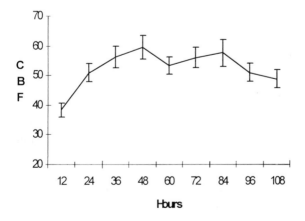

accompanying obvious or occult injury to other organ systems. In the elderly or in very young children, scalp lacerations accompanying the head injury may produce sufficient hemorrhage to result in hypotension. In most cases, however, injuries associated with the hypotension involve the chest, abdomen, pelvis, or uncontrolled bleeding from major vascular injuries in the extremities. The patient should be adequately resuscitated with crystalloid fluid and packed red blood cells. Concern about aggravation of brain edema as the result of volume resuscitation with crystalloid solutions has not been borne out in patients with multiple injuries. Furthermore, there is incontrovertible evidence of the harmful effects of shock on patients with brain injury. Chesnut et al have documented a 150 percent increase in mortality in patients who are hypotensive following severe brain injury. Hypoxia was also shown to be deleterious, but not to the same extent as hypotension. The same study showed that there was no effect of multiple systemic injuries on brain injury if one controlled for the effects of hypoxia and hypotension.[47]

Sepsis   Sepsis may arise from central or systemic sources and both may adversely affect cerebral function. Central causes usually are the result of meningitis or, less commonly, cerebral abscess, subdural empyema, or extradural abscess. All arise as a result of breaching of the normal sterile intracranial space, the usual cause being basal skull fracture with persistent CSF leakage. Parenchymal abscesses are usually the result of penetrating wounds. All cases in which there is potential contamination of the intracranial contents require close observation, debridement and closure of compound depressed skull fractures, and operative repair of CSF fistulae in cases of basal skull fracture with persistent (beyond a few days) CSF leakage. Normally, otorrhea ceases spontaneously. Rhinorrhea often requires open repair. Use of prophylactic antibiotics is controversial. In the author's unit, they are not used for fear of promoting the growth of resistant organisms.

Systemic infection usually arises within a few days of injury in patients with persistent unconsciousness. The usual sources are lung and urinary tract. The patient's neurologic state may be transiently worsened by the effects of sepsis and/or by the associated fever (Chap. 12). Reversal of the neurologic deterioration is the rule with successful management of the systemic infection. The differential diagnosis of fever in these patients includes pulmonary embolism and, less commonly, febrile reactions to prophylactic anticonvulsants.

Electrolyte Disorders   Fluid and electrolyte disorders frequently complicate severe traumatic brain injury, and, less often, may complicate lesser degrees of injury. The most common of these is the syndrome of inappropriate antidiuretic hormone secretion (SIADH). As the result of the retention of excessive amounts of free water, the serum sodium concentration may fall to levels sufficiently low to produce worsening in the level of consciousness or to precipitate seizure activity (see Chap. 17).

Diabetes insipidus occurs as the result of loss of secretion of antidiuretic hormone from the posterior pituitary gland. Patients have excessive diuresis, with a resultant increase in serum osmolarity and serum sodium. The diuresis is severe enough to produce hypotension. In the context of blunt head injury, diabetes insipidus is rare, other than as a preterminal event. Presumably, this is a result of the deep central location of the hypothalamus and pituitary gland and the relative lack of involvement of this area in all but the most severe injuries.

DIFFERENTIAL DIAGNOSIS

Brain injury due to trauma is seldom difficult to diagnose, other than as the result of unwitnessed injuries, or when a minor fall and bump on the head is the result of some other catastrophic illness, such as cardiac arrest, subarachnoid hemorrhage, or ischemic stroke. In the latter circumstances, modern imaging with CT scanning has gone a long way toward sorting out the differential diagnosis because of the often characteristic findings of traumatic brain injury versus other forms of intracranial pathology.

Unwitnessed Coma

Diagnostic difficulties frequently arise when a patient is brought into the emergency room having been found unconscious, without witnesses to the events preceding the disturbance of consciousness. In such cases, the differential diagnosis includes drug or alcohol intoxication or metabolic coma. Diabetics may be suffering from either hypoglycemic or hyperglycemic coma. In the former circumstance, administration of 50 g of intravenous glucose may be lifesaving and is not harmful should the patient be suffering from coma of some other etiology. It should be followed by thiamine administration to prevent Wernicke's encephalopathy in potentially nutritionally deprived patients.

Physical examination of the head may reveal signs of head trauma, such as scalp or facial lacerations or bruising. Particular patterns of bruising indicate basal skull fracture rather than simple direct trauma to the face or scalp. These consist of uni- or bilateral periorbital ecchymosis (raccoon eyes, Fig. 6-6) or bruising over the mastoid (Battle's sign). The former occurs in fractures of the orbital roof (anterior fossa floor) when blood tracks through the loose orbital connective tissue until it is stopped by the attachment of the orbital periosteum at the margins of the bony orbit. This gives the characteristic raccoon appearance which is distinguished from an ordinary black eye by the fact that the bruising does not extend beyond the orbital rim onto the cheek or forehead. Battle's sign occurs when bleeding from a petrous bone fracture tracks through the overlying scalp, producing a bruise over the mastoid. The bruising remains localized over the mastoid process as there is no subgaleal space into which the blood may disperse, unlike over the vault of the skull. Fractures of the vault bleed beneath the galea aponeurotica, the latter being easily separable from the underlying pericranium. The resulting subgaleal hematoma produces a swollen, boggy area of scalp overlying the fracture. In cases of temporal bone fracture, there may be otorrhagia or otorrhea, alerting the examiner to the presence of the basal skull fracture. Rhinorrhea may occur with fractures of the anterior fossa floor.

Care should be taken not to move the patient's head during the initial examination and resuscitation of the patient if there is any suspicion of trauma. Cervical spine fractures occur in association with head injury and cannot be confidently ruled out in an unconscious patient without a minimum of a lateral, anteroposterior (AP), and open-mouth odontoid cervical radiographs. In one series of 775 motor vehicle crash patients, the incidence of cervical spinal fractures in patients with disturbed consciousness was 13 percent.[48] If endotracheal intubation is required prior to obtaining cervical spine film, gentle in-line traction should be maintained on the cervical spine during the intubation procedure. Immobilization of the spine with a rigid collar and sandbags should be maintained until appropriate radiographic views can be obtained. Cervical cord injury (central cord syndrome) may occur in the absence of a spinal fracture. Typically, the injury results from a hyperextension injury in a patient with a spinal canal narrowed by cervical spondylosis. Clinical signs of a hyperextension injury include bruising of the chin or forehead.

The neurologic examination of an unconscious patient with head injury is brief. In the vast majority of such patients, lesions requiring surgical intervention can only be reliably diagnosed with a CT scan, and the examination of myotatic

Figure 6-6

Raccoon eye on patient's left. This is a sign of fracture of the anterior fossa floor.

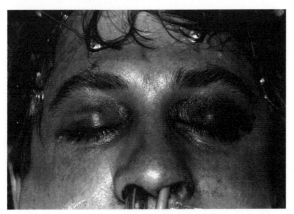

reflexes, plantar responses, etc., has no bearing on management decisions, nor any role in determining prognosis. The level of consciousness is the single most important feature of the examination and is ascertained using the parameters of the GCS. Discrepancies in the motor response between left and right sides, elicited as part of the GCS, should be noted. A brief examination of brainstem function is then carried out. The commonly elicited signs are pupillary size and reaction, corneal responses, and the gag reflex. The latter is often apparent from the patient's response to airway instrumentation. Examination of extraocular movement is useful but is often hampered by the inconvenience and time delay of caloric testing and the contraindication to oculocephalic testing in patients where there is the possibility of cervical spine injury. The pupillary responses are extremely useful in cases of coma of unknown etiology. In cases of drug intoxication or metabolic coma, pupillary reaction to light is usually spared, even when there is complete flaccidity on motor examination, with loss of gag and corneal responses. In contradistinction, traumatic or other coma resulting from structural lesions impairs brainstem function in an orderly rostral-caudal fashion, i.e., pupillary response is lost before corneal or gag responses. Unilateral pupillary dilatation is always the result of a structural lesion and, for the reasons indicated above, is a surgical emergency. The one exception is mydriasis resulting from local ocular trauma, and the latter is usually evident on checking the patient history and upon general physical examination.

Serial patient examinations are important to detect changes in patient neurologic status over time. Fortunately, the brevity of the neurologic examination in the unconscious patient easily permits re-examination on a frequent basis. Primary impact injury results in a stable or improving neurologic examination. Deterioration in level of consciousness implies the presence and evolution of secondary injury processes and mandates a search for the cause and subsequent initiation of appropriate treatment.

A full history and neurologic examination is required in the patient who is known to have been unconscious or to have suffered a significant blow to the head, but who is alert and cooperative at the time of examination. Signs of subtle diffuse impairment, such as mild confusion or personality change (often noted by families), or evidence of focal dysfunction on examination will indicate the need for CT scanning and/or admission to hospital. Those patients who have suffered only a brief loss of consciousness, and who have a completely normal neurologic examination, may be discharged home with a responsible caregiver.

Multiple Trauma

While the diagnosis of traumatic brain injury in cases of multiple trauma is usually straightforward, the challenge lies in correctly prioritizing the diagnosis and therapy of the various injuries. Management of the airway and respiration, and diagnosis and treatment of lesions producing hypotension take precedence over management of the brain injury. While this is a truism, it is surprising how often this principle is overlooked or ignored, presumably because the head injury is often very obvious and injuries that may produce respiratory embarrassment or shock are often initially occult. In centers where neurosurgical consultation is not available, there may be inordinate haste to transfer the patient to a neurosurgeon, without first attending to more pressing injuries.

The general physical examination of a head-injured patient with disturbed consciousness is difficult and often unreliable due to lack of patient cooperation and an altered response to painful stimuli. This is particularly true when examining the abdomen for signs of peritoneal irritation. These may be absent in conditions that normally produce peritonitis. On the other hand, motor posturing may be associated with contraction of the abdominal musculature, which may resemble abdominal guarding in the absence of intra-abdominal pathology. Other than in very obvious circumstances (i.e., shock with a distended abdomen), it is usually necessary to rely on imaging (ultrasound, CT) or other studies (diagnostic peritoneal lavage) to make the diagnosis of intra-abdominal hemorrhage.

Investigations/Imaging

In the unconscious patient, the diagnostic investigation of choice is an unenhanced CT scan of the brain. It is the best imaging modality for detecting acute intracranial bleeding. While magnetic resonance imaging (MRI) may be more sensitive to white matter change resulting from diffuse injury, the latter does not affect the early management of the patient.[49] Additionally, special ventilators and other equipment are required in the MRI suite, making this investigation particularly difficult and inconvenient in critically ill patients.

The most important reason for obtaining a scan is to diagnose those patients with an operable acute intracranial hematoma. These are either extradural, subdural, or intracerebral, and the various types frequently coexist in the same patient, the most common combination being an acute subdural hematoma associated with a cerebral contusion (see Fig. 6-3). The CT findings for each type are quite characteristic. Extradural hematomas (Fig. 6-7) have a convex inner margin. This is the result of the hematoma having to strip the pericranium off the inner table at the margins of the hematoma. For this reason, the hematoma is always thickest in the middle and tapers at the margins where the pericranium remains attached to the skull. Using bone windows, one can often diagnose the overlying skull fracture. In contradistinction, an acute subdural hematoma (Fig. 6-8) occurs within a potential space (between the dura and arachnoid) so that the blood spreads out easily over a large part of or the entire hemisphere. The hematoma has a concave inner margin as it conforms to the shape of the underlying brain. Occasionally, there may be significant hemorrhage along the falx cerebri, or over the surface of the tentorium. Contusions have a typical appearance consisting of an admixture of blood (high signal intensity) and necrotic, edematous brain (low signal intensity) (Fig. 6-9). If bleeding within a contusion continues, the appearance may take on that of a confluent intracerebral hematoma.

In addition to the presence or absence, and location, of traumatic intracranial hematomas, other important information is evident from the CT scan. This includes the amount of midline shift (measured at the septum pellucidum), the presence or absence of subarachnoid hemorrhage, and whether or not the ambient cisterns are patent or compressed. Compressed ambient cisterns suggest the likelihood of raised ICP. This CT finding is associated with poor patient outcome, as is the presence of subarachnoid hemorrhage.[50]

The role of plain skull films in head injury has assumed progressively less importance with the widespread availability of CT scanning. The diagnostic procedure of choice in an unconscious patient is the CT scan, and treatment and CT scanning of such patients should never be delayed

Figure 6-7

Acute left extradural hematoma. Note the convex inner margin, the obliteration of the ipsilateral ventricle, and the shift of the contralateral ventricle away from the midline.

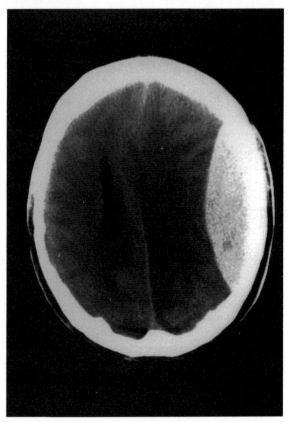

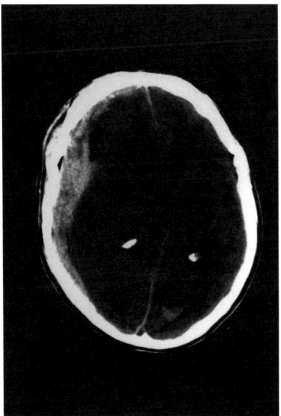

Figure 6-8

Acute right subdural hematoma. The hematoma conforms to the surface of the brain and spreads over virtually the entire hemisphere.

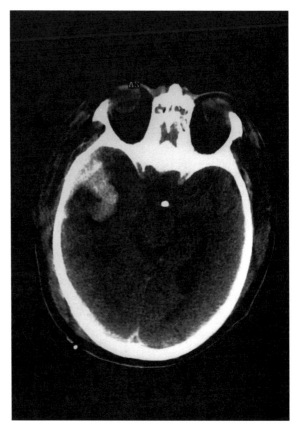

Figure 6-9

Right temporal contusion. The irregularly shaped core of hyperdense intracerebral blood is surrounded by low-density necrotic brain tissue.

in order to obtain plain skull films. Along the same lines, indirect findings of intracranial mass, such as a shifted pineal gland, are irrelevant in the CT era. Anyone in whom there is suspicion of an intracranial mass requires a scan. The value of skull radiography lies solely in the diagnosis of skull fracture, and occasionally to help in the localization of intracranial foreign bodies such as missile fragments. The latter are often obscured on CT scans by metallic artifacts and localization of foreign bodies in three-dimensional space is often easier using an AP and lateral skull film than is localization from axial imaging (Fig. 6-10).

Plain skull radiography has been advocated as a screening investigation in patients who have

suffered a head injury with disturbed consciousness, but who are conscious and have a normal neurologic examination at the time of assessment. The likelihood of intracranial bleeding in such a patient is in excess of 200-fold greater in an adult with a skull fracture than it is in a patient without a fracture of the skull.[40]

Cerebral angiography is indicated in cases where major extracranial vessel injury is suspected. Dissection of the carotid artery with partial or complete occlusion may result from injury to the artery at the skull base (Fig. 6-11). The vertebral arteries are less commonly involved (Fig. 6-12). Arterial injury should be suspected in cases where profound focal deficits are present or evolve in the

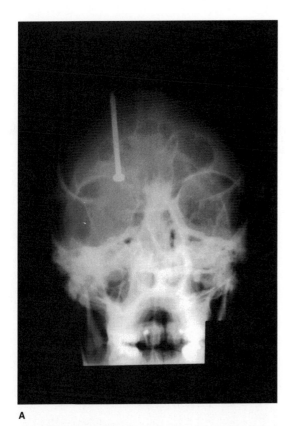

A

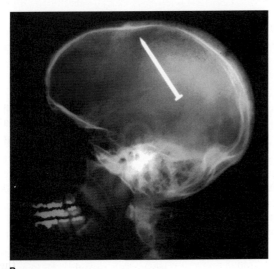

B

Figure 6-10

A. *Anteroposterior and* B. *lateral plain skull films are useful for localization of intracranial metallic foreign bodies in three dimensions in order to assist in removal.*

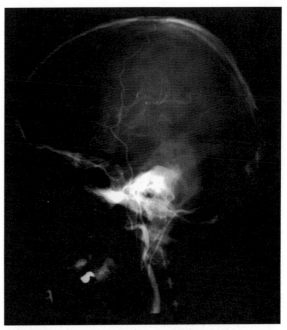

Figure 6-11

Traumatic right internal carotid artery dissection following moderate (GCS 9) head injury. The patient developed delayed hemiplegia at 2 days postinjury. The CT scan was initially negative at the onset of the hemiplegia. The internal carotid artery tapers to a narrow "string" at the level of C1 and ends at the skull base.

absence of an explanatory traumatic lesion on CT scan (e.g., hematoma, depressed fracture fragment). The development of focal symptoms may be delayed. If a repeat CT scan does not show a delayed hematoma, angiography should be carried out to rule out vascular injury. Anticoagulation in patients without hemorrhage may prevent evolution of dissection with partial occlusion to complete thrombosis of the artery.

MANAGEMENT

Respiratory and Cardiovascular

Securing an airway, preventing aspiration, and assuring adequate gas exchange are of paramount importance in unconscious head-injury patients. Patients who are comatose (GCS ≤ 8) require

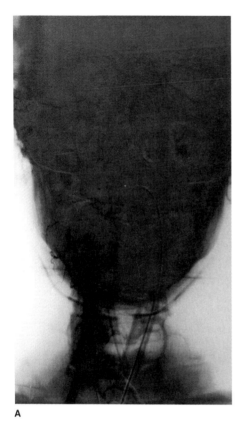
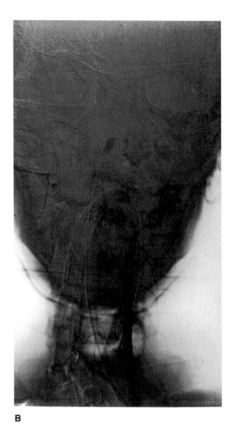

A

B

Figure 6-12

A. and B. Bilateral vertebral artery occlusions in a patient with an admission GCS of 12 and delayed deterioration in the level of consciousness with a normal CT scan at 24 h postinjury. When he recovered consciousness, multiple lower cranial nerve palsies and ataxia were obvious on clinical examination.

endotracheal intubation for airway patency, protection from aspiration, and tracheal toilet regardless of the presence or absence of other indications for intubation. In emergent circumstances, intubation is normally carried out via the oral or nasal routes, and depends to a large extent on individual skill and preference. Nasal-tracheal intubation is best avoided when there is extensive facial fracturing, extensive fracturing of the skull base, or for prolonged periods of time, the latter being due to a propensity to cause pyogenic sinusitis. In all cases where intubation is carried out prior to radiography of the cervical spine, in-line traction on the spine should be applied by an assistant, during the intubation, in order to prevent motion

of the cervical spine. Tracheotomy is normally reserved for patients with prolonged coma in whom the need for ventilation, airway protection, and pulmonary toilet exceeds or is expected to exceed 10 to 14 days. Occasionally, emergency tracheotomy is required when endotracheal intubation cannot be carried out via the oral or nasal routes, usually as a result of severe facial injury. Patients with a GCS of 9 or 10 often appear to be ventilating adequately, but, frequently, these patients cannot properly protect themselves from aspiration, nor can they effectively clear their pulmonary secretions. Unless rapid recovery of consciousness is anticipated it is better to err on the side of safety and intubate these patients as well. Many intubated patients will require mechanical ventilation, in addition to intubation, to prevent hypercarbia from central depression of ventilation and to prevent and treat hypoxemia. Common causes of hypoxemia include atelectasis, pneumonia, and other airspace disease. Atelectasis can be minimized by the use of positive end expiratory pressure (PEEP) ventilation. There is often concern about the effect of PEEP on ICP. In patients with increased intracranial elastance (decreased compliance), one may see elevation of ICP with the application of greater than 10 mmHg of PEEP.[51] The effect is mediated by alteration in venous pressure. In this author's experience, commonly used levels of PEEP (5 to 10 mmHg) do not usually cause problems with ICP, and any effect can be detected with ICP monitoring. The potential deleterious effects of PEEP on ICP have to be weighed against the harmful effects of pulmonary atelectasis and reduced gas exchange.

The next order of priority in the treatment of the head-injured patient is the establishment of intravenous access and the restoration of normal blood pressure in patients who are hypotensive. A 50-g bolus of glucose should be given to patients with coma of unknown etiology. Use of large amounts of glucose-containing solutions may precipitate hypophosphatemia (Chap. 13). Blood for diagnostic testing and blood typing should also be taken at this juncture. Patients who are hypotensive should be vigorously resuscitated with saline or Ringer's lactate, and packed red blood cells, and a search for the cause of the hypotension should be made. The usual causes are hemorrhage into the abdomen, pelvis, or chest. Tension pneumothorax may also produce profound hypotension, as well as obstruction of cerebral venous return with severe elevation of ICP. This combination is particularly damaging in patients with brain injury.

Patients with isolated brain injury are often hypertensive and tachycardic due to increased circulating catecholamines associated with head injury, and such patients normally do not require treatment for the hypertension. Hypertension may be useful as a protective response to maintain adequate cerebral perfusion, and its treatment early after injury is inappropriate until the nature of the intracranial pathology, ICP, and cerebral perfusion pressure are known. Once the patient has been stabilized, severe systemic hypertension may occasionally require treatment. Patients with systemic hypertension as a result of intracranial pathology may be very sensitive to vasodilators and these drugs should be used initially in lower than normal doses and only when intra-arterial pressure monitoring is available. Elevation of the pulse to 100 to 120 beats per minute is not uncommon following head injury, and, given that this most commonly occurs in young healthy patients, ordinarily does not require treatment. The same catecholamine response may be potentially harmful in older patients with coronary artery disease, and treatment of hypertension and tachycardia in this group of patients may be indicated. Beta blockers lower cardiac work, blood pressure, and pulse, and are the agents of choice in this population.[52]

Surgical

Once a secure airway, adequate respiration, and treatment of hypotension have been assured, the next item of priority is the diagnosis and treatment of intracranial hemorrhage. Normally, the diagnosis is made with a CT scan. In exceptional circumstances in which there is obvious evolution of an intracranial hemorrhage (witnessed significant deterioration of level of consciousness, i.e., greater than 2 points on the GCS and the development of unilateral pupillary dilatation), one may elect to proceed directly to operation for a presumed surface hematoma. This occurs very uncommonly, and valuable time can be wasted making exploratory burr holes in patients in whom the presence of an evolving hematoma is not clear-cut. The other circumstance in which one may have to bypass the CT scan occurs when a patient with a severe head injury, or a mild or moderate injury with localizing signs, has to be taken to the operating room for treatment of life-threatening systemic injuries. In this circumstance, surgical diagnosis of intracranial hematoma may have to be carried out. Techniques for doing this are discussed at the end of this section.

In the usual circumstance, one performs a CT scan to enable diagnosis and localization of intracranial hematomas. This greatly simplifies surgical planning and enables one to accurately place craniotomy incisions. One normally operates in the presence of surface hematomas or intracerebral contusions of sufficient size to produce shift of the midline structures (at the septum pellucidum) of 5 mm or more. This rule of thumb may be modified in the presence of deep-seated intracerebral hematomas in critical areas of the brain, or smaller surface clots that are felt to be primarily responsible for deterioration in the level of consciousness or focal symptoms. Occasionally, surface clots may continue to enlarge in patients who are scanned very early (usually within 1 h) after injury, and one may elect to operate on a small surface hematoma in this circumstance. Midline shift cannot be used as an indication for operation in the presence of bilateral hematomas of roughly equal size and mass effect. In that circumstance, surgical decision making is based on judgement regarding the size of the hematomas and the patient's clinical condition. Acute intracranial hematomas are of jelly-like consistency and must be evacuated through a craniotomy. They cannot be removed through burr holes. The craniotomy must be large enough to allow identification of the source of bleeding and its definitive treatment. With the exception of well-localized extradural hematomas, this normally means a large frontotemporal craniotomy "trauma flap" allowing access to the usual contusion sites, temporal and frontal, and the bridging veins at the sagittal area and at the junction of the transverse and sigmoid sinuses (termination of the inferior anastomotic vein of Labbé). Often, small surface contusions are hidden by an overlying acute subdural hematoma, and, occasionally, brain swelling following evacuation of a surface clot may mandate removal of a swollen, contused temporal or frontal lobe. Formal lobectomy is normally required when operating on isolated cerebral contusions of sufficient size to require operative intervention. Local debridement and arrest of hemorrhage from small contusions may be adequate in cases of operation for acute subdural hematoma associated with contusion, if the brain is slack following removal of the surface clot.

In the circumstances described above, in which one does not have time to obtain a CT scan because of the requirement for immediate life-saving surgery for systemic injuries, two strategies are available for diagnosing operable intracranial hematomas. The first is to carry out bilateral exploratory burr holes. Burr hole exploration is time consuming and frequently unproductive when there are no localizing signs, such as a unilateral dilated pupil or major discrepancies in the motor examination between sides. Additionally, the procedure is of no value in diagnosing an intracerebral hematoma or contusion even when there are focal signs. A single burr hole is indicated when there is progressive profound deterioration in the level of consciousness associated with focal signs. This type of deterioration is virtually always associated with a surface hematoma. A better alternative in less clear-cut cases is to insert a ventriculostomy tube, as is normally done for ICP monitoring. One then injects 5 to 10 cm^3 of air into the ventriculostomy tube and obtains an AP film of the skull. Deviation of the septum pellucidum on the resultant ventriculogram of greater than 5 mm from the midline indicates the likely presence of a surgical lesion.[38] The advantages of this technique are that a single burr hole (or twist drill hole) is required and the surgeon can diagnose intracerebral as well as surface hematomas using this technique. The major disadvantage is that the ventricle can be difficult to cannulate if it is shifted and/or compressed. Facility with ventricular catheterization, even under the difficult circumstances described above, can be anticipated with experience.

Compound depressed fractures of the cranial vault require debridement and watertight closure of the dura mater to prevent the development of meningitis or brain abscess. Indriven bone, hair, bits of scalp, and foreign bodies within the brain should be removed to prevent abscess formation. In the case of missile wounds, it is not necessary to remove small bullet fragments deep within the brain.[53,54] Large foreign bodies may migrate through the brain subsequently, and should be removed (Fig. 6-10). Intracranial hematomas associated with penetrating injury should be dealt with according to the principles outlined above. Entrance and exit wounds should be debrided and closed.

Basal skull fractures with rhinorrhea (and less commonly otorrhea) may require surgical exploration and closure of the CSF fistula in cases associated with large skull defects or persistent CSF leakage. Rhinorrhea from anterior fossa fractures often occurs in association with extensive facial fracturing, and repair of the CSF fistula may be undertaken at the time of facial fracture repair. Dural defects too large to be sutured are patched with autologous tissue grafts (from the pericranium, temporalis fascia, or fascia lata). In cases of CSF fistula in which meningitis has already occurred, surgery should be postponed until the meningitis has been cleared up with appropriate antibiotic therapy. Similarly, in patients with significant accompanying brain injury who do not require craniotomy for management of an acute hematoma, repair of the CSF fistula is best delayed for several days until brain swelling has subsided, due to the amount of brain retraction necessary to properly visualize and repair a fistula.

Intracranial Pressure Monitoring and Treatment

Management of raised ICP begins with resuscitation of the patient and control of the airway and respiration. Hypercarbia from inadequate ventilatory effort will produce cerebral vasodilatation and increase in cerebral blood volume. The latter increases the ICP, and adequate ventilation of the patient may make a dramatic difference in ICP. Perfusion pressure (mean arterial blood pressure [MABP] – ICP) should be maintained by volume replacement in patients who are hypotensive. In emergent situations, mannitol (0.5 to 1 g/kg of 20% solution) should be given for those patients who are known or suspected to harbour an intracranial mass lesion. If a traumatic hematoma is subsequently identified, it should be evacuated as soon as possible. Two absolute contraindications to the

use of mannitol are hypotension and anuria. In the case of patients with shock (compensated or uncompensated), the diuresis produced by mannitol will further deplete the patient's extracellular fluid volume and further compromise their hemodynamic status.

Monitoring of ICP is frequently carried out in patients with severe head injury (GCS $\leq$ 8), or in less severely injured patients under special circumstances. Routine monitoring of ICP in severely injured patients has become the de facto standard of care in most North American academic neurosurgical units. Typical indications for monitoring in less severely injured patients include monitoring following removal of mass lesions when significant brain swelling is observed at operation or anticipated postoperatively, or when a patient is unable to be clinically examined because of the use of large doses of sedative drugs and/or neuromuscular blockade (for respiratory management).

The contents of the cranium are incompressible, so that pressure recorded from the subarachnoid space is equivalent to that in the parenchyma or within the ventricular system. Pressure gradients do, however, develop across dural partitions, so that the pressure monitored from the subdural or subarachnoid space over one hemisphere may differ from that in the opposite side. For this reason, ICP monitoring should normally be carried out on the side with the greatest demonstrable structural pathology. Technology exists to monitor pressure within the subarachnoid space, epidurally, subdurally, within the cerebral parenchyma, or within the ventricular fluid. Transduction of the pressure wave may be carried out within the catheter itself[55] or within a transducer that is fluid-coupled to the subarachnoid, subdural or intraventricular spaces. Fluid coupling cannot be carried out within the parenchyma or extradurally. The oldest monitoring systems involve external transduction of a fluid-coupled system, the gold standard of which is monitoring the intraventricular fluid pressure. Externally transduced systems have the advantage of allowing rezeroing of the pressure measurement, and the latter ensures continued accuracy of the monitor over prolonged periods. The major disadvantage is that loss of fluid coupling results in loss of accurate pressure measurement. This happens with displacement of the catheter out of the ventricle, or due to brain swelling with obliteration of the subarachnoid or intraventricular spaces. Loss of fluid coupling is apparent from loss of the normal ICP waveform. In practice, loss of subarachnoid pressure readings occurs far more frequently than loss of intraventricular pressure measurements. The latter normally occurs with repeated drainage of the ventricular catheter and accurate readings can usually be restored by cessation of drainage and/or by irrigation of the catheter with 1 cm^3 of fluid. Another major advantage of ventricular pressure monitoring is the ability to drain CSF in order to treat ICP. The major disadvantages are higher incidence of infection (particularly with monitoring beyond 5 days) and the potential for intracerebral hemorrhage on insertion.

The level of ICP at which treatment should be initiated has been estimated empirically at 20 to 25 mmHg. The duration of elevation should exceed 5 min, and elevations of short duration due to obvious patient agitation or movement can normally be ignored. The initial treatment should consist of adequate sedation of ventilated patients as struggling against the endotracheal tube will elevate intrathoracic pressure, decrease venous return, and elevate ICP. It is frequently necessary to paralyze patients pharmacologically with neuromuscular blockers in order to adequately control intrathoracic pressure due to patient agitation or posturing. If a ventricular catheter is in place, small amounts of CSF should be drained intermittently to lower ICP. Continuous drainage of the ventricles is not appropriate because the ventricles will soon collapse and further drainage will no longer be possible. Furthermore, in fluid-coupled systems the pressure cannot be read while the catheter is draining, and one can find oneself in the situation of no longer lowering ICP because of ventricular collapse, and not knowing what the ICP really is because the pressure cannot be read with the catheter open for drainage.

Vigorous hyperventilaton to control ICP is best avoided. A controlled randomized trial has shown that patients who are hyperventilated to a level of approximately 25 mmHg have a worse outcome than patients who are moderately hyperventilated, i.e., 35 mmHg. The adverse effect of profound hyperventilation is most likely mediated by cerebral vasoconstriction and induction of cerebral ischemia. Another contributing factor may be a disturbance in acid-base balance due to depletion of bicarbonate ions.[56]

If sedation and intermittent drainage of CSF (where possible) are not effective in controlling ICP, mannitol may be used in doses of 100 to 200 mL of 20% solution. The smallest dose that produces an adequate effect on the ICP should be used, as repeated doses are likely to be necessary. As mannitol is nephrotoxic in high concentrations, it should not be given when serum osmolarity is $\geqslant$ 320 mosmol/L. At 350 mosmol/L, progressive renal failure occurs.[57] Administration of mannitol produces profound diuresis. Systemic dehydration is not necessary for mannitol to effectively lower ICP. Therefore, the ability to use mannitol repeatedly can be increased by replacing that portion of the patient's urine output estimated to result from the administration of mannitol with an appropriate crystalloid solution. In cases where mannitol is being used repetitively on a very frequent basis (e.g., 2 to 3 hourly), and urine output is being partially replaced, central venous or pulmonary artery catheterization may be necessary to adequately monitor and manage patient extracellular fluid volume. Frequent monitoring of electrolytes and serum osmolarity is also essential.

When mannitol is ineffective or can no longer be used because of unacceptably high serum osmolarity, barbiturates may be used to control ICP. The usual agent is pentobarbital given intravenously in 50-mg boluses. The pentobarbital is given until the ICP is brought down to an acceptable level or until there is an unacceptable level of hypotension. The latter is an extremely common side effect of barbiturate use. Pulmonary artery pressure monitoring is normally necessary for barbiturate coma in order to maintain optimal left heart filling pressures, cardiac output, and systemic blood pressure. Treatment with vasopressors may be necessary. Barbiturates have been shown to be less effective than mannitol for controlling raised

ICP.[58] They do not improve outcome when given prophylactically to patients in coma.[59] Nevertheless, they have been shown to bring ICP under control in some patients who are refractory to other treatment measures.[60]

In the past, decompressive craniectomy had been advocated as a measure for controlling refractory ICP. With further follow-up, it was found that this technique usually succeeded only in increasing the incidence of survival with severe disability or in a persistent vegetative state.[61] Consequently, most surgeons feel that decompressive craniectomy is contraindicated. In very rare instances of refractory ICP in patients in lighter grades of coma (i.e., GCS > 5), the technique may be useful as a method of last resort.

Measurement of ICP does not, in itself, give any information about the compliance state of the brain. This is due to the exponential relationship between pressure and volume. Thus, two patients (or the same patient at two different points in time) may respond quite differently to small increments or decrements in intracranial volume. In order to measure brain compliance, it is necessary to manipulate CSF volume and to measure the effect on pressure. This has been recognized for some time and a number of measures have been proposed. The most commonly described measure of compliance is the pressure volume index (PVI). The PVI is measured by injecting 1 cm^3 of saline or withdrawing a cubic centimeter of CSF from the ventricular catheter and calculating the logarithm (base 10) of the change in pressure over the volume increment (or decrement). The resulting number is the volume required to change the ICP by a factor of 10. In normal adult patients, this number is 25 mL. A PVI of 13 or below signifies dangerously low compliance and indicates the likelihood of uncontrollable ICP.[62] Treatment of brain compliance rather than ICP has been advocated as a means of averting dangerous elevations of ICP. Treatment of intracranial compliance has not gained widespread acceptance, likely as a result of the inconvenience of calculating the measurement, the requirement for ventricular cannulation, the necessity of manipulating intracranial volume, and, perhaps most importantly, the lack of convincing demonstration

of a difference in patient outcome based on management of compliance rather than ICP.

More recently, the emphasis on ICP management has shifted away from maintenance of ICP below an arbitrary level to support of adequate CPP. The latter is thought to be at 60 to 70 mmHg or above. One author has advocated treating raised ICP by using vasopressors to increase the mean arterial blood pressure.[63] This both protects CPP, and, in patients with intact pressure autoregulation, the increase in mean arterial blood pressure results in cerebral vasoconstriction and a consequent lowering of ICP.

While ICP monitoring and aggressive treatment of raised ICP in severely head-injured patients has become routine in a great many centers, the impact of such aggressive management of raised ICP on critically ill patients has never been unequivocally shown. While there is clearly an association between high ICP and poor outcome, causation has not be proven.[64] The alternative to the hypothesis that uncontrolled ICP causes brain damage is that raised or uncontrollable ICP is simply a reflection of the volume of the damaged brain. Two nonrandomly controlled clinical trials have purported to show a beneficial effect of monitoring and aggressive treatment of raised ICP on patient outcome.[65,66] In one series, the controls were historical, and, in another, control patients were treated in different hospitals where there were presumably differences in other aspects of patient management apart from the monitoring and treatment of ICP. Serial measurement of evoked potentials has not shown a clear-cut relationship between ICP elevation and evoked potential deterioration, and, in this author's own series of patients, uncontrollable ICP frequently followed the complete disappearance of hemispheric evoked potential activity by a few hours to 1 or 2 days. This suggests that, in many cases, uncontrollable ICP is indeed the result, rather than the cause, of massive cerebral damage.[67]

Attempts have been made to identify patients at particular risk for development of raised ICP, and clinical features and intracranial pathology seen on CT scan. Patients with mass lesions and other CT abnormalities, low GCS, and low blood pressure seem particularly at risk for raised ICP.[68] While this strategy identifies patients at risk for raised ICP, it does not necessarily identify those who might derive the most benefit from its aggressive treatment. Clearly, a patient with massive brain injury is very likely to have raised ICP, but it remains to be proven that successful control of ICP in such a patient will translate into functional recovery.

Other Physiologic Monitoring

The other intracranial physiologic parameters that may be measured/monitored in comatose head-injury patients are cerebral blood flow and metabolism, and brain electrophysiology. The latter is commonly carried out with evoked potentials or with some type of signal processing of the electro-encephalogram (EEG).

Cerebral Blood Flow and Metabolism   The relationship between cerebral blood flow (CBF), oxygen extraction, and the cerebral metabolic rate of oxygen ($CMRO_2$) is described by the following equation:

$$CMRO_2 = CBF \times AVDO_2 \div 100$$

where $AVDO_2$ is the transcranial arterial-venous oxygen difference in volumes percent (vols.%), and CBF is measured in milliliters per 100 g of brain tissue per minute. The $AVDO_2$ can be measured in patients by inserting a central venous catheter upward into the internal jugular vein until it reaches the jugular bulb. At this location, the blood sampled from the catheter contains almost exclusively blood from the intracranial circulation. Blood can be drawn simultaneously from an intra-arterial catheter. The difference in oxygen content (mL O_2/100 mL blood) is the $AVDO_2$ in vols.%. Cerebral blood flow can be measured by nitrous oxide washout (using the same arterial and internal jugular catheters), radioactive xenon washout (using external collimators over the head), "cold" xenon inhalation with CT scanning, or newer technology involving laser doppler flowmetry or thermal diffusion. The latter two techniques involve placing small probes over the cerebral

cortex and flow measurement is limited to the cortex immediately under the probe. There may be technical difficulties maintaining accurate readings. The major advantages are the ability to carry out multiple readings over hours or days in an intensive care setting. Nitrous oxide flow measurements are quite labour intensive and give flows averaged from the entire brain. No regional or local resolution is possible. The main limitation to the number of possible studies is the amount of work involved. The measurements can be readily carried out in the intensive care unit (ICU). Radio-active xenon studies may also be carried out in the ICU using portable equipment, and these do give some spatial resolution to the flow information. This depends on the number and placement of external collimators. The number of studies that can be repeated in a single patient is limited by radiation concerns. "Cold" xenon CT scanning yields the most accurate information about regional flow and no radiation exposure is involved. The requirement for CT scanning rules out its use in the ICU or the use of frequent measurements.

The older literature generally failed to show significant global ischemia in patients following head injury.[45] Often CBF measurements were carried out 24 h or more following injury. More recent work by Bouma et al[46] has shown that if the initial CBF measurements are conducted within 12 h of injury, then there is a significant incidence of ischemia and this is often associated with a poor outcome. Blood flow tends to return to normal or supranormal levels by 24 h and beyond in patients who survive. Other than avoidance of hyperventilation and appropriate resuscitation for reduced intravascular volume, there are currently no effective treatments for those patients identified as suffering from global or regional ischemia. It is unclear whether induction of hypertension is helpful in this circumstance.[69] Given the amount of expense and effort necessary to measure cerebral blood flow at this time, and the hitherto small impact of such measurement on patient management, it is likely that, for the time being, direct measurement of CBF will remain in the province of specialized units as a tool for clinical investigation.

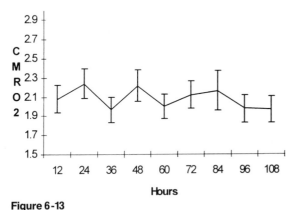

Figure 6-13

The CMRO_2 in a series of 52 patients following severe closed head injury. The measurement is relatively constant over the initial few days postinjury. The units of measurement (ordinate) are mL per 100 g brain tissue per min.

The difficulty in measuring CBF directly has led to the search for surrogate measures of the adequacy of cerebral blood flow. Recall from the equation above that $CMRO_2$ is the product of CBF and $AVDO_2$. Given the assumption of relative constancy of $CMRO_2$, and this seems borne out by empirical measurement[46] (Fig. 6-13), the $AVDO_2$ will vary inversely with CBF. The $AVDO_2$, or simply the jugular oxygen saturation, can be measured relatively easily with a catheter placed in the jugular bulb. Fiber-optic catheters are available that will produce a constant readout of jugular oxygen saturation. Investigators have found that clinical events that might reasonably be expected to lower CBF, such as episodes of raised ICP, hypoxia, and hypotension, are frequently reflected in a falling jugular O_2 saturation.[70] The number of episodes of jugular desaturation have also been found to correlate well with patient outcome.[70] Technical improvements continue to be made in this monitoring technology, and it is likely to become more widespread with improved reliability and lower costs.

Electrophysiologic Monitoring An objective, reliable measure of neurologic function in severely head-injured patients is desirable to monitor patient progress, or lack thereof, the impact of secondary insults on neurologic function, and to measure the immediate effect of therapeutic interventions. This need arises both as a result of the relative paucity and insensitivity of measurable clinical responses in the deeper grades of coma, and because of the frequent use of sedatives and neuromuscular blockers that further reduce the level of measurable clinical response. Ideal attributes would include sufficient sensitivity to detect important change in patient status, the generation of reasonable volumes of data, data interpretation by nonexperts, minimal impact of commonly used doses of sedative and analgesic drugs on the monitored parameter, and low random variability of the monitored parameter so that observed changes in the parameter have a high likelihood of indicating meaningful clinical change in the patient. Available electrophysiologic measures meet these requirements to differing degrees in head-injury patients. None possess all of the above attributes.

Electroencephalogram The EEG has been employed in the investigation of traumatic coma virtually since its inception. Coma is generally associated with slowing of the background frequencies, with the amount of slowing generally proportionate to the depth of coma.[71] Special electroencephalographic patterns of coma exist (alpha coma, spindle coma) and there is considerable debate as to whether these have any special prognostic significance. Generally, it is felt that alpha coma carries a particularly bad prognosis, and spindle coma—the presence of intermittent sleep spindles—is associated with a good prognosis. Variability of any kind in the background frequencies, whether spontaneous or induced by external stimulus, is associated with a better prognosis than the absence of such variability. In the era preceding the development of modern CNS imaging techniques (CT, MRI), much emphasis was placed on the correlation of EEG abnormalities with structural lesions such as subdural hematoma. The development of CT, and then MRI, has rendered this particular aspect of EEG diagnosis irrelevant.

The major technical difficulties associated with use of conventional EEG as a monitoring tool for comatose patients involve the tremendous amount of data generated and the requirement for expert interpretation of the data at the bedside. Unfortunately, the latter consideration plagues a good deal of electrophysiologic monitoring. Modern techniques of digitization of multiple-channel EEG at the bedside, with transmission across data lines to the electroencephalographer, may mitigate this concern to some extent. A number of authors have attempted to deal with the problems of data reduction and simplification of EEG output. One of the earliest techniques was the cerebral function monitor. The EEG record is recorded from one channel, and by means of bandpass filtering, amplitude compression, and slowing the trace speed of the recording apparatus, a manageable tracing of many hours of electrical activity is produced.[72] The successfully detected change in cerebral function is associated with such dramatic events as cardiac arrest and recovery from barbiturate overdose.[72] Less obvious changes in cerebral activity may be less well reflected in the cerebral function monitor.[73]

A more recent and more widely accepted form of data compression is power spectrum analysis of the EEG. The latter is a mathematical transformation of the EEG (or other wave phenomenon) from the time to the frequency domain. The result is the description of a complex wave phenomenon, such as the EEG, as the amount of amplitude at each of the component frequencies measured over a given epoch of time, typically 2 to 4 s. The development, miniaturization, and constant improvement of computer hardware has permitted the widespread availability, at reasonable cost, of computerized EEG monitoring equipment for what was formerly a very computationally demanding technique. Power spectral analysis is most useful for characterizing background frequencies and will miss transients. The ability to analyze the morphology of EEG waves is also sacrificed so that a seizure discharge occurring at a given frequency may not appear any different than background activity at that same frequency. Various graphic displays have evolved to present the frequency information, usually on a video terminal. The most frequently used measure has

been the compressed spectral array pioneered by Bickford.[74] Interpolation of frequency data between electrode positions allows the development of topographic maps of amplitude and frequency data.

A number of authors have shown a relationship between compressed spectral patterns and outcome from coma. As with conventional EEG, the amount of slowing in the background of the EEG is related to the depth of coma. Within several days of injury, there is a very good correlation between the dominant frequencies in the EEG and Glasgow Coma Score[75] and outcome can be predicted to a fair degree of accuracy from patterns observable on the compressed spectral array. In general, slow monotonous records are associated with a worse prognosis than fast, changeable records.[76] Unfortunately, the analysis referred to above was carried out in a retrospective fashion, and, in this study and others,[77,78] the degree of outcome prognostication accuracy based on the frequency content of the EEG does not exceed that achievable from the clinical parameters of patients' age and GCS on admission to hospital. In the author's experience, it is much harder to discern the status of a patient at given point in time while monitoring is ongoing with EEG power spectral analysis than with somatosensory evoked potentials (SSEPs). This author also finds that the temporal course of the EEG power spectrum measured over several days after injury is much less useful, both in predicting outcome and in identifying meaningful trends in individual patients, than are SSEPs. Other authors have noted the prognostic superiority of SSEPs over EEG.[79] The problem may lie in the fact that the EEG is primarily a measure of cortical neuronal activity, whereas the pathology in diffuse head injury is primarily in the white matter of the cerebral hemispheres. Measurement of coherence and phase properties of the EEG may address this deficiency.[77]

Evoked Responses Investigators have had considerably more success in establishing a relationship between evoked potentials and outcome from head injury. Perhaps more importantly, evoked potentials have been shown to change in clinically meaningful ways when monitored over time.[80,81] Of the commonly measured evoked potentials—auditory, SSEPs, and visual—SSEPs have been shown to bear the greatest relationship to patient outcome. Visual evoked potentials are not as good as SSEPs for outcome prediction, but they are useful for diagnosing suspected injury to the optic apparatus in a comatose patient. Brainstem auditory evoked potentials (BAEPs) are the least useful for outcome prognostication.[82] The BAEPs clearly predict poor outcome when absent beyond wave I. Absence of wave I indicates endorgan damage and this does not necessarily reflect damage to CNS pathways.[83] Unfortunately, in this author's experience with severe head-injury patients, this technical problem is distressingly frequent. While the presence of BAEPs is a necessary condition for good outcome, it is not a sufficient condition.[83] This is presumably related to the limitation of BAEPs to establishing the functional integrity of the brainstem, but not the cerebral hemispheres. Abnormalities in BAEPs are clearly correlated with clinical signs of brainstem nuclear dysfunction (pupillary areactivity, corneal and oculocephalic abnormalities) but not with the GCS.[84] In the author's experience with patients whose evoked potentials deteriorate, complete loss of cortical SSEP activity generally precedes loss of brainstem peaks.

Sweep times for SSEPs typically vary from about 50 to 250 ms. The most significant feature(s) of the SSEP is subject to debate. Outcome has been well correlated with central conduction time, number of peaks, longest latency activity in the SSEP, total amplitude in the SSEP, and more complex subjective grading systems. Certainly, features of the SSEP that are dependent upon early latency components are the most reproducible, both within and among individuals. The central conduction time (cervicomedullary junction to primary somatosensory cortex) is one such measure that has been extensively employed and clearly distinguishes between survivors and nonsurvivors from head injury. Loss of all cortical activity bilaterally in the SSEP is uniformly associated with death or survival in a severely debilitated state. However, it is the intermediate and

long latency activity (70 ms and beyond) that best distinguishes functional status among survivors. This appears to be true both in head-injury patients[81,82] and in patients suffering from post-arrest hypoxic/anoxic coma.[85]

As noted above, SSEPs frequently change over time. In one series, about half of patients who died from head injury, and were not moribund at the outset of monitoring, showed progressive deterioration of SSEP waveforms.[81] Newlon et al had previously hypothesized that such deterioration was the result of secondary insults, such as raised ICP or ischemic/hypoxic insults.[80] In the author's experience, progressive deterioration of evoked potentials was usually not associated with obvious secondary insult while the patients were being monitored. Deterioration was often unassociated with raised ICP, and, when patients did succumb to raised ICP, this most often followed the disappearance of SSEPs. Other investigators have also observed a lack of relationship between raised ICP and evoked potential deterioration.[86] Deterioration is frequently seen in association with a drop in $AVDO_2$, raising the possibility of disordered oxidative metabolism as a significant contributor to the observed decline in SSEPs.[87]

The prognostic capability of evoked potentials is roughly equivalent to the commonly measured clinical features (age, GCS, pupillary reactivity),[82,83] so that evoked potential monitoring does not confer any special prognostic advantage in a patient who is accessible to clinical examination. It does, however, provide important information about patient status in patients who are pharmacologically paralyzed and sedated to facilitate respiratory or ICP management. In this situation, one frequently relies on SSEP management to guide therapy. For instance, in patients who have lost cortical SSEP activity, this author will not employ heroic measures to control refractory ICP, i.e., barbiturate coma or decompressive craniectomy. The labour intensity and requirement for bedside expertise necessary to continuously monitor SSEPs prevents widespread use of the technique. However, one-time measurement of SSEPs may be practical for many units caring for patients with severe head injury in circumstances when patients may not be accessible to clinical examination and early information about prognosis is required.

Management of Complications

Seizures Posttraumatic epilepsy is common following serious head injury, occurring in up to 20 percent of patients within 1 year of admission to hospital with a serious head injury.[88] Certain injury features make seizures more likely, such as intracerebral hematoma, depressed skull fracture with cortical laceration, the severity of injury, and, most importantly, early posttraumatic epilepsy. The latter may be extremely detrimental to patients as seizure activity may significantly increase the metabolic demands on cells that are already compromised by injury. Steps should be taken immediately to control the seizure with intravenous benzodiazepines. The patient should be protected from further seizure activity by parenteral loading with phenytoin (1 g over an hour in an adult) and maintenance on an appropriate daily dose (usually 300 mg/day). Blood levels of phenytoin (or other anticonvulsants) should be checked periodically and the dosages adjusted as necessary to maintain therapeutic blood levels.

Postictally, there may be profound depression of consciousness, beyond that caused by the head injury. This may occasionally cause some confusion, with progressive deterioration in consciousness associated with an expanding hematoma. Usually, one can elicit a history of seizure activity from witnesses and, unless the seizure has been prolonged, the patient will recover to some degree from the postictal state, whereas a patient with an expanding hematoma will continue to deteriorate. The confusion may be further compounded by the fact that the onset of a delayed intracerebral hematoma is frequently heralded by a seizure. In this circumstance, the patient does not recover to the previous level of consciousness, and the patient should be investigated with CT.

The issue of the use of prophylactic anticonvulsants remains controversial, with no convincing evidence being available that they reduce the incidence of late posttraumatic epilepsy. There is evidence to suggest that prophylactic phenytoin does reduce the incidence of posttraumatic seizures in the first week postinjury (3.6 percent treated versus 14.2 percent untreated),[88] and this justifies early prophylactic use because of the extra morbidity and increased length of hospital stay often associated with early seizures. For the longer term, many neurosurgeons continue to use prophylactic anticonvulsants for patients with severe head injury (i.e., patients with GCS $\leqslant$ 8) and for patients with depressed skull fractures with cortical laceration, in spite of the lack of compelling evidence for doing so.

Infection

Systemic Sepsis Pulmonary sepsis is frequent in patients who are comatose beyond a few days. Its incidence can be kept to a minimum by avoidance of aspiration by early intubation and frequent suctioning, positional change, and chest physiotherapy, once patients are intubated. In patients who are unresponsive or anticipated to be unresponsive beyond about 2 weeks postinjury, tracheostomy should be carried out to meet the needs of patients for ongoing pulmonary toilet. Colonization of the respiratory tract with nosocomial organisms is very frequent and use of antibiotics should be reserved for those patients with established infection as indicated by clinical or radiographic signs of pneumonia, fever, and leukocytosis.

Because of the necessity for catheter drainage of the bladder, there is a similar propensity in comatose patients to develop urinary tract sepsis. Again, colonization of the bladder is frequent and treatment should be reserved for patients with systemic signs of infection.

Central Nervous System Central nervous system sepsis is fortunately relatively uncommon in patients with head injury. The commonest site of infection is the ventricular system when a ventricular drain is used. The incidence of infection is proportional to the length of time the ventricular catheter is in place. The incidence of infection begins to rise rapidly after the fifth day in place. The incidence also increases in proportion to the amount of manipulation of the drain. Daily cultures of the CSF from the drainage bag may give some idea as to the most probable organism infecting the drain. However, this fluid is subject to contamination with airborne bacteria at the bedside, and confirmation of the presence of infection and the responsible agent should always be made with freshly drawn ventricular CSF and/or culture of the catheter tip from within the ventricle. Treatment is carried out with an antibiotic to which the organism is sensitive and which is capable of crossing the blood-brain barrier. At the outset, culture results may not be available and treatment with a broad-spectrum cephalosporin capable of crossing the blood-brain barrier is most appropriate.

For meningitis due to CSF leak, the meningitis should be completely treated with the appropriate intravenous antimicrobial, and then the offending fistula should be closed. Development of parenchymal abscess at the site of a penetrating wound will require appropriate microbial therapy and drainage, and possible eventual excision of the abscess capsule. The sequence and number of treatments depends on the maturity of the abscess and the response to simple drainage procedures. Monitoring response to therapy with serial CT scans has greatly simplified the management of this unusual complication.

Fever In addition to the direct and indirect effects of microbial disease on the injured brain, hyperthermia associated with sepsis is detrimental The interplay between these factors can be seen clinically with frequent deterioration of a global nature, or aggravation of focal deficits with the onset of fever, and mitigation of the deficits with control of the fever. A similar demonstration of the adverse effects of hyperthermia occurs when monitoring ICP. Often, a stubborn increase in ICP in a febrile patient may be completely resolved by cooling the patient to a normal or slightly below normal temperature. More aggressive levels of hypothermia are now undergoing therapeutic trials for management of the primary brain injury and

have been demonstrated to be safe and potentially efficacious.[89]

The differential diagnosis of a febrile comatose patient includes recurrent pulmonary emboli and a febrile reaction to commonly used prophylactic anticonvulsants (usually phenytoin). The former can be diagnosed by pulmonary angiography or a ventilation/perfusion lung scan. The latter may require a trial of a different anticonvulsant or the cessation of anticonvulsants.

Fluid and Electrolyte Disorders The commonest disorder seen following closed head injury is SIADH. Excessive free water is retained at the distal renal tubule and collecting ducts, and this is manifested by a drop in the patient's serum sodium (see Chap. 13). Normally, the drop is modest (to ~130 mmol/L) and treatment with moderate fluid restriction (1 L/day) is sufficient to reverse the decrease in serum sodium. Occasionally, the drop in serum sodium is refractory to fluid restriction and treatment with demeclocycline hydrochloride (a tetracycline antibiotic that produces nephrogenic diabetes insipidus) may be useful in this situation. If the sodium drops much below 120 mmol/L, the patient may have significant aggravation of their neurologic disturbance and/or suffer seizures. Treatment with hypertonic saline may be required. During sodium replacement with hypertonic saline, the serum sodium should be carefully monitored and the initial amount used should not exceed one-half of the calculated sodium deficit.

Diabetes insipidus is the other commonly observed neuroendocrine abnormality following head injury. It is ordinarily a preterminal event, and the usual context for treatment is the avoidance of cardiovascular collapse due to severe extracellular volume contraction, pending the declaration of brain death and organ donation. Desmopressin acetate is used for treatment.

Hydrocephalus True hydrocephalus is an uncommon complication of head injury. When it does occur, it is of the communicating variety and presumably results from an absorptive defect from hemorrhage at the time of injury. The patient's condition can be seen to deteriorate and signs of raised ICP may develop, such as unilateral or bilateral sixth nerve palsy. In order to avoid futile shunting procedures, it is important to distinguish this form of hydrocephalus from the hydrocephalus ex vacuo that accompanies cerebral atrophy following very severe injury. In the former case, the CT shows obliteration of the convexity sulci and sylvian cisterns, whereas these structures are enlarged in ex vacuo hydrocephalus. Often, the onset is delayed for weeks or months following injury.

Nutrition

Patients who have suffered a severe head injury enter a catabolic state with a net loss of nitrogen.[90] The latter is at least partly due to an increase in circulating catecholamines. The caloric expenditure rate may be extremely high in cases where there is uncontrolled posturing, and may reach levels commonly found with severe systemic trauma, such as large burns. Sedation or neuromuscular blockade attenuates that part of the response due to excessive muscle activity. It is possible to reduce the nitrogen loss of patients in coma from head injury by enteral or parenteral nutrition, although it is not possible to eliminate the state of net nitrogen loss on a consistent basis.[90] Parenteral nutrition is not demonstrably superior to enteral nutrition via a nasogastric tube, so the former should be avoided unless enteral nutrition is not possible. Usually, enteral feeding can be started within a day or two of injury, and should not be postponed beyond 2 to 3 days. Drugs to improve gastric motility (e.g., metoclopramide), or insertion of a feeding tube beyond the pylorus (under radiographic control), may enhance patients' tolerance for enteral feeding.

PROGNOSIS

The outcome from head injury depends primarily on the level of consciousness of the patient at the outset of injury and the age of the patient. These findings are consistent across a number of series. Not surprisingly, patients with deeper levels of coma fare worse than those with milder levels of disturbance of consciousness. The predictive value of the GCS and age of the patient is valid across the entire range of head injury severity. Other indices of cerebral function may be highly predictive of some outcomes but not terribly useful across the full spectrum of injury. One example is the presence of bilaterally absent pupillary reactions. This predicts death with a high degree of certainty, but the converse situation, where the pupils are reactive, has no bearing on the quality of survival. The presence of operable (large size) intracranial mass lesions worsens the prognosis of head-injury patients, as does the presence of multiple systemic injuries. The latter factor operates via the agency of hypotension and/or hypoxia. Uncontrollable ICP is associated with a poor outcome, but levels of ICP are not otherwise predictive of outcome. Features on the CT scan, apart from mass lesion, that tend to predict poor outcome are subarachnoid hemorrhage and obliteration of the basal cisterns.

Evoked potentials and EEG have also been correlated with outcome, and multimodality evoked potentials have been found to marginally improve clinical predictions when used in conjunction with clinical measures, but are, of themselves, not clearly superior to clinical measurement.[14,82] This is not that surprising given that electrophysiologic measures and clinical measures are largely measuring the same thing (i.e., neurologic function). In the context of prognosis, evoked potentials find their greatest utility in patients who, for a variety of reasons, cannot be properly assessed clinically. Such use may prevent unnecessarily heroic attempts to save the patient.

Different clinical features at, or shortly after, admission have been used in combination to predict outcome from head injury. Prediction is usually made using logistic regression techniques.[91] An alternate technique employs bayesian probability statistics.[92] A recent paper examining the impact of the provision of calculated outcome probabilities for treating physicians in a neurosurgical ICU found a reduction in inappropriate therapeutic heroics without any increase in mortality nor any reduction in the number of head-injury survivors with reasonable quality outcomes.[93] In another application, actual outcomes can be compared with predicted outcomes, retrospectively, as a quality control measure.[94]

The weakness of statistical prediction of outcome is that while quite accurate predictions can be made about large groups of patients, based on probability of inclusion of a patient with certain clinical characteristics at hospital admission into a certain outcome group, one can never be certain of the outcome in a given patient at the outset of treatment. With the passage of time, outcome predictions can be made with a greater degree of certainty. Patients who do succumb to their injuries usually do so within the first week or two after injury. Death within 48 h is usually due to uncontrollable ICP. Beyond 1 to 2 weeks, the usual causes of death are sepsis and other systemic complications of injury.

Outcome from the Coma Data Bank in the United States shows that the mortality rate for severe head injury, i.e., patients admitted to hospital in coma, is 36 percent. About 27 percent of patients are able to return to normal employment, social, and educational pursuits. A further 16 percent function completely independently but have not resumed their former level of activity, 16 percent are severely disabled (i.e., cannot function independently), and 5 percent survive in a persistent vegetative state.[95] This data has come to be used as a benchmark for outcome from severe injury, although some caution must be exercised in interpreting the data as outcome for series of head injury is quite dependent on case mix (e.g., mean age, incidence of mass lesions) within the series.[7]

Major improvements in the outcome from head injury are unlikely in the absence of effective treatments for primary impact injury. Current research in this area revolves primarily around the areas of neurotransmitter excitotoxicity, protection from the effects of oxygen free-radical species, the role of ionic calcium in axonal injury, and the treatment of severe brain injury with moderate hypothermia.

Even in the absence of a therapeutic breakthrough for primary impact injury, clinicians can have a significant effect on head injury mortality in individual patients by careful attention to the diagnosis and treatment of secondary insults before they cause significant clinical deterioration. In large series of patients with severe injuries, there are a substantial number of patients who "talk and die," and, therefore, presumably have not suffered overwhelming impact injury, and who succumb to potentially preventable or treatable secondary injury.[96,97]

REFERENCES

1. Frankowski RF, Annegers JF, Whitman S: Epidemiological and descriptive studies: Part I: The descriptive epidemiology of head trauma in the United States, in Povlishock JT, Becker DP (eds): *Central Nervous System Trauma Status Report 1985.* Richmond, William Byrd Press, 1985, pp 33–43.
2. Max W, MacKenzie EJ, Rice DP: Head injuries: costs and consequences. *J Head Trauma Rehabil* 6(2):76, 1991.
3. Kraus JP, Peek C: The impact of two related prevention strategies on head injury reduction among nonfatally injured motorcycle riders, California, 1991–1993. *J Neurotrauma* 12(5):873, 1995.
4. Thompson RS, Frederick PR, Thompson DC: A case-control study of the effectiveness of bicycle safety helmets. *New Engl J Med* 320(21):1361, 1989.
5. Sorenson SR, Kraus JF: Occurrence, severity, and outcomes of brain injury. *J Head Trauma Rehabil* 6(2):1, 1991.
6. Cooper KD, Tabaddor K, Hauser WA, et al: The epidemiology of head injury in the Bronx. *Neuroepidemiology* 2:70, 1983.
7. Shedden PM, Moulton RJ, Sullivan I, et al: Effect of population characteristics on head injury mortality. *Pediatr Neurosurg* 91(16):203, 1990.
8. Kelly DF: Alcohol and head injury: an issue revisited. *J Neurotrauma* 12(5):883, 1995.
9. Flamm ES, Demopoulos HB, Seligman ML, et al: Ethanol potentiation of central nervous system trauma. *J Neurosurg* 46:328, 1977.
10. Bullock R, Hanneman CO, Murray L, Teasdale GM: Recurrent hematomas following craniotomy for traumatic intracranial mass. *J Neurosurg* 72:9, 1990.
11. Crockard HA, Brown FD, Johns LM, Mullan S: An experimental cerebral missile injury model in primates. *J Neurosurg* 46:776, 1977.

12. Hammon WM: Analysis of 2187 consecutive penetrating wounds of the brain from Vietnam. *J Neurosurg* 34:127, 1971.

13. Teasdale G, Jennett B: Assessment of coma and impaired consciousness. A practical scale. *Lancet* 2:81, 1974.

14. Narayan RK, Greenberg RP, Miller JD, et al: Improved confidence of outcome prediction in severe head injury. A comparative analysis of the clinical examination, multimodality evoked potentials, CT scanning, and intracranial pressure. *J Neurosurg* 54:751, 1981.

15. *The Abbreviated Injury Scale.* 1990 Revision. Des Plaines, Association for the Advancement of Automotive Medicine, l990.

16. Russell WR, Smith A: Post-traumatic amnesia in closed head injury. *Arch Neurol* 5:4,1961.

17. Levin HS, O'Donnell VM, Grossman RG: The Galveston orientation and amnesia test. A practical scale to assess cognition after head injury. *J Nerv Ment Dis* 167(11):675, 1979.

18. Schwartz ML, Stuss DT, Carruth F, et al: The course of post traumatic amnesia. *J Neurotrauma* 12(3):352, 1995.

19. Gennarelli TA, Thibeault LE: Biological models of head injury, in Povlishock JT, Becker DP (ed.): *Central Nervous System Trauma Status Report 1985.* Richmond, William Byrd Press, 1985, pp 391–404.

20. Ommaya AK, Gennarelli TA: Cerebral concussion and traumatic unconsciousness. Correlation of experimental and clinical observations on blunt head injuries. *Brain* 97:633, 1974.

21. Holbourn AHS: The mechanics of brain injuries. *Brit Med Bull* 3:147, 1945.

22. Gurdjian ES: Recent advances in the study of the mechanism of impact injury of the head—a summary. *Clin Neurosurg* 19:1, 1972.

23. O'Brien PK, Norris JW, Tator CH: Acute subdural hematomas of arterial origin. *J Neurosurg* 41:435, 1974.

24. Gennarelli TA, Thibeault LE: Biomechanics of acute subdural hematoma. *J Trauma* 22(8):680, 1982.

25. Strich SJ: Shearing of nerve fibres as a cause of brain damage due to head injury. A pathological study of twenty cases. *Lancet* 2:443, 1961.

26. Adams JH, Mitchell DE, Graham DI: Diffuse brain damage of immediate impact type: Its relationship to 'primary brain-stem damage' in head injury. *Brain* 100:489, 1977.

27. Povlishock JT, Becker DP, Cheng CLY, Vaughan GW: Axonal change in minor head injury. *J Neuropath Exp Neurol* 42(3):225, 1983.

28. Povlishock JT: Pathobiology of traumatically induced axonal injury in animals and man. *Ann Emerg Med* 22(6):980, 1993.

29. Adams JH, Graham DI, Gennarelli TA, Maxwell WL: Diffuse axonal injury in non-missile head injury. *J Neurol Neurosurg Psychiatry* 54:481, 1991.

30. Katamaya Y, Becker DP, Tamura T, Hovda DA: Massive increases in extracellular potassium and the indiscriminate release of glutamate following concussive brain injury. *J Neurosurg* 73:889, 1990.

31. Hovda DA, Lee SM, Smith ML, et al: The neurochemical and metabolic cascade following brain injury: moving from animal models to man. *J Neurotrauma* 12(5):903, 1995.

32. The European Study Group on Nimodipine in Severe Head Injury: A multicenter trial of the efficacy of nimodipine on outcome after severe head injury. *J Neurosurg* 80:797, 1994.

33. Baker AJ, Moulton RJ, MacMillan VH, Shedden PM: Excitatory amino acids in cerebrospinal fluid following traumatic brain injury in humans. *J Neurosurg* 79:369, 1993.

34. Ross DT, Graham DI, Adams JH: Selective loss of neurons from the thalamic reticular nucleus following severe human head injury. *J Neurotrauma* 10(2):151, 1993.

35. Bazan NG, Rodriguez de Turco EB, Allan G: Mediators of injury in neurotrauma: Intracellular signal transduction and gene expression. *J Neurotrauma* 12(5):791, 1995.

36. Bracken MB, Shepard MJ, Collins WF, et al: A randomized controlled trial of methylprednisolone or naloxone in the treatment of acute spinal cord injury. *New Engl. J. Med* 322(2):1405, 1990.

37. Muizelaar JP, Marmarou A, Young HF, et al: Improving the outcome of severe head injury with the oxygen radical scavenger polyethylene glycol-conjugated superoxide dismutase: a phase II trial. *J Neurosurg* 78:375, 1993.

38. Becker DP, Miller JD, Ward JD, et al: The outcome from severe head injury with early diagnosis and intensive management. *J Neurosurg* 47:491, 1977.

39. Gutman MB, Moulton RJ, Sullivan I, et al: Risk factors predicting operable intracranial hematomas in head injury. *J Neurosurg* 77:9, 1992.

40. Teasdale GM, Murray G, Anderson E, et al: Risks of acute traumatic intracranial haematoma in children and adults: implications for managing head injuries. *Br Med J* 300:363, 1990.

41. Bullock R, Butcher SP, Chen M, et al: Correlation of the extracellular glutamate concentration with extent of blood flow reduction after subdural hematoma in the rat. *J Neurosurg* 74:794, 1991.

42. Marmarou A, Shulman K, Lamorgese J: Compartmental analysis of compliance and outflow resistance of the cerebrospinal fluid system. *J Neurosurg* 43:523, 1975.

43. Chan KH, Miller JD, Dearden NM, et al: The effect of changes in cerebral perfusion pressure upon middle cerebral artery blood flow velocity and jugular bulb venous oxygen saturation after severe brain injury. *J Neurosurg* 77:55, 1992.

44. Graham DI, Adams JH, Doyle D: Ischaemic brain damage in fatal non-missile head injuries. *J Neurolog Sci* 39:213, 1978.

45. Obrist WD, Langfitt TW, Jaggi JL, et al: Cerebral blood flow and metabolism in comatose patients with acute head injury. *J Neurosurg* 61:241, 1984.

46. Bouma GJ, Muizelaar JP, Choi SC, et al: Cerebral circulation and metabolism after severe traumatic brain injury: the elusive role of ischemia. *J Neurosurg* 75:685, 1991.

47. Chesnut RM, Marshall LF, Klauber MR, et al: The role of secondary brain injury in determining outcome from severe head injury. *J Trauma* 34(2):216, 1993.

48. MacDonald RL, Schwartz ML, Mirich D, et al: Diagnosis of cervical spine injury in motor vehicle crash victims: How many x-rays are enough? *J Trauma* 30(4):392, 1990.

49. Snow RB, Zimmerman RD, Gandy SE, Deck MDF: Comparison of magnetic resonance imaging and computed tomography in the evaluation of head injury. *Neurosurgery* 18(1):45, 1986.

50. Eisenberg HM, Gary HE, Aldrich EF, et al: Initial CT findings in 753 patients with severe head injury: a report from the NIH Traumatic Coma Data Bank. *J Neurosurg* 73:688, 1990.

51. Apuzzo MLJ, Wiss MH, Petersons V, et al: Effect of positive end expiratory pressure ventilation on intracranial pressure in man. *J Neurosurg* 46:227, 1977.

52. Robertson CS, Clifton GL, Taylor AA, Grossman RG: Treatment of hypertension associated with head injury. *J Neurosurg* 59:455, 1983.

53. Carey ME, Young HF, Mathis JL: The neurosurgical treatment of craniocerebral missile wounds in Vietnam. *Surg Gynecol Obstet* 135:386, 1972.

54. Brandvold B, Levi L, Feinsod M, George ED: Penetrating craniocerebral injuries in the Israeli involvement in the Lebanese conflict, 1982–1985: analysis of a less aggressive surgical approach. *J Neurosurg* 72:15, 1990.

55. Crutchfield JS, Narayan RK, Robertson CS, Michael LH: Evaluation of a fiberoptic intracranial pressure monitor. *J Neurosurg* 72:482, 1990.

56. Muizelaar JP, Marmarou A, Ward JD, et al: Adverse effects of prolonged hyperventilation in patients with severe head injury: a randomized clinical trial. *J Neurosurg* 75:731, 1991.

57. Becker DP, Vries JK: The alleviation of increased intracranial pressure by the chronic administration of osmotic agents, in Brock M, Dietz H (eds); *Intracranial Pressure*. New York, Springer-Verlag, 1972, pp 309–315.

58. Schwartz ML, Tator CH, Rowed DW, et al: The University of Toronto head injury treatment study: a prospective, randomized comparison of pentobarbital and mannitol. *Can J Neurol Sci* 11:434, 1984.

59. Ward JD, Becker DP, Miller JD, et al: Failure of prophylactic barbiturate coma in the treatment of severe head injury. *J Neurosurg* 62:383, 1985.

60. Eisenberg HM, Frankowski RF, Contant CF, et al: High-dose barbiturate control of elevated intracranial pressure in patients with severe head injury. *J Neurosurg* 69:15, 1988.

61. Cooper PR, Rovit RL, Ransohoff J: Hemicraniectomy in the treatment of acute subdural hematoma: a re-appraisal. *Surg Neurol* 5:25, 1976.

62. Maset AL, Marmarou A, Ward JD, et al: Pressure-volume index in head injury. *J Neurosur* 67:832, 1987.

63. Rosner MJ, Daughton S: Cerebral perfusion pressure management in head injury. *J Trauma* 30(8):933, 1990.

64. Miller JD, Becker DP, Ward JD, et al: Significance of intracranial hypertension in severe head injury. *J Neurosurg* 47:503, 1977.

65. Bowers SA, Marshall LF: Outcome in 200 consecutive cases of severe head injury treated in San Diego County: a prospective analysis. *Neurosurgery* 6(3):237, 1980.

66. Saul TG, Ducker TB: Effect of intracranial pressure monitoring and aggressive treatment on mortality in severe head injury. *J Neurosurg* 56:498, 1982.

67. Konasiewicz SJ, Moulton RJ, Shedden PM: Somatosensory evoked potentials and intracranial pressure in severe head injury. *Can J Neurol Sci* 21:219, 1994.

68. Narayan RK, Kishore PR, Becker DP, et al: Intracranial pressure: to monitor or not to monitor? A review of our experience with severe head injury. *J Neurosurg* 56:650, 1982.

69. Muizelaar JP, Becker DP, Lutz HA, Newlon PG: Cerebral ischemia after severe head injury: its role in determining clinical status and its possible treatment, in Villani R, Papo M, Giovanelli M, Gaini SM, Tomei G (ed): *Advances in Neurotraumatology.* Amsterdam, Excerpta Medica, 1982, pp 92–98.

70. Sheinberg M, Kanter M, Robertson CS, et al: Continuous monitoring of jugular venous oxygen saturation in head-injured patients. *J Neurosurg* 76:212, 1992.

71. Stockard JJ, Bickford RG, Aung MH: The electroencephalogram in traumatic brain injury, in Vinken PJ, Bruyn GW (eds): *Handbook of Clinical Neurology,* vol 23, *Injuries of the Brain and Skull,* part I. Amsterdam, Elsevier, 1975, pp 317–367.

72. Maynard D, Prior PF, Scott DF: Device for continuous monitoring of cerebral activity in resuscitated patients. *Br Med J* 4:545, 1969.

73. Levy WJ, Shapiro HM, Maruchak G, Meathe E: Automated EEG processing for intraoperative monitoring: a comparison of techniques. *Anesthesiology* 53(3):223, 1980.

74. Bickford RG: Computer analysis of background activity, in Remond E, (ed): *A Didactic Review of Methods and Applications of EEG.* Amsterdam, Elsevier, 1977, pp 215–232.

75. Moulton RJ, Marmarou A, Ronen J, et al: Spectral analysis of the EEG in craniocerebral trauma. *Can J Neurol Sci* 15:82, 1988.

76. Bricolo A, Turazzi S, Faccioli F, et al: Clinical application of compressed spectral array in long-term EEG monitoring of comatose patients. *Electroenceph Clin Neurophysiol* 45:211, 1978.

77. Thatcher RW, Cantor DS, McAlaster R, Geisler F, Krause P: Comprehensive predictions of outcome in closed head-injured patients. The development of prognostic equations. *Ann NY Acad Sci* 620:82, 1991.

78. Karnaze DS, Marshall LF, Bickford RG: EEG monitoring of clinical coma: the compressed spectral array. *Neurology* (NY) 32:289, 1982.

79. Hutchinson DO, Frith RW, Shaw NA, et al: A comparison between electroencephalography and somatosensory evoked potentials for outcome prediction following severe head injury. *Electroenceph Clin Neurophysiol* 78:228, 1991.

80. Newlon PG, Greenberg RP, Hyatt MS, et al: The dynamics of neuronal dysfunction and recovery following severe head injury assessment with serial multimodality evoked potentials. *J Neurosurg* 57:168, 1982.

81. Moulton R, Kresta P, Ramirez M, Tucker W: Continuous automated monitoring of somatosensory evoked potentials in posttraumatic coma. *J Trauma* 31 (5):676, 1991.

82. Lindsay KW, Carlin J, Kennedy I, et al: Evoked potentials in severe head injury—analysis and relation to outcome. *J Neurol Neurosurg Psychiatry* 44:796, 1981.

83. Lindsay K, Pasaoglu A, Hirst D, et al: Somatosensory and auditory brain stem conduction after head injury: a comparison with clinical features in prediction of outcome. *Neurosurgery* 26(2):278, 1990.

84. Barelli A, Valente MR, Clemente A, et al: Serial multimodality-evoked potentials in severely head-injured patients: diagnostic and prognostic implications. *Crit Care Med* 19(11):1374, 1991.

85. Madl C, Grimm G, Kramer L, et al: Early prediction of individual outcome after cardiopulmonary resuscitation. *Lancet* 341:855, 1993.

86. Garcia-Larrea L, Artru F, Bertrand O, et al: The combined mointoring of brain stem auditory evoked potentials and intracranial pressure in coma. A study of 57 patients. *J Neurol Neurosurg Psychiatry* 55:792, 1992.

87. Moulton RJ, Shedden PM, Tucker WS, Muller PJ: Somatosensory evoked potential monitoring following severe closed head injury. *Clin Invest Med* 17(3):187, 1994.

88. Temkin NR, Dikmen SS, Wilensky AJ, et al: A randomized, double-blind study of phenytoin for the prevention of post-traumatic seizures. *New Engl J Med* 323(8):497, 1990.

89. Marion DW, Obrist WD, Carlier PM, et al: The use of moderate therapeutic hypothermia for patients with severe head injuries: a preliminary report. *J Neurosurg* 79:354, 1993.

90. Clifton GL, Robertson CS, Grossman RG, et al: The metabolic response to severe head injury. *J Neurosurg* 60:687, 1984.

91. Stablein DM, Miller JD, Choi SC, Becker DP: Statistical methods for determining prognosis in severe head injury. *Neurosurgery* 6(3):243, 1980.

92. Jennett B, Teasdale G, Braakman R, et al: Predicting outcome in individual patients after severe head injury. *Lancet* 1:1031, 1976.

93. Murray LS, Teasdale GM, Murray GD, et al: Does prediction of outcome alter patient management? *Lancet* 341:1487, 1993.

94. Moulton R, Tucker W, Sullivan I, et al: Development of an audit tool for preventable death from head injury. *Ann Roy Coll Physicians and Surgeons of Canada.* 25(4):188, 1992.

95. Marshall LF, Gautille T, Klauber MR, et al: The outcome of severe closed head injury. *J Neurosurg* (suppl) 75:S28, 1991.

96. Rose J, Valtonen S, Jennett B: Avoidable factors contributing to death after head injury. *Br Med J* 2:615, 1977.

97. Marshall LF, Toole BM, Bowers SA: The National Traumatic Coma Data Bank, Part 2: patients who talk and deteriorate: implications for treatment. *J Neurosurg* 59:285,1983.

Chapter 7

IMPAIRED CONSCIOUSNESS ASSOCIATED WITH NEOPLASIA

G. Bryan Young

This chapter will discuss impaired consciousness in patients with primary brain tumors or with systemic cancer. In the United States, there are about 17,000 primary brain tumors discovered each year.[1] Systemic cancer is much more common, with over 1 million new cases each year in the United States.[1] Table 7-1 gives a more comprehensive listing. Some alteration in mental status or seizures occurred in about 16 percent of cases of systemic cancer seen in a large cancer center.[2] Seizures and metabolic or toxic encephalopathies account for much of the morbidity of cancer. At least 11 percent of children with cancer develop acute mental status changes, either from complications of the cancer or from its treatment.[3] Such problems can usually be managed; even if the symptoms and signs from tumors or structural complications cannot be completely reversed, they can often be relieved.

PRIMARY BRAIN TUMORS

Primary brain tumors produce impaired consciousness by the following mechanisms: (1) mass effect from the tumor, edema, or hemorrhage; (2) strategic location; (3) epileptic seizures; (4) meningeal spread; (5) complication of therapy; and (6) remote effects, usually hormonal. These will be discussed individually.

Mass Effect

The pathogenesis of impaired consciousness that is due to the secondary mass effect at a distance from a tumor in the supra- and infratentorial compartments is discussed in Chap. 4. With acutely expanding masses, there is a correlation between the degree of impairment of consciousness and the amount of lateral shift in the supratentorial compartment. This is not as apparent with slowly growing neoplasms (Chap. 4). As noted in Chap. 4, the volume of the mass is important, but the acuity of the volume change and the location of the mass are more salient. With rapidly enlarging masses, there is also less time for adaptive mechanisms to reduce the intracranial pressure (ICP). Causes of rapid evolution of a pre-existing mass effect include hemorrhage into a tumor, cerebral edema, and necrosis of the tumor with swelling or rapid growth.[4]

Table 7-1

Neoplasms

Primary tumors	New cases in USA in 1993	No. deaths in USA in 1994	Percentage with intracranial tumor at autopsy at MSKCC	Estimated total no. of deaths with intracranial tumor
Lung	172,000	153,000	34	52,020
Breast	183,000	46,300	30	13,890
Colon and rectum	149,000	56,000	7	3,920
Urinary organs	78,800	21,900	23	5037
Melanoma	32,000	6900	72	4968
Prostate	200,000	38,000	31[a]	11,780
Pancreas	27,000	25,900	7	1813
Leukemia	28,600	19,100	23[b]	4393
Lymphoma (non-Hodgkin)	45,000	21,200	16[b]	3392
Female genital tract	75,300	25,200	7	1764
Brain and CNS	17,500	12,600	100	12,600
All sites	**1,208,000**	**538,000**	**24**	**129,120**

[a] Largely skull and dura.
[b] Largely leptomeningeal.
Abbreviations: CNS = central nervous system; MSKCC = Memorial Sloan-Kettering Cancer Center.
Source: From Posner,[4] with permission.

Location of Tumor

Some tumors are located in or near centers for alertness (see Figs. 1-1 and 1-2). Several configurations may pertain. Low-grade tumors may infiltrate structures without causing severe dysfunction of the structure, e.g., infiltrative tumors of the brainstem and supratentorial lesions in childhood. Pituitary or hypothalamic tumors may enlarge and compress the rostral brainstem, or hypothalamic or thalamic structures. This is more likely with acute expansion, namely, pituitary apoplexy. Intraventricular or periventricular tumors may produce acute obstruction to intracranial cerebrospinal fluid (CSF) circulation. Thalamic tumors that invade or compress the reticular formation of the rostral brainstem or the thalamus, or that affect both frontal lobes, produce various degrees of obtundation, coma, stupor, vegetative state, akinetic mutism (see Chap. 2), or an evolving spectrum of impaired cognitive functioning (see Figs. 7-1 and 7-2).

Seizures

Seizures are discussed in the section on seizures in patients with cancer, below.

Meningeal Spread

The main features of meningeal seeding from primary brain tumors are similar to those for systemic cancer, discussed later in this chapter. Meningeal spread occurs with medulloblastoma, ependymoma, malignant gliomas (especially after surgery), choroid plexus papilloma, pineal tumors, and, sometimes, with malignant meningioma. With most primary brain tumors, neoplastic meningitis is associated with relentless progression to coma and death.

Complications of Cancer Therapy

Operations for primary brain tumors are followed by neurologic and medical complications in a

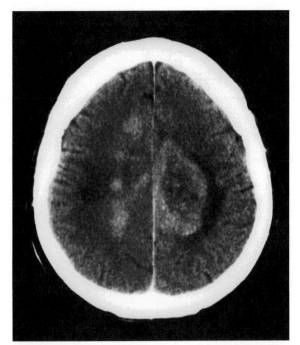

Figure 7-1

A T1-weighted MRI scan of an adult patient with a malignant glioma that spread across the corpus callosum and also invaded the ventricular walls. The patient showed impaired alertness and arousability. He was confused and disoriented after brief arousal.

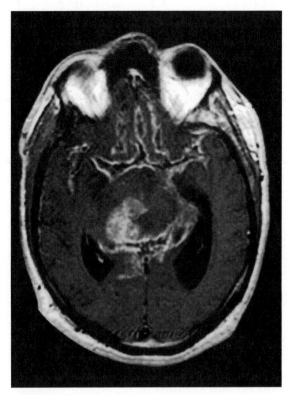

Figure 7-2

An MRI scan showing a thalamic astrocytoma. The patient developed progressively impaired alertness as the tumor infiltrated the thalamus bilaterally.

moderate proportion of patients. Fadul and colleagues assessed morbidity and mortality from operations for supratentorial gliomas at the Memorial Sloan-Kettering Cancer Center and the New York Hospital.[5] Overall, 74 percent of cases showed no change, or improved, while 26 percent had neurologic deterioration. Short-term neurologic deterioration from hemorrhage or herniation was more common in those patients with superficial lesions who had incomplete resections than in those who had larger resections. Patients with deep midline or bilateral lesions were also more likely to deteriorate postoperatively, usually from hydrocephalus or hemorrhage, than those with superficial, lateralized lesions. All herniations occurred within 3 days of surgery. Neurologic complications outnumbered medical complications by 10 : 1. Medical problems were more common in patients with low preoperative Karnofsky scores, and included pneumonia (3.3 percent), deep venous thrombosis (2.3 percent), and pulmonary embolism (1.5 percent). Myocardial infarctions and gastrointestinal bleeding each occurred in less than 1 percent of patients The syndrome of inappropriate diuretic hormone secretion (SIADH) occasionally follows craniotomy for tumor (4 percent of children in one series).[6]

Other complications are discussed later, under the complications of systemic cancer.

IMPAIRED CONSCIOUSNESS IN SYSTEMIC CANCER

Posner's authoritative monograph, *Neurological Complications of Cancer,*[4] gives the combined perspectives of a neurologist and oncologist. Nervous system complications of cancer are common, serious, frequently difficult to diagnose, but often treatable. They are clinically important and are increasing in incidence and prevalence. Further, they give biologic insights into the relationship between the brain and systemic cancer.

Approximately 25 to 40 percent of patients with cancer and 85 percent of terminally ill cancer patients suffer from delirium.[7,8] Brain dysfunction in patients with systemic cancer can result from a myriad of factors, either acting singly or in combination in the individual patient. With many cancers, e.g., lung or breast cancers, brain metastases are by far the most common causes of coma. With systemic disease, however, metabolic or toxic effects from metastases from other organs, from drugs and their impaired clearance, and from superimposed coagulation disorders or infections (related to the disease or its treatment) need to be considered as factors in the genesis of coma. Elderly cancer patients are especially likely to suffer encephalopathies.[9]

Metastatic Cancer

Metastases constitute the most common mechanism by which cancer affects brain function.[10] Consciousness may be compromised by metastases to the brain parenchyma or to the meninges.[4,11–14] Occasionally, metastases to neighboring structures, such as the pituitary or the subdural or epidural spaces, affect the brain directly by acute expansion or by causing compression, such as with hemorrhage into such tumors, or indirectly with complications such as a CSF leak (see Fig. 7-3).

Pathogenesis of Impaired Consciousness from Brain Metastases

As with other brain lesions, impaired consciousness relates to the sites of involvement and their acuity. Metastatic tumors also disrupt the blood-brain barrier. As tumors grow, they promote angiogenesis with capillaries that are distinct from normal brain capillaries[4]:

1. Tumor capillaries lack the tight junctions that form the main structural component of the

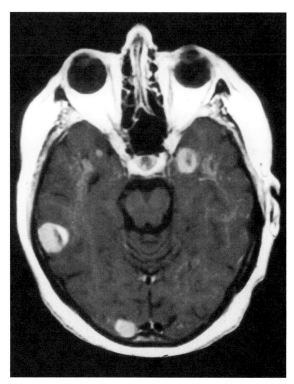

Figure 7-3
An MRI scan showing multiple brain metastases from a malignant melanoma.

blood-brain barrier. Tight junctions form a physical barrier to the direct diffusion of polar (non lipid soluble) solids between the blood and brain compartments.

2. Brain capillaries do not allow much vesicular transport and lack the fenestrations found in tumor and systemic capillaries.

3. The sodium-potassium pump is more active in brain than in tumor capillaries. This requires more energy production and, thus, greater numbers of mitochondria.

4. Brain capillaries have special carrier systems for the transport of certain substances, e.g., glucose and L-amino acids. Also, there may be special endothelial enzyme systems that convert chemicals and drugs, such as L-DOPA, before releasing them into the brain compartment.

As a consequence, capillaries in and around brain tumors are "leaky," resulting in more tissue fluid (vasogenic edema), with increased tissue pressure initially near, and then remote from, the tumor. Interference with CSF circulation may lead to more edema and raised ICP. Increased interstitial fluid alters diffusion between brain cells and capillaries. The breakdown in the blood-brain barrier alters the chemical milieu of the brain cells and exposes them to toxic substances from which they are usually protected.

Clinical Features of Central Nervous Systems Metastases

Confusion, often heralded by headache, is by far the most common symptom.[15,16] Impairment of consciousness may occur if several metastases are strategically placed so as to affect the projection pathways of the ascending reticular activating system (ARAS), e.g., bifrontal metastases with edema. However, it is more common that mass lesions impair consciousness by secondary intracranial shifts, as discussed in Chap. 4. Much of the mass effect relates to vasogenic cerebral edema. Hydrocephalus may also produce impairment of consciousness. Increasing headache is a common premonitory symptom before herniations or severe hydrocephalus develop. When the headache is focal, it has localizing value; however, diffuse headache may accompany either focal or multifocal lesions, diffusely raised ICP, or hydrocephalus.

Headaches due to raised ICP characteristically are present on awakening or are precipitated or worsened by Valsalva maneuvers, such as in coughing or sneezing, but occur in less than one-third of patients.[17] The headaches gradually worsen over days. Usually, but not always, neurologic signs accompany such headaches.[17,18] The signs reflect the site of the lesions; hemiparesis is the most common feature.[14] The signs also gradually become more marked with time.

Intermittent impairment of consciousness may be due to seizures (discussed later).

A differential diagnosis for metastatic brain tumors is given in Table 7-2.

Table 7-2
Differential diagnosis of brain metastases

I. Primary brain tumors: especially gliomas or meningiomas

II. Cerebrovascular disease: see Table 7-3
    A. Cerebral hemorrhage
        1. Intratumoral
        2. Vascular anomaly
    B. Cerebral embolism
        Nonbacterial endocarditis
        Tumor
    C. Cerebral thrombosis
        1. Arterial
        2. Venous

III. Infections
    A. Abscess — especially with Hodgkin disease and lymphoma
    B. Viral infection — progressive multifocal leukoencephalopathy

IV. Side effects of chemotherapy
    A. Methotrexate leukoencephalopathy
    B. Radionecrosis

V. Other disorders
    A. Related to cancer — paraneoplastic syndromes
    B. Not related to cancer

Source: Modified from Posner,[4] p. 91, with permission.

Investigations

The diagnostic test of choice is magnetic resonance imaging (MRI) with infusion of gadolinium. This procedure is more sensitive than the computed tomography (CT) scan and, if normal, effectively excludes parenchymal metastases in any part of the brain, except perhaps multiple miliary or leptomeningeal metastases.[4] A CT scan with contrast is usually adequate, but is marred by bony artifacts in the posterior fossa and temporal regions.

If symptomatic patients have a type of cancer that is known to metastasize to the brain, metastases are likely if multiple lesions are found on radiologic studies. A single nodule creates difficulty; although the mass could be a metastasis, about 11 percent of the time it represents another condition, e.g., a cerebral abscess or a meningioma.[19] Often, in such circumstances, it is better to perform a stereotaxic needle biopsy or to remove the lesion surgically. In patients without known cancer who have "suspicious lesions" on MRI or CT scans, it is best to look first for a primary tumor and additional secondary deposits.[20]

Management

Brain metastases that cause a change in alertness require stabilization using corticosteroids to reduce the edema and mass effect. A typical initial dose of dexamethasone or its equivalent is 16 mg per 24 h. This step affords some clinical relief of symptoms, improves survival, and safeguards, to a large extent, the edema that can be anticipated from brain radiotherapy. Corticosteroid treatment should be continued until radiotherapy is completed, then tapered off if possible. Symptomatic therapy with anticonvulsants should be given to patients following seizures.

Once the diagnosis is reasonably secure, the choice of treatment is guided by the patient's neurologic status and the extent of systemic disease.[14] Although the prognosis for patients with single or multiple brain metastases is poor, considerable improvement in quality of life is possible with corticosteroid and radiotherapy and the judicious use of surgery. Neurologic improvement can be expected in at least two-thirds of patients.[15,21–23]

LEPTOMENINGEAL METASTASES (CARCINOMATOUS AND LYMPHOMATOUS MENINGITIS)

The spread of metastatic cancer to the subarachnoid space can affect the brain in a number of ways, depending on the extent, location, and pattern of the involvement. The overall incidence of neoplastic meningitis is between 0.8 and 8 percent of patients with cancer.[12,24] The most common malignancies involved are leukemia (especially acute lymphocytic type), non-Hodgkin lymphoma, breast and lung cancer, and melanoma.[12] Some uncommon tumors, such as retinoblastoma and embryonal rhabdomyosarcoma, have a high rate of spread to the meninges.[25] Metastases usually occur late in the course of systemic cancer, often accompanying relapse in other parts of the body.[4] Longer survival in patients with systemic cancer increases the risk of meningeal metastases. Occasionally, meningeal spread can be an initial manifestation of systemic cancer.

Pathophysiology

Tumors reach the meninges either by direct extension from pre-existing parenchymal tumors, along nerve roots into the subarachnoid space, or by hematogenous spread involving the arachnoid vessels or the choroid plexus.

Meningeal cancer may affect the brain in various ways, depending on the pattern of spread. If there is obstruction to CSF circulation, hydrocephalus or raised ICP results. Even when hydrocephalus is present, it is not always the cause of the encephalopathy, as the latter may fail to clear with shunting. Multifocal parenchymal lesions or extensive perivascular lesions may result from the spread of tumor into the brain along the subpial Virchow-Robin spaces. Ischemia can result from compression of vessels in the Virchow-Robin space, often with the effect of tissue edema that alters the composition of the extracellular fluid and impairs diffusion from capillaries.[26] Vascular involvement or a secondary hypercoagulable state may also cause cortical vein thrombosis.[27] Other mechanisms of diffuse or multifocal brain dysfunction are: (1) metabolic dysfunction in the brain (selective reduction in glucose metabolism of underlying brain);[28,29] (2) deafferentation or disconnection due to mechanical disruption of association, commissural, or projection of white matter fibers; and (3) immunologic response: increased cytokine production in the CSF or plasma (uncertain role).[4]

Clinical Features

A progressive, nonfluctuating impairment of concentration, memory, or cognitive function, or depressed consciousness occurs in 25 to 33 percent of patients with meningeal cancer.[4] The possible mechanisms are discussed above. Most commonly, this mimics the encephalitic syndrome with meningeal signs and seizures (Chap. 11) or metabolic encephalopathy (Chap. 13). Episodic loss of consciousness usually relates to seizures, but bouts of raised ICP may account for some cases.[4]

With either syndrome, there may be superimposed focal signs, such as hemiparesis or aphasia. Signs of cranial nerve dysfunction are helpful diagnostically. These are often late, but are common. Ocular muscle paresis from a third or sixth nerve palsy is perhaps the most common. Other cranial nerve deficits include: optic neuropathy, trigeminal neuropathy, facial palsy, deafness, hypoglossal palsy, and ninth or tenth nerve palsy with dysphagia or hoarseness. Palsies of cranial nerves III, IV, VI, and the ophthalmic division of V suggest invasion of the cavernous sinus. Deafness suggests lymphomatous involvement of nerve VIII.

Spinal symptoms and signs occur in at least 50 percent of patients with leptomeningeal cancer.[4] These include: neck stiffness, Kernig's sign, radicular pain, depressed reflexes locally (from nerve root involvement), bladder dysfunction, back pain, dermatomal sensory loss, and lower motor neuron signs. A cauda equina syndrome is common, but *signs* of spinal cord compression or invasion are relatively infrequent.

Investigation

The most useful test is CSF analysis. A CT or MRI brain scan should be obtained first to exclude an asymmetric mass lesion or acute hydrocephalus, and to reduce the risk of decompensation following lumbar puncture. Often, it is possible to reduce the risk by treatment with corticosteroids for several days. Cytologic analysis is the principal test of value (Fig. 7-4). At least 4 mL of CSF should be mixed with an equal volume of 50% absolute alcohol and sent immediately to the cytology laboratory. The use of immunohistochemistry and flow cytometry can be useful in meningeal lymphomatosis. The yield with the first spinal tap is about 50 percent.[4]

Biochemical tumor markers in the CSF are occasionally helpful in specific situations.[30] These

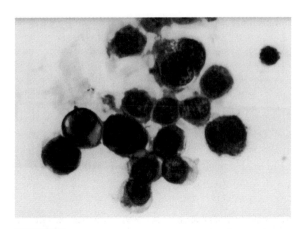

Figure 7-4
A CSF sample positive for malignant cells from a mucus-producing adenocarcinoma. Malignant cytologic features include enlarged nuclear-to-cytoplasmic ratio, multinucleated cells, and mitotic figures. Also note the intracytoplasmic mucus appearing as clear regions.

are rarely present in the CSF, even in widespread metastatic disease that does not involve the central nervous system (CNS), so that an elevated-CSF-to-serum ratio of certain chemicals is supportive of meningeal metastases.[31] However, parenchymal metastases allow increased permeability of the blood-brain barrier, resulting in high titers of serum markers passing from the plasma into the CSF. Carcinoembryonic antigen (CEA) in carcinomas of the breast, colon, ovary, bladder, and lung, and CA-125 and CA15-3 breast cancer gene (BRCA) in ovarian and breast carcinoma, respectively, may be found in CSF.[4] β-Glucuronidase, lactic acid dehydrogenase, and β_2-microglobulin elevations in CSF help to confirm the spread of some solid tumors and hematologic malignancies to the meninges and also assist in the assessment of therapy.[32–35]

Scanning by CT or MRI, with or without enhancement, can be helpful in showing diffuse or multifocal meningeal enhancement (Fig. 7-5). The demonstration of hydrocephalus is supportive. Contrast enhancement of the basal cisterns or cortical convexities with hydrocephalus, without a mass lesion, is the most typical CT finding.[32] These features, however, are not specific for

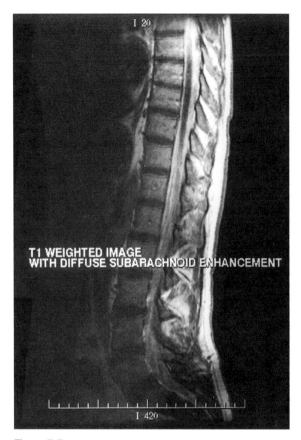

Figure 7-5
A gadolinium-enhanced MRI showing diffuse sub-arachnoid enhancement in the spinal canal due to neoplastic meningitis. The MRI can be helpful in confirming neoplastic meningitis. Often, this is manifest as "studding" of the cauda equina by metastatic nodules.

meningeal cancer. The MRI demonstration of enhancing deposits on the cauda equina roots is more specific.

Biopsy of the meninges is rarely necessary, but may be of value when other diagnostic measures fail.

Differential Diagnosis

The main differential diagnosis is CNS infection, producing either an encephalitic, meningoencephalitic picture or a predominantly meningitic picture. Bacterial infections are more likely than metastases to cause fever and a "toxic" picture, and are less likely to cause multiple cranial nerve and radicular palsies. Chronic fungal, candida infections and tuberculous meningitis may, however, closely mimic leptomeningeal metastases.

Management

In some advanced situations, in which drowsiness or coma as a consequence of meningeal cancer accompanies widespread systemic disease, palliative care, without an attack on the tumor, may be the best approach. For more definitive therapy, the usual approach is radiation treatment directed to symptomatic areas of known bulky disease (e.g., cranial lesions or cauda equina) plus intrathecal chemotherapy. Direct injection of methotrexate or cytarabine, usually with an Ommaya reservoir (a sealed capsule, embedded in the scalp, connected to a catheter inserted into a brain ventricle), is commonly used. Care should be taken that there is no obstruction to CSF circulation at the foramina or within the ventricular system before the intraventricular route is used. Systemic chemotherapy may be useful when the blood-CSF barrier has been largely disrupted by metastases.

Ventriculoperitoneal shunting is performed in some patients who are severely symptomatic, especially those with severe, intractable headaches, severe papilledema with threatened loss of vision, stupor or coma, and repeated plateau waves. Seeding of the peritoneal cavity is usually not a concern.[4]

Global brain dysfunction may improve dramatically with shunting, radiation therapy, or antineoplastic therapy, but patients with advanced disease, fixed focal deficits, and cranial nerve palsies are unlikely to improve.[32] Optimal therapy of the systemic disease is important, as the latter is often the determining factor in the patient's outcome.

Prognosis

Treatment may allow symptomatic relief and improvement in the quality of life, but patients usually succumb to their cancer. Occasionally, long-term survivors are found, especially those with meningeal leukemia or lymphoma. These groups should, therefore, be treated vigorously, with close follow-up and retreatment with chemotherapy if necessary.

DURAL METASTASES

Impaired consciousness from a single large metastasis, or multiple metastases, may relate to brain compression and shift from the mass or indirectly from associated subdural hemorrhage or effusion.[4,36,37] Some subdural effusions may be malignant. Metastases to the skull dura may arise from local extension from the skull or by hematogenous spread.[4,38] Carcinomas of the lung, prostate, and breast are the most common. Others include Hodgkin disease, gastric carcinoma, leukemia, pancreatic cancer, and plasmacytoma.

SECONDARY VASCULAR DISORDERS

Incidence and Significance

Cerebrovascular complications are not uncommon in cancer patients (see Table 7-3). An autopsy series revealed cerebrovascular lesions in 15 percent of such patients, of whom 50 percent were symptomatic in life.[39] Cerebrovascular complications can be divided into hemorrhagic and thrombotic-embolic states, but both hemorrhages and thromboses may occur simultaneously, e.g., in disseminated intravascular coagulation, hemorrhage into infarction, and with cortical vein thrombosis.

Bleeding produces single or multifocal mass lesions that compress or destroy brain tissue, or lead to vasospasm and ischemia. Such hemorrhages may be intraparenchymal, subdural, or subarachnoid in location. Hemorrhage within a brain tumor is the most common cause of intraparenchymal bleeding in patients with solid

Table 7-3
Neurovascular complications in systemic cancer

Disorders	No. of patients	No. of symptomatic patients[a]
Cerebral hemorrhage	244	138 (57%)
Intracerebral hematoma		
Intratumoral	60	47 (78%)
Secondary to coagulopathy	88	57 (65%)
Hypertensive	9	8 (89%)
Subdural hematoma	63	16 (25%)
Subarachnoid hemorrhage	24	10 (42%)
Cerebral infarction	256	117 (46%)
Atherosclerosis	73	17 (23%)
Intravascular coagulation	39	28 (72%)
Nonbacterial thrombotic endocarditis	42	32 (76%)
Septic occlusion	33	22 (67%)
Tumor embolus	12	4 (33%)
Venous occlusion	33	6 (18%)
Miscellaneous	24	8 (33%)
Total	**500**	**255 (51%)**

[a] Percentage (%) in this column = no. of symptomatic patients/number of patients in group × 100.
Source: Adapted with modification from Graus et al,[39] with permission.

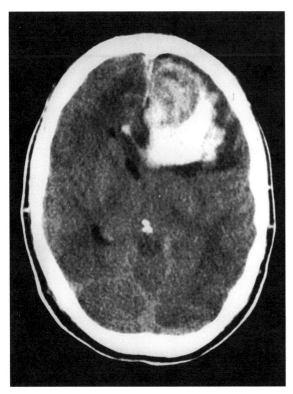

Figure 7-6

A CT scan showing hemorrhage into a single metastasis from a malignant melanoma. The patient showed impaired alertness and attention, as well as a mild right hemiparesis.

neoplasms.[40] Bleeding into metastatic tumors (especially lung, breast, and renal tumors, malignant melanoma, and choriocarcinoma) is more common than hemorrhage into primary brain tumors (see Fig. 7-6). Hemorrhages are usually intraparenchymal, but they can occur in the subdural space, especially with dural metastases from lymphoma, leukemia, and carcinomas.[40,41] On CT or MRI scans, there is frequently an adjacent bony metastasis or an area of dural tumor enhancement.

Thrombocytopenia is a serious risk factor for hemorrhage when the platelet count falls below 10,000 per cubic millimeter. This occurs primarily in myeloproliferative disorders, when there is replacement of bone marrow by tumor, as complications of chemotherapy or after radiotherapy, or when disseminated intravascular coagulation complicates promyelocytic leukemia or other malignancies.[42]

Thrombotic complications, due to a hypercoagulable state, are more common in patients with widespread cancer. Septic emboli should be suspected in patients who are immunosuppressed and who develop embolic complications, especially in the face of pulmonary or other acute infections.

Malignant angioendotheliomatosis (intravascular lymphoma or intravascular malignant lymphomatosis) is a rare cause of multifocal ischemic lesions.[43] It consists of the malignant proliferation of neoplastic B cells within small blood vessels. This may cause thromboembolic phenomena or even disseminated intravascular coagulation that can affect the brain with multiple small or single large infarcts.[44] Alternatively, deficits can result from extension of the lymphoma into the brain parenchyma.[45] The clinical picture can, thus, vary from that of single focal vascular lesions to multifocal deficits or to an apparently diffuse encephalopathy. The author has seen instances of coma developing over several days due to bilateral white matter ischemia. Systemic symptoms, from involvement of other organs or skin, may be associated with a secondary metabolic encephalopathy.[46]

Intravascular lymphoma is rarely diagnosed during life. Most patients become acutely ill and die rapidly. Occasionally, antemortem cases are diagnosed if tissues (and their blood vessels) are examined pathologically. Some patients respond favorably to high-dose corticosteroids and chemotherapy.[47] Some may need specific therapy for disseminated intravascular coagulation (DIC) seizures, or other secondary problems.

Clinical Features

Unlike patients with mundane cerebrovascular disorders, those patients with cancer are more likely to present with an encephalopathy or global dysfunction.[40] The clinical features relate to the site(s), size, time course and nature of the underlying vascular complications, as discussed in Chap. 14. Hemorrhage into primary tumors is likely to be solitary. However, hemorrhage into metastases, or thrombotic and embolic complications may be single, multifocal, or clinically diffuse. Multifocal or diffuse disease may resemble a metabolic encephalopathy if there are bilateral lesions without herniation or brainstem or cranial nerve involvement. For example, the initial neurologic signs of 32 patients with nonbacterial thrombotic endocarditis were focal in 18 cases: hemiparesis, aphasia, visual field defects or cortical blindness, focal seizures, or brainstem symptoms.[4] Nine patients had a diffuse picture with confusion, lethargy, or coma, while five had a multifocal presentation.

Vascular complications should be considered when patients with brain tumors or widespread systemic cancer develop sudden neurologic symptoms or stepwise deficits. The general physical examination is occasionally helpful: septic emboli may cause hemorrhagic skin lesions, especially with pseudomonas infections.[4] Multifocal deficits raise the possibility of emboli if metastases are excluded by neuroimaging.

Investigations

Neuroimaging will often reveal the type of vascular lesion: hemorrhagic or ischemic. The pattern of lesions may define the process, e.g., cortical vein thrombosis or emboli. Scans should be done without contrast, then with contrast, to exclude hemorrhage into a tumor. For acute hemorrhage, CT scans are more sensitive that are MRI scans.

Hematologic evaluation includes a complete blood count, including platelets, and screening for coagulation disorders if necessary. A blood smear may give support to a microangiopathic process. A coagulation profile, including the international normalized ratio (INR) and partial thromboplastin time, may be helpful in hemorrhages. A screen for disseminated intravascular coagulation (reduced platelet count, a positive smear for fragmented red blood cells, elevated prothrombin time and partial thromboplastin time, decreased fibrinogen titer, and increased fibrin degradation products) should be carried out if multifocal ischemia is a consideration.

Blood cultures may be helpful in septic embolism. Chest film and echocardiographs (transesophageal, if necessary) may give supportive evidence for the source and type of emboli.

Management

Decisions regarding treatment are dependent on the stage of illness and the possibility of reversibility that would allow some quality of life for the patient, as well as consideration of the wishes of the patient. The treatment of specific disease entities is discussed in other areas of this book or in relevant references, e.g., *Harrison's Principles of Internal Medicine*.

INFECTIONS

Central nervous system and systemic infections constitute a major group of problems in patients with systemic cancer; in one series, 60 percent of cancer patients died from infections.[48]

Pathogenesis

Mechanisms for impaired consciousness are those discussed in Chap. 11. Risk factors that are present in over 85 percent of CNS infections in cancer patients include: Hodgkin disease or non-Hodgkin lymphoma, leukopenia, long-term use of immunosuppressive drugs, and a communication between the CNS and the epithelial surface, such as a ventricular drain or recent neurosurgery.[4] These risk factors may be combined. Certain organisms are favored in certain types of malignancy; these are listed in Table 7-4.

Systemic infections or sepsis are also common. Predisposing factors are immunosuppression (affecting polymorphonuclear leukocytes, lymphocytes, or immunoglobulin synthesis) from chemotherapy or radiation, or from systemic malignancy, especially lymphomas and leukemias. Occasionally, natural barriers to infection, e.g., mucosal surfaces, may be breached or compromised. Sepsis can affect the brain indirectly, as discussed in the section on septic encephalopathy (Chap. 12).

Table 7-4
Infections in cancer patients

Predisposing factor	CNS site	Bacteria	Fungi	Parasites	Viruses
T-lymphocyte or mononuclear phagocyte defects	Meningitis or meningoencephalitis	Listeria monocytogenes	Cryptoccocsus Coccidioides Histoplasma	Toxoplasma Strongyloides	Varicella-zoster Papovavirus (PML) Cytomegalovirus
	Brain abscess or encephalitis	Nocardia Listeria	Cryptococcus Histoplasma	Toxoplasma	Cytomegalovirus Herpes simplex
Neutrophil defects	Meningitis	[a] Enteric bacilli Pseudomonas aeruginosa E. coli K. pneumoniae Listeria Strep. pneumoniae Staph. aureus	Candida sp.		
	Meningoencephalitis	As above[a]	Aspergillis sp.		
	Abscess	As above[a]	Mucoraceae Candida sp.		
Splenectomy or B-cell abnormalities	Splenectomy	[b] Strep. pneumoniae H. influenzae N. meningitidis			Echovirus Cocksackie B
	Hypogammaglobulinemia	As above[b]			
CSF-surface communication	Meningitis	[c] Enteric bacilli Staph. aureus Coagulase-negative staph Propionobacter acnes	Candida	Trichomonadida	
	Meningoencephalitis	As above[c]	Candida		
	Abscess	As above[c]	Candida		

Abbreviations: Staph/staph = Staphylococcus; H = Haemophilus; E = Eschericheria; Strep = Streptococcus; N = Neisseria; K = Klebsiella; Listeria = Listeria monocytogenes; PML = progressive multifocal leukoencephalopathy.
Source: Modified from Posner,[4] with permission.

The pattern of bacterial infections in cancer patients, especially those who are immunosuppressed, is changing. Gram-positive infections are becoming more common; emerging infections with antibiotic-resistant organisms, e.g., methicillin-resistant *Staphylococcus aureus* and resistant enterobacter species, are now more common than pseudomonas infections. Prolonged myelosuppression, e.g., after bone marrow transplantation, and the use of venous access devices, e.g., Hickman catheters, are contributing factors.

Clinical Features

The clinician needs a high index of suspicion, as manifestations of infections in cancer patients may be different from other populations. Headache, meningismus, and fever may be absent, with an impaired inflammatory responses due to the cancer or its treatment. Manifestations of the infection can easily be attributed mistakenly to other causes, e.g., metastases or side effects of chemotherapy or radiotherapy.

A short list of diagnostic possibilities depends on the clinical setting (Table 7-4). The time course is most helpful. Acute meningitic symptoms (<5 days duration) suggest a pyogenic meningitis, while a subacute progression (>10 days) is more typical of a fungal or tuberculous meningitis, or possibly a viral infection such as progressive multifocal leukoencephalopathy (PML).[49] Infections following neurosurgical procedures are commonly caused by gram-negative organisms, or, more recently, gram-positive organisms, specifically *Staphylococcus* spp.

The pattern of clinical signs and symptoms may also help.[49] Focal signs suggest space-occupying lesions, such as one or more abscesses, cerebritis, PML, or vasculitis secondary to meningitis or preceding varicella infection. Cranial nerve involvement is common with meningitis due to tuberculosis, fungi, or *Listeria monocytogenes* infection.[49] Involvement of cranial nerves III, IV, VI, and the ophthalmic division of V strongly suggests cavernous sinus involvement, often from fungi or gram-negative bacteria.[49]

Herpes zoster-associated meningoencephalitis occurs as a complication in about 12 percent of patients who have both systemic cancer and cutaneous herpes zoster infections.[50] This is more common in those patients who have zoster involvement of the ophthalmic division of the trigeminal nerve.[50] Patients typically present with confusion, headache, and somnolence. Cerebrospinal fluid contains lymphocytes (up to 200 per cubic millimeter), increased protein, and normal glucose concentrations. Patients often respond well to acyclovir.[50]

Progressive multifocal leukoencephalopathy may cause impaired consciousness and function because of the fairly aggressive destruction of confluent regions of brain white matter, effectively causing disconnection.

Investigations

In cancer patients, it is probably best to do a CT or MRI of the head and to check the platelet count before performing a lumbar puncture to exclude meningitis. Amelioration of brain swelling (using corticosteroids or mannitol) and thrombocytopenia (by platelet transfusions for counts under 50,000 per cubic millimeter) allows the spinal tap to be performed in affected patients. A CSF white blood cell count of more than 100 cells per cubic millimeter is suggestive of a bacterial meningitis.[49] This may be lower if the patient is leukopenic. The glucose concentration is reduced in bacterial and tuberculous meningitis as well as in some fungal infections. In differential diagnosis, neoplastic meningitis can also cause lymphocytic pleocytosis, hypoglycorrhachia, and protein elevation. Table 11-1 gives a list of causes of lymphocytic meningitis. Among infections in cancer patients, lymphocytic meningitis mainly occurs with *Cryptoccocus neoformans, Listeria monocytogenes, Aspergillus fumigatus, Nocardia asteroides,* or viral infections.

Scanning by MRI or CT, especially with contrast enhancement, provides evidence for meningeal or dural disease. Neither method may allow differentiation of abscesses from tumors, or sufficient microbiologic information to allow for definitive antimicrobial therapy to be decided. This information is often available through blood or

CSF cell counts, chemical [including polymerase chain reaction (PCR)] analysis, and cultures.

Angiography may be needed if mycotic aneurysms are suspected, e.g., when bacteremia is accompanied by embolic stroke or intracranial hemorrhage. Any progressive CT or MRI lesion that is not responding to therapy, in a patient for whom treatment is worthwhile, should be biopsied. Examples might include: (1) suspect toxoplasmosis that fails to respond to 2 to 3 weeks of appropriate therapy, (2) the differentiation of herpes simplex encephalitis from other lesions, and (3) a non-specific ring-enhancing single mass lesion.

Treatment

The management of specific infections is discussed in Chaps. 11 and 12. Some caveats concerning cancer patients include the following:

1. With raised ICP, the volumes of free water administered need to be limited.

2. Neutropenic patients require especially vigorous treatment and monitoring to prevent superinfections, especially urinary tract sepsis.

3. Opportunistic infections are the major concern. Steps should be taken to reduce the risk in patients with immunologic deficiencies. Patients should be carefully monitored and symptoms of headache, lethargy, altered mental status, focal signs, or any combination of these, should trigger investigation to exclude a primary CNS or systemic infection. This investigation may include CSF analysis for meningitis, biopsy for parenchymal lesions (e.g., PML), or PCR techniques in the CSF or blood, to detect nucleic acid of the agent.[51]

4. Investigation and early institution of broad-spectrum treatment, based on the best clinical judgment and available microbiologic and other laboratory tests, should be vigorous.

5. Apparently successful treatment of a CNS or systemic infection should be followed by continued vigilance for late sequelae or recurrence of infection.

6. It is wise to keep current in the treatment of infections, which changes almost yearly.

Therapeutic strategies are emerging for disorders that were previously considered to be untreatable.[52,53]

DRUG, METABOLIC, AND NUTRITIONAL FACTORS

Metabolic encephalopathy in cancer patients occurs mainly as a result of vital organ dysfunction, and abnormal products secreted by the tumor or as the result of treatment, such as chemotherapy or radiotherapy or due to other concomitant medications.[4] Malnutrition can be caused by the disease or its treatment. These are collectively common complications; Posner estimates that about 15 percent of patients admitted to the Memorial Sloan-Kettering Cancer Center were suffering from a metabolic encephalopathy.[4] Most of the time the cause is multifactorial; drugs and single or multiple organ failure were the main contributors. Old age is probably a risk factor.

Advanced systemic cancer can lead to anorexia, accelerated catabolism, and reduced intake of essential micronutrients and vitamins. If nutritionally deficient cancer patients are given carbohydrate without thiamine supplementation, they are at risk for Wernicke's encephalopathy. Although this is occasionally documented, Wernicke's encephalopathy is probably underrecognized in this context.[54]

Specific Toxic and Metabolic Causes

Drugs

Medication effects should always be considered in the differential diagnosis when a cancer patient develops neurologic deterioration. Drug effects often need to be differentiated from direct or remote effects of the cancer itself, and from other complications such as infection, depression, seizures, or unrelated conditions.

There are a number of mechanisms by which drugs used in cancer patients may adversely alter brain function. Those drugs most commonly associated with an acute confusional state in cancer patients are opioids, and, less commonly, benzodiazepines, corticosteroids, and histamine receptor blockers. Chemotherapeutic agents themselves may cause any one of the following (1) a direct drug-related toxic effect on the brain, (2) a drug-induced intracranial hemorrhage from thrombocytopenia or altered coagulation, (3) CNS infection by producing immunosuppression, or (4) a psychologic effect on the patient.[55,56] In addition, there may be adverse effects from interactions between chemotherapeutic agents and other drugs.

Some of the toxic effects on the nervous system are irreversible, while others are reversible. Most effects are serious and require either discontinuation of the drug or a dose reduction.

Some drugs produce characteristic encephalopathic features. These are profiled briefly in the following sections.

Methotrexate Methotrexate (MTX) is a competitive inhibitor of the enzyme dihydrofolate reductase and it blocks synthesis of DNA, RNA, and proteins by limiting folate availability. High-dose ($>1 \, \text{g/m}^2$) intravenous MTX may cause a transient encephalopathy with an acute confusional state, coma, and/or seizures in 15 percent of treated patients.[55] It may also produce a stroke-like picture with hemiparesis. This is often delayed until several days after the second or third treatment. The condition is reversible and is unlikely to recur with subsequent lower-dose MTX therapy. Intrathecal MTX may produce an acute encephalomyelopathy that may be fatal. Intraventicular injections can also produce a toxic encephalopathy if there is outflow obstruction; inadvertent intracerebral injection produces an acute encephalopathy with focal features.[57]

A chronic, irreversible leukoencephalopathy is also associated with methotrexate.[4] This is characterized by reduced activity, an apathetic demeanor, and lack of spontaneity. In more extreme cases, patients are frankly abulic or have akinetic mutism, and upper motor neuron deficits. Scanning by CT and MRI reveals diffuse white matter change, while positron emission tomography (PET) shows a diffuse decrease in glucose metabolism in the deep white matter.[58] Pathologically, the condition is a disseminated necrotizing leukoencephalopathy.[59,60] The necrotizing white matter lesions are seen mainly in patients who had brain radiation in combination with intrathecal methotrexate; a synergistic effect is probable.

Less common encephalopathies include diffuse parenchymatous degeneration with gliosis and axonal dystrophy, diffuse and focal subpial necrosis of gray matter, mineralizing microangiopathy and dystrophic calcification, and a multifocal, nonnecrotizing axonopathy in the cerebral white matter.[61] The clinical pictures of encephalopathy with these varied pathologies did not differ greatly; in each, synergistic effect of intrathecal methotrexate and radiotherapy is possible.

Cisplatin Cisplatin has a variety of cellular effects. It may cause an encephalopathy, mainly with intra-arterial (sometimes used in head and neck cancer) or high-dose intravenous chemotherapy. Cortical blindness or a generalized encephalopathy with or without seizures may result. Ocular toxicity has also been described.[62] Systemic administration may be complicated by metabolic disturbances, including hypomagnesemia, hypocalcemia, and water intoxication from overhydration; or SIADH with brain swelling, hyponatremia, and seizures may occur as systemic complications.[63,64] Increased brain edema can be fatal, especially in patients who already have mass effects from an intracranial tumor. A large fiber axonal sensory neuropathy is probably the most common neurologic complication.

Cytarabine(Ara-C) This antimetabolite, affecting pyrimidine metabolism, is used systemically for the treatment of acute lymphoblastic and leukemia and non-Hodgkin lymphoma, and intrathecally for leukemic and lymphomatous meningitis.[65] It has been reported to cause a necrotizing encephalopathy when given intrathecally, in combination with radiotherapy. Not all cases received methotrexate intrathecally. A myelopathy may also occur.[65] In regimes requiring high intravenous doses, Ara-C is sometimes associated with an acute reversible encephalopathy consisting of generalized convulsions or complex partial seizures. Irreversible cerebellar degeneration and axonal polyneuropathy are probably more common. The Ara-C crosses the blood-brain barrier fairly readily; its neurotoxicity, which is dose dependent, is increased by prolonged high serum concentrations related to dosing or to hepatic or renal failure, which cause impaired drug clearance. Regimes with lower dosing may be as successful and have less risk of neurotoxicity.[66]

Nitrosoureas   Carmustine (BCNU), lomustine (CCNU), and semustine (methyl-CCNU), are alkylating agents that bind DNA. In addition, cellular damage is enhanced by the inhibition of intracellular peroxide detoxification.[67] High-dose (600 to 800 mg/m^2) intravenous administration may be associated with transient confusion and seizures. Intracarotid BCNU for glioma patients may produce an early, reversible encephalopathy, but it is also occasionally followed several weeks later by permanent dysfunction in the ipsilateral cerebral hemisphere, with necrosis, swelling, and dystrophic axonal calcification.[68] This is reported in patients who have not been irradiated and is reproduced by intracarotid injection in dogs.[69] Monocular blindness ipsilateral to the injected carotid artery also occurs. The disorder is usually not helped by corticosteroids and appears to be largely a direct neurotoxic effect of the BCNU.

L-Asparaginase   L-Asparaginase acts by catalyzing the hydrolysis of asparaginine to aspartic acid and ammonia, thereby depriving cells of asparaginine. It may cause a reversible encephalopathy that is dose dependent. Cortical vein or sinus thrombosis, and cerebral hemorrhage or infarction may occur as vascular complications.

Isofamide   Isofamide, an alkylating agent, may cause a reversible encephalopathy with disorientation, confusion, and somnolence.

Procarbazine   Procarbazine, a weak monoamine oxidase inhibitor that acts mainly as an alkylating agent, may cause a mild reversible encephalopathy when used systemically. High-dose intravenous or intra-arterial administration may produce a severe encephalopathy.

Chlorambucil   This alkylating agent may produce a reversible encephalopathy with seizures.

Biologic Response Modifiers   These naturally occurring compounds augment the inflammatory response against tumors. They include cytokines and interferons. Interleukin-2 commonly causes cerebral edema with a patchy or diffuse pattern of increased blood-brain barrier permeability. This is usually a mild, transient encephalopathy with focal or generalized dysfunction. Alpha interferon has been reported to cause an acute, reversible confusional state with hallucinations and sometimes seizures.[55]

Bone Marrow Transplantation

The immunosuppression and myelosuppression associated with bone marrow transplantation is associated with both early (within 6 weeks) and late (after 6 weeks from transplantation) neurologic, complications.[70] Among 168 patients with Hodgkin disease who had undergone bone marrow transplants, early complications occurred in about one-third of the patients and usually related to pulmonary complications with encephalopathy secondary to sepsis or respiratory failure. Others suffered seizures, psychiatric symptoms, and cerebral hemorrhage. Overall, early complications are reversible in about three-quarters of cases. Late complications are less common and include encephalopathy and intracerebral hemorrhage.

Overall, the incidence of neurologic complications may be somewhat higher than with bone marrow transplants for Hodgkin disease; approaching one-half the patients in some series.[70,71] Dysrhythmias of the EEG and visual evoked response abnormalities are common when looked for; these can be reversible. Leukoencephalopathies are uncommon, but do occur.[71] Infectious complications, especially if patients are depleted of T cells, include bacteremia (with encephalopathy) and systemic fungal infections that may directly invade the CNS.[72]

Hypoxemia, Global Ischemia, Hypoglycemia, and Hyperglycemia

Hypoxemia may relate to pneumonia, pulmonary metastases, or severe anemia. Severe hypotension or cardiac arrest may produce global ischemia. Isolated hypoglycemia is an uncommon cause of impaired consciousness in cancer. Fasting hypoglycemia may be found with severe hepatic damage from metastases (impaired glucose synthesis), reduced insulin antagonism (as found in adrenal or pituitary failure from metastases), increased glucose utilization by large tumors such as retroperitoneal sarcomas, and secretion of insulin-like hormones. In severely debilitated patients, starvation may be the cause. Some drugs, e.g., pentamidine, may produce hypoglycemia.

Hyperglycemia may be due to the accentuation of diabetes mellitus by the stresses or medication, e.g., corticosteroids, associated with cancer or its treatment. Occasionally, anti-insulin antibodies are produced in patients with myeloma.[73]

Sepsis

See Chap. 12.

Electrolytes, Calcium, and Magnesium

The clinical aspects of disturbances, diagnosis, and management of fluid and electrolyte disturbances are discussed in Chap. 13. Hyponatremia, which occurs in about 1 percent of cancer patients, is usually due to increased secretion of antidiuretic hormone, e.g., by small-cell lung cancer, or by drugs.[4] It is rarely the sole cause of encephalopathy in these patients, but it commonly contributes to the encephalopathy in patients with multifactorial encephalopathy.[74] Hypernatremia or hyperosmolality occurs less commonly, mainly in very ill patients.[75] It may relate to impaired thirst activity or obtundation, the inability to swallow fluids, or from excess water excretion or insensible loss with fever. Diabetes insipidus may result from cancer spread to the pituitary or hypothalamus, especially if there is exogenous corticosteroid replacement.

Hypercalcemia frequently accompanies cancer with bony metastases or in tumors that produce parathormone-like secretions—mainly associated with either small-cell lung cancer or breast cancer.[76] Less commonly, increased vitamin D-like substances secreted by the tumor, cytokine release, decreased renal excretion, or gastrointestinal absorption of calcium is responsible.[77] Hypocalcemia is unusual and a rare cause of encephalopathy in cancer patients.[4]

Hypomagnesemia may occur with cisplatin treatment, but this rarely causes an encephalopathy.[4] Hypermagnesemia is rare; it may occur with renal failure and magnesium administration.

Hypophosphatemia may result from reduced dietary intake, and certain parenteral or nonparenteral hyperalimentation, but it is not usually directly related to the cancer or specific anticancer treatment.

Organ Failure

The brain may be affected by an indirect secondary mechanism related to organ failure related to the cancer. Hepatic and pulmonary insufficiencies commonly produce an encephalopathy in cancer patients. Hyperammonemia associated with tumor lysis may cause a syndrome that resembles hepatic encephalopathy.[4]

Nutritional Deficiency Syndromes

Nutritional deficiency may develop if patients have insufficient intake of vitamins, or with malabsorption. Wernicke-Korsakoff syndrome (see Chap. 13) affects some patients during vigorous treatment for leukemia or lymphoma.[78] Any malnourished patient who develops an encephalopathy, especially with ocular movement problems, should be treated with thiamine. Also, vitamin supplementation should be given to any patient at risk of becoming malnourished.

Vitamin B_{12} deficiency has been described in patients with malabsorption secondary to radiation therapy for bladder cancer.[79]

Carcinoid syndrome is sometimes associated with pellagra. Carcinoid syndrome, consisting primarily of autonomic flushing and diarrhea, relates, at least in part, to increased serotonin production by the tumor.[80] Since serotonin synthesis requires niacin as a cofactor, the niacin may be depleted or insufficiently synthesized. Niacin deficiency is thought to be responsible for pellagra. Besides dermatitis and diarrhea, pellagra consists of mental changes, most commonly an agitated delirium. Emotional changes are also common. At least 35 percent of patients with pellagra have altered level of consciousness.[4]

Clinical Signs of Drug, Nutritional, and Metabolic Encephalopathies

The features are described in Chaps. 13, 15, and 16.

Management of Drug, Nutritional, and Metabolic Encephalopathies

Management hinges on an accurate diagnosis; prompt investigation is crucial. Structural lesions (multiple metastases, leptomeningeal cancer, or multifocal vascular insults) and seizures are commonly considered whenever cancer patients become confused or lose awareness. Metabolic factors and systemic or CNS infections must also be considered. Besides specifically targeted investigation, it is reasonable to perform an electroencephalogram (EEG) on any acutely confused cancer patient. This can give an immediate indication about the underlying process. The EEG is especially useful in detecting seizure activity; nonconvulsive status epilepticus may be otherwise unsuspected.

The specific tests and treatments for infectious, inflammatory, and metabolic causes can be found in Chaps. 3, 11, 12, and 13.

RADIOTHERAPY

Radiotherapy (RT) is beneficial in the treatment of primary and secondary brain tumors, as well as in the prevention of metastases or CSF seeding of secondary and primary brain tumors.[81] It can,

however, be followed by neurologic complications in many patients, depending on survival. The effects of radiation are often synergistic with those of chemotherapy.

Pathophysiology

The vascular endothelium is affected, with increased capillary permeability. Damage to groups of endothelial cells may lead to thromboses or, later, to multiplication of surviving cells with resultant plugging of the vessel and ischemia.[82] Neuronal and glial nucleic acid damage, lipid and protein alteration, activation of apoptotic controlling mechanisms, and immunologic activation (hypersensitivity vascular injury) have also been proposed to play secondary roles.[83–85] Indirectly, hypothyroidism may follow irradiation that involves the supraclavicular nodes and the adjacent thyroid gland.[86]

Clinical Syndromes

Acute Encephalopathy   This is found mainly in individuals with large brain tumors or raised ICP and it manifests within a few hours of their first RT treatment.[87] The syndrome almost certainly relates to increased permeability of the blood-brain barrier. It is more common with large dose fractions (>400 cGy) than conventional dose fractions (200 to 300 cGy).

In mild cases, patients experience increased headache, nausea, vomiting, somnolence, and worsening of pre-existing deficits. With more swelling, impairment of consciousness occurs with the appearance of herniation syndromes (see Chap. 4).

Corticosteroids are beneficial in the established syndrome. Acute encephalopathy may also be prevented or lessened by treating the patient with dexamethazone for at least 48 h before RT is started.

Most patients do well; the syndrome itself is usually completely reversible.[88]

"Early-Delayed Encephalopathy"   This deterioration begins between 2 weeks and 4 months following RT. The clinical manifestations are similar to those described for the acute encephalopathy. Like the acute form, the condition is usually reversible; in this case, within 6 months. Early-delayed encephalopathy is more difficult to differentiate from tumor regrowth. As with the acute syndrome, corticosteroids are beneficial.

A "radiation somnolence syndrome" consists of somnolence, often accompanied by headache, nausea, vomiting, raised ICP with papilledema, and decreased level of consciousness. It occurs mainly in children and does not necessarily involve a CNS tumor. It probably relates to a diffuse increase in blood-brain barrier permeability caused by the radiation, although immunologically mediated demyelination is also feasible. It usually resolves completely in 3 to 6 weeks without treatment.[4]

"Focal encephalopathy" may follow a high dose of RT delivered to a cranial structure such as an eye or ear tumor. The brainstem is often affected. Symptoms begin 8 to 11 weeks after the course of RT. Brainstem findings commonly include ataxia, nystagmus, and variable ophthalmoplegia. Although most patients recover in 6 to 8 weeks, some lapse into coma and die.[89] Some patients have widespread CNS demyelination with loss of oligodendroglia or dystrophic calcification in neuronal clusters and white matter axons. The blood vessels usually appear normal. Occasionally, the brainstem may be involved, with a clinical presentation of increasing somnolence, nystagmus, ataxia, cranial nerve deficits and, finally, deep stupor and respiratory insufficiency.[85,90] The brainstems of children, e.g., treated with radiation for brainstem gliomas, may be especially susceptible to radiation necrosis in this "early-delayed" period.[91]

"Late-Delayed Encephalopathy" Late-delayed encephalopathy, or radionecrosis, begins several months to years after the RT treatment. This, the main serious adverse effect of radiotherapy of the brain, is usually associated with vascular damage and regional necrosis of CNS tissue in the region of the radiation. The initial focal signs are the same as with the original tumor if this is in the field of radiation. Rarely the region is at a distance from the original lesion. The main differential diagnosis is recurrence of the tumor. Radiation necrosis can also be a complication of RT of extracranial tumors, such as head and neck cancers, in which the brain is included in the radiation field. The differential diagnosis here is direct extension of the tumor through the skull base or brain metastases. Radiation necrosis is also a recognized complication of repeat cranial irradiation, radiosurgery, and brachytherapy treatments of brain tumors and vascular malformations.

Neuroimaging with CT or MRI may not differentiate between necrosis and tumor. The diagnosis is made by demonstrating that the tissue is necrotic. This should be possible with nuclear medicine scanning with pyrophosphate, SPECT (single photon emission computed tomography), or PET with examination of blood flow or regional glucose metabolism. The mass effect can produce herniation and is best treated by surgical resection.

Diagnosis of Radiation-Induced Encephalopathy

To determine whether it is feasible that radiation produced the clinical picture observed, the clinician should determine the following: (1) if the signs or radiologic lesion correlate with the region irradiated, (2) the dose of radiation, (3) the total dose of radiation and the volume irradiated, and (4) the time between the RT and the onset of clinical symptoms.[4]

Management of Radiation Necrosis

Corticosteroids may help control associated cerebral edema. Anticoagulation has been proposed to be helpful, as well.[92] Surgical decompression is necessary if the mass effect is compromising function or if herniation is likely.

REMOTE EFFECTS OF CANCER

Paraneoplastic Limbic Encephalitis

Paraneoplastic limbic encephalitis (PLE) is a rare complication of small-cell cancer of the lung and occasionally of other tumors.[93,94] A similar syndrome can occur without underlying neoplasia.[95]

Pathology and Pathogenesis

Inflammatory changes are usually restricted to the limbic system and the insular cortex, although other deep gray matter structures may be involved, or extension into the white matter may occur.[96] Perivascular lymphocytic cuffing, microglial reaction, and neuronal loss with reactive gliosis are the microscopic findings.

The condition is due to inflammation within limbic structures. It is most likely an autoimmune phenomenon, but there is not conclusive evidence for this.[97] Most patients have anti-Hu antibodies in the serum.[98] In patients who die with paraneoplastic encephalitis, tissue-bound anti-Hu IgG is found in the neuronal nuclei of hippocampal and dentate gyrus neurons, bound to a 35- to 40-kDa nucleoprotein.[99,100] The role of the antibody in the production of the disorder is, however, uncertain. There is an imperfect correlation of the antibody in or attached to neurons with clinical and neuropathologic findings. The antibodies may not be essential for all cases or may be an epiphenomenon; indeed, the immunopathogenesis may be cell-mediated.[99]

Clinical Presentation

Patients develop subacute (days to weeks) symptomatology due to dysfunction in the limbic system, including profound memory disturbance, and personality and affective changes, often with agitation, hallucination, insomnia, and temporal lobe seizures (the latter may be complex partial or secondary generalized). Disinhibition, confusion and cognitive impairment may occur. The condition often is associated with subacute sensory neuropathy, although each occurs independently.[101]

Investigations

The EEG shows focal abnormalities (slowing, with or without epileptiform activity) in the temporal lobes. The CSF typically shows several to 100 mononuclear inflammatory cells per cubic millimeter. Neuroimaging is usually normal, but altered signal, reversible enhancement or T2-weighted MRI changes (Fig. 7-7) are found in the medial temporal lobe structures and sometimes in the brainstem.[102–104] A proportion (incidence not well defined) of patients have anti-Hu antibodies in their serum.[105]

Treatment

Patients rarely have spontaneously improved or recovered with treatment of the underlying cancer. Seizures can be treated and prevented with antiepileptic drugs. Immunosuppression, corticosteroids, plasmapheresis (to remove circulating antineuronal antibodies), high-dose intravenous immunoglobulin (IVIG), and other immunologically directed therapies are usually ineffective.

Encephalomyelitis

A similar brainstem or diffuse encephalomyelitis has also been described as a paraneoplastic syndrome.[4] With rostral brainstem involvement, alertness may be affected.[106] Multiple cranial nerve palsies (any cranial nerve may be affected), hypoventilation, dysphagia, myoclonus, and motor deficits may occur. Movement disorders, including chorea, dystonia, and parkinsonism, sometimes occur. The CSF usually shows inflammatory changes. The syndrome is probably immuno-mediated. Some patients with encephalitis and small-cell lung cancer have anti-Hu antibodies.[107] These IgG antibodies appear to be produced intrathecally and become attached to neuronal nuclei. Their role in the pathogenesis of this and other paraneoplastic syndromes remains unclear.

SEIZURES IN PATIENTS WITH CANCER

Seizures in patients with cancer may be due to brain or meningeal metastases, chemotherapy-related metabolic disturbance, infections, or, less commonly, a direct effect of the drug.

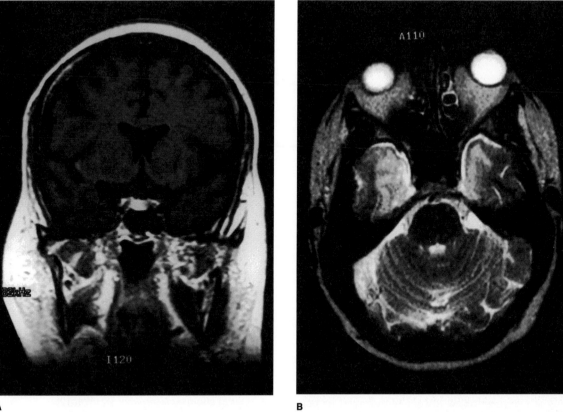

A   B

Figure 7-7

A. *A coronal T1-weighted MRI showing in the mesial-inferior temporal regions in a patient with limbic encephalitis. There was no enhancement with gadolinium. B. Another patient with limbic encephalitis. A T2-weighted MRI shows abnormal signal in both mesial-temporal regions, being more marked on the patient's right (left side of photograph).*

Focal Seizures and Structural Lesions

The association of cancer or brain tumors with seizures depends on the location of the lesions, the type of cancer/tumor, and possibly the patient's age. Seizures account for 60 percent of acute mental status changes in children with cancer.[3] Focal seizures (simple, complex, or secondary generalized) occur with brain tumors, typically when the cerebral cortex is directly infiltrated or deafferented. Low-grade primary brain tumors are more likely to cause seizures than high-grade tumors: 48 percent of low-grade gliomas and oligodendrogliomas are associated with seizures, compared with an incidence of 9 to 30 percent of glioblastoma cases.[108] Metastatic tumors, because of their proximity to the cerebral cortex, are commonly associated with seizures. Tumors with recent or remote hemorrhage are more epileptogenic than those without bleeding. Frontal lobe lesions are more commonly responsible for status epilepticus than lesions in other sites. It is common for convulsive status epilepticus to be the presenting symptom of a frontal lobe tumor. Nonconvulsive status epilepticus, either complex partial, simple partial, or generalized, can also occur.

Strokes, either embolic or thrombotic, arterial or venous, may be associated with focal or multifocal seizures.

Leptomeningeal cancer is commonly associated with seizures.

Metabolic Disorders and Drugs

Metabolic encephalopathies are one source of seizures: hyponatremia (e.g., with SIADH), hypoglycemia (e.g., with retroperitoneal sarcomas), hypophosphatemia (e.g., with leukemias and lymphomas), hypomagnesemia (e.g., with cisplatin therapy), and nonketotic hyperglycemia (e.g., in predisposed patients on corticosteroids).[4] These are discussed in greater detail in Chap. 13.

Seizures may occur as complications of the following chemotherapeutic agents: methotrexate, high-dose etoposide, cisplatin, vincristine, asparaginase, nitrogen mustard, carmustine, cyclosporine, dacarbazine, busulfan, cyclosporine,[109] mitronidazole, and misonidazole.[4] Some antibiotics such as imipenim and high-dose penicillin (usually in association with renal impairment) may also produce seizures. Seizures may rarely occur with α-interferon therapy.[110] Occasionally, myoclonus may complicate meperidine therapy, especially in patients with renal failure.[111] Seizures may sometimes follow abrupt withdrawal of benzodiazepines, barbiturates, or antiepileptic drugs.

Miscellaneous and Uncertain Etiologies

Occasionally, seizures may be due to CNS or systemic infection related to immunosuppression. Some antimicrobials, e.g., imipenim and in penicillin, may cause seizures in themselves at high doses or in association with renal failure.

Drislane has described a group of patients with neoplasms who developed nonconvulsive status epilepticus (NCSE) without any of the above etiologies.[112] These presented with an acute confusional state. It is unclear whether these were related to the cancer (e.g., a remote effect) or whether they occurred by chance. In the general hospital from which these came, 10 of 54 patients (19%) with EEG-proven NCSE had cancer. The nonconvulsive seizures showed generalized sharp and slow wave complexes on EEG.

Antiepileptic drug therapy improved the mental status in those patients who were vigorously treated. However, all ultimately died of various complications of cancer or sepsis.

Although the explanation of the NCSE in these patients remains in doubt, it is probably worthwhile to request an EEG in patients with cancer who develop an acute confusional state. If seizures are found, patients are likely to benefit from antiepileptic drug therapy.

REFERENCES

1. Boring CC, Squires TS, Tong T, et al: Cancer statistics 1994. *CA Cancer J Clin* 44:7, 1994.
2. Clouston PD, DeAngelis LM, Posner JB: The spectrum of neurological disease in patients with systemic cancer. *Ann Neurol* 31:268, 1992.
3. Di Mario FJ Jr, Packer RJ: Acute mental status changes in children with systemic cancer. *Pediatrics* 85:353, 1990.
4. Posner JB: *Neurological Complications of Cancer.* Philadelphia: FA Davis, 1995.
5. Fadul C, Wood J, Thaler H, et al: Morbidity and mortality of craniotomy for excision of supratentorial gliomas. *Neurology* 38:1374, 1988.
6. Blumberg DL, Sklar CA, Wisoff J, David R: Abnormalities of water metabolism in children and adolescents following craniotomy for a brain tumor. *Child's Nerv Syst* 10:505, 1994.
7. Zimberg M, Berenson S: Delirium in patients with cancer: nursing assessment and intervention. *Oncol Nurs Forum* 17:529, 1990.
8. Massie MJ, Holland J, Glass E: Delirium in terminally ill cancer patients. *Am J Psychiatry* 140:1048, 1983.
9. Weinrich S, Sarna L: Delirium in the older person with cancer. *Cancer* 74:2079, 1994.
10. Lassouw GM, Twinjnstra A, Schouten LJ, van de Pol M: The neuro-oncology register. *Neuroepidemiology* 11:261, 1992.
11. Delattre JY, Krol G, Thaler HTM et al: Distribution of brain metastases. *Arch Neurol* 45:741, 1988.
12. Posner JB, Chernik NL: Intracranial metastases from systemic cancer. *Adv Neurol* 19:575, 1978.
13. Pickren JW, Lopez G, Tsukada Y, et al: Brain metastases: an autopsy study. *Cancer Treatment Symp* 2:295, 1983.

14. Patchell RA: Brain metastases, in Patchell RA (ed): *Neurologic Clinics (Neurologic Complications of Systemic Cancer)*. Philadelphia, Saunders, vol 9, 1991, pp 817–824.

15. Sculier J-P, Feld R, Evans WK, et al: Neurologic disorders in patients with small cell lung cancer. *Cancer* 60:2275, 1987.

16. Dethy S, Piccart MJ, van Houtte P, Klastersky J: History of brain and epidural metastases from breast cancer in relation with disease evolution outside the nervous system. *Eur Neurol* 35:38, 1995.

17. Forsyth P, Posner J: Headaches in patients with brain tumors: a study of 111 patients. *Neurology* 43:1078, 1993.

18. Pepin EP: Cerebral metastases presenting as migraine with aura. *Lancet* 336:127, 1990.

19. Patchell RA, Tibbs PA, Walsh JW et al: A randomized trial of surgery in the treatment of single metastases to the brain. *N Eng J Med* 322:494, 1990.

20. Bentson JR, Steckel RJ, Kagan AR: Diagnostic imaging in clinical cancer management. *Invest Radiol* 23:335, 1988.

21. Moser RP, Johnson ML: Surgical management of brain metastases: How aggressive should we be? *Oncology* 3:123, 1989.

22. Cairncross JG, Kim JH, Posner JB: Radiation therapy for brain metastases. *Ann Neurol* 7:529, 1980.

23. Rosner D, Takuma N, Warren WL: Chemotherapy induces regression of brain metastases in breast carcinoma. *Cancer* 58:832, 1986.

24. Gonzalez-Vitale JC, Garcia-Brunuel R: Meningeal carcinomatosis. *Cancer* 37:2906, 1976.

25. Bigner SH, Johnson WW: The cytopathology of cerebrospinal fluid. II. Metastatic cancer, meningeal carcinomatosis and primary central nervous system neoplasms. *Acta Cytol* 25:461, 1981.

26. Alcolado R, Weller RO, Parrish EP, et al: The cranial arachnoid and pia mater in man: anatomical and ultrastructural observations. *Neuropathol Appl Neurobiol* 14:1, 1988.

27. Averback P: Primary cerebral venous sinus thrombosis in young adults: the diverse manifestations of an under-recognized disease. *Ann Neurol* 3:81, 1978.

28. Hiesiger EM, Picco-Del Bo A, Lipschutz LE, et al: Experimental meningeal carcinomatosis selectively depresses local cerebral glucose utilization in the rat brain. *Neurology* 39:90, 1989.

29. Hiesiger EM, Picco-Del Bo A, Lipschutz LE, et al: Experimental meningeal carcinomatosis selectively depresses local cerebral glucose utilization in the rat brain. *Neurology* 39:90, 1989.

30. Schold SC, Wasserstrom WR, Fleisher M, et al: Cerebrospinal fluid biochemical markers of central nervous system metastases. *Ann Neurol* 8:597, 1980.

31. Jacobi C, Reiber H, Felegenhauer K: The clinical relevance of locally produced carcinoembryonic antigen in cerebrospinal fluid. *J Neurol* 233:358, 1986.

32. Gossman SA, Moynihan TJ: Neoplastic meningitis, in Patchell RA (ed): *Neurologic Clinics (Neurologic Complications of Systemic Cancer)*. Philadelphia, Saunders, vol 9, 1991, pp 843–856.

33. van Zanten AP, Twijnstra A, Ongerboer de Visser BW, et al: Cerebrospinal tumor markers in patients treated for meningeal malignancy. *J Neurol Neurosurg Psychiatry* 54:119, 1991.

34. Twijnstra A, van Zanten AP, Nooyen WJ, Ongerboer de Visser BW: Sensitivity and specificity of single and combined tumor markers in the diagnosis of leptomeningeal metastases from breast cancer. *J Neurol Neurosurg Psychiatry* 49:1246, 1986.

35. Oschmann P, Kaps M, Volker J, Dorndorf W: Meningeal carcinomatosis: CSF cytology, immunocytochemistry and biochemical tumor markers. *Acta Neurol Scand* 89:395, 1994.

36. Bergmann M, Puskas Z, Kuchelmeister K: Subdural hematoma due to dural metastases: case report and review of the literature. *Clin Neurol Neurosurg* 94:235, 1992.

37. Kamada K, Isu T, Houkin K, et al: Acute aggravation of subdural effusion associated with pachymeningitis carcinomatosa: case report. *Neurosurgery* 29:464, 1991.

38. Minette SE, Kimmel DW: Subdural hematoma in patients with systemic cancer. *Mayo Clin Proc* 64:591, 1989.

39. Graus F, Rogers LR, Posner JB: Cerebrovascular complications in patients with cancer. *Medicine* 64:16, 1985.

40. Rogers LR: Cerebrovascular complications in cancer patients, in Patchell RA (ed): *Neurologic Clinics (Neurologic Complications of Systemic Cancer)*. Philadelphia, Saunders, vol 9, 1991, pp 889–899.

41. Belmusto L, Begelson W, Owens G, et al: Intracranial extracerebral hemorrhages in acute lymphocytic leukemia. *Cancer* 8:1079, 1964.

42. Ey FS, Goodnight SH: Bleeding disorders in cancer. *Semin Oncol* 17:187, 1990.

43. Glass J, Hochberg FH, Miller DC: Intravascular lymphomatosis. A systemic disease with neurologic manifestations. *Cancer* 71:3156, 1993.

44. Stahl RL, Chan W, Duncan A, Corley CC Jr: Malignant angioendotheliomatosis presenting as disseminated intravascular coagulopathy. *Cancer* 68:2319, 1991.

45. Torenbeek R, Scheltens P, Strack van Schijindel RJ, et al: Angiotropic intravascular large-cell lymphoma with massive cerebral extension. *J Neurol Neurosurg Psychiatry* 56:914, 1993.

46. Curtiss JL, Wharnock ML, Conrad DJ, Helfend LK, Boushey HA: Intravascular (angiotropic) large cell lymphoma (malignant angioendotheliomatosis with small vessel pulmonary vascular obstruction and hypercalcemia. *West J Med* 155:72, 1991.

47. Demirer T, Dail DH, Aboulafia DM: Four varied cases of intravascular lymphomatosis and a literature review. *Cancer* 73: L1738, 1994.

48. Hooper DC, Pruitt AA, Rubin RH: Central nervous system infection in the chronically immunosuppressed. *Medicine* 61:166, 1982.

49. Pruitt A: Central nervous system infections in cancer patients' in Patchell RA (ed): *Neurologic Clinics (Neurologic Complications of Systemic Cancer)*. Philadelphia, Saunders, vol 9, 1991, pp 867–888.

50. Hughes BA, Kimmel DW, Aksamit AJ: Herpes zoster-associated meningoencephalitis in patients with systemic cancer. *Mayo Clin Proc* 68: 652, 1993.

51. Aksamit AJ Jr.: Nonradioactive in situ hybridization in progressive multifocal leukoencephalopathy. *Mayo Clin Proc* 68:899, 1993.

52. Dalsgaard Hansen NJ, Madsen C, Stenager E: Progressive multifocal leukoencephalopathy. *Ital J Neurosci* 17:393, 1996.

53. Moreno S, Miralles P, Diaz MD, et al: Cytarabine therapy for progressive multifocal leukoencephalopathy in patients with AIDS. *Clin Infect Dis* 23:1066, 1996.

54. Engel PA, Grunnet M, Jacobs B: Wernicke-Korsakoff syndrome complicating T-cell lymphoma: unusual or unrecognized? *South Med J* 84:253, 1991.

55. Macdonald DR: Neurologic complications of chemotherapy, in Patchell RA (ed): *Neurologic Clinics (Neurologic Complications of Systemic Cancer)*. Philadelphia, Saunders, vol 9, 1991, pp 955–967.

56. Macdonald DR: Neurotoxicity of chemotherapeutic agents, in Perry MC (ed): *The Chemotherapy Source Book*, 2nd ed. Baltimore, Williams and Wilkin, 1996, pp 745–765.

57. Packer RJ, Zimmerman RA, Rosenstock J, et al: Focal encephalopathy following methotrexate therapy. Administration via a misplaced intraventricular catheter. *Arch Neurol* 38:450, 1981.

58. Milaytake S, Kikuchi H, Oda Y, et al: A case of treatment-related leukoencephalopathy: sequential MRI, CT and PET findings. *J Neuro-Oncol* 14:143, 1992.

59. Norrel H, Wilson CB, Slagel DE, Clark DB: Leukoencephalopathy following administration of methotrexate in the treatment of primary brain tumors. *Cancer* 33:923, 1974.

60. Skullerud K, Halvorsen K: Encephalopathy following intrathecal methotrexate treatment in a child with acute leukemia. *Cancer* 42:1211, 1978.

61. Shibutani M, Okeda R, Hori A, Schipper H: Methotrexate-related multifocal axonopathy. *Acta Neuropathol* 79:333, 1989.

62. Cattasneo MT, Filipazzi V, Piazza E, et al: Transient blindness and seizure associated with cisplatin therapy. *J Cancer Res Clin Oncol* 114:528, 1988.

63. Bellin SL, Selim M: Cisplatin-induced hypomagnesemia with seizures. A case report and review of the literature. *Gynecol Oncol* 30:104, 1988.

64. Ritch PS: Cis-dichlorodiammineplatinum II-induced syndrome of inappropriate secretion of antidiuretic hormone. *Cancer* 61:448, 1988.

65. Baker WJ, Royer GL, Weiss RB: Cytarabine and neurologic toxicity. *J Clin Oncol* 9:679, 1991.

66. Peters WCT, Willemze R: Cytarabine and CNS toxicity. *J Clin Oncol* 10:169, 1992.

67. Smith BH, Greenwood MA, Cummins CJ, et al: Non-nuclear cytotoxic actions of DNA cross-linking and/or alkylating agents in glioma-derived cell lines, in Walker MD, Thomas DGT (ed): *Biology of Brain Tumors*. Martinus Nijhof, 1986.

68. Rosenblum MK, Delattre J-Y, Walker RW, Shapiro WR: Fatal necrotizing encephalopathy complicating treatment of malignant gliomas with intra-arterial BCNU and irradiation: a pathological study. *J Neuro-Oncol* 7:269, 1989.

69. DeWys WD, Fowler EH: Report of vasculitis and blindness after intracarotid injection of 1,3-bis(2-chloroethyl)-1-nitrosourea (BCNU; NSC-409962) in dogs. *Cancer Chemother Rep* 57:33, 1973.

70. Snider S, Bashir R, Bierman P: Neurologic complications after high-dose chemotherapy and autologous bone marrow transplantation for Hodgkin's disease. *Neurology* 44:681, 1994.

71. Diener HC, Ehninger G, Schmidt H, et al: Neurologische Komplikationeen nach Knochenmarktransplantation. *Nervenzart* 62:221, 1991.

72. Pirsch JD, Maki DG: Infectious complications in adults with bone marrow transplantation, and T-cell depletion of donor marrow. Increased susceptibility to fungal infections. *Ann Intern Med* 104:619, 1986.

73. Redmon B, Pyzdrowski KL, Elson MK, et al: Hypoglycemia due to an insulin-binding monoclonal antibody in multiple myeloma. *N Eng J Med* 326:994, 1992.

74. Tuma R, DeAngelis LM: Acute encephalopathy, in patients with systemic cancer. *Ann Neurol* 32:288, 1992.

75. Snyder NA, Fiegal DW, Arieff AI: Hypernatremia in elderly patients. A heterogenous, morbid and iatrogenic entity. *Ann Intern Med* 107:309, 1987.

76. Theriault RL: Hypercalcemia of malignancy: pathophysiology and implications for treatment. *Oncology* 7:47, 1993.

77. Warrell RP Jr: Etiology and current management of cancer-related hypercalcemia. *Oncology* 6:37, 1992.

78. De Reuck J, Sieben G, De Coster W, et al: Prospective neuropathologic study on the occurrence of Wernicke's encephalopathy in patients with tumors in the lymphoid-hemopoietic systems. *Acta Neuropathol Suppl* 7:356, 1981.

79. Kinn A-C, Lantz B: Vitamin B12 deficiency after irradiation for bladder carcinoma. *J Urol* 131:888, 1984.

80. Moertel CG, Lvols LK, Rubin J: A study of cyproheptadine in the treatment of metastatic carcinoid tumor and the malignant carcinoid syndrome. *Cancer* 67:33, 1991.

81. Lischner M, Feld R, Payne DG, et al: Late neurological complications after prophylactic cranial radiation in patients with small-cell lung cancer: the Toronto experience. *J Clin Oncol* 8:215, 1990.

82. Hopewell JW, Wright EA: The nature of latent cerebral irradiation damage and its modification by hypertension. *Br J Radiol* 43:161, 1970.

83. Lavey RS, Johnstone AK, Taylor JM, et al: The effect of hyperfractionation on spinal cord response to radiation. *Int J Radiat Oncol Biol Phys* 24:681, 1992.

84. Carson DA, Ribeiro JM: Apoptosis and disease. *Lancet* 341:1251, 1993.

85. Lampert PW, Davis RL: Delayed effects of radiation on the human central nervous system: "early" and "late" delayed reactions. *Neurology* 14:912, 1964.

86. Bruning P, Bonfrer J, De Jong-Bakker M, Nooyen W, Bergers M: Primary hypothyroidism in patients with irradiated supraclavicular lymph nodes. *Br J Cancer* 51:659, 1985.

87. Young DF, Posner JB, Chu F, et al: Rapid-course radiation therapy of cerebral metastases: Results and complications. *Cancer* 4:1069, 1974.

88. Sheline G, Wara WM, Smith V: Therapeutic irradiation and brain injury. *Rad Oncol Biol Phys* 6:1215, 1980.

89. Monro P, Wair WG: Radiation effects on the human central nervous system 14 weeks after x-radiation. *Acta Neuropathol* 11:267, 1968.

90. Kleinschmidt-Demasters BK: Necrotizing brainstem leukoencephalopathy six weeks following radiotherapy. *Clin Neuropath* 14:63, 1995.

91. Packer RJ, Zimmerman RA, Kaplan A, et al: Early cystic/necrotic changes in hyperfractionated radiation therapy in children with brain stem gliomas. *Cancer* 71:2666, 1993.

92. Glantz MJ, Burger PC, Friedman AH, et al: Treatment of radiation-induced nervous system injury with heparin and warfarin. *Neurology* 44:2020, 1994.

93. Bakheit AMO, Kennedy PGE, Behan PO: Paraneoplastic limbic encephalitis: clinico-pathological correlations. *J Neurol Neurosurg Psychiatry* 53:1084, 1990.

94. Deohare S, O'Connor P, Ghazarian D, Bilboa JM: Paraneoplastic limbic encephalitis in Hodgkin's disease. *Can J Neurol Sci* 23:138, 1996.

95. Brierley JB, Corsellis JAN, Hierons R, et al: Subacute encephalitis of later adult life mainly affecting the limbic areas. *Brain* 83:357, 1960.

96. Corsellis JA, Goldberg GJ, Norton AR: "Limbic encephalitis" and its association with carcinoma. *Brain* 91:481, 1968.

97. Posner JB, Dalmau J: Clinical enigmas of paraneoplastic neurologic disorders. *Clin Neurol Neurosurg* 97:61, 1995.

98. Honnorat J, Antoine JC: Value of detection of anti-nervous system antibodies in neurologic paraneoplastic syndrome. *Rev Med Interne* 15:124, 1994.

99. Dalmau J, Furneaux HM, Rosenblum MK, Graus F, Posner JB: Detection of the anti-Hu antibody in specific regions of the nervous system and tumor

from patients with paraneoplastic encephalomyelitis/sensory neuropathy. *Neurology* 41:1757, 1991.

100. Heidenriech F, Schober R, Brinck U, Hartung HP: Multiple paraneoplastic syndromes in a patient with antibodies to neuroproteins. *J Neurol* 242:210, 1995.

101. Graus F, Elkon KB, Cordon-Cardo C, Posner JB: Sensory neuropathy and small cell lung cancer: anti-neuronal antibody that also reacts with the tumor. *Am J Med* 80:45, 1986.

102. Burton GV, Bullard DE, Walther PJ, et al: Paraneoplastic limbic encephalopathy with testicular carcinoma. A reversible neurological syndrome. *Cancer* 62:2248, 1988.

103. Dalmau J, Graus F, Rosenblum MK, et al: Anti-Hu-associated paraneoplastic encephalomyelitis/sensory neuropathy. A clinical study of 71 patients. *Medicine* 71:59, 1992.

104. Dirr LY, Elster AD, Donofrio PD, et al: Evolution of brain MRI abnormalities in limbic encephalitis. *Neurology* 40:1304, 1990.

105. Dalmau J, Furneaux HM, Rosenblum MK, et al: Detection of the anti-Hu antibody in specific regions of the nervous system and tumor from patients with paraneoplastic encephalomyelitis/sensory neuropathy. *Neurology* 41:1757, 1991.

106. Reddy RV, Vakili ST: Midbrain encephalitis as a remote effect of a malignant neoplasm. *Arch Neurol* 38:781, 1981.

107. Dalmau J, Furneaux HM, Rosenblum MK, et al: Detection of the anti-Hu antibody in specific regions of the nervous system and tumor from patients with paraneoplastic encephalomyelitis/sensory neuropathy. *Neurology* 41:1757, 1991.

108. LeBlanc FE, Rasmussen T: Cerebral seizures and brain tumors, in Vinken PJ, Bruyn GW (eds): *Handbook of Clinical Neurology*. Amsterdam, North Holland, vol 15, 1974, pp 295–301.

109. Gieron MA, Barak LS, Estrada J: Severe encephalopathy associated with ifosamide administration in two children with metastatic tumors. *J Neuro-Oncol* 6:29, 1988.

110. Meyers CA, Obbens EA, Sheibel RS, Mosper RP: Neurotoxicity of intraventricularly administered alpha-interferon for leptomeningeal disease. *Cancer* 68:88, 1991.

111. Kaiko RF, Foley KM, Grabinski PY, et al: Central nervous system excitatory effects of meperidine in cancer patients. *Ann Neurol* 13:180, 1983.

112. Drislane FW: Nonconvulsive status epilepticus in patients with cancer. *Clin Neurol Neurosurg* 96:314, 1994.

Chapter 8

IMPAIRED CONSCIOUSNESS AND DISORDERS OF TEMPERATURE

G. Bryan Young

HYPERTHERMIA

Humans are homeothermic animals who regulate their internal body temperature within narrow limits (36 to 37.5°C in the 24-h cycle). While a core temperature of 37°C allows us a certain degree of independence from the environment, it is at the upper end of the limits of thermal viability. The high metabolic rate, production of free radicals, and optimal enzyme activity at 37°C require an efficient system of thermoregulation to prevent a destructive rise in temperature. The hypothalamus plays a key role in monitoring temperature and maintaining thermal homeostasis by physiologic and behavioral modifications. Increased heat flow to the skin and increased sweating are the two physiologic methods of dissipating heat, while peripheral vasoconstriction and shivering (increasing metabolic production of heat) are methods of reducing heat loss and raising body temperature. Avoidance of exposure to heat and drinking cool liquids are behavioral adaptations to prevent excessive body temperature.

Temperature measurement remains a "vital sign." In fever, the hypothalamic set point is elevated to a higher value. Fever has been associated with disease since at least the time of Hippocrates (about 400 B.C.). The differential diagnosis of fever related to encephalopathy is given in Chap. 12. In most cases, fever, or temperature $T = >38.5°C$, is due to activation of prostaglandin E_2, which resets the hypothalamic autoregulatory set point, by various endogenous pyrogens.

In hyperthermia, the hypothalamic set point is normal, but there is a problem with heat generation or heat dissipation. Table 8-1 gives a classification of hyperthermia based on excessive heat production, problems with heat dissipation, and problems with the central regulatory function of the hypothalamus.

Excessive heat is generated in malignant hyperthermia, a dominantly inherited defect in calcium transport resulting in increased muscle activity.[1,2] Attacks are often triggered by medications, especially general anesthetics. The latter leads to increased metabolism in the large skeletal muscle mass and causes dangerous elevations in body temperature. A somewhat similar end result may occur with abrupt loss of central dopaminergic activity from neuroleptic drugs (neuroleptic malignant syndrome) or the sudden cessation of antiparkinsonian drugs in patients with severe

Table 8-1

Causes of hyperthermia

Disorders of heat production
Exertional hyperthermia
Heatstroke (exceptional)
Malignant hyperthermia of anesthesia
Neuroleptic malignant syndrome
Lethal catatonia
Thyrotoxicosis
Pheochromocytoma
Salicylate intoxication
Drug abuse (especially cocaine and amphetamines)
Delirium tremens
Status epilepticus (especially convulsive type,
　　occasionally with complex partial seizures)
Generalized tetanus

Disorders of diminished heat dissipation
Heatstroke (classic)
Extensive use of occlusive dressings
Dehydration
Autonomic dysfunction
Use of anticholinergic medications
Neuroleptic malignant syndrome[a]
Cervical spinal cord lesions (+ hot environment)

Disorders of hypothalamic function
Neuroleptic malignant syndrome[a]
Cerebrovascular accidents
Encephalitis
Sarcoidosis and granulomatous infections
Trauma

[a]Mixed mechanisms.
Source: Adapted from Simon.[35]

Parkinson disease.[3–6] Similarly, epileptic seizures, the increased activity of delirium tremens, tetanus, and malignant catatonia are associated with increased muscular activity and excessive heat production. Increased metabolism also occurs with hyperthyroidism. The sympathetic overactivity of pheochromocytoma and certain drugs (cocaine and amphetamines) decrease heat loss because of vasoconstriction, but may also be associated with increased muscular activity and a resetting of the hypothalamus.

　　Lesions of, or drug effects on, the anterior hypothalamus may impair heat-dissipating mechanisms. Because of impaired hypothalamically

mediated vasodilatation and sweating, patients with cervical cord lesions or autonomic neuropathy are especially prone to hyperthermia in a hot environment.

　　Temperature elevation is itself a threat to the nervous system and to the body in general. This section will concentrate on heat illness in its own right. In the purest sense, it relates to environmental heat stress, but endogenous problems such as malignant hyperthermia are also important.

Definition

Heatstroke refers to central nervous dysfunction related to hyperthermia due to high environmental temperatures, with or without exertion. Because heatstroke is the main hyperthermic condition that directly relates to impaired consciousness, it will be emphasized.

　　Hyperthermia may also result from the other disorders listed in Table 8-1.

Incidence

The incidence of severe hyperthermia is highest in hot, summer months. During a summer heat wave in the United States, the death rate due to hyperthermia may exceed 1200 persons.[7] The elderly poor are the most vulnerable. Clusters of cases may occur during military exercises, fun runs, and other activities in hot weather.

Clinical Features

The principal manifestations of heatstroke are listed in Table 8-2.

　　Pyrexia and prostration are the most important and common manifestations. The rectal temperature is usually greater than 41.1°C. The pulse is increased, blood pressure is usually low, and the respirations are shallow. The skin is typically warm and dry (no sweating). Petechiae may be present on the skin and mucous membranes.

　　Initially, there is a mild impairment of cognitive function, including judgment, followed by a more profound acute confusional state. This may progress to a delirium with agitation, increased sympathetic nervous activity, and hallucinations.

Table 8-2

Manifestations of heatstroke

System	Manifestation
Central nervous system	Confusional state (delirium)
	Seizures (status epilepticus)
	Oculogyric crisis
	Stupor
	Coma
	Cerebellar damage
	Hemiplegic episodes
Cardiovascular	Tachycardia
	Hypertension
	Hypotension (shock)
	Acute left heart failure
Pulmonary	Hyperventilation
	Pulmonary edema
	Pulmonary infarction
Renal	Acute nephropathy
	Chronic interstitial nephritis
Hematologic	Pupura, bleeding into various organs, including CNS
Gastroenterologic	Diarrhea and vomiting
	Hematemesis and melena
Endocrine	Hypoglycemia
Musculoskeletal	Muscles contracted and rigid, myoglobinuria

Source: Hart and Sutton,[36] with permission.

Further progression may lead to impairment of alertness with somnolence, stupor, or coma. Convulsive seizures may occur with markedly elevated temperatures. Bouts of oculogyric crises or decerebrate rigidity may occur.

Pupils are usually small, but reactive. Corneal and oculocephalic responses are intact.

Pathophysiology and Pathology

In experimental animals, temperatures above 42°C cause decreased cerebral metabolism and slowing of the electroencephalogram (EEG).[8]

Hyperpyrexia may impair neurologic function by a number of mechanisms. Interleukin-1 and other cytokines may have a direct effect on the central nervous system in those conditions in which they are generated (see "Sepsis-Associated Encephalopathy," Chap. 12).

The brain concentration of extracellular glutamate, an excitotoxic neurotransmitter, is directly related to temperature. Excessive amounts may cause an encephalopathy, including seizures.

Systemic abnormalities may also play a role in contributing to the encephalopathy. This applies to hypoglycemia, hypophosphatemia, extreme electrolyte disturbances, uremia, and other end-organ damage.

Hemorrhages may occur in various organs, including the brain. These and microscopic infarctions relate to endothelial damage and disseminated intravascular coagulation. Areas showing maximal damage include the cerebellar cortex, cerebral cortex, thalamus, and striatum.[9]

In a number of conditions associated with hyperthermia, especially the neuroleptic malignant syndrome and acute dopamine deficiency in treated parkinsonian patients, it has been proposed that activation of *N*-methyl-D-aspartate (NMDA) receptors, upon which glutamate acts, plays a role in the disorder itself.[10]

Laboratory Features

Hemoconcentration, electrolyte abnormalities (potassium is initially decreased and then increased in late stages), acid-base disturbances (respiratory alkalosis in early stage and metabolic acidosis late), hypoglycemia, hypocalcemia, hypophosphatemia, hypomagnesemia, myoglobinuria, elevated muscle enzymes, proteinuria, and microscopic hematuria are common. Thrombocytopenia and leukocytosis are frequent. Disseminated intravascular coagulation is a potentially serious complication. Hepatic dysfunction and renal failure are among the first evidences of multiorgan failure; these may contribute significantly to the encephalopathy.

Management

Prevention People who are most at risk for heatstroke are the very young, the very old, the obese, and those who are lacking in acclimatization.[11] Other predisposing conditions include autonomic neuropathy (especially in diabetes mellitus), the use of anticholinergic drugs, skin diseases associated with impaired sweating, and the use of diuretics. Such individuals should exercise caution: i.e., avoid running in hot, humid weather; seek shade, adequate hydration, and air conditioning.

Treatment   Treatment should begin on-site with cooling therapy and hydration with intravenous fluids. Removing clothing, and cooling with a fan and a fine, warm spray is a simple effective method of instituting prompt therapy that can prove life-saving.[12]

Meticulous electrolyte, cardiovascular, and neurologic monitoring is necessary as soon as the patient reaches medical care.

Cooling is important. Cooling of the brain is difficult unless the blood going to it is also cooled. Ice-water baths may be necessary in a severe case. Phenothiazines help to reduce shivering and antipyretics may assist in resetting the hypothalamus if the problem relates to fever as described above.

Kornhuber and colleagues (1993) recommend the use of NMDA antagonists for neuroleptic malignant syndrome and akinetic hyperthermic parkinsonian crisis related to abrupt withdrawal of dopaminergic agents.[10] Such drugs include amantadine and memantine.

Antiepileptic drug therapy involves standard therapy for status epilepticus (see Chap. 17).

Outcome

The outcome is often an all-or-none phenomenon; patients usually either die or recover completely. Neurologic sequelae include mental disorder, pancerebellar ataxia, central weakness, and flaccid quadriplegia.[13] Other problems include heat sensitivity and a persisting inability to perspire despite anatomically normal sweat glands.[14] Mortality in some series is 50 percent.[15]

HYPOTHERMIA

Definition

Hypothermia is defined as a body temperature below 35°C. Severe cases are much less common than those of hyperthermia, but hypothermia is even more of a medical emergency as it often reflects very serious underlying disorders.

Clinical Significance

In hospitals admitting from inner cities, patients who collapse indoors from hypothermia are usually the elderly, living alone, who have an underlying systemic illness and fall to the floor in poorly heated residences.[16] In contrast, hypothermic patients admitted from outside their place of residence are younger. Those from cities are often acutely intoxicated alcoholics.[16] Those exposed during recreational activities (skiing, hiking, etc.) are usually younger and in previously good health. More profound hypothermia resulting from prolonged exposure to very cold temperatures is more likely in the latter group, however.

Classification

Hypothermia can be divided into accidental, primary, and secondary (Table 8-3). Cases of idiopathic hypothermia, sometimes spontaneous and episodic, have been reported.[17] However, these are usually not severe or protracted.

Hypothermia is also classified by severity as mild (32 to 35°C body temperature), moderate (28 to 32°C), and severe (<28°C). This is shown in Table 8-4, along with the associated physiologic changes. Hypothermia may also be acute (minutes), subacute (hours), and chronic (days), depending on the time of development.

Hypothermia may also be thought of in terms of the following causes: (1) excessive heat loss: cold weather or immersion in cold water; (2) abnormal heat conservation and reduced heat production: hypothyroidism, hypoglycemia (substrate depletion), hypopituitarism, hypoadrenalism, uremia, spinal cord transection above T1, peripheral neuropathy, autonomic neuropathy and use of certain drugs (alcohol, barbiturates, and neuroleptics); and (3) defective heat regulation: hypothalamic lesions including Wernicke's encephalopathy, strokes, tumors, head trauma, and congenital abnormalities (e.g., Shapiro syndrome).

Table 8-3
Classification of hypothermia

Type	Cause	Examples
Accidental	Exposure to extreme cold	Outdoor activities; falls with immobilization in cold indoors
Primary	Hypothalamic disorder affecting thermoregulation	Hypothalamic lesion, Wernicke's encephalopathy, spontaneous cyclic hypothermia, congenital CNS abnormalities
Secondary	Underling cardiovascular, neurologic or endocrine disease. Mental illness, drug abuse, alcoholism, and malnutrition may contribute	Quadriplegia, severe parkinsonism, autonomic neuropathy,[a] hypothyroidism, adrenal insufficiency, hypopituitarism, Wernicke's encephalopathy, advanced sepsis, alcohol or drugs, multiple sclerosis[a,b]

[a] Affecting efferent outflow.
[b] Hypothalamic involvement.

Table 8-4
Severity classification of hypothermia

Level of hypothermia	Body temperature range	Physiologic effects
Mild	36.5–32°C	Catecholamine release; peripheral vasoconstriction; increased ventilatory rate; cold-induced diuresis; confusion, faulty judgment; shivering, hyporeflexia
Moderate	32–28°C	Decreased metabolic rate, decreased oxygen consumption, enzyme suppression, sympathetic nervous reduction, hyporeflexia, coagulopathies, decreased ventilation rate, stupor
Severe	28–20°C	Metabolic acidosis, increased cardiac irritability, ventricular fibrillation, severe hypotension, decreased or absent ventilation, hyperkalemia, coma
Profound	<20°C	Asystole, mimics brain death, flat EEG

Pathophysiology

Hypothermia is due to a disturbance in the net regulation of heat production and heat loss, weighted towards the latter. This can result from defective homeostatic regulation, reduced metabolism (including diminished cellular metabolism and shivering), or increased loss from exposure to extreme cold or an impaired cardiovascular response, especially loss of vasomotor tone.

Acute hypothermia is usually the result of submersion in cold water, subacute hypothermia often results from exposure to cold air, while chronic hypothermia relates to underlying disease with disordered or insufficient autoregulation.

Metabolic processes slow, and cerebral blood flow diminishes, by about 6 percent for each 1°C decrease in body temperature. At 28°C, the metabolic rate falls to half normal. At less than 25°C, the patient looks dead and has asystole.

With severe hypothermia of 25°C, there is loss of cerebrovascular autoregulation.[18] Cerebral blood flow declines in a pressure-passive manner along with a fall in systemic blood pressure. The EEG synaptic activity fails.

Both intrinsic and extrinsic coagulation systems are affected in hypothermia.[19] Platelet function becomes ineffective because thromboxane B_2 is inhibited. Fibrinolytic activity is increased and a heparin-like substance is released. Reduced activity of enzymes necessary to initiate and maintain platelet-fibrin clots results in a net increase in bleeding tendency. These features produce a disseminated intravascular coagulation-like syndrome but with a marked hemorrhagic tendency. This can be aggravated in the hypothermic trauma patient who may require massive transfusions for blood loss.

Clinical Features

Clinical features of mild hypothermia include shivering, tachycardia, tachypnea, diuresis, and peripheral cyanosis. It is important to feel the temperature of the trunk. In hypothermia, the trunk and normally warm regions such as the axillae and groins are cold. A low-reading thermometer should be used to take a rectal temperature. The patient with chronic hypothermia may resemble a patient with hypothyroidism, having puffy facies, slow hoarse speech, and mental changes. The skin has a doughy consistency. Neurologic features include dysarthria, ataxia, and amnesia.

With worsening, the pulse gets weaker and slower, shivering ceases, respirations are slow and shallow, and the patient becomes very pale. Deep tendon reflexes are increased above 32°C; hyporeflexia occurs between 26 and 32°C, and areflexia is present below 26°C. Confusion worsens, sometimes to delirium, and muscular rigidity develops. Further deterioration leads to stupor or coma. Coma does not usually occur above 28°C; other causes for coma should be sought if the patient is comatose with a core temperature of $> 28°C$. The pupils may become fixed to light, and the heart may develop ventricular fibrillation without palpable pulse or audible heart beat.

The clinical context of the hypothermia is often the best clue to the underlying cause. Environ-mental exposure to cold, or a history or findings of a high cervical cord lesion, polyneuropathy, or hypothryroidism are usually obvious. The patient who presents with hypothermia in the summer usually has a serious illness, e.g., Wernicke's encephalopathy (even if ocular movement abnormalities are not present), sepsis, drug overdose (e.g., neuroleptics, high-dose barbiturates) or, sometimes, combinations of causes.[20]

Laboratory Features

The EEG develops evolutionary changes, with generalized slowing beginning at 30°C, then it changes to a burst-suppression pattern by 20 to 22°C, and becomes flat at 18°C.[21] Evoked responses are less affected. At 29°C, wave forms are delayed by 33 percent, but are still identifiable. Latencies become lengthened progressively to unrecordable levels as 19°C is approached, and waveforms may disappear altogether.[22,23] Barbiturates and hypoxia modify the evoked responses to hypothermia.[24] Transcranial motor evoked responses increase in amplitude and latency to reach a maximum at 28°C.[25] This effect is modified by anesthesia and carbon dioxide concentration.

A series of cardiac abnormalities occurs with progressive hypothermia: obscured P waves; prolonged PR, QRS, and QT intervals; atrial fibrillation; and ventricular dysrhythmias. Ventricular fibrillation may develop at $\leq 28°C$.

Serum potassium should be checked, as hyperkalemia is a common accompaniment.[26] A coagulation screen should probably be performed.[27]

Tests to confirm or exclude diagnostic impressions for the underlying cause are usually necessary, but are context-dependent (see above).

Management

Prevention of hypothermia involves dressing warmly in cold weather, avoiding adverse weather, maintaining adequate nutrition, maintaining adequate indoor temperatures, and regular checks on elderly patients in cold weather. Patients with quadriplegia, who cannot conserve heat by vasoconstriction or increase heat production by shivering, are especially at risk of hypothermia if exposed to cold environmental temperatures.[28]

As a general policy, patients found in an acute hypothermic situation should not be pronounced dead until they are assessed after rewarming to at least 33°C core temperature. It is also important not to give up prematurely in resuscitative efforts. There are no reliable outcome scores or predictors.

Rewarming should be carried out expectantly, watching for serious cardiac arrhythmias, afterdrop (a drop in core body temperature associated with conduction of heat away from the core during the rewarming of surrounding cold tissues and the associated vasodilatation), and hypotension.

Simple rewarming techniques should begin in the field. These include removing wet, cold clothing, covering with warm, dry blankets, and administering warmed intravenous fluids.

Active internal rewarming using intravenous fluids and warmed medical air (core rewarming) should be carried out only when the temperature is < 32°C. The temperature should be increased to 40 to 42°C to prevent afterdrop. However, it is safest to perform vigorous rewarming in an intensive care unit (ICU) setting, because of cardiovascular instability/complications. Other methods of increasing core temperature more rapidly include the use of cardiopulmonary bypass, and continuous arteriovenous rewarming or irrigation of the gastrointestinal tract or body cavities.[29] Monitoring core temperature with an esophageal temperature probe or pulmonary artery catheter should be considered for more accurate measurement of "core" temperature. Cardiovascular support in the ICU is required.[30,31]

In frail, elderly individuals, the rewarming should be performed gradually to avoid cardiovascular collapse: a rate of no more than 0.5°C/hour has been recommended.[32]

Treatment of the underlying cause should be in concert with rewarming. The administration of thiamine, antibiotics, or drug antagonists need not wait for correction of temperature.

Outcome/Prognosis

An overall mortality associated with hypothermia is about 17 percent.[33] This involves all ages, etiologies, and classifications of hypothermia. Those with extreme hyperkalemia (mean serum potassium of 14.5 mmol/L) are always in cardiopulmonary arrest and have a poor prognosis for successful resuscitation.[26] Markedly elevated serum ammonia is also a marker of cell lysis.[34]

REFERENCES

1. Britt BA, Kalow W: Malignant hyperthermia: a statistical review. *Can Anaesth Soc* 17:293, 1970.
2. Nelson TE, Flewellen EH: Current concepts: the malignant hyperthermia syndrome. *N Eng J Med* 309:445, 1983.
3. Gratz SS, Levinson DF, Simpson GM: The treatment and management of neuroleptic malignant syndrome. *Prog Neuropsychopharmacol Biol Psychiatry* 16:425, 1992.
4. Susman VL, Addonizio G: Recurrence of neuroleptic malignant syndrome. *J Nerv Ment Dis* 176:234, 1988.
5. Pfeiffer RF, Sucha EL: "On-off"-induced lethal hyperthermia. *Mov Disord* 4:338, 1989.
6. Di Rosa AE, Morgante L, Corcaci MA, et al: Functional hyperthermia due to central dopaminergic impairment. *Funct Neurol* 3:211, 1988.
7. Heatstroke—United States, 1980. *MMWR Morb Mortal Wkly Rep* 30:277, 1981.
8. Meyer JS, Handa J: Cerebral blood flow and metabolism during experimental hyperthermia (fever). *Minn Med* 50:37, 1967.
9. Malmud N, Haymaker W, Custer RP: Heat stroke: a clinicopathologic study of 125 fatal cases. *Mil Surgeon* 99:397, 1946.
10. Kornhuber J, Weller M, Riederer P: Glutamate receptor antagonists for neuroleptic malignant syndrome and akinetic parkinsonian crisis. *J Neurol Transm Park Dis Dement Sect* 6:63, 1993.
11. Sutton JR, Bar-Or O: Thermal illness in fun running. *Am Heart J* 100:778, 1980.
12. Kielblock AJ: Strategies for the prevention of heat disorders with particular reference to the efficacy of body cooling procedures, in Hales JRS, Richards D (eds): *Heat Stress.* Amsterdam, Excerpta Medica, 1987, pp 489–497.

13. Salem SN: Neurological complications of heat stroke in Kuwait. *Ann Trop Med Parasitol* 60:393, 1966.

14. Fog M: General acquired anhidrosis: report of a case and investigation of heat regulation and circulation. *JAMA* 107:2040, 1936.

15. de Mari M, Lamberti P, Simone F, et al.: Intravenous administration of lisaride in the treatment of neuroleptic malignant syndrome. *Funct Neurol* 6:285, 1991.

16. Woodhouse P, Keatinge WR, Coleshaw SR: Factors associated with hypothermia in patients admitted to inner city, hospitals. *Lancet* 2:1201, 1989.

17. Kloos RT: Spontaneous periodic hypothermia. *Medicine* 74, 268, 1995.

18. Bracker MD: Environmental and thermal injury. *Clinics Sports Medicine* 11:419, 1992.

19. Rohrer MJ, Natale AM: Effect of hypothermia on the coagulation cascade. *Crit Care Med* 20:1402, 1992.

20. MacDonnell JE, Wrenn K: Hypothermia in the summer. *Southern Med J* 84:804, 1991.

21. Prior PF: *The EEG in Acute Cerebral Anoxia.* Amsterdam, Excerpta Medica, 1973.

22. Markand ON, Warren CH, Moorthy SS, Stoetling RK, King RD: Monitoring of multimodality evoked potentials during open heart surgery under hypothermia. *Electroenceph Clin Neurophysiol* 59:432, 1984.

23. Strain GM, Tucker TA, Graham MC, O'Malley NA: Brain-stem auditory evoked potentials in the alligator. Effects of temperature and hypoxia. *Electroenceph Clin Neurophysiol* 67:68, 1987.

24. Janssen R, Hetzler BE, Creason JP, Dyer RS: Differential impact of hypothermia and pentobarbital on brain-stem auditory evoked responses. *Electroenceph Clin Neurophysiol* 80:412, 1991.

25. Broniong JL, Heizer ML, Baskin DS: Variations in corticomotor and somatosensory evoked potentials: effects of temperature, halothane anesthesia and partial pressure of CO_2. *Anesth Analg* 74:643, 1992.

26. Schaller MD, Fischer AP, Perret CH: Hyperkalemia. A prognostic factor during severe hypothermia. *JAMA* 264:1842, 1990.

27. The effect of hypothermia on the incidence of delayed traumatic intracerebral hemorrhage. *Neurosurgery* 34:252, 1994.

28. Altus P, Hickman JW, Nord HJ: Accidental hypothermia in a healthy quadriplegic patient. *Neurology* 35:427, 1985.

29. Fritsch DE: Hypothermia in the trauma patient. *AACN Clin Issues* 6:196, 1995.

30. Oung CM, Ebglish M, Chiu RC, Hinchey EJ: Effect of hypothermia on hemodynamic responses to dopamine and dobutamine. *J Trauma* 33:671, 1992.

31. Elder PT: Accidental hypothermia, in Shoemaker W, et al (eds): *Textbook of Critical Care*, Philadelphia, WB Saunders, 1989, pp 101–109.

32. Collins K: Hypothermia: the elderly person's enemy. *Practitioner* 239:22, 1995.

33. Klein DG: Physiologic response to traumatic shock. *AACN Clin Issues Crit Care Nursing* 3:305, 1990.

34. Hauty MG, Esrig BC, Hill JG, Long WB: Prognostic factors in severe accidental hypothermia: evidence from the Mt. Hood tragedy. *J Trauma* 27:1107, 1987.

35. Simon JF: Hyperthermia. *N Eng J Med* 328:483, 1993.

36. Hart LE, Sutton JR: Environmental considerations for exercise. *Clin Cardiol* 5:246, 1987.

Chapter 9
ELECTRICAL INJURIES

G. Bryan Young

DEFINITION AND CLASSIFICATION

Electrical injuries of the brain can be due to lightning strikes or alternating current (AC) injuries. Often, the brain is indirectly affected, especially by an anoxic-ischemic insult due to cardiac arrest.

LIGHTNING STRIKE

Lightning strikes are the leading cause of weather-related fatalities in the United States. Approximately 300 people are struck yearly; about one-third of these die.[1] There is marked geographic and seasonal variation. The incidence of thunderstorms is higher in North America than in Europe and higher in the eastern seaboard of the United States than in the west.[2,3]

Lightning strikes generate currents of more than 25,000 A, with voltages up to 1000 kV. Temperatures may exceed 2750°C.[4] Usually, lightning occurs during storms, and typically the tallest-standing structures that conduct electricity are hit preferentially. About 30 percent of victims of lightning strike die and up to 70 percent have permanent sequelae.[5]

Pathogenesis

Lightning must directly strike the head to have a direct effect on the brain; arm-to-arm transmission does not affect the brain.[6] The degree of damage relates to the intensity of current.[7] The nervous system carries more current than other tissues in electrocution; electrical conductivity is highest in the cerebrospinal fluid and the blood vessels. Hence vascular injuries may predominate. Lightning is a single, massive countershock that suddenly depolarizes the heart, rather than causing fibrillation.[8]

A number of possibilities for electrical effects on the nervous system have been proposed:

1. A direct heating effect of the current: this may especially damage Purkinje cells.[9]

2. A direct electrolytic effect from the electrical charge.

3. The mechanical effect of the lightning strike.

4. Intense vasoconstriction resulting in acute hypertension.

Seizures may result from direct insult to nervous tissue, either with direct or indirect current. Indirectly, the seizures may result from vascular complications, e.g., cortical vein thrombosis, anoxic-ischemic insult, or as a late complication of tissue damage.

The nervous system may be indirectly affected if the electrical impulse passes through the heart, causing cardiac arrest, or if the respiratory system is compromised for a sufficient period of time, resulting in secondary hypoxemia or cardiovascular compromise. Acute myocardial necrosis may result.[1] Disseminated intravascular coagulation may develop as a delayed complication.[10] Damage to blood vessels may lead to stroke. Head injury from falls or seizures may also occur.

Clinical Effects

Effects of lightning on the brain can be direct or indirect. It may be difficult in some situations to separate primary central nervous system (CNS) lightning damage from secondary effects of the arrest: i.e., hypoxic-ischemic encephalopathy.

Direct lightning injury to the head may cause either immediate or delayed CNS effects. Immediate effects include transient loss of consciousness, seizure, amnesia of variable duration, or transient or residual paresis. Patients often recover completely, but recurrent or delayed loss of consciousness related to vasomotor syncope has been described.[11] Deafness may occur as a residual complication. If the patient remains unconscious, worsens, or develops focal signs, a more serious complication (such as anoxic-ischemic encephalopathy, stroke, or intracranial hemorrhage) should be suspected. Recovery followed by relapse into unconsciousness may represent cerebral edema, or hemorrhage into the brain parenchyma, or subdural or epidural space.[4]

A complication that indirectly affects the brain is reversible ventilatory failure. Patients can initially appear dead yet recover completely, if supported (lightning stroke or lightning paralysis).[12] Focal deficits may also completely reverse.

Delayed effects include a progressive parkinsonian syndrome, stroke, cerebellar ataxia, or motor system disease, including "robotic speech."[13] Cortical vein thrombosis as a delayed neurologic complication has resulted from electrocution with AC at 800 V.[14]

Basal ganglia hemorrhage, seen on computed tomography (CT) or magnetic resonance imaging (MRI) head scans, has been reported in some survivors.[15] The patient described by Ozgun and Castillo[15] was lethargic, but ataxic with upgoing plantar responses. He made a complete recovery from the CNS aspect. Ischemic stroke, diffuse cerebral edema with later cerebral and cerebellar atrophy, and cortical venous thrombosis may transpire with their attendant clinical pictures.[16]

On general examination, there are often cutaneous burns where metal (e.g., bracelets, necklaces, and zippers) has touched the skin. Direct burns and exit wounds, e.g., on the feet, may reflect the direct entry and exit of the lightning. Red streaking may be found on the limbs, chest, or neck. A tympanic membrane may be perforated from the sound blast at the time of the lightning strike.

Investigations

Scanning of the head by CT or MRI may be helpful in detection of cerebral edema, looking for cortical venous thrombosis (checking for hemorrhage) and ischemic stroke.

Comatose patients might also have an EEG to exclude nonconvulsive seizures, especially if seizures had been present earlier.

Management

Prevention is the most important measure. Outdoor hikers and campers should take shelter during electrical storms, to prevent exposure. They should avoid hilltops, high trees, or wire fences. If caught outdoors, people should temporarily discard any metal objects such as golf clubs, rifles, and even hearing aids. Indoors, properly installed electrical equipment and attention to the relation of the equipment user to the electrical ground are key steps in avoiding electrocution.[17]

In cases of electrocution, cardiopulmonary resuscitation should be started and continued for at least 4 h, even if the vital signs are absent, including apnea and loss of cranial nerve reflexes. Some surprising recoveries have occurred with continued resuscitative efforts. The respiratory center may fail for several hours, only to recover after assisted ventilation for several hours. On restoration of cardiac activity and blood pressure, tachycardia and hypertension can develop; these can usually be managed with a beta blocker. Fluid replacement, treatment of burns, management of myoglobinuria and secondary renal failure, and correction of metabolic acidosis are often required.

Management involves supportive care for the clinical issues: unconsciousness, seizures, brain swelling, hemorrhage, cortical vein thrombosis, apnea, etc. Each of these should be treated as mentioned in appropriate parts of this book.

ALTERNATING CURRENT INJURIES

Alternating current injuries are at least five times as common as those from lightning[8] Two-thirds of such accidents occur in those with occupations that expose individuals to high-voltage power lines (e.g., linemen) and one-third occur with low-voltage domestic currents in the home.[17]

Alternating currents under 200 V (domestic currents) may fibrillate the heart but do not directly affect the respiratory center. Currents greater than 1000 V tend to affect the respiratory center but not the heart and intermediate voltages affect both.[17]

Alternating current injuries to the brain are not common. Secondary cardiac arrests, however, commonly affect the brain. The affected muscles go into tetanic spasm that causes the victim grabbing an electrical source to be unable to relax the grip, resulting in the current continuing to pass through the body.

Immediate deaths result from respiratory arrest due to impairment of the respiratory center, prolonged tetanus of the respiratory muscles, or cardiac arrest. Delayed deaths may result from cerebral edema or medical complications, e.g., renal failure.

Management

Prevention is that of electrical safety measures: grounding of power supply, permanent switches on the hot side of household currents, grounding of electrical apparatus, and avoidance of grounding of individuals using electrical appliances, especially outdoors.[17]

With electrocution, the patient should be separated from the electrical source by turning of the power supply or by separating the victim from the electrical contact using a nonconducting device like a belt or wooden stick. Resuscitation should be conducted as described for lightning injuries.

REFERENCES

1. Langley RL, Dunn KA, Esinhart JD: Lightning fatalities in North Carolina. *NC Med J* 52:281, 1991.
2. Duclos PJ, Sanderson LM: An epidemiological description of lightning-related deaths in the United States. *Int J Epidemiol* 19:673, 1990.
3. Lynch MJG, Shorthouse PH: Injuries and death from lightning. *Lancet* 1:473, 1949.
4. Stanley LD, Suss RA: Intracerebral hematoma secondary to lightning strike: case report and review of the literature. *Neurosurgery* 16:686, 1985.
5. Craig SR: When lightning strikes. Pathophysiology of lightning injuries. *Postgrad Med* 79:109, 1986.
6. Sances A, Myklebust JB, Szablya JF, et al: Current pathways in high voltage injuries. *IEEE Trans Biomed Eng* 30:118, 1983.
7. Langworthy OR: Abnormalities produced in the central nervous system by electrical injuries. *J Exp Med* 51:943, 1930.
8. Cooper MA: Electrical and lightning injuries. *Emerg Med Clin North Am* 2:489, 1984.
9. Freeman W, Dumoff E: Cerebellar syndrome following heat stroke. *Arch Neurol Psychiat* 51:67, 1944.
10. Ekoe JM, Cunningham M, Jacques O, et al: Disseminated intravascular coagulation and acute myocardial necrosis caused by lightning. *Intens Care Med* 11:160, 1985.
11. Alexander L: Electrical injuries of the nervous system. *J Nerv Ment Dis* 94:622, 1941.
12. Taussig HB: "Death" from lightning and the possibility of living again. *Ann Intern Med* 68:1345, 1968.
13. Gilbert GJ: Lightning-induced robotic speech. *Neurology* 44:991, 1994.
14. Patel A, Lo R: Electric injury with cerebral venous thrombosis. Case report and review of the literature. *Stroke* 24:903, 1993.
15. Ozgun B, Castillo M: Basal ganglia hemorrhage related to lightning strike. *Am J Neuroradiol* 16:1370, 1995.
16. Cherington M, Yarnell P, Lammereste D: Lightning strikes: nature of neurological damage in patients evaluated in hospital emergency departments. *Ann Emerg Med* 21:575, 1992.
17. Patten BM: Lightning and electrical injuries. *Neurol Clin* 10:1047, 1992.

Chapter 10
BURN ENCEPHALOPATHY

G. Bryan Young

INCIDENCE

Over 2.5 million Americans have medical attention annually for burns; of these, 100,000 are hospitalized and 12,000 die.[1] Most burns are thermal, due to flash or flame. Thermal burns primarily involve the skin, but can cause, usually indirectly, a multitude of systemic and central nervous system (CNS) effects. The latter are listed in Table 10-1.

The incidence of CNS complications of burns is uncertain, but the likelihood increases with burns of large surface area, or a burn infection with *Pseudomonas aeruginosa* and *Candida* species, or *Staphylococcus aureus* endocarditis or bacterial endocarditis as a complication.[1] In some series,[2,3] burn encephalopathy is more common in children, but in others, children and adults are equally affected.[1] At least 30 percent of hospitalized burns patients develop features of delirium. Of fatal cases, over half have CNS complications.[1]

CLINICAL FEATURES

Delirium in burns patients may be characterized by agitation, hallucinations, and coarse tremor.[3–6] Patients may deteriorate to coma. Seizures, focal or generalized, are more common in children than in adults, where they may reflect vascular complications, hyponatremia, or hypoxia.[7]

The onset of the neurologic features from the burn injury is variable; it may be weeks afterwards, when the fever and metabolic derangements have settled. Early encephalopathy and seizures often relate to anoxia or electrolyte disturbance; later encephalopathy more commonly relates to septic complications (including vascular lesions, multiorgan failure, and CNS infection).[2]

The differential diagnosis depends on the clinical appearance and context. The following conditions may mimic "burn encephalopathy": cerebral vein thrombosis, anoxic-ischemic encephalopathy [including (acutely) carbon monoxide intoxication], osmotic demyelination syndrome, nonketotic hyperglycemia, and Wernicke's encephalopathy.

Table 10-1
Complications of thermal burns

Complication	Clinical features
Systemic inflammatory response syndrome, with or without infection	"Septic encephalopathy"
Osmolality changes	Hypernatremia—central pontine/extrapontine myelinolysis
	Hyponatremia—seizures

PATHOLOGY AND PATHOGENESIS

The neuropathologic findings show wide variation, likely reflecting different pathologic mechanisms, despite a similar clinical picture suggestive of a diffuse encephalopathy.[1] There are similarities to septic encephalopathy (Chap. 12), but anoxia, large ischemic lesions, and disseminated intravascular coagulation (DIC) are more common with burns.

The mechanisms for burn encephalopathy are not mutually exclusive. Most cases qualify as metabolic encephalopathies, often secondary to multiorgan failure. Metabolic encephalopathies outnumber vascular and infective mechanisms, even in fatal cases.[1] Anoxic encephalopathy, in contrast to most septic patients, is common in autopsied burns patients.[1] This can relate to anoxic hypoxia, carbon monoxide poisoning, or anoxic-ischemic mechanisms. Hyperplasia of protoplasmic astrocytes is common and often relates to renal failure.[1]

About 20 percent of fatal cases reveal CNS infections.[1] Over 75 percent of CNS infections are due to either *Candida* species, *Pseudomonas aeruginosa*, or *Staphylococcus aureus*. Microabscesses or septic infarcts at autopsy are more common with candida and *Staphylococcus aureus* bacteremia.[1] Meningitis is caused most commonly by *P. aeruginosa*. The patients with CNS infections had systemic inflammatory response syndrome (Chap. 12) and extensive, deep burns. All the cases of bacterial CNS infections, but only half the patients with candida infections, had positive blood cultures. Candida-infected patients, however, presented later and were preceded by documented bacterial infection.

Cerebral infarcts occur in 18 percent of cases.[1] In contrast to septic patients, some of the infarcts are macroscopic. These relate to septic arterial occlusions, and often from *Candida* or *Aspergillus* species.[1] Others are due to meningitis, infected emboli from endocarditis, or an arteritis without endocarditis or meningitis, DIC, or septic shock.[1] Septic infarcts always occur after the first week.[1] In one-third of patients, such infarcts are related to atherosclerosis, atrial fibrillation, or other causes found in the general population.

Cortical vein thrombosis occurred in 2 of 20 children with burn encephalopathy.[2]

Some patients develop severe cerebral edema with resultant compromise of intracranial circulation. The edema may relate to anoxia with early presentation or to the later development of "toxic encephalopathy" (Chap. 12).[1,2]

Intracranial hemorrhages occur about one-third as frequently as infarcts and usually relate to DIC with thrombocytopenia.[1] Blood cultures are usually positive in patients who develop intracranial hemorrhages. Hypotension is common.

Some patients develop central pontine myelinolysis.[1,8] This is thought to be due to increases in serum osmolality, whether from a hyponatremic value or an increase to hypernatremic concentrations from previously normal osmolality.

Iatrogenic causes of coma include some cases of electrolyte disturbances, and the side effects of drugs from the administration of sedatives, analgesics, antibiotics, anticonvulsants, etc. The free fraction of the serum concentration of drugs can change considerably after burns injury.[9–11] Since albumin is often decreased after burns injury, the free fraction of drugs that are normally bound to albumin, e.g., phenytoin, increases. Those drugs that bind to the acute phase reactant, α_1-acid glycoprotein—which increases with burns and infection, show greater protein binding and lower percentage free fraction. The net total concentration that is measured needs to be reinterpreted, even though the drug handling by the body and the absolute free concentration of the drug do not change.

INVESTIGATION

Because of the varied pathogenetic mechanisms for burn encephalopathy and the similarity of clinical presentation, ancillary laboratory tests are often necessary. The following are suggested:

1. Blood cultures.

2. DIC screen.

3. Complete blood count (CBC) and platelet count.

4. Electroencephalogram (EEG): particularly to examine for seizures, to estimate the severity of the encephalopathy, and to monitor sedative drug effects. Note that in burn encephalopathy, EEG abnormalities correlate poorly with reversibility and prognosis.[4]

5. Computed tomography (CT) scan of head: to exclude ischemic or hemorrhagic lesions and to check for brain swelling.

6. Lumbar puncture: especially in comatose patients with no contraindications to lumbar puncture (burns or infections of overlying skin; coagulopathy; or massive, especially asymmetric, brain swelling or mass effect). Patients are usually encephalopathic before developing meningitis. Blood cultures positive for *P. aeruginosa* increase the probability of meningitis.

7. Biochemistry: serum electrolytes, lactate, urea, creatinine, calcium, magnesium, osmolality, proteins (including albumin), bilirubin, and alkaline phosphatase. Metabolic disturbances, especially electrolyte imbalance, are likely causes of early encephalopathy.

ADDITIONAL MANAGEMENT

Drug history should be examined: narcotics and sedatives are commonly used and may have cumulative effect, especially with decreased clearance with hepatic or renal failure. Infection is unlikely without a total body surface area burn of under 30 percent.[1] In patients who are candidates for meningitis, it is best to do a lumbar puncture; if this is not feasible, the patients should be covered for *Pseudomonas aeruginosa* meningitis and other organisms revealed in systemic or wound cultures.

Vigorous treatment is indicated unless there is incontrovertible evidence of irreversible anoxic-ischemic damage or brain death from swelling. Most of the children who survived severe burns injury had little-to-no neurologic sequelae, despite stormy courses.[2] The case for adults may not be quite as favorable.

REFERENCES

1. Winleman MD, Galloway PG: Central nervous system complications of thermal burns. A postmortem study of 139 patients. *Medicine* 71:271, 1992.
2. Antoon AY, Volpe JJ, Crawford JD: Burn encephalopathy in children. *Pediatrics* 50:609, 1972.
3. Mohnot D, Snead OC III, Benton JW Jr: Burn encephalopathy in children. *Ann Neurol* 12:42, 1981.
4. Andreasen NJC, Hartford CE, Knott JR, Canter A: EEG changes associated with burn delirium. *Dis Nerv Syst* 38:27, 1977.
5. Rosenbloom C, Kravath R: Neurological disturbances following minor burns. *Lancet* II: 1423, 1969.
6. Sanders R: Neurological disturbances and minor burns. *Lancet* II: 1133, 1969.
7. Hughes JR, Cayaffa JJ, Boswick JA Jr: Seizures following burns of the skin. Electroencephalic recordings. *Dis Nerv Ment Dis* 36:443, 1975.
8. McKee Winkelman M, Banker B: CPM in severely burned patients. Relationship to serum hyperosmolality. *Neurology* 38:1211, 1988.
9. Martyn JAJ, Abernethy DR, Greenblatt DJ: Plasma protein binding of drugs after severe burn injury. *Clin Pharmacol Ther* 35:535, 1984.
10. Pugh CB: Phenytoin and phenobarbital protein binding alterations in a uremic burn patient. *Drug Intell Clin Pharm* 21:264, 1987.
11. Stanford GK, Pine RH: Postburn delirium associated with the use of intravenous lorazepam. *J Burn Care Rehabil* 9:160, 1988.

Part 3

IMPAIRED CONSCIOUSNESS AND INFLAMMATORY CONDITIONS

Chapter 11

INFECTIONS OF THE CENTRAL NERVOUS SYSTEM

Charles F. Bolton

Infection of the central nervous system (CNS) is a prime consideration in any patient presenting with impaired consciousness or coma. A wide variety of infecting organisms may be responsible and the clinical manifestations are extremely varied. Many conditions of the nervous system of noninfective origin, such as neoplasms, may simulate those of CNS infection. In addition to the diagnostic difficulty, treatment is particularly challenging, and effective methods are still being worked out. Moreover, this book emphasizes early diagnosis and treatment, before consciousness is seriously affected (Chap. 1). The book by Scheld et al[1] and the monograph by Tyler and Martin[2] provide comprehensive discussions of the subject, and the recent volume by Hacke[3] provides essential discussions of management of CNS infection in the neurocritical care unit. Imaging studies have become of prime importance, not only in diagnosis, but also in monitoring treatment and understanding the pathogenesis. In this regard, the account by Zimmerman[4] is valuable. Nonetheless, at an early stage, the results of imaging studies may be equivocal, and the electroencephalogram (EEG) is a valuable investigative tool whenever CNS infection is suspected as a cause of stupor and coma.[5] Finally, polymerase chain reaction (PCR) investigation of the cerebrospinal fluid (CFS) has revolutionized early and accurate diagnosis of many types of CNS infections.

This chapter will emphasize the mechanisms of coma in CNS infection, the general approach to a patient with such a disorder, and the general principles of treatment, and, finally, brief discussions of specific disease entities. The only exception is bacterial meningitis, which will be discussed in some detail, not only because of its prevalence, but also because it illustrates the pathophysiology of brain dysfunction in CNS infection, and there has been much interesting work on the topic in recent years. Because of its increasing worldwide prevalence, emphasis will be given to opportunistic infections associated with immune deficiency in the acquired immunodeficiency syndrome (AIDS) and organ transplantation. Subacute bacterial endocarditis, septic encephalopathy, and postinfectious immunologically mediated encephalitis are discussed elsewhere (Chap. 12). Chronic infections, such as those caused by slow viruses, e.g., Creutzfeldt-Jakob disease, and which cause dementing illness before affecting consciousness, will not be discussed.

MECHANISM OF COMA IN CENTRAL NERVOUS SYSTEM INFECTION

Depressed levels of consciousness, at times progressing to coma, are relatively common clinical manifestations of CNS infection. Fifty percent of patients with acute meningitis have a depressed level of consciousness.[6] Once stupor or coma develop, the complication rate rises, and, even in the modern era of intensive care management, the mortality rate for pneumococcal meningitis may be as high as 30 percent.[7]

The mechanisms of depressed level of consciousness in coma due to infection are remarkably complex and still not completely worked out. The microbial agent or its toxins may directly involve brain parenchyma. This mechanism is most likely to occur with virus infection. But, the mechanisms described below, particularly in bacterial meningitis, are likely of equal or greater importance. These mechanisms are complex and involve disturbances of the microvasculature and larger cerebral arteries, and result in altered cerebral metabolism, altered cerebral blood flow, cerebral edema, increased intracranial pressure ICP, focal cerebral lesions (including mass lesions with resulting tentorial or foramen magnum herniation), and hydrocephalus. Seizures, perhaps subclinical, also contribute to coma in some CNS infections.

Disturbance of the Microvasculature

Any severe infection in the body will induce an equally severe systemic response, termed sepsis. More recently, the term systemic inflammatory response syndrome (SIRS) was designed to indicate that not only infection, but also noninfectious illnesses, e.g., severe trauma, burns, and pancreatitis, may cause a similar clinical picture.[8] Central nervous system infection of a primary nature will thus induce this syndrome within the microvasculature of the CNS, and bacterial meningitis is particularly likely to do so, since the offending organisms are in close contact with the microvasculature. Thus, in bacterial meningitis, the bacteria in the subarachnoid space, including their presence in the Virchow-Robin perivascular spaces, disturb the microcirculation throughout the parenchyma by the induction of SIRS.

In SIRS, cellular and humoral responses are activated.[9] The chief mediators of the humoral response, the cytokines, are activated locally, and include interleukins-1, 2, and 6, tumor necrosis factor-alpha, arachidonic acid, coagulation factors, free oxygen radicals, and proteases. The cellular response involves lymphocytes, monocytes, and neutrophils. These cellular and humoral factors interact with themselves, and with adhesion molecules, the latter of which are elevated in the blood of patients with sepsis.[10] They adhere to leukocytes, platelets, and endothelial cells and induce "rolling neutrophils" and fibrin-platelet aggregates which obstruct capillary flow. Increased capillary permeability induces local tissue edema. Activation of nitric acid, now known to be the endovascular relaxing agent (or, formally, the endothelium-derived relaxing factor),[11] causes arteriolar dilatation, which may further slow capillary flow. Thus, essential nutrients fail to reach the organ parenchyma. For example, despite adequate oxygenation via mechanical ventilation, there is a severe oxygen debt at the parenchymal level, resulting in multiple organ dysfunction, including the brain.[12] However, brain metabolism has not been adequately studied in either children or adults with meningitis. The encephalopathy may be due to abnormalities related to reduced substrate delivery, increased metabolic demands, or ineffective substrate utilization.

Disturbance of Larger Vessels

In bacterial meningitis, purulent material in the meninges directly bathe the cortical pial arteries, vessels in the basal subarachnoid space, and larger vessels such as the carotid arteries and branches of the circle of Willis, as well as their perforating branches.[13] This results in structural thickening of the vessel wall and also in vasospasm. Which of the two is most important is still not known with certainty. This vasculitis, which may affect arteries or veins, results in arterial or venous infarctions of various sizes and locations.

Patterns of Cerebral Blood Flow in Meningitis

Using xenon,[14] it has been shown that, in adults, cerebral blood flow is normal within the first 24 h in patients with meningococcal meningitis. However, in the rat pneumococcal meningitis model, Pfister et al[15] found a 135 percent increase in cerebral blood flow at 1 h and a 211 percent increase at 6 h after infection. This was associated with marked increase in ICP due to hyperemia. Soon after this, cerebral blood flow begins to decrease and, in some patients, this appears to be quite substantial, reflecting the severity of the disease.[16] These patterns of cerebral blood flow relate to prognosis. Of patients with normal cerebral blood flow, 77 percent were normal or had mild neurologic sequelae. In contrast, 80 percent of those with low cerebral blood flow had severe neurologic complications.[17]

Focal neurologic deficits may be due to cerebrovascular lesions, including inflammation or thrombosis of cerebral arteries, veins, and sinuses, as well as embolic occlusion. There may be local areas of reduced cerebral blood flow, even in patients with normal generalized blood flow. These local areas may be associated with structural brain injury, or larger areas of hypoperfusion may be associated with the later development of severe atrophy. Regional edema with moderate hyperemia suggests luxury perfusion or loss of coupling between cerebral blood flow and metabolism.[12]

Cerebral Edema and Raised Intracranial Pressure

The development of brain edema results from an interaction of various disturbances of the microcirculation, direct toxic effects on brain parenchyma, and obstruction to CSF flow. The injury to the vascular endothelium alters the blood-brain barrier permeability and causes vasogenic edema.[19] Endotoxins cause cytotoxic edema while interstitial edema is induced by obstruction to CSF outflow resistance.

Cerebral edema is a critical factor affecting morbidity and mortality in children with meningitis.[20,21] The granulocyte inflammatory response is less important than the effects of bacterial wall products that stimulate the release of various endothelial factors, such as interleukin-1, which increases blood-brain barrier permeability.[22a] This concept was supported by

a study by Horwitz et al,[20] which reported 18 children with bacterial meningitis in whom there was no correlation between the CSF cell count and cerebral herniation. The presence of edema correlates with increased CSF protein, perhaps a reflection of the inflammatory response and altered blood-brain barrier permeability. Hyponatremia, which occurs in one-third to one-half of children with bacterial meningitis, secondary to antidiuretic hormone release, also contributes to cerebral edema formation.[20]

Although brain edema contributes to the development of increased ICP, other factors, such as increased CSF volume or intracranial blood volume, might be of equal significance.[22b,23] Early computed tomography (CT) scan results in children indicate that one of the earliest findings is increased CSF volume in the ventricular and subarachnoid spaces.[24,25] As already noted, regional edema with moderate hyperemia suggests luxury perfusion or loss of coupling between cerebral blood flow and metabolism.[18] Early cerebral hyperemia could precipitate an increase in ICP.[26] This is an important issue. If a component of elevated ICP is due to increased blood volume, then hyperventilation should be effective treatment. However, if increased ICP is due to increased CSF volume, then either removal of CSF, or other treatments aimed at decreasing CSF volume, would need to be considered. This is difficult to test clinically, since the relation between brain edema, CSF volume, and intracranial blood volume affecting ICP are variables that cannot be simply or noninvasively measured.

In animal studies, dexamethasone reversed the development of brain edema with increased ICP at 24 to 26 h after acute inoculation with the offending organism.[27] In humans, dexamethasone prevents hearing loss and improves neurologic outcome.[28–30]

However, a recent study[31] using magnetic resonance imaging (MRI) did not find any decrease in brain water content in those children with bacterial meningitis who were treated with dexamethasone. Moreover, one recent MRI study, performed 2 to 5 days after the onset of therapy, found no correlation between the presence of edema and outcome in 31 children with bacterial meningitis.[32] Nonetheless, it has long been known that the presence of cerebral edema is associated with transtentorial herniation and increased mortality.[20,21,33] Thus, while dexamethasone improves overall outcome, its usefulness for the acute management of raised ICP is still controversial.

Cerebral Perfusion Pressure

Continuous ICP monitoring in childhood bacterial meningitis indicates that morbidity and mortality are greatest in those children in whom the cerebral perfusion pressure (CPP) is less than 30 to 50 mmHg.[34–36] In those children who did not survive, a decrease in CPP was related less to systemic hypotension than to increased ICP. Several studies[35,36] have clearly demonstrated that ICP is maximally elevated within the first 24 to 48 h. In 106 patients, Dodge and Swartz[37] found that CSF pressure averaged 307 mm of CSF (range of 50 to 600 mm) at the time of initial lumbar puncture. Minns et al[38] observed that ICP was elevated in 33 of 35 children with proven bacterial meningitis. McMenamin and Volpe[39] found that ICP was at a maximum early on, and that this correlated with reduced Doppler cerebral blood flow (CBF) velocity in the middle cerebral artery in the presence of a relatively constant arterial blood pressure. Overall, these studies suggest that ICP is maximally increased within the first 24 to 48 h of hospitalization, rather than later in the course, and that this may be due to hyperemia, vasodilatation, and increased cerebral blood flow.

Autoregulation

While studies in infants and children are limited,[14,40] studies in older children and adults demonstrate impaired autoregulation.[14] This has been further supported with studies in the rat model of meningitis, which showed a loss of autoregulation over a maximum arterial pressure of between 40 and 120 mmHg.[41] It has been postulated[35,36] that poor outcome is due to impaired autoregulation and decreased CPP, causing decreased cerebral blood flow, although cerebral

blood flow was not measured in any of several studies that have been carried out.

Cerebral Flood Flow and P_{CO_2} Reactivity

It is known that acute, severe head injury in children and adults—such as trauma, asphyxia, and strangulation—blunts the CBF/P_{CO_2} reactivity. In seven children with meningitis,[17] hyperventilation significantly reduced rather than increased CBF, and, in two children, it fell below the ischemic thresholds in several brain regions. Ashwal et al[18] found that approximately 30 percent of children had baseline values that were already reduced. Assuming that the majority of children with meningitis maintain CBF/P_{CO_2} reactivity, it is possible that hyperventilation in such patients could further reduce below CBF ischemic thresholds.

Hydrocephalus

The CT appearance of communicating hydrocephalus is an enlargement of the entire ventricular system, including the fourth ventricle, with paraventricular lucencies surrounding the frontal horns. The latter represents transependymal movement of CSF from the ventricular system into the brain parenchyma as a result of blockage in the normal CSF reabsorption pathways. The development of an obstructive hydrocephalus secondary to blockage of CSF flow by exudate at the foramina of Magendie and Luschka has a CT appearance of dilated lateral, and third and fourth ventricles. If there is nonvisualization of the fourth ventricle, the obstruction is likely at the aqueduct.

The development of hydrocephalus may require placement of a ventricular drain or shunt and, in some cases, this may be necessary even when active infection is present.

Formation of Mass Lesions

Subdural hygromas may form over the surface of the brain. These are particularly common in young children. In most cases, such subdural collection usually subsides spontaneously and no treatment is required; in the long run, this may be of little consequence. In a few instances, hygromas may progressively enlarge and act as a significant mass lesion. When brain abscesses occur in association with meningitis, the meningitis is likely to be secondary to the abscess. Abscesses also may act as a mass lesion, contribute to increased ICP, and ultimately cause tentorial herniation. Surgical excision or aspiration should be performed.

Transtentorial herniation (see Chap. 4) may occur in advanced herpes simplex encephalitis due to swelling of one or both temporal lobes.

Seizures

Seizures may complicate various CNS infections (see Chap. 17).

A decreased level of consciousness may also be due to recurring seizures, some of which may be subclinical. Thus, there may be a role for serial or continuous EEG recordings to monitor this possibility. Jordan found nonconvulsive seizures in one-third of patients with CNS infections who had EEG monitoring.[42–44]

EARLY MANAGEMENT OF SUSPECTED CENTRAL NERVOUS SYSTEM INFECTION

Background

These management issues are very important, since it is known that the earlier the treatment is started in bacterial meningitis or in herpes simplex encephalitis, the more likely it is for a complete recovery. In patients who present with what this author proposes be called the "acute meningitis-encephalitis syndrome": symptoms are fever, headache, and confusion in adults; or fever, lethargy, and vomiting in children. The traditional concern has been the presence of bacterial meningitis, and it has been recommended that a lumbar puncture should be carried out on an emergency basis to establish that diagnosis and then treatment should be started immediately, without waiting for the results of cultures, due to the danger of a delay in treatment. However, it has been recognized that

there is some risk to this protocol. Tentorial herniation may be precipitated by the lumbar puncture when there is either a cerebral edema, secondary to the meningitis, or a mass lesion, such as an abscess or a swollen temporal lobe from herpes simplex encephalitis. Also, delaying antibiotic or antiviral prescription until investigative tests are done may increase the incidence of sequelae.

Two illustrative case reports will be discussed here.

Case 1: An intraventricular abscess presenting as acute bacterial meningitis and mimicking a tumor on neuroimagery

A 64-year-old farmer was well until the day before admission, when he developed mild headache and low-back pain. On the morning of admission, he was unresponsive to a telephone call and his son found him in bed, drowsy and confused. Examination in an outlying emergency department showed that his temperature was 37.4°C and his neck was stiff. Antibiotic treatment was started and immediate transfer to a tertiary care hospital was arranged. On examination in the emergency department there, he was mildly agitated and disorientated to date and place. There was neck stiffness typical of meningitis and some limitation of straight leg raising, bilaterally. The remainder of the neurologic examination was normal and, in particular, there were no focal neurologic signs. The peripheral white blood cell count was mildly elevated at 11.9×10^9 per liter.

The features were so typical of acute bacterial meningitis that there was initial discussion as to whether to proceed immediately to a lumbar puncture. However, an emergency CT head scan was arranged, which revealed an isodense brain lesion in the right lateral ventricle, involving the trigone and body. There was enhancement of ependyma over the right lateral ventricle and a more enhancing mass in the region of the right choroid plexus. Because of occlusion of the foramen of Monro, the right temporal horn was enlarged. The differential diagnosis in the report mentioned possible ependymoma, glioma, and lymphoma. The patient was admitted to the neuro-observation unit and prescribed mannitol and decadron therapy. He subsequently underwent stereotactic brain biopsy but interpretation of the biopsy was difficult. He died 1 week after admission. Autopsy revealed an intraventricular brain abscess rather than a brain tumor.

Despite the later difficulties in establishing the diagnosis before death in this patient, the main lesson here is that the initial clinical picture was that of acute bacterial meningitis, and only the initial CT scan disclosed a mass lesion which precluded a lumbar puncture because of the risk of precipitating tentorial herniation. Moreover, in such patients, antibiotic coverage should be given until a diagnosis can be clearly established.

Thus, while there has been disagreement regarding protocol,[45] it has been recommended that a CT head scan be carried out first. An abnormal CT scan was present in one-third of children[46] and one-half of adults[47] with meningitis. In adult patients who died of bacterial meningitis, one-third had evidence of cerebral or cerebellar herniation.[47] Modern imaging techniques will provide essential information on cerebral edema, areas of breakdown in the blood-brain barrier, sites of cerebral infarction, abscesses, subdural collections, hydrocephalus, tentorial or foramen magnum herniation, and images that suggest specific diseases i.e., herpes simplex encephalitis.[4]

Case 2: Primary intracerebral hemorrhage presenting as bacterial meningitis

A 7-year-old female developed fatigue, confusion headache, vomiting, and photophobia over several hours. Examination in the emergency department of an outlying hospital demonstrated a stiff neck, even though body temperature was normal. Acute bacterial meningitis was suspected and a lumbar puncture was performed. It revealed grossly bloody CSF. Nonetheless, antibiotic treatment was started, but she continued to be lethargic and, ultimately, confused and disorientated. Approximately 12 h after onset, her pupils

became dilated and fixed and she showed decorticate posturing. She was given dexamethasone and mannitol, and was intubated and ventilated. With this treatment, the left pupil became normal but she remained deeply comatose. She was transferred to a children's hospital where an emergency CT head scan showed hemorrhage in the left cerebral hemisphere, with intraventricular extension. The patient was pronounced brain dead 2 days after her first symptom. Examination of the brain at autopsy revealed an arteriovenous malformation involving the left parietal region.

Thus, again, a CT scan performed initially would have identified the mass lesion and avoided the risky performance of a lumbar puncture.

The delay involved in having a CT head scan performed before starting definitive treatment for meningitis is often unacceptable. The wait for a CT head scan in this author's hospital caused delay in treatment beyond 2 hours in three-quarters of the patients requiring lumbar puncture for suspected bacterial meningitis (Pringle CE, Austin TW, Moulin DE, unpublished data).

A diagnostic concern is the fact that the typical picture of bacterial meningitis may not be present. Fever is not invariably present, nor is a stiff neck. Conversely, in a typical picture of bacterial meningitis, the acute lesion may be a brain abscess or a noninflammatory condition, such as a posterior fossa tumor in a child or a tumor anywhere within the ventricular system at any age. The performance of a lumbar puncture in either instance would entail the risk of tentorial or cerebellar herniation, sometimes with rapid development of coma.

A final point relates to treatment. In the early stages, it may be difficult to differentiate between bacterial meningitis and herpes simplex encephalitis. Both may be characterized by fever, headache, and decreased levels of consciousness, these occurring in at least 75 percent of patients with herpes simplex encephalitis.[48] Empiric emergency treatment should be started in both of these conditions.

Management of the Acute Meningitis-Encephalitis Syndrome

Because of the above concerns, the author's hospital recommends the following management of the suspected acute meningitis-encephalitis syndrome (Fig. 11-1). When the patient is being seen in an outlying center or emergency department, it is wise to recommend over the telephone that empiric treatment be given before transfer to the tertiary care center for further definitive investigations and treatment. However, the empiric treatment should not be given before a blood culture and glucose level have been arranged. [Occasionally, the organism may initially be identified at other sites; i.e., skin (Fig. 11-2)]. Moreover, if the patient is in a stuporous or comatose state, all measures to ensure airway protection and maintenance of hydration and blood pressure should be instituted in the outlying hospital, and these must be maintained during transportation. After the patient has arrived in the emergency department, an initial general and neurologic assessment should be carried out. Then, the patient should be transferred to the CT or MRI suite to determine the presence of cerebral edema, mass lesions, early tentorial herniation, ventricular obstruction, etc. If any of these conditions is present, transfer to the intensive care unit (ICU) should be arranged. An attempt should be made to reduce edema by intravenous mannitol and hyperventilation in the early stages of bacterial meningitis. If this fails, or if there is a mass lesion, a neurosurgical consultation should be sought. Craniotomy, ventilation, etc., may be necessary. If there appears to be no risk for performing a lumbar puncture, it should be then performed immediately. The CSF should be tested with Gram's stain and specific tests for bacterial antigens (particularly latex agglutination), and also for herpes simplex using PCR (if available). If results of Gram's stain testing or PCR are positive, specific therapy should be started. If negative, empirical treatment should be continued for 5 days and then stopped if bacterial meningitis or herpes simplex encephalitis seems unlikely.

There is a good rationale for such management. Blood cultures are positive in up to 71 percent of cases of pneumococcal meningitis, 53 percent of meningococcal meningitis, and 45% of *Haemophilus influenzae* meningitis.[49] They may be important in determining antibiotic sensitivity if antibiotics have been started prior to a lumbar puncture. The institution of antibiotic therapy will not alter the CSF abnormalities of high cell count, low glucose, or high protein for at least 24 h,[50] and possibly not for several days.[51] Antibiotic therapy will not sterilize the CSF for at least several hours. Diluting the CSF in the laboratory to remove the antibiotic effect results in positive cultures, even after 12 h of treatment.[52] Similarly, tests for bacterial antigens in the CSF by the latex agglutination test are relatively unaffected in the first few hours of treatment.[53–55] Whether prior antibiotic treatment reduces the yield of positive CSF culture is controversial,[56] the evidence, in the opinion of the author of this chapter, being insufficient to argue against prior antibiotic treatment. Moreover, PCR testing of the CSF is relatively unaffected by antibiotic treatment.[56] The otherwise excellent review of acute bacterial meningitis by Tunkel and Scheld[57] failed to recommend prior antibiotic treatment for bacterial meningitis or treatment of possible herpes simplex encephalitis, methods which are strongly endorsed by the author of this chapter.

In untreated patients with bacterial meningitis, Gram's stain of the CSF is positive in 60 to 89 percent of cases,[49,58,59] and cultures of CSF are positive in 80 to 90 percent of cases at 48 h.[58]

Lumbar Puncture

In performing a lumbar puncture, measurements of CSF pressure are often inaccurate and time-consuming. The color of the CSF in successive tubes should be noted. Cells should be tested in the first and fourth specimens to help determine the possibility of a traumatic tap. Cells, glucose, protein, and Gram's stain tests (Fig. 11-3) should be performed on an emergency basis. Cultures should be sent for all potential bacterial or fungal pathogens. If cryptococcal meningitis is suspected, an India ink stain should be performed.

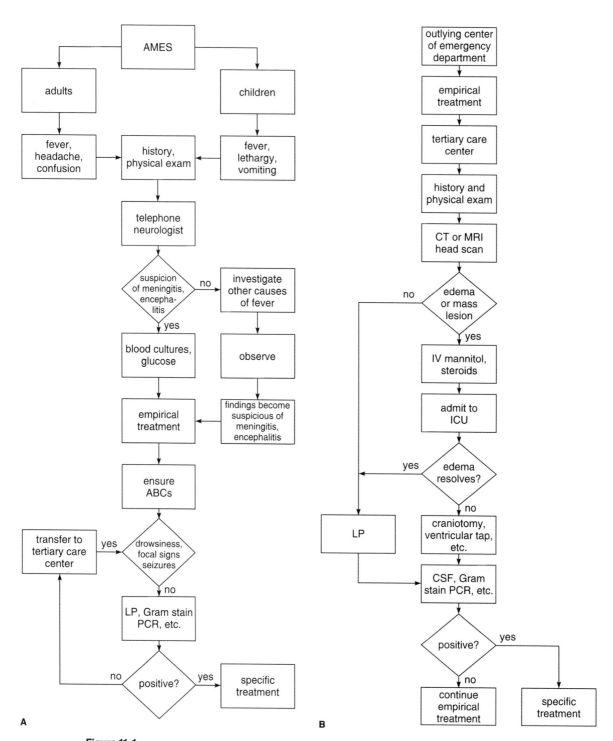

Figure 11-1

Management of the acute meningitis–encephalitis syndrome (AMES). A. Management in outlying center or emergency department. B. Management in tertiary care center. LP = lumbar puncture. (From Bolton,[147] with permission.)

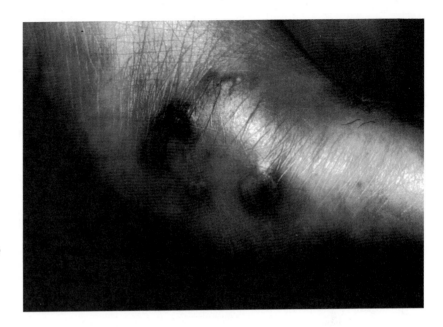

Figure 11-2

Skin lesions at the base of the great toe in staphylococcal septicemia and meningitis. Culture at this site identified the organism.

The CSF is normally clear, and contains no more than 5×10^6 leukocytes per liter (0 to 30×10^6 in neonates), a glucose level of 2.2 to 4.4 mmol/L (i.e., two-thirds of a simultaneously taken blood glucose level), and a protein level of 150 to 450 mg/L (<1000 at 0 to 3 months of age). The typical CSF findings in various types of infective meningitis and carcinomatous meningitis are shown in Table 11-1.

Figure 11-3

Meningococci in a Gram stain of CSF. (From Bolton,[147] with permission.)

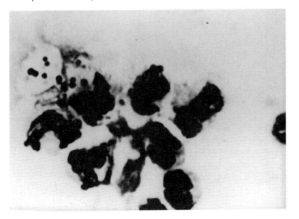

In addition to testing for pyogenic organisms, the CSF should be tested for herpes simplex encephalitis. Specimens should be sent for PCR, which is positive in the first 10 days of onset. Negative PCR results may be obtained within the first 48 h. Early treatment with acyclovir will not cause a negative PCR result for at least 10 days. Because of the success of PCR in diagnosis, brain biopsy is now rarely indicated.[60,61]

Empiric Treatment of the Acute Meningitis-Encephalitis Syndrome

The empiric treatment for bacterial meningitis is as follows. In adults with normal renal function, cefotaxime should be prescribed, 2 g intravenously over 4 h, which will cover all three of the common pathogens, *Streptococcus pneumoniae, Neisseria meningitidis* and *H. influenzae*, and most enteric gram-negative organisms. Penicillin may be used as first-line empiric therapy in areas of the world in which the incidence of penicillin-resistant organism is low.[62] In situations where penicillin-resistant *Strep. pneumoniae* is suspected, or if *Listeria monocytogenes* is a concern (i.e., in an immunosuppressed patient), vancomycin, 1 g intravenously

Table 11-1

Cerebrospinal fluid findings in meningitis

Meningitis	Pressure (mmH₂O)	Leukocytes (per cubic millimeter)	Protein (mg/dL)	Glucose (mg/dL)
Acute bacterial	Usually elevated	Several hundred to more than 60,000; usually a few thousand; occasionally fewer than 100 (especially meningococcal or early in disease); polymorphonuclear cells predominate	Usually 100 to 55 occasionally more than 1000	5 to 40 in most cases (in the absence of hyperglycemia)
Tuberculous	Usually elevated; may be low with spinal block in advanced stages	Usually 25 to 100; rarely more than 500; lymphocytes predominate except in early stages polymorphonuclear cells may account for 80% of cells	Nearly always elevated; usually 100 to 200; may be much higher if dynamic block	Usually reduced; less than 45 in three-quarters of cases
Cryptococcal	Usually elevated	0 to 800; average 50; lymphocytes predominate	Usually 20 to 500; average 100	Reduced in most cases; average 30 (in absence of hyperglycemia)
Viral	Normal to moderately elevated	5 to a few hundred; but may be more than 1000 particularly with lymphocytic choriomeningitis; lymphocytes predominate but may be more than 80% polymorphonuclear cells in first few days	Frequently normal or slightly elevated; less than 100; may show greater elevation in severe cases	Normal (reduced in one-quarter of cases of mumps, herpes simplex, CMV)
Syphilitic (acute)	Usually elevated	Average 500; usually lymphocytes; rarely polymorphonuclear cells	Average, 100	Normal (rarely reduced)
Cysticercosis	Often increased, low with spinal block	Increased mononuclear cells and polymorphonuclear cells with 2 to 7% eosinophilia in about one-half of cases	Usually 50 to 200	Reduced in 1/5 cases
Sarcoid	Normal to considerably reduced	0 to fewer than 100 mononuclear cells	Slight to moderate elevation	Reduced in one-half of cases
Carcinomatous	Normal or elevated	0 to several hundred mononuclear cells plus malignant cells	Elevated often to high levels	Normal or reduced (low in 75% of cases)

The CSF immunoglobulins are generally increased in all of the above infections. They are also increased in multiple sclerosis and in carcinomatous meningitis. In sarcoid, the IgG index is often increased with normal oligoclonal bands.

The CSF immunoglobulins are assessed by the IgG index: $\dfrac{\text{IgG (CSF)} \times \text{albumin (serum)}}{\text{IgG (serum)} \times \text{albumin (CSF)}}$; the normal index is less than about 0.65.

The presence of oligoclonal bands (with gel electrophoresis) is also a measure of abnormally increased CSF immunoglobulins. *Source*: From Fishman,[137] p. 257, with permission.

over 12 h, should be given until culture and sensitivity are available. In the event of life-threatening penicillin allergy, chloramphenicol, 2 g intravenously over 6 h, should be instituted. Therapy can later be adjusted according to the results of CSF and blood cultures. The current recommendation for the length of the therapy is 10 to 14 days.[63]

Empiric treatment of herpes simplex encephalitis should also be started. Acyclovir, 10 mg/kg intravenously over 8 h, with each infusion lasting 1 h. should be given. This treatment should be continued until later imaging or microbiologic studies have excluded herpes simplex encephalitis. If the PCR is negative, the treatment should be discontinued after 5 days; if positive, it should be continued for 10 days.

The role of corticosteroids in bacterial meningitis or herpes simplex encephalitis is controversial. Two recent, double-blind placebo-controlled studies of children with bacterial meningitis (mostly *H. influenzae*), found that the administration of dexamethosone for the first 4 days of treatment resulted in statistically significant decreases in the incidence of hearing loss and other neurologic complications.[29,30] No equivalent study has been carried out in adults. Its value in herpes simplex encephalitis has not been established, and some have postulated an increased risk of spread of the infection.

If edema will not resolve, or there is a significant mass lesion, neurosurgical consultation should be sought.

BACTERIAL MENINGITIS

Bacterial meningitis is a prime consideration in any patient, child or adult, presenting in a state of altered consciousness. However, despite modern methods of management, the case fatality rate of meningitis in infants and children approaches 5 percent, with as many as 20 percent of survivors experiencing long-term sequelae.[64,65] The mortality rate in adults with pneumococcal meningitis may be 30 percent or more.[7] Neurologic sequelae and death are primarily due to delays in treatment, and

are more frequent as the level of unconsciousness deepens. Improved outcome depends largely on early and accurate diagnosis.[66] Thus, bacterial meningitis will be covered extensively in this chapter, stressing management at an early stage, in addition to the later stages of stupor and coma.

Clinical Presentation

This occurs in two main ways: (1) gradual onset over a day or more, often preceded by febrile illness; or (2) acute onset, with rapidly developing cerebral edema, transtentorial herniation, and coma. This latter fulminant form is most often associated with meningococcal meningitis and a high mortality rate.[67]

In neonates and young infants, the findings are often subtle and include fever, lethargy, respiratory distress, jaundice, disinterest in feeding, vomiting, and diarrhea. Fever is an unreliable indicator, being present in only 50 percent of infected infants. There may be irritability, poor muscle tone, and a bulging fontanelle. Seizures occur in 40 percent of newborn infants with meningitis.[67] Half of the patients may not have a fever.[74] A change in an older child's affect or state of alertness is an important sign, whereas stiff neck, Kernig and Brudzinski signs, seizures, bulging fontanelle, and coma occur less commonly and develop later in the course of the illness.[67]

In older children and adults, fever, headache, photophobia, nausea, vomiting, mental confusion, lethargy, and excessive irritability are commonly observed. Unfortunately, prior antibiotic therapy may modify the physical and CSF findings, causing delay in diagnosis.

Meningococcal meningitis occurs in both children and adults, but is rare in infants. It should be suspected in epidemics of meningitis when the evolution is extremely rapid; if there is a measles-like, petechial or purpuric skin eruption, large ecchymoses and lividity of the skin and the lower parts of the body; or when there is circulatory collapse.

Pneumococcal meningitis occurs predominantly in adults and is less likely in small children and infants. It is often preceded by an infection in the lungs, ears or sinuses, and, rarely, by endocarditis. It should be suspected in patients suffering from alcoholism, sickle cell disease or basal skull fracture, or in those following splenectomy or organ transplantation, or when there are multiple recurrences of bacterial meningitis following head trauma.

Haemophilus influenzae, type B, is responsible for most cases in children and is rarely present in adults and infants. It often follows upper respiratory tract and ear infections in young children.

Listeria monocytogenes has emerged as an important cause of bacterial meningitis, particularly in infants or the elderly, debilitated patients or those with immunosuppression secondary to transplantation, those receiving therapy for cancer, or those with connective tissue disease. Alcoholism and high steroid treatment are also predisposing factors.

The classic signs of meningitis may be minimal in the elderly; in debilitated patients, simply a low-grade fever without headache or nuchal rigidity. Stiff neck or positive Kernig's or Brudzinski's signs may be absent in the very young, the very elderly, or those who are severely obtunded.

Petechiae and purpura are frequently associated with meningococcemia but may appear with other bacterial, viral, or rickettsial diseases.[68,69] Purpura, when seen with hypothermia and shock, is usually accompanied by disseminated intravascular coagulation, and represents a poor prognostic sign.[29]

Seizures occur in 30 percent of patients. Focal seizures have a worse prognosis than primary generalized seizures. They may be due to inappropriate antidiuretic hormone and low sodium. They may also be caused by cerebritis, subdural effusion, vascular thrombosis, or abscess formation.[67] They are seen most frequently in association with pneumococcal or listeriosis infection.[49,70]

Papilledema is rarely seen and, if present, suggests venous sinus thrombosis, subdural effusion, or brain abscess.[67] A dilated, unresponsive pupil in a child with bacterial meningitis may be due to increased ICP with impending herniation, but may also be caused by local inflammation of the third cranial nerve, without increased ICP.[71] Focal neurologic signs, such as hemiparesis, quadriparesis, facial palsy, endophthalmitis, and visual field defects, occur in 15 percent of patients. Stupor and coma, and focal neurologic signs are associated with a poor prognosis if present before the start of therapy.[66]

In children, subdural effusions may occur in up to 34 percent of the cases,[49] but this is rare in adults.[70]

Hyponatremia may occur in up to one-third of bacterial meningitis patients, usually due to the syndrome of inappropriate antidiuretic hormone secretion (SIADH). As many as three-quarters of patients with tuberculous meningitis may develop SIADH.[59]

Bacterial meningitis occurs in 20 percent of children with a septic arthritis. In patients with recurrent meningitis, the presence of a fluid-filled or persistently draining middle ear should suggest the possibility of CSF fistula. If the disease is caused by staphylococci, enteric gram-negative organisms, or anaerobes, a congenital dermal sinus tract should be suspected.[72]

A variety of complications can occur during the course of bacterial meningitis. Early ones are cerebral edema, septic shock, disseminated intravascular coagulation, myocarditis, hyponatremia, and seizures.[142] Later ones are subdural effusion, empyema, and hydrocephalus. Neurologic complications include cranial nerve palsies, hemiparesis or quadriparesis, muscular hypertonia, ataxia, permanent seizure disorder, cortical blindness, transverse myelitis, cerebral or spinal cord infarction, pericardial effusion, and polyarteritis. Brain abscess is a rare complication and, when present, has likely preceded the meningeal infection.[67]

Mortality rates vary, depending on the infectious organism. They are higher in cases of pneumococcal meningitis (26 percent), followed by meningococcal meningitis (10 percent) and *Haemophilus influenzae* (6 percent).[73]

Laboratory Investigations

These investigations should follow the algorithm for investigating patients suspected to have acute

CNS infection (Fig. 11-1). The peripheral white blood cell count is often not helpful, except that a low count, below 3000 per cubic centimeter, suggests severe disease and a poor outcome.[67]

Blood cultures are positive in more than 80 percent of previously untreated cases of bacterial meningitis.[67] [The organism may initially be identified from other sites: i.e., the skin, particularly in cases of meningococcemia or staphyloccal septicemia (Fig. 11-2).] Blood should be drawn prior to obtaining CSF, because equilibrium between serum and CSF glucose generally takes between 30 min and 2 h, and the stress of a lumbar puncture may raise the serum glucose.[66,67]

The lumbar puncture remains the definitive test for bacterial meningitis. The following are typical findings: the protein concentration exceeds 100 mg/dL; the glucose concentration is below 30 mg/dL; and the CSF/serum glucose ratio is < 0.31. Gram stain discloses bacteria in 90 percent of the patients (Fig. 11-3). If antibiotics have been given, the chances of a positive culture are reduced to 40 percent. An elevated C-reactive protein may distinguish bacterial from viral meningitis. The CSF findings in different types of meningitis are shown in Table 11-1, as well as those in nonmeningitis cases.

However, this "typical" picture may vary according to a variety of circumstances. In neonates, there may normally be 32 white blood cells (60 percent polymorphs) per cubic millimeter. A white cell count of <1000 cells per cubic millimeter may be found in the early stages of bacterial meningitis, partially treated meningitis, overwhelming bacterial meningitis due to pneumococci, and in patients who are leucopenic or immunosuppressed.[74] The CSF protein concentration will be elevated in a traumatic lumbar puncture at the rate of approximately 1 mg/dL for every 1000 red blood cells. The glucose may be lowered, at times, by hypoglycemia, subarachnoid hemorrhage, and viral meningitis. In nonpurulent meningitis, a low CSF glucose concentration suggests partially treated meningitis or tuberculosis.[75]

Further tests on the CSF may be helpful, particularly in cases of partially treated meningitis.

These tests include countercurrent immunoelectrophoresis (CIE), latex particle agglutination, and enzyme-linked immunosorbent assays (ELISA). Latex agglutination is more sensitive than CIE and is now used in most laboratories; it can be used to detect the polysaccharide antigens HIB (*Haemophilus influenzae*, type 8), *Staph. pneumoniae*, *N. meningitidis*, and group B streptococci.[67] Unfortunately, a positive test is helpful but a negative test does not exclude bacterial disease. Polymerase chain reaction (PCR) has proven valuable in the diagnosis of meningococcal meningitis.[56,143]

The results of CSF analysis may be equivocal, failing to distinguish between bacterial and aseptic meningitis. Thus, in aseptic meningitis, the white blood cell count is less than 1000 cells per cubic millimeter (with 70 percent lymphocytes), the CSF glucose is normal, and the Gram stain and latex agglutination test are negative. Despite the likelihood of this being aseptic meningitis, the author recommends that the patient be prescribed empiric antibiotic treatment after appropriate cultures have been obtained. Antibiotics may be discontinued if the cultures are sterile after 72 h.[67]

A CT head scan,[144] utilizing the bone window technique, may reveal areas of primary infection near the base of the brain, such as purulent sinusitis or mastoiditis. A brain abscess or subdural empyema will be readily apparent. The complicating factors of venous sinus thrombosis, hydrocephalus or infarction of the brain parenchyma, are usually also evident with CT scan. Scanning by MRI often reveals more detailed evidence of parenchymal damage, and, in the early stages, marked enhancement of the meninges (Fig. 11-4). Scanning by MRI is more effective than by CT for cortical (versus sinus) vein thrombosis and brainstem lesions (e.g., in listeriosis, menocytogenese).

Cerebral angiography is indicated in instances of focal deficits or seizures, or in progressive lowering in the level of consciousness when other causes of coma have been excluded. The angiography may show arterial or venous occlusions.

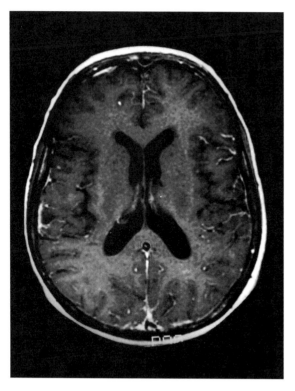

Figure 11-4

This adult female presented in coma. An initial T2-weighted MRI scan was normal. However, the post-gadolinium image shows marked enhancement of the meninges over both hemispheres. Subsequent investigations identified pneumococcal meningtis. (From Bolton,[147] with permission.)

Differential Diagnosis of Bacterial Meningitis

A wide variety of conditions must be considered.[76] In viral meningitis, there are the classic signs of headache, fever, and stiff neck, but the level of consciousness is normal, as is mental functioning, in general. The CSF count ranges between 50 to 1000 white blood cells per cubic millimeter, with mainly lymphocytes. The CSF concentration is only mildly elevated and the glucose concentration is normal. If the brain is affected at the same time by the virus, the level of consciousness may be decreased and there may be focal neurologic signs and seizures.

In encephalitis due to herpes simplex virus, type 1, there may be several days of simple headache and a gradually developing, mild confusional state. Then, more clear-cut evidence of frontal or temporal lobe disease develops, manifested as clear-cut personality change and impaired memory. In some cases, the illness may progress rapidly to a comatose state. One patient, a young medical student, developed symptoms and signs over a long weekend and was found in a comatose state by his classmates when they returned to his apartment after the weekend. Recurring seizures occur in nearly 50 percent of patients.[77] On CSF examination, the pressure is elevated and the white blood cell count ranges from 50 to 500 cells per microliter, mainly lymphocytes. A more typical feature is the presence of red blood cells or frank xanthochromia. The protein concentration is elevated and the glucose concentration may be normal or moderately reduced. The EEG is quite helpful diagnostically in showing focal slow-wave abnormalities, mainly in the temporal lobes, and often with asymmetry and periodic lateralized epileptiform discharges (PLEDs). These discharges characteristically recur every 1 to 5 s.

Rocky Mountain spotted fever is caused by *Rickettsia rickettsii* which is transmitted to humans by ticks. It may be manifest as focal signs; decreased levels of consciousness leading to coma and seizure activity. The rash is typically maculopapular or purpuric, diffuse, and involving the palms and soles. It may be difficult to distinguish from the rash of meningococcal infection, except that it does not involve the mucous membranes. The diagnosis may be made between the fourth and tenth day by biopsy of the skin lesion, which shows the organism by using the immunofluorescence antibody test. The CSF typically shows <100 cells per cubic millimeter or the cells may be absent, the glucose concentration is normal, and the protein level is only mildly to moderately elevated.

In Lyme disease, due to *Borrelia buradorferi*, the onset is subacute with only mild CSF pleocytosis, mild protein elevation, and normal glucose. Antibodies against the offending organism may be detected in the CSF. Testing of CSF by PCR may be positive.[78]

Fungal meningitis characteristically develops in a chronic fashion. The CSF reveals increased white blood cells and protein and low glucose. An India ink examination may reveal the cryptococcal organism in 50 percent of the cases. The organism may be cultured from the CSF, but repeated lumbar punctures and cultures are often necessary. The detection of fungal antigen in the serum and CSF and complement-fixing antibodies may further assist the diagnosis.

Brain abscess (see Case 1) and subdural empyema may both present in a similar manner to bacterial meningitis. Only CT or MRI scanning will clearly demonstrate the lesion.

A number of noninfective conditions should always be considered in the differential diagnosis. Foremost among these is intracranial hemorrhage, either subarachnoid or primary intracerebral hemorrhage due to ruptured arteriovenous malformations (see Case 2), or berry or mycotic aneurysms. The headache characteristically develops suddenly in a matter of minutes, but otherwise, the clinical features may be quite similar to bacterial meningitis. In these circumstances, it is wise to do a CT head scan before a lumbar puncture because of the risk of an intracranial mass lesion or tonsillar herniation. The CT scan will usually reveal if there is a subarachnoid or intracerebral hemorrhage. In about 10 percent of the cases of subarachnoid hemorrhage, the CT scan is negative and the diagnosis must then be made by lumbar puncture and the finding of red blood cells and/or xanthochromia in the CSF.

In the neuroleptic malignant syndrome, there is fever, generalized rigidity of the body, decreased level of consciousness, autonomic instability, and marked elevation of the serum creatinine phosphokinase. Adrenal crisis may be associated with fever, confusion, collapse, and hypotension.

Treatment

Antibiotic Therapy After blood cultures are performed, antibiotics should be given prior to performing a lumbar puncture if a delay in diagnosis is anticipated, either to obtain a head CT scan or to transport the patient to another facility (Fig. 11-1). If the CT scan indicates cerebral edema, mannitol, 0.25 g/kg, should be given intravenously, just before the lumbar puncture. Ideally, antibiotics should be administered within 30 min of encountering the patient. Talan et al[145] found that a 4-h delay ocurred when a CT scan preceded the lumbar puncture or if the physician waited for the lumbar puncture results prior to administering antibiotics. If antibiotics were withheld until the patient was admitted to the inpatient ward, the delay averaged 4.5 h.

Empiric treatment in adults is: cefotaxime, 2 g intravenously over 4 h; ampicillin 2 g intravenously over 4 h. Chloramphenicol should be used if there is a history of penicillin allergy. This therapy should be later adjusted (Table 11-2) based on the results of the CSF and blood culture.

In children with bacterial meningitis, antibiotics should be administered in the appropriate dosages (Table 11-3). Neonatal meningitis should be treated initially with ampicillin, an aminoglycoside, or a cephalosporin. Ampicillin should be used in infants up to 4 weeks old to provide adequate coverage for both *Listeria* spp. and enterococcus. In infants and children, either a cephalosporin or ampicillin plus chloramphenicol is appropriate initial therapy. Ceftriaxone is preferred to cefuroxime. Few adverse reactions are associated with the use of cephalosporins.

Supportive Measures

If possible, children and adults should be managed in an ICU to counteract seizures, apnea, septic shock, and other complications. Supplemental oxygen by mask or oxygen tent may be necessary. However, mechanical ventilation is only rarely required.[79] Hyponatremia (serum sodium <135 mmol/L) may occur due to inappropriate secretion of antidiuretic hormone. Thus, excessive intravenous fluid administration should be avoided. Intravenous fluids of 5% dextrose/0.2 normal saline should be infused at a rate of two-third maintenance.[79] In cases of septic shock, increased fluid administration should be applied; e.g., 10 to 20 mL/kg bolus of isotonic sodium chloride or

Table 11-2
Recommended treatment of bacterial meningitis according to organism isolated

Meningeal pathogen	Antibiotic
N. meningitidis	Penicillin G or ampicillin
Strep. pneumoniae	Penicillin G or third-generation cephalosporin[a]
H. influenzae type b	Third-generation cephalosporin[a]
Streptococci (group B)	Penicillin G or third-generation cephalosporin[a]
Enterobacteriaceae	Third-generation cephalosporin[a]
Pseudomonas aeruginosa	Ceftazidime plus aminoglycoside[b]
Staph. aureus (methicillin sensitive)	Oxacillin
Staph. aureus (methicillin resistant)	Vancomycin
Coagulase-negative staphylcocci	Vancomycin
L. monocytogenes sulfamethoxazole	Ampicillin (plus aminoglycoside[b])

[a] Cefotaxime or ceftriaxone—in areas where penicillin-resistant pneumococci have been encountered, vancomycin is recommended.
[b] Gentamicin or tobramycin.
Source: From Pfister and Roos,[76] with permission.

lactated Ringer's solution. In cases of anemia, whole blood or packed red blood cells may be required. In rare instances, hemodynamic monitoring and pressor agents, such as dopamine and dobutamine, may be necessary to counteract shock. Patients who are in refractory hemodynamic shock or suffering from respiratory distress syndrome may benefit from extracorporeal membrane oxygenation (ECMO), or "heart-lung" machine therapy. In a recently reported series, three-quarters of such severely affected patients with meningococcal sepsis survived.[80]

Seizures should be treated with intravenous benzodiazepines, and phenobarbital and dilantin for long-term control.[79] Elevated ICP can usually be managed initially with elevation of the head of the bed and fluid restriction. If there is development of pupillary dilatation, bradycardia, apnea, decreased responsiveness, or signs suggesting raised ICP, mannitol should be administered, 0.5 to 2 g/kg over 30 min, and repeated as necessary. Cerebral herniation may be seen within hours of admission, evidenced by unilateral or bilateral pupillary dilatation, decorticate or decerebrate posturing, apnea, hyperventilation, Cheyne-Stokes respiration, or loss of oculocephalic response. Immediate intubation, hyperventilation, and mannitol infusion may be life-saving.[79]

However, if mechanical ventilation is required, the prognosis may be poor. Thus, of 32 children given such treatment,[81] 50 percent had a Glasgow Coma Scale of <8 and 30 percent ultimately died. Twenty percent were left with severe functional deficits.

In case of a primary infected focus at the base of the skull, especially with a bony defect or direct communication with CSF space, surgical drainage of the sinus or mastoid should be instituted as promptly as possible. Until such drainage has been effected, improvement may fail to occur.

Isolation Procedures Patients with meningococcal meningitis should be isolated for the first 24 h after the onset of the antibiotic therapy. Isolation is not required in other CNS infections.

Treatment in Advanced Cases At a more advanced stage, when coma and focal neurologic signs are present, more aggressive management may be indicated: serial imaging studies, ICP monitoring, the use of mannitol, steroids, and so forth. While the value of such measures is

Table 11-3

Empiric antibiotic dosing in bacterial meningitis according to age[a]

	Dose
Neonates, age 0–7 days, weight > 2 kg	
Amikacin	10 mg/kg IV q12h
Ampicillin	50 mg/kg IV q8h
Cefotaxamine	50 mg/kg IV q12h
Ceftazidime	30 mg/kg IV q8h
Ceftriaxone	50 mg/kg IV q24h
Gentamicin	2.5 mg/kg IV q12h
Neonates, age > 7 days, weight > 2 kg	
Amikacin	10 mg/kg IV q8h
Ampicillin	50 mg/kg IV q6h
Cefotaxime	50 mg/kg IV q8h
Ceftazidime	50 mg/kg IV q8h
Ceftriaxone	75 mg/kg IV q24h
Gentamicin	2.5 mg/kg IV q8h
Older infants and children	
Ampicillin	200 mg/kg per day IV, divided q6h
Cefotaxime	200 mg/kg per day IV, divided q6h
	100 mg/kg per day IV q12h or
Ceftriaxone	80 mg/kg IV or IM 1/day
Chloramphenicol	100 mg/kg per day IV, divided q6h

[a] In areas where penicillin-resistant *S. pneumococci* have been encountered, give vancomycin.
Abbreviations: IV = intravenously; IM = intramuscularly; q12h = over 12 h, etc.
Source: From Nelson[138] and Pichichero,[139] with permission.

controversial, increasing attention is being given this topic, as discussed by Ashwal et al.[18] In relation to increased ICP and reduced cerebral blood flow, monitoring of ICP is not routinely-carried out in adults or children with bacterial meningitis, nor have criteria been established to determine who might benefit from monitoring. Monitoring ICP may be considered in infants and children in whom there is clinical or neuroimaging evidence of moderate to marked increased ICP. The CPP is calculated as CPP = MABP – ICP (where MABP = mean arterial blood pressure). Changes in transcranial Doppler are late events. Measurement of jugular venous oxygen saturation (JVO_2) is potentially useful[82] but its role in bacterial meningitis has not yet been demonstrated.

If the initial CT or MRI is normal, in the author's opinion it is unlikely that cerebral blood flow will be reduced to ischemic levels, and hyperventilation is likely to safely reduce elevated ICP for the first 24 to 48 h before its effect diminishes. These patients, presumably seen early in the course of infection, without cerebral edema, have raised ICP primarily due to an increase in cerebral blood flow and cerebral blood volume, as well as an increase in CSF volume. It should be realized, however, that it is still uncertain if this group of patients requires treatment as control studies examining this issue have yet to be performed.

The second group of patients, those children who have cerebral edema upon CT or MRI scanning, are unlikely to have cerebral hyperemia and more likely to have normal or reduced cerebral blood flow. In such patients, hyperventilation may reduce the increased ICP at the expense of significantly reducing cerebral blood flow. In some patients, this may approach ischemic thresholds. Early use of diuretics, such as furosemide, or osmotic dehydrating agents, such as mannitol are recommended, providing that the circulatory blood volume is protected. Corticosteroids may also be of value in this situation. Although mannitol is effective in reducing ICP, it is less effective when disruption of the blood-brain barrier occurs in meningitis. Some studies suggest that mannitol reduces ICP by other mechanisms, such as vasoconstriction.[83] If monitoring and treatment of increased ICP associated with cerebral edema are to be performed, they should be instituted very early in the course.

Those patients with increased ventricular or subarachnoid CSF volume with normal ICP do not require treatment since spontaneous resolution of this abnormality will occur as the infection is treated. However, in patients in whom ICP is elevated, consideration should be given for decreasing CSF volume and pressure by one or more of the conventional therapies, as available. As there is some risk in removal of CSF by lumbar puncture and there are potential complications from performing a ventricular tap or ventriculostomy, the clinical decision must take into account many factors. Potential candidates include those with increased ICP, signs of mass effect or impending herniation on neuroimaging, and those with markedly reduced cerebral blood flow or infarction. Less invasive therapies, such as decreasing CSF production with acetazolamide or digoxin, or decreasing CSF outflow resistance by decreasing the inflammatory response by the use of steroids, may be of some benefit. However, since these therapies have delayed action, they may be ineffective.

Subdural effusions are common in children, but recent studies have found that there is no substantial increase in the long-term risk for neurologic or development deficits, seizures, or hearing loss.[27,84] Thus, no specific treatment is usually indicated and the lesions resolve spontaneously. In rare circumstances, the subdural fluid may expand or become infected and cause local cerebral symptoms requiring drainage and culture of the fluid.

If neuroimaging reveals infarction, several approaches can be considered. Hyperventilation could worsen the situation by causing local vasoconstriction. Diuretics may initially improve local cerebral blood flow but do not appear to affect the long-term neurologic sequelae.[85,86] Diuretics also could worsen focal ischemic tissue injury by decreasing brain interstitial volume and blood volume. While barbiturates or hypothermia might be considered in this situation, their value has not been proven and there may be some risk in increasing the chances of long-term infection. Dexamethasone may also reduce cerebral edema and improve vasculitis, particularly in pneumococcal meningitis in adults. It has clearly been shown to be beneficial in children with meningitis and, in this instance, should be given intravenously in a dosage of 0.15 mg/kg every 6 h for 4 days. Intravenous H_2 receptor antagonist should be given to prevent gastric ulceration.

While controversial, intravenous heparin may be potentially beneficial in preventing infarction from either venous or arterial thrombosis.[87] Both bacterial and venous cerebrovascular complications account for high mortality rates and long-term sequelae, particularly in pneumococcal meningitis.[88,89] Studies by Haring et al[90] of cerebral blood flow velocity using the transcranial Doppler sonographic technique indicates that there is a high risk of developing brain ischemia in the first 5 days of bacterial meningitis. This probably reflects hemodynamic changes secondary to vasculitis.[37] There may also be damage to the endothelium, activating the endogenous coagulation cascade and converting prothrombin into thrombin. Thus, heparin as a thrombin antagonist should counteract these changes and prevent cerebral ischemia and infarction.

Heparin has the side effects of mild thrombocytopenia and causes intravascular coagulation from heparin-induced reduction of antithrombin III activity. Thus, platelets and antithrombin III activity should be monitored regularly. In the experience of Haring et al,[87] this treatment was found to be successful in bacterial meningitis, particularly pneumococcal meningitis, and has had no adverse complications. In particular, CT head scans, have shown no evidence of hemorrhage as a complication in the 41 patients treated by this method. However, the results of the studies of Haring et al have not been subject to a controlled trial.

Outcome

Predictors of an unfavourable outcome are: (1) large numbers of bacteria in the CSF and the presence of a low cell count; (2) age over 40 years; (3) underlying conditions such as splenectomy or endocarditis; (4) gram-negative organisms or pneumococci; and (5) a long interval between the onset of symptoms and treatment.

TUBERCULOSIS

Mycobacterium tuberculosis and *M. bovis* may affect any part of the body, but the CNS is involved in approximately 10 percent of cases.[91–93] Tuberculosis remains as a serious and prevalent illness throughout the world. In industrialized countries, tuberculosis occurs mainly among the poor, drug addicts,[94] immigrants from other countries and the aboriginal population, and immunosuppressed patients. Although there has been a steady decrease in the incidence of tuberculosis over the past century, the number of reported cases has dramatically increased in the past decade, not only because of AIDS, but also because multiple-drug-resistant organisms are unfortunately now developing. When such organisms infect AIDS patients, the response to treatment is often poor.[95] However, in non-AIDS patients, the response to appropriate chemotherapy of supposed drug-resistant organisms was quite good.[96]

Clinical Features

The CNS may be involved as meningitis, a diffuse encephalopathy, or focal disorders such as tuberculomas or brain abscesses.

Tuberculous meningitis may develop in a more insidious fashion in which fever or meningeal signs may or may not be present. The manifestations may be simply a slowly progressive, diffuse encephalopathy, often with multifocal features. Occasionally, the onset is much more rapid and typical of acute bacterial meningitis. If untreated, both forms may go on to coma with decerebrate posturing, hypothalamic disturbances, and death. There may be the acute onset of focal dysfunction due to cerebral infarction secondary to arteritis, and seizures are also fairly common.

A diffuse encephalopathy occurs in children without evidence of meningitis and this is thought to be an immune-mediated response manifest as edema of the white matter. The onset is acute, with seizures, coma, and decerebrate posturing.[97]

Tuberculomas present as typical space-occupying lesions with various manifestations dependent upon the location. If in the posterior fossa, there may be cerebellar and brainstem signs with evidence of obstructive hydrocephalus. Tuberculomas may expand during treatment. A tuberculous abscess presents as focal signs with increased ICP. Pathologically, the tuberculous abscess lacks a granulomatous capsule.

Investigations

Because of the possibility of hydrocephalus or focal mass lesions, CT or MRI scans should be carried out in advance of the lumbar puncture. The CSF is characteristically clear or opaque and under increased pressure. Cells are increased, mainly lymphocytes, with variable reduction in the glucose but an increase in the CSF protein concentrations. Unfortunately, acid-fast bacilli are found in the CSF in only 30 percent of patients.[97] The organism may be cultured in 75 percent of patients but the final result may not be obtained for several weeks. Several other methods of more immediate investigation have been tried but the results are variable or are not widely available: i.e., measurements of tuberculostearic acid, dot immunobinding, and ELISA. The PCR is now the definitive method of early diagnosis[98] and may be positive for up to 3 weeks after the start of treatment.[99] The PCR was positive in the CSF in 92 percent of cases whereas microscopy using Ziehl-Neelsen staining was positive in only 17 percent. Later culture was positive in 75 percent. However, a negative PCR does not exclude the diagnosis.[100]

Intradermal skin tests may be helpful but, if positive, are not clear evidence of recent infection. Skin tests may be falsely negative in 40 percent of patients, even those who are not immunosuppressed. The tuberculin test may become positive during treatment. Chest film may show findings suspicious of tuberculosis but it is abnormal in only 50 percent of patients. If chest lesions are present, diagnostic thoracocentesis or pleural biopsy should be considered. Tuberculosis should also be looked for in gastric secretions, and sputum and urine should be stained for acid-fast bacilli and sent for culture.

On CT scanning,[101] obstructive hydrocephalus is found in 80 percent of patients. Contrast enhancement may reveal basal meningeal enhancement. Imaging by MRI may give better visualization of granulomatous changes within the basilar cisterns[102] With imaging, it may be difficult to distinguish tuberculomas from tumors, or tuberculous abscesses from bacterial abscesses.

Brain biopsy may be considered in immunocompromised patients in whom the diagnosis of tuberculous meningitis is difficult and in whom delay of treatment may be harmful.[97] Biopsy should also be considered in cases of possible tuberculoma.

Treatment

Treatment should be started immediately in any suspected case, even though the organism has not been clearly identified, either by acid-fast stains or by culture. Treatment should continue until the results of culture are positive or negative and the clinical situation has clarified itself. Treatment consists usually of a three-drug combination of isoniazid, rifampin, and ethambutol, carried on for a period of 3 to 4 months, followed by isoniazid and rifampin for up to 21 months. Other drugs, such as pyrazinamide and streptomycin, may also be utilized. A peripheral neuropathy can be prevented by giving pyridoxine whenever isoniazid is used. While corticosteroids have been tried, to prevent adhesions and arteritis, they have never been clearly shown to be effective. Although corticosteroid treatment may be useful in patients who already have hydrocephalus or who have mass lesions with surrounding edema, intraventricular and intrathecal hyaluronidase may be tried to reduce arachnoiditis.[97] Seizures should be treated appropriately, keeping in mind that the metabolism of phenytoin is blocked by isoniazid and, thus, phenytoin toxicity may occur. Hydrocephalus may need to be treated by ventriculoatrial or ventriculoperitoneal shunts. Mass lesions should also be dealt with surgically, except for tuberculomas, which may be treated conservatively and monitored with CT scanning.[97]

Protection of airways, and ventilator support, fluid management, and other general measures will be necessary in the more seriously ill or comatose patient.

Prognosis

Central nervous system tuberculosis can be a devastating illness, with mortality rates reaching 30 percent, and up to 50 percent of patients surviving having varying degrees of residual nervous system damage.[103,104]

BRAIN ABSCESS

Bacterial abscesses generally develop in four stages.[105, pp. 407–417; 106] Following inoculation of the site, days 1 to 3 show a microscopic picture of an "early" or diffuse cerebritis. From days 4 to 9, the picture is that of a more organized, or "late" cerebritis. Early capsule formation is noted from days 10 to 13, and late capsule formation after 2 weeks. Generally, the single thick-walled abscesses are due to contiguous spread, while the thin-walled variety, especially if multiple, are associated with hematogenous spread. Contiguous spread occurs with traumatic injury, surgery, and sinus infections. Contiguous spread from sinusitis or otitis is still the most common cause of brain abscess. Frontal and ethmoidal sinus infections are associated with frontal lobe abscesses, infections in the maxillary sinuses with temporal lobe abscesses, and mastoid sinus disease with cerebellar, temporal, and occipital infections. Sinusitis of the ethmoid or sphenoid sinuses may be associated with temporal or frontal abscesses. Brain abscesses which develop due to blood-borne bacteria are associated with congenital right-to-left intracardiac shunting, immunosuppressive drug use, AIDS, and immune suppression occurring as a result of trauma. The most common bacteria associated with abscesses are streptococci (aerobic and beta-hemolytic), *Staph. aureus*, pneumococcis, enterococcis, bacteroides species and anaerobic streptococcus. Careful anaerobic technique is necessary to allow growth from abscess tissue.

Brain abscesses present in four ways: (1) as focal findings which progress rapidly to a diffuse picture with elevated ICP; (2) as a diffuse depression of cerebral function with little or no focality but elevated ICP; (3) as a diffuse destructive lesion with multiple deficits; and (4) as a small, discrete lesion with focal deficits and little or no elevation of ICP.

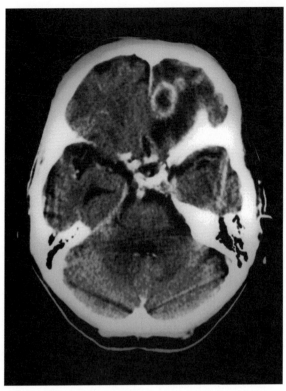

Figure 11-5

This adult female presented with stupor and fever. A CT scan showed extensive edema in the inferior left frontal lobe plus a 1.5-cm ring-enhancing lesion and a smaller daughter brain abscess just adjacent to it, measuring 7 mm.

Fever, usually low grade and seen in approximately 50 percent of cases, nausea and vomiting, and a diffuse alteration in mental status are seen to varying extent in approximately half the cases.

Lumbar puncture seldom yields useful information and should be avoided because of the risk of herniation (see Case 2). Scanning by CT (Fig. 11-5) has significantly decreased the time taken to diagnosis in these cases, enabling earlier definitive therapy to be started. It is also of value in determining the progress of medical therapy or the degree of surgical success in aspiration or excision. Scanning by MRI gives even better resolution and provides early identification of subdural abscess or additional meningeal involvement. Surgical

therapy consists of drainage or excision. Definitive identification of the organism(s) may be obtained via proper culture. Devitalized tissue and cavity fluid may be removed or reduced in volume, which may reduce elevated ICP.

Shahzadi et al[107] found stereotactic management to be highly effective, even in comatose patients. In cases of multiple abscesses, stereotactic aspiration of a large abscess plus antibiotic treatment was successful.

Excision is associated with a lower recurrence rate than aspiration. Aspiration may be performed via CT or other stereotactically guided technique; the anesthetic risks are fewer, with less systemic stress to the patient, and it may be performed more than once in a patient who remains unstable.

Abscesses which occur in contiguity with extradural infections are treated at the same time. Empiric antibiotic coverage is begun based upon Gram-stain results unless the etiology is already known; coverage usually includes ceftriaxone, vancomycin, and metronidazole. The antibiotics are continued for 4 to 8 weeks, with CT scans performed weekly or when needed as dictated by the patient's condition.

Medical therapy is reserved for those patients who, for medical reasons, are not able to undergo aspiration or excision, or where the abscesses are smaller and thinner-walled in the cerebritic stage. The organism will have been identified via blood or aspirate culture. Antibiotic therapy is maintained for 6 to 8 weeks and serial CT scans are performed to monitor the efficacy of therapy.

Management in an ICU is often necessary for maintenance of ICP, acceptable CPP, control of seizures, and provision of adequate systemic support.

Epidural Abscess

This is frequently associated with suppurative sinusitis or with trauma or prior surgical intervention. Streptococcus and *Staph. aureus* are the most frequently encountered organisms. There are findings of sinusitis with associated osteomyelitis and soft tissue scalp or facial swelling. Plain skull film, radionuclide bone scanning, and CT or MR scanning are usually diagnostic. Craniect-omy is indicated, although some advocate craniot-omy if no osteomyelitis is present.

Subdural Empyema

This is an exudative, spreading, purulent collection in the subdural space, not contained by a mem-brane.[105, p. 414;108] It arises from an extracranial infection transmitted through an emissary vein. The dura and overlying bone appear uninvolved. When the infection arises in a sinus, an epidural abscess may also be encountered. In pediatric cases, the infection may develop from an infected subdural effusion. The acute presentation is one of rapid onset and progression. Headache, fever, nausea, vomiting, and neck stiffness are observed. There may be a history of sinusitis or prior oto-laryngologic surgery. However, the patient may present with progressive neurologic deficit(s) or surgery. In the pathogenesis of size and focal signs, cortical vein thrombosis has been involved (at least for some cases). In the subacute form, there is usually a relatively long history of headache and fever, and a prior cranial procedure. There is usually some degree of membrane formation. The infantile form usually develops in a patient with a postmeningitic subdural effusion; the organism is frequently *H. influenzae*. Seizures, fever, vomiting, progressively altered consciousness, and evidence of an intracranial expanding mass are presenting signs. Scanning by CT, including scans of the skull base utilizing the bone window technique, is diag-nostic in the acutely ill patient. Scanning by MRI may also be valuable.

The treatment is burr holes and irrigation, with large flaps (free or osteoplastic), and debride-ment. The ICU management is critical, since the patient frequently presents in an obtunded state and is rarely improved immediately after surgery. Brain swelling is often marked, and the ICP may be elevated in spite of the craniectomy. The ICP is controlled via the methods described previously, although care must be taken to avoid techniques which may worsen the underlying ischemia. Empiric antibiotic treatment is prescribed, as above. The cortical damage frequently results in a

focus, or foci, for seizures. Continuous EEG mon-itoring may be necessary to aid diagnosis of sei-zures, which may be subclinical, and to monitor treatment. Scanning by CT is performed, usually within 24 h postoperatively, and is repeated at weekly intervals during the course of antibiotic therapy. Recurrent collections usually require a full reopening of the operative site.[105, p. 413]

MYCOPLASMA PNEUMONIAE

The CNS is affected in 0.1 percent of patients who suffer this primarily respiratory infection.[109] Ence-phalitis is the most frequent manifestation, but cases of meningitis, myelitis, polyradiculitis, and stroke have been reported. The onset of these manifestations is usually acute, with impaired con-sciousness, coma, psychosis, ataxia, convulsions, and pareses. Severe, fatal cases occur. The patho-physiology is unknown. *Mycoplasma pneumoniae* has never been isolated from brain tissue, but it has been recovered from CSF. Besides direct invasion by *M. pneumoniae* into the brain, neurotoxic or autoimmune reaction within the brain tissue is suspected. At neuropathologic examination, edema, demyelination, and microthrombi have been described. Diagnostic methods may reveal the pathophysiology of CNS manifestations asso-ciated with *M. pneumoniae* infection. The diagnosis is made by throat culture (positive in 65 percent of cases) and elevation of antibody titers in the serum and CSF, although such elevations may be non-specific. While treatment with erythromycin and tetracycline may be effective for the primary infec-tion, the prognosis for CNS manifestations is uncertain. The effect of plasma exchange is also uncertain.

HERPES VIRUS ENCEPHALITIS

The following herpes viruses can cause severe nervous system infections: herpes simplex virus 1 (HSV-1), herpes simplex virus 2 (HSV-2), cyto-megalovirus (CMV), varicella-zoster virus (VZV), Epstein-Barr virus (EBV), human herpesvirus 6, and simian herpesvirus B. Latency is characteristic of all of these viruses and there may be provocative stimuli, such as surgery on the trigeminal ganglia or emotional upset, fever, and exposure to ultraviolet light. Latent virus has been isolated from the trigeminal, sacral, and vaginal ganglia in humans.

Herpes Simplex Encephalitis

This is the commonest viral illness of the brain to require intensive management. The subject has been comprehensively reviewed by Meyding-Lamade et al.[48] It has an incidence of approximately 1 in 250,000 to 1 in 300,000.[61] It typically occurs throughout the year, and untreated has a mortality of 70 percent. In adults and older children, the encephalitis is caused by HSV-1; HSV-2 causes a benign lymphocytic meningitis. In the newborn, HSV-2 causes a diffuse encephalitis with or without systemic infection.

There is usually a prodrome of up to 4 days, during which the patient experiences headache and fever. Then, alteration of consciousness, memory loss, personality changes, confusion, or olfactory hallucinations supervene. Focal neurologic signs such as hemiparesis, aphasia, and, later, focal or generalized seizures may then develop. Signs of meningeal irritation are usually present. Papilledema may occur as a result of raised ICP.

The differential diagnosis[146] involves any disease in which there is rapidly increasing edema and focal involvement of the temporal and frontal lobes. These include abscesses, subdural hematoma, bacterial meningitis, venous sinus thrombosis and Reye syndrome, and also hemorrhagic post-infectious leukoencephalopathy. It should be noted that alteration of consciousness in herpes simplex encephalitis occurs in up to 100 percent of the cases.[48] Seizures occur in 60 percent of cases.[48] In the investigation of herpes simplex encephalitis, the CT scan looks normal until day 4. After that, hypodense areas appear most commonly in the temporal lobe and insular region, and then may involve the opposite side and, finally, the frontobasilar regions. There may be a space-occupying effect to these lesions. Hemorrhage is rarely seen on CT scan.[110] Scanning by MRI will

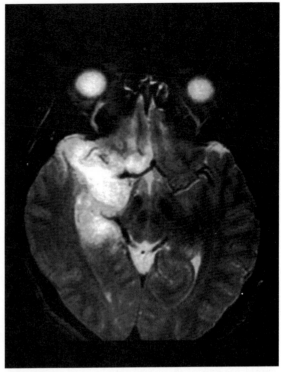

Figure 11-6

This adult male suffered herpes simplex encephalitis. In this T2-weighted image of an MRI scan, one sees dramatically increased signal throughout the right temporal lobe, extending into the insula and inferior frontal lobe. (From Bolton,[147] with permission.)

reveal abnormalities earlier, possibly as early as day 4, and is more sensitive in detecting lesions in the involved areas (Fig. 11-6). Signal changes indicating early hemorrhage may also be present. Edema can be detected by the MRI scan, as well as the later developing necrosis.[111]

The EEG is abnormal (Fig. 11-7) in 84 percent of the cases. It may show the nonspecific changes of spike and slow wave. More specific are PLEDS initially, from one temporal lobe and then from both temporal lobes. There may also be rhythmic, triphasic waves or delta waves at 1 to 2 per second. If PLEDS occur later, they have a poor prognostic implication.[112,113]

Lumbar puncture should be performed, but may be withheld in the presence of a mass lesion

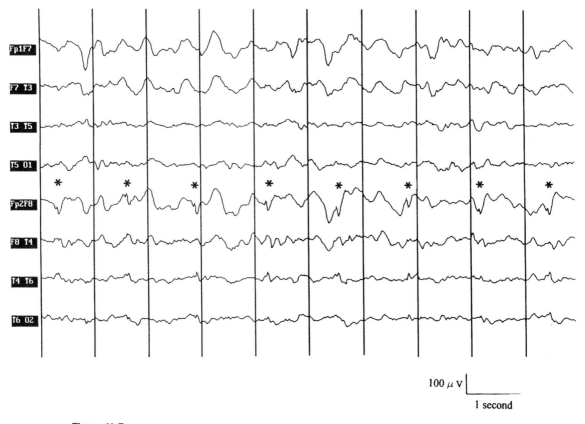

100 μ V ⌐
_____
1 second

Figure 11-7
This EEG was performed on the fourth day of an illness characterized by fever, head-ache, confusion, and recurrent complex partial seizures. There is bilaterally slow back-ground with medium-voltage delta waves in the frontal and anterior temporal regions (first, second, third, and fourth channels), and PLEDs under the asterixes in the right anterior–mid temporal region (F8-T4). These discharges occurred in a regular pattern with an interval of just over 1 s. The MRI and CSF results were compatible with herpes simplex encephalitis. (From Bolton,[147] with permission.)

that might precipitate tentorial herniation. Empirical treatment is started with acyclovir and antibiotics as outlined in the earlier discussion. If a lumbar puncture can be performed safely, the white blood cell count is elevated early on and is usually predominantly lymphocytes, with counts being 50 to 500 per cubic millimeter. The counts may go as high as 2000 per cubic millimeter. There may be erythrocytes and even xanthochromia. The CSF protein is elevated from 0.5 to 2.5 mg/L. Positive oligoclonal bands almost always develop.[114]

Polymerase chain reaction (PCR) has now become the method of accurately diagnosing herpes simplex encephalitis.[115,116] It is positive within the first 10 days from onset and is usually positive in the earliest stages of the disease. However, negative PCR results may be obtained when intrathecally synthesized antibodies are detectable, suggesting that neutralization of the virus by specific antibodies has occurred during the course of the infection. Similar effects can be seen following the administration of acyclovir, which has caused disappearance of the herpes simplex virus.[60] However, this will not occur until after 10 days of treatment with acyclovir.

Because of the specificity and sensitivity of PCR testing, brain biopsy is now rarely indicated.

Treatment

Acyclovir is now the drug of choice and should be given as early as possible in the course of the disease, even in patients where the results of investigation and other PCR testing are not yet available.[48] As indicated earlier, the author recommends that patients with fever and mental confusion, where there is any possibility of bacterial meningitis or herpes simplex encephalitis, should be given immediate treatment for these conditions before any investigations are launched. With regard to treatment for herpes simplex virus, acyclovir should be given intravenously as 10 mg/kg every 8 hours, with each infusion lasting over 1 hour. This treatment should continue for at least 10 days. In patients who have renal failure, the dosage should be reduced appropriately. The side effects of acyclovir are rare and include phebitis, nausea, hematuria, and hypotension. Obstructive nephropathy and encephalopathy may occur with very high dosages. In the event that acyclovir may not be effective, adenine arabinoside may be used at a dosage of 15 mg/kg as a constant intravenous infusion over 12 to 24 h. The side effects include thrombophlebitis, hypokalemia, and inappropriate secretion of antidiarrhetic hormone.

Raised ICP should be treated aggressively by maintenance of the airway (endotracheal intubation and mechanical ventilation if necessary), positioning, analgesia, sedation, prevention of seizures, controlled hyperventilation, hyperosmolar agents, and diuretics. The use of steroids is controversial. Seizures should be treated with phenytoin, initially 250 mg intravenously over 10 min and thereafter as an infusion of 750 mg over a period of 45 min. It should then be given daily as either 125 or 250 mg tid, depending upon serum levels.

Low-dose heparin can be given safely to prevent deep vein thrombosis (despite MRI evidence of intraparenchymal hemorrhage due to vascular necrosis).

The encephalitis should be monitored closely, in an ICU setting if the patient is deeply comatose and has significant respiratory and possibly cardiac compromise. To prevent edema, fluid limitation, diuresis, and hyperosmolar therapy may be needed. Brain function, particularly in comatose patients, can be monitored by continuous or serial regular EEG examinations. Serial CT scans are not helpful and may be hazardous because of worsening during transportation to the CT suite.

Untreated, herpes simplex encephalitis carries a mortality rate of 70 percent and almost invariable, severe mental deficiencies in those who survive, particularly severe memory loss and personality change. However, with successful and early treatment with acyclovir, the mortality rate is only 20 percent, with 40 percent of the patients recovering completely. Reasonably good results can also be obtained with arabinoside. Results of treatment are more likely to be ineffective in patients who are elderly, who are comatose, or when treatment has been given late in the illness.

Herpes Zoster Encephalitis

This may occur in two forms, one in association with chicken pox as the primary infection—a meningoencephalitis which may have the features of Reye syndrome. The second form is an encephalitis-complicating herpes zoster, occurring when a latent virus has been reactivated. Herpes zoster encephalitis may be accompanied by granulomatous angiitis which contributes to the distinctiveness and severity of the encephalitis. Patients who are immunosuppressed, including the elderly and those with AIDS, are more likely to develop this complication. It has a mortality rate of 30 percent and a significant morbidity.

In children with chicken pox, the differential diagnosis of Reye syndrome is usually entertained. The encephalitis comes on 1 to 2 weeks after the rash appears, although, occasionally, it may antedate the appearance of the rash. However, in children, a post-varicella cerebellitis that does not produce coma is the usual picture.

The EEG shows generalized abnormalities with diffuse slowing of a nonspecific nature. The CT head scans are usually unhelpful but MRI imaging may show early changes. Cerebrospinal fluid examination is typical of a viral CNS infection. The herpes zoster virus may be cultured from the CSF. However, as in herpes simplex encephalitis, PCR analysis of CSF is now the definitive method of diagnosing herpes zoster encephalitis, meningitis and myelitis.[117,118]

The treatment is the same as for herpes simplex encephalitis, but cases are still too few to gauge the effects of this treatment.

OTHER VIRAL INFECTIONS

Coxsackie and ECHO Virus Infections

Infection of the CNS by enteroviruses (EV) is of major epidemiologic importance.[119, p. 468] In the United States, about half of the annual 40,000 to 60,000 cases of aseptic meningitis and up to 10 percent of a probable 20,000 cases of encephalitis are likely to be caused by an EV agent, mainly the Coxsackie or enterocytopathogenic human orphan (ECHO) viruses.

As with most viruses, serious CNS involvement is a complication of hematogenous spread in the course of a systemic disease, and, in the case of EV infection, the prognosis may be limited by cardiac (Coxsackie) or hepatic (ECHO) rather than by cerebral involvement. Males, athletes, and B-cell-deficient patients are more likely to develop clinically relevant EV infection.

In temperate climates, epidemics occur mainly in summer and early autumn. Almost all cases present—after a variable incubation period of 5 to 10 days—with high fever up to 40°C; this is accompanied by nonspecific symptoms and signs such as rhinitis, pharyngitis, nausea, vomiting, exanthema, lymphadenopathy, arthralgia, or myalgia.

In adults and older children, CNS involvement is rare. Headache, photophobia, and nuchal rigidity are the common findings in this age group, suggesting the diagnosis of meningitis, and are often accompanied by hypersomnia and increased irritability. These symptoms are usually self-limited.

The picture is that of aseptic meningitis. A well-known complication is SIADH, while febrile seizures may be found in young children. Focal signs are rarely found. Nonpolio EVs are responsible for nearly all cases of paralytic poliomyelitis not caused by polio viruses and have frequently been found to cause cerebellar ataxia. They can also mimic the clinical presentation of herpes simplex or arbovirus infection.

In neonates, neurologic and multiorgan involvement with EV infection is associated with significant acute morbidity and mortality. Nuchal rigidity, convulsions, or bulging of the anterior fontanelle may be seen, but the prognosis is also influenced by extracerebral manifestations, such as hepatic, adrenal, or intestinal necrosis or myocarditis. The clinical picture in the newborn may be indistinguishable from bacterial sepsis with multiorgan failure and disseminated intravascular coagulation.

Diffuse brain edema on cranial CT scan or MRI is a common finding in neonatal EV infection, whereas focal lesions are rare. The EEG frequently shows diffuse slowing or dysrhythmia and is helpful to differentiate from herpes simplex encephalitis, where progressive temporal lobe involvement is usually seen. The EEG may also help to identify patients with a high risk for seizures. There is usually a moderate leukopenia and lymphocytosis or only slightly elevated white blood cell counts and thrombocytopenia. Moderate to marked CSF pleocytosis of 10 to 1000 cells per cubic millimeter (predominantly mononuclear cells) are the most typical finding in acute EV infection of the CNS, but considerably higher numbers have been described. Granulocytes may dominate the picture in early infection, but they are usually replaced by mononuclear cells within 2 days. The CSF glucose and protein concentrations are mostly not markedly altered, but a wide range of values, mimicking tuberculous meningitis, have been reported. Low CSF glucose is more frequently found than high CSF protein. It is possible to recover virus from the throat, feces, and blood, even before the onset of symptoms, while CSF culture will yield positive results soon after the onset of neurologic symptoms in aseptic meningitis, but less frequently in other

CNS manifestations. Respiratory specimens will be positive only for 1 to 2 weeks after clinical onset, indicating acute infection. Culture of EV has an overall detection sensitivity of only 65 to 75 percent and a frequent delay in the availability of results (3.7 to 8.2 days, mean, for CSF growth). Blood and CSF recovery provide the strongest causative links between clinical disease and the virus detected. In the future, more rapid diagnosis will be made by PCR. Serologic evidence of EV infection is obtained either from serum (high IgM levels or fourfold rise in IgG titers) or from CSF-antibody detection (elevated specific antibody of IgG ratio in the CSF, elevated IgG to albumin index in CSF/serum), but it may be falsely positive during the acute phase of febrile illness and does not allow rapid diagnosis in the case of acute infection. However, its sensitivity for the confirmation of a suspected disease is high. In suspected cases, B-cell defects or agammaglobulinemia should be considered. Administration of high doses of gamma globulin has shown positive effects in such cases and may prove useful in neonates. Since no specific therapy for EV infection is available, the main aim is to provide optimal supportive care and protect the patient from potentially harmful medication, which may have been considered due to the often difficult differential diagnosis. Management in a critical care unit is rarely necessary. However, CNS involvement is most likely to be complicated by elevated ICP, seizures, or electrolyte disturbance due to SIADH. Wherever possible, a CT scan should be obtained before lumbar puncture to detect elevated ICP, which may lead to herniation of the cerebellar tonsils during or after lumbar puncture. Measurement via epidural or intraventricular catheters may be necessary to monitor therapy. The possibility of SIADH should be considered if consciousness deteriorates, and fluid and electrolyte balance may require meticulous care. Extracerebral complications are usually due to cardiac or hepatic failure.

An EV infection with neurologic involvement is common but usually benign. Only neonates, very young children, or B-cell-deficient patients more frequently have a poor or fatal outcome—mostly due to nonneurologic, multiorgan complications.

Arboviral Infections

Togaviruses, bunya viruses, reoviruses, and the tick-borne complex are transmitted by ticks or mosquitos.[119, p. 477;120] Human cases show a peak incidence between July and October. Central European encephalitis (CEE), Russian spring-summer encephalitis, St. Louis encephalitis, California encephalitis, Colorado tick fever, and Japanese B encephalitis are all caused by these viruses.

The incubation period of CEE lasts 2 to 28 days, with a period of 7 to 14 days most often observed. The first stage of the disease lasts 1 to 8 days and correlates with the stage of viremia. Nonspecific clinical symptoms and signs include fever, malaise, headache, and fatigue. After this first stage, a fever-free interval of 1 to 20 days follows. The patients are free of symptoms during this period. In the second stage of the disease, symptoms and signs may develop. Neurologic abnormalities include meningitis (56 percent), meningoencephalitis (34 percent), meningomyelitis (4.5 percent), or meningoencephalomyelitis (4.9 percent). In children and young adults, the course of CEE is usually milder than in adults, with a predominance of meningitis. With increasing age, especially in patients over 60 years, severe clinical courses with paralytic symptoms may develop. Approximately two-thirds of persons infected with CEE virus have an inapparent infection with viremia, or have only the first stage of the disease with nonspecific symptoms. The mortality is approximately 1 percent of patients who have neurologic manifestations. Neurologic sequelae are found in 7 percent of the patients.

Diagnosis is based upon the detection of CEE-IgM antibodies in the serum by enzyme-linked immunoassay. Serum IgM and IgG antibodies can be detected at the time of hospital admission. The CSF reveals a lymphocytic pleocytosis of up to 1600 cells per cubic millimeter, and the protein concentration is elevated to 50 to 200 mg/dl.

No specific treatment exists for arthropod-borne encephalitides. Therefore, supportive care is essential in the management of patients infected with arboviruses. A vaccine is available for some of these viruses, e.g., Japanese B encephalitis or CEE, for prevention of human infection. Active immunization is recommended for persons visiting or living in areas known to be endemic for CEE.

Rabies

Rabies is a worldwide disease which is still very common in developing countries (e.g., about 50,000 cases per annum in India) but has become rare in central Europe and the United States, where less than five cases occur per year.[121] But, even today, rabies is an invariably fatal illness in a nonimmunized patient. In contrast to most other virus species, rabies is spread to the CNS neurogenically (axoplasmatic flow in peripheral neurons).

Infection is usually caused by direct contact with saliva or other infectious material, most frequently as a result of a bite, notably from skunks, foxes, raccoons, bats, wolves, jackals, and small carnivores. Domestic dogs and cats account for 90 percent of cases worldwide. Rodents, squirrels, guinea pigs, gerbils, rabbits and hares can all be lethally infected with rabies virus; however, they are not considered significant reservoirs for transmission—in fact, virus transmission to man by bites from these species is considered extremely unlikely. Similarly, bites by herbivores other than bats (horses, cows, deer, etc.) represent no significant risk.[119,p.481] Intact skin provides protection from infection, while injured skin and intact mucosa may permit viral acquisition.

The incubation period varies between 20 and 90 days (range of 4 days to several years in single cases). Local pain, and paresthesia and itching, followed by fasciculations at the site of infection, often precede generalized symptoms, which might be explained by viral involvement of dorsal root ganglia after spread via the peripheral nerve. Flu-like symptoms including fever, increased irritability, or apathy are the first signs in most patients, before more specific symptoms occur.

Most cases show the furious form of rabies with the characteristic symptoms of intermittent hydrophobia and aerophobia. These consist of life-threatening spasms of the diaphragm, sterno-cleidomastoid muscles, and the accessory muscles of inspiration, which may lead to a general increase in extensor tone and spasms. Typically, these symptoms are initiated by attempts to drink water and are accompanied by panic and terror. Episodes of generalized arousal and excitation, with sometimes bizarre neuropsychiatric symptoms, hyperesthesia, and vegetative disturbance may alternate with symptom-free intervals with entirely normal neurostatus. Due to the general brain involvement in furious rabies, a wide range of abnormalities are seen. Meningism, cranial nerve involvement, and upper and lower motoneuron symptoms, as well as involuntary movements, seizures, or characteristic limbic disinhibition, can be found. Autonomic symptoms, such as hypersalivation, changes in heart rate and blood pressure, fever, or sweating, can contribute to dangerous electrolyte disturbances, sometimes complicated by SIADH, and respiratory and cardiac failure. Death invariably occurs within a week in the natural course of furious rabies and can be prolonged for up to several months by ICU treatment.

Paralytic rabies occurs less frequently, but is typical for infections acquired from bat bites in Latin America. After the nonspecific prodromata, the bitten limb becomes paralytic and painful and may develop paresthesia or fasciculations, reflecting the fact that the spine is the predominant site of infection (Table 11-2). Progression to para- or tetraparesis is followed by the involvement of respiratory muscles and cranial nerve palsy, which leads to death within several days or weeks (longer under critical care unit conditions).

If the animal from which the infection was acquired is available for examination, the diagnosis can be established by histologic examination of a CNS specimen using immunofluorescence. In man, confirmation of the diagnosis is obtained from skin (preferably from the nape of the neck) or brain biopsies using immunofluorescence. Viral culture in neuroblastoma cells, requiring only 2 to 4 days, yields positive results from saliva and throat swabs at the onset of clinical symptoms, a few days later from the CSF or brain biopsy, but not from blood. Neutralizing antibodies against rabies appear in the serum about 7 days after the onset of symptoms, and, several days later, also in the CSF, where intrathecal IgG synthesis can be found. Vaccination or passive immunization against rabies makes interpretation difficult, but high CSF/serum IgG levels suggest the presence of rabies infection.

The CSF pleocytosis is usually mild with normal glucose and slightly elevated protein levels of 50 to 200 mg/dL. There are no specific laboratory findings in rabies.

While animal control and pre-exposure prophylaxis for risk groups have helped to make rabies a rare disease in central Europe and the United States, postexposure measures before the onset of clinical symptoms are essential. Immediate, thorough wound cleaning and disinfection should be followed as soon as possible by active and passive immunization. If these measures have not been performed properly, or are delayed for more than 7 days, about 15 to 60 percent of people exposed to a rabid animal will develop the clinical picture of rabies. Critical care unit management may be the only hope of achieving survival in single cases. Convulsions, cerebral edema, respiratory and cardiac problems, gastrointestinal bleeding, ileus, and electrolyte disturbance are the most common life-threatening problems encountered in the course of rabies. To counter overexcitability and vegetative crises, heavy analgesia, sedation, and early intubation and tracheotomy are essential. Close monitoring of cardiac function is as important as careful fluid balance and electrolyte checks. Diabetes insipidus and SIADH are known complications of rabies and require therapy.

HUMAN IMUNODEFICIENCY VIRUS INFECTION AND ASSOCIATED OPPORTUNISTIC INFECTIONS

The nervous system is often severely affected in patients with the human immunodeficiency virus (HIV).[122,123] Patients suffer from internal complications, such as *Pneumocystis carinii* pneumonia or generalized cytomegalovirus infection, and

therefore need interdisciplinary intensive care. Thus, management in the ICU may be necessary.

Spectrum of Human Immunodeficiency Virus Neurologic Manifestations

Neurologic complications of AIDS usually occur in the advanced stages, although they can also develop at earlier stages. It is possible to differentiate between primary, i.e., directly HIV-induced, and secondary neurologic manifestations. At the time of HIV seroconversion, acute HIV meningoencephalitis develop in about 1 percent of all cases, leading to progressive loss of consciousness, and seizures, at times requiring management in a critical care unit. Chronic AIDS encephalopathy, also called AIDS dementia complex, is usually not accompanied by impaired consciousness.

Among the secondary neuromanifestations, toxoplasmosis is the most common cause of neurologic illness. However, other opportunistic pathogens, e.g., *Cryptococcus neoformans, Mycobacteria,* or *Listeria monocytogenes* may cause serious neurologic disease. Furthermore, CNS lymphoma may lead to emergency situations, such as seizures, progressive stroke hemiparesis, or elevated ICP. Among those patients with known HIV-1 infection admitted to critical care units in the United States, more than two-thirds have respiratory failure due to infections (*Pneumocystis carinii*, cytomegalovirus, *Toxoplasma, Mycobacterium avium-intracellulare, Cryptococcus, Aspergillus,* gram-negative organisms), tumors (Kaposi's sarcoma, lymphoma), lymphoid interstitial pneumonitis, sedative overdose, and asthma. Seizures occur in about 13 percent of seropositive ICU patients and may require management in a critical care unit. Typical CSF findings in the various CNS diseases associated with AIDS are shown in Table 11-4.

Management of patients in hospital is invasive and raises the risk of infection for nurses and doctors. Since it may not be known if a patient has AIDS, and testing is not universally mandatory, all health care personnel should practice universal precautions when handling blood and body fluids from all patients. In addition to these

Table 11-4

Cerebrospinal fluid findings in acquired immunodeficiency syndrome patients with central nervous system disease

Disease	No. of patients	CSF findings (mean)		
		Protein (mg/dL)	Glucose (mg/dL)	WBCs[a] (cells/mm³)
HIV encephalopathy	100	62	53	3
Secondary viral encephalitis	28	95	63	64
Progressive multifocal leukoencephalopathy	8	69	46	4
Toxoplasmosis	53	97	58	6
Cryptococcosis	68	82	43	49
Primary CNS lymphoma	25	81	57	9

[a] WBCs = white blood cells.

Source: From Fishman,[137] p. 284. Modified from Levy RM, Bredesen DE: Central nervous system dysfunction in acquired immunodeficiency syndrome, in Rosenblum ML et al (eds): *AIDS and the Nervous System.* New York, Raven Press, 1988.

precautions, the indication for any invasive procedure should be checked thoroughly. Wooden toothpicks, which can be discarded after use, are preferred to reusable pins in the neurologic examination of any patient.

If, despite all precautions, a member of the staff suffers a needle-stick injury from contaminated material, bleeding from the wound should be encouraged. The wound should then be cleansed and disinfected with 70 percent alcohol and prophylactic zidovudine therapy given as 5 and 250 mg daily for 2 weeks. HIV seroconversion may occur after needle-stick injury. In spite of these measures, the needle-stick injury carries a risk of seroconversion of about 0.5 percent.

Acute Human Immunodeficiency Virus Meningoencephalitis

Acute HIV meningoencephalitis is due to HIV itself, and occurs in about 1 percent all HIV patients before or during HIV seroconversion. Patients have nonspecific acute to subacute encephalitic signs and symptoms, such as headache, fever, progressive alteration in mental status, and seizures. The diagnosis is difficult and may be linked to HIV only retrospectively. The HIV antigen in blood and CSF is normally detectable, whereas HIV antibodies may develop days to

weeks later. Therefore, repeated HIV serology tests should be performed in suspected cases. Polymerase chain reaction may show the presence of the HIV genome in the CSF.[124] Inflammatory signs in the CSF and general changes in the EEG are nonspecific. Neither CT scans nor MRIs show any abnormalities. Management in a critical care unit may be necessary. Intravenous acyclovir is given in case of herpes simplex encephalitis. Whether zidovudine is effective is not known.

The prognosis is good, with complete remission within days to weeks.

Central Nervous System Toxoplasmosis

Central nervous system toxoplasmosis is the usual reason for severe illness in HIV patients and may require management in a critical care unit. It occurs in 10 to 20 percent of AIDS patients and results from reactivation of dormant bradyzoites in persons who have previously had toxoplasmosis (20 to 90 percent in the general population).

The CNS toxoplasmosis develops subacutely within days to several weeks.[125] The clinical picture depends on the site of the intracranial granulomas. It can consist of a progressive organic brain syndrome (>70 percent), focal neurologic deficits (hemiparesis [>60 percent], aphasia, extrapyramidal signs, hemianopsia, or cerebellar hemiataxia), and/or generalized or focal seizures (>30 percent). Less than half of the patients have fever. Differential diagnosis includes CNS lymphoma and progressive multifocal leukoencephalopathy.

Neuroimaging is of great diagnostic value. Characteristic CT or MRI findings in patients with CNS toxoplasmosis are multiple hypodense brain lesions with ring enhancement and perifocal edema. Ninety percent of toxoplasmosis lesions may be seen on CT with contrast administration, but enhanced MRI can demonstrate lesions that are not reliably seen on CT, particularly those in the posterior fossa. It is not possible to distinguish toxoplasmosis from lymphoma. In some cases, both can be present simultaneously. Areas infected with toxoplasmosis show early normalization during treatment. Lymphoma should be suspected if there is no change or even growth of the lesion upon repeated imaging 1 week after the start of treatment.

Lumbar puncture and specific toxoplasmosis serology is usually not helpful. The CSF shows nonspecific inflammation (Table 11-4). Serologic tests will reveal low or moderately elevated specific IgG titers, due to earlier *Toxoplasma gondii* primary infection. The IgM titers are usually not elevated. However, in some cases, active infection is indicated by rise in IgM titer, a fourfold rise in IgG titer, or a stable IgG titer greater than 1024. Toxoplasmosis PCR testing may improve diagnostic accuracy in the future. In vivo diagnosis of toxoplasmic infection can be achieved by identification of the organism in tissue sections obtained at biopsy. Organisms may be seen with Wright-Giemsa or hematoxylin-eosin stains, or by immunoperoxidase staining techniques using antibodies specific to *Toxoplasma* antigens. However, *T. gondii* may be difficult to detect in vivo, and intraperitoneal injection of infected material into nude mice may be necessary.

Electroencephalography will show general slowing and often focal or paroxysmal changes.

If CNS toxoplasmosis is suspected, empiric anti-*Toxoplasma* therapy should be started immediately. Clinical remission will begin within a few days and normalization of CT and MRI scans can be expected within 4 weeks. Table 11-5 sets out an effective drug regimen which will lead to clinical improvement in 90 percent of all cases. Daily administration of folinic acid is necessary to avoid thrombocytopenia. Alternatively, clindamycin may be given intravenously, which may be preferable in acute treatment, if the patient is not able to swallow, or if the patient shows allergic or toxic adverse reactions to sulfonamides. Patients with significant cerebral edema respond well to

Table 11-5

Treatment recommendations in human immunodeficiency virus-associated opportunistic infections

Infection	Recommended treatment (doses per day)
CNS toxoplasmosis	1. 50–100 (–150) mg pyrimethamine 2. (2–) 4–6 (–8) sulfadiazine 3. 15 mg folinic acid
CNS cryptococcosis	1. 0.3–0.6 mg/kg amphotericin B (in 5% glucose, over 6–8 h) 2. 75–150 mg/kg flucytosine (four divided doses) 3. 400 mg fluconazole
Progressive multifocal leukoencephalopathy	No therapy available
CNS tuberculosis	1. 5 mg/kg isoniazid 2. 10 mg/kg rifampicin 3. 15–25 mg/kg ethambutol 4. 15–30 mg/kg pyrazinamide
CNS listeriosis	6–12 g ampicillin (three to four divided doses)

Source: From Enzensberger and Royal,[122] p. 505, with permission.

corticosteroid treatment (prednisone, 50 mg). Seizures respond to routine anticonvulsant therapy. About 80 percent of patients treated for CNS toxoplasmosis will relapse if the drug therapy is stopped. Therefore, treatment of this opportunistic infection is lifelong. If there is no clinical improvement within 2 weeks, stereotactic brain biopsy should be performed. Biopsy may yield an alternative histologic diagnosis of the lesions examined, e.g., lymphoma or other infections.

The degree of disturbance of consciousness upon admittance, and the initiation of therapy, is directly related to prognosis. About 80 percent of patients with successfully treated CNS toxoplasmosis will have neurologic defects. The average survival time after CNS toxoplasmosis is about 6 to 12 months.

Cryptococcal Meningitis

Cryptococcal meningitis is the most prevalent fungal infection in patients with AIDS. Bird feces are a common reservoir, and in patients with AIDS the cryptococcus is normally acquired by inhalation.[126] Up to 10 percent of the AIDS patients in France, Belgium, and the United States suffer from cryptococcosis.

Patients usually have insidious onset of fever, malaise, and headache. Only 30 percent have neck stiffness. Cranial CT or MRI scans are usually not helpful. The CSF shows only a minimal inflammatory response (Table 11-4). India ink staining will reveal the cryptococci, with their typical light halo, in 80 percent of patients. The organism may be cultured on special media and cryptococcal antigen titers in CSF and blood are positive in more than 90 percent of patients. Testing of CSF by PCR may be positive.[127]

Treatment is by amphotericin B with flucytosine (Table 11-5). It is important to monitor renal function because of the nephrotoxic side effects of amphotericin B. Flucytosine may induce lymphopenia and thrombopenia as side effects. Fluconazole is very well tolerated and can be given in combination (400 mg daily), especially in patients with significant adverse reactions to amphotericin B or flucytosine. Therapy should be monitored by lumbar punctures and cryptococcal antigen titers in CSF and blood, and isolation of the microorganisms in culture. After successful treatment for 4 to 8 weeks, permanent maintenance therapy with fluconazole, at a reduced dosage (200 mg daily), has to be given orally to avoid relapse.

The prognosis is closely related to the progression of the underlying disease and the level of consciousness at the beginning of treatment. If the patient is still alert at the start of therapy, remissions of more than 2 years are possible.

Progressive Multifocal Leukoencephalopathy

Progressive multifocal leukoencephalopathy (PML) is a subacute demyelinating disease of the CNS in patients who are immunosuppressed.[128] It is caused by a reactivation of the JC virus in 2 percent of patients with AIDS. About 70 percent of all persons in the general population have been exposed to the virus.

The onset of PML is insidious. There is progressive loss of mental faculties and focal development of neurologic deficits. The differential diagnosis includes all the focal secondary HIV neuromanifestations, CNS toxoplasmosis, CNS lymphoma, mycobacterial CNS infection, etc.

The disease is suspected if CT or MRI scans show single or multiple white matter lesions without contrast enhancement and without a major mass effect.

The EEG shows nonspecific focal or general changes. The CSF analysis shows nonspecific inflammatory signs (Table 11-4). Identification of the virus from the urine is sometimes possible by electron microscopy. The JC virus can now be detected in the CSF by PCR.[129]

There is still no successful treatment. The disease normally leads to death within months but spontaneous remission has also been seen in patients with less severe immunosuppression.

Other Infections

Central nervous system tuberculosis has been reported in as many as 1 to 2 percent of patients with AIDS. Listeriosis of the CNS is a rare complication. When encountered, treatment is described in Table 11-5.

Ethical Issues of Critical Care For HIV-1 Seropositive Patients

Physicians treating patients in ICUs are often faced with decisions of whether to withhold or terminate treatment of the severely ill. The patient's wishes should always guide the doctor's decisions (see Chap. 24 on "Ethics"); if the patient desires or refuses intensive diagnostic and therapeutic measures, a number of medical measures must be considered in each individual case. Asymptomatic HIV patients with HIV-independent diseases will usually be treated like HIV-negative patients. In case of severe AIDS, other factors, such as the duration of the disease, the patient's general state, the presence of a wasting syndrome, or other life-threatening non-CNS manifestations of AIDS, will influence the decisions. Whether resuscitation, mechanical ventilation, or surgery are still indicated or not depends on a variety of individual factors. The general prognosis of AIDS patients dependent on mechanical ventilation, according to treatment results published by several intensive care centers, is poor.[122]

OPPORTUNISTIC INFECTIONS FOLLOWING ORGAN TRANSPLANTATION

The mortality and morbidity in posttransplant patients are due to a variety of conditions that continue to complicate the posttransplant state and reduce survival for renal transplant patients to 45 percent at 10 years.[130] The incidence of these complications remains relatively high, even into the second decade (Table 11-6).

In assessing the posttransplant patient, the diagnosis may be established by the typical symptoms and signs of the primary disease, e.g., a typical skin lesion such as herpes zoster. However, in many instances, the history and physical findings will give no clue as to the nature of the condition,

Table 11-6

Complicating and clinical results in the second decade of renal transplantation

Complications/results	(N = 57)	
	Number	(%)
Infection	24	(42)
Malignancy	9	(16)
Vascular disease	9	(16)
Hypertension	24	(42)
Aseptic necrosis	6	(11)
Cataracts	19	(33)
Death rate	7	(12)
Graft loss	7	(12)

Data from The University of Minnesota.
Source: From Rao,[140] with permission.

including any central nervous system involvement. Thus, comprehensive investigations are almost always indicated, and admission to a hospital is required.

Central nervous system involvement is probably common and usually presents a difficult differential diagnosis (Table 11-7). If the organ transplant was recent, a medication effect, such as complication of cyclosporine treatment, or the phenomenon of rejection encephalopathy, should be considered. Then, infection should be thoroughly investigated. Blood, urine, and, if indicated, other specimens should be cultured for viruses, bacteria, and fungi. Serologic studies should also be performed for specific changes in antibody titer, including HIV. For example, the diagnosis of cytomegalovirus is established by a fourfold or greater seroconversion in cytomegalovirus antibody titers. It should be noted here that all types of infections—viral, bacterial, or fungal—if left unchecked, will ultimately produce systemic symptoms not due to direct invasion of organisms, which has been recognized as a septic syndrome. This may ultimately be complicated by multi-organ failure. The systemic response often includes both encephalopathy and a critical illness polyneuropathy.

Table 11-7
The differential diagnosis of nervous system complications following organ transplantation

Condition/organism	Time after transplant	Neurologic manifestations	Cerebrospinal fluid	CT head scan	Treatment
Cyclosporin complications	0–3 months	Tremor, ataxia, seizures confusion, coma, paraplegia	Normal, or mild increase in protein and lymphocytic reaction	Normal, or white matter edema	Stop cyclosporin, give parenteral magnesium
Septic encephalopathy	0–3 months	Diffuse encephalopathy, mild or severe	Normal, or mildly increased protein	Normal	Treat sepsis and multiple organ failure
Clinical illness polyneuropathy	0–3 months	Failed weaning from ventilator, axonal polyneuropathy	Normal, or mildly increased protein	Normal	Treat sepsis and multiple organ failure
Rejection encephalopathy	1–3 months	Headache, confusion and convulsions	Increased pressure	Normal or edema	Give steroids, manage hypertension and fluid balance
Cerebrovascular disease	Any time	Sudden onset of focal cerebral deficit	Normal, or signs of subarachnoid hemorrhage	Relatively specific for subdural hematoma infarction, or hemorrhage	Conservative
Viruses					
Cytomegalovirus	1–4 months	None	Normal	Normal	Prophylaxis only
Epstein-Barr	2–6 months	None, or rare B-cell lymphoma	Normal	Normal, or rare B-cell lymphoma	Prophylaxis only
Herpes simplex	Any time	Encephalitis—rare	Increased WBC, RBC, and protein: normal or decreased glucose	Areas of decreased density, occasional small hemorrhages in frontal and temporal lobes	Acyclovir

Varicella-zoster	Any time	Encephalitis—rare	Increased WBC and protein; normal glucose	?	Acyclovir
HIV	Any time	Encephalopathy, myelopathy, peripheral neuropathy	Variable	Variable, depending on type of infection or malignancy	None
JC	Any time	Progressive multifocal leukoencephalopathy	Normal	Areas of decreased density with no enhancement	None
Bacteria					
Listeria monocytogenes	1–3 months (?)	Acute meningitis	Increased WBC (mainly neutrophils) and protein decreased glucose	Normal, or generalized edema	Penicillin and tobramycin
Mycobacteria	Any time	Subacute and chronic meningitis or focal signs	Increased WBC (mainly lymphocytes) and protein: decreased glucose	Normal, or hydrocephalus	Isoniazid, rifampin
Fungi					
Cryptococci	1–8 months	Mild, chronic Meningitis	Increased WBC and protein: decreased glucose	Normal, or hydrocephalus	Amphotericin B
Coccidioides	1–8 months	Chronic meningitis	Increased WBC and protein; decreased glucose	Normal, or hydrocephalus	Amphotericin B

Abbreviations: WBC = white blood cells; RBC = red blood cells.
Source: Adapted from Bolton and Young,[141] with permission.

In investigating the CNS, the EEG is often of great value. It may rule in or out an organic disease, the EEG being normal in mental depression and nonorganic psychoses. The CT head scan is of even more value. It may reveal the relatively specific findings of subdural hematoma, infarction, or hemorrhage. The CT head scan may also aid in identifying lesions due to immunosuppression. *Toxoplasma gondii* and *Nocardia asteroides* may produce ring-enhancing lesions, although if immunosuppression has been great, such enhancement may be lost. Lymphomas tend to produce multiple, periventricular, solidly enhancing lesions. Progressive multifocal leukoencephalopathy produces nonenhancing hypodense areas near the ventricles.[144] However, such signs are not invariably specific, and brain biopsy is often necessary. At a minimum, the CT head scan will rule out a mass lesion, which would contraindicate the performance of a subsequent lumbar puncture. Lumbar puncture is also contraindicated in any bleeding tendency, i.e., low platelet levels, anticoagulant treatment, or aspergillosis. If a lumbar puncture is performed, adequate amounts of fluid should be taken for all the tests that are necessary. Removal of such amounts is of no concern since, even after the needle is withdrawn, fluid will continue to leak for some hours from the puncture site. Cerebrospinal fluid determinations of white blood cell count and differential and of glucose should be carried out immediately, since these elements deteriorate rapidly in the test tube. Fluid should be studied by a Gram stain for bacteria and by India ink stain for *C. neoformans*. The fluid should then be subject to comprehensive culture for bacteria, including aerobic and anaerobic organisms, and for fungi. If mycobacterial infection is a possibility, it will be necessary to do an acid-fast stain for mycobacteria and to send the fluid for culture for *M. tuberculosis*. Most opportunistic infections can now be detected by PCR (see "Introduction," Table 11-7). Finally, CSF should be sent for identification of malignant cells.

In many instances, a precise diagnosis of CNS infection is not possible and empiric therapy should be started. *Listeria monocytogenes* is the most likely cause of bacterial meningitis and should be treated with penicillin and tobramycin. If there is a strong suspicion of a specific fungal, parasitic, or tubercular infection, therapy may have to be started empirically.

In a disturbing number of instances, the diagnosis may still be in doubt. For example, all microbiologic studies may have initially been negative and no malignant cells found in the CSF. A CT head scan may show single or multiple lesions of a nonspecific nature. In this case, brain biopsy may be necessary. The neuropathologist and microbiologist should be notified in advance of this procedure and be prepared to study the tissue comprehensively.

Treatment will depend upon the underlying condition (Table 11-7).

ACUTE DISSEMINATED ENCEPHALOMYELITIS

Acute disseminated encephalomyelitis (ADEM)[131] is an autoimmune inflammation of the CNS, causing multifocal demyelination. It follows a variety of precipitating events, including infections with viruses or bacteria, immunization, or drugs. Viruses most likely to produce this rare illness are measles, rubella, and varicella-zoster. The brain is often involved, and, hence, there is usually altered consciousness, seizures, and other signs of cerebral dysfunction.

However, the pattern of abnormality in ADEM is quite variable, with varying combinations of diffuse encephalitis, brainstem or cerebral dysfunction, myelitis, and peripheral nerve or cranial nerve involvement. These various manifestations may come and go in the same patient over time.

The precipitating event, which occurs 1 to 3 weeks before the onset of neurologic symptoms, may consist of general malaise, fever, and evidence of involvement of either the gastrointestinal or upper respiratory tract. Members of the family or community may have exposed the patient to infection. Other precipitating events are immunization or medications such is sulfa drugs. In some instances, no antecedent event will be discovered.

Cerebral involvement is characterized by headache, fever, stiff neck, and vomiting, as well as dysfunction of any of the cranial nerves, hemiparesis, focal or generalized seizures, depressed level of consciousness, and even coma.

It may be particularly difficult to differentiate ADEM from acute viral encephalitis, Reye syndrome, metabolic and electrolyte disturbances, intracranial mass lesions, and various types of intracranial hemorrhages.

In investigation, a CT head scan should be performed on an emergency basis. If there is no risk of tentorial herniation, a lumbar puncture should then be carried out, and the results will usually give positive evidence of bacterial or fungal infection. Findings in the CSF are often similar in ADEM and acute viral infections, with increased white blood cells and a mildly increased protein level. The glucose concentration is not usually depressed in ADEM.

Acute multiple sclerosis (MS) involving the cerebrum may be a difficult differential. Patients with ADEM often have more widespread, multifocal CNS disturbances than those with MS. Optic neuritis is usually bilateral in ADEM and unilateral in MS. Transverse myelitis in ADEM is often complete in a few days, and is associated with aflexia. In MS, it is usually incomplete, develops over a longer period, and is associated with hyperreflexia.

Up to 10 percent of patients die during the acute phase of ADEM and 30 percent recover fully, the remainder have residual deficits.

Parainfectious, acute cerebral ataxia or acute transverse myelitis may occur independently or appear concomitantly with the manifestations of ADEM.

Acute hemorrhagic leukoencephalopathy (AHL) is a particularly rare form of ADEM. The precipitating circumstances are similar to ADEM, although the time between the precipitating event and AHL may be short as 4 days. Patients experience headache, general malaise, fever, depressed level of consciousness, vomiting, and neck stiffness. Hemiparesis is observed in 50 percent of cases. Acute hemorrhagic leukoencephalopathy should be suspected in patients with infection followed by rapidly evolving hemispheric dysfunction, fever, and leukocytosis. The differential diagnosis is broad and includes cerebral abscess, dural sinus thrombosis, etc. Patients usually become comatose within a few days and 70 percent die from tentorial herniation.

Neuroimaging is quite valuable in investigation.[132] Within 5 to 14 days, CT scans will reveal low-density lesions in the white matter, similar to those seen in MS, except they tend to be smaller. Occasionally, CT and MRI scans are normal. Contrast enhancement occurs in the lesions in 25 percent of patients. There may be midbrain edema. With clinical improvement, there is complete or partial resolution of the low-density lesions and disappearance of contrast enhancement. There is, however, no correlation between the abnormalities on CT and the clinical outcome. The MRI will show, on T2-weighted images, lesions similar to those in MS. As in MS, the contrast enhancement may disappear after treatment with steroids. In general, acute MRI abnormalities in ADEM are more extensive and symmetric than those in MS. The MRI abnormalities may persist for 2 years, in spite of complete clinical recovery. In transverse myelitis, the demyelinating lesions may be seen within 1 week.

The CSF shows increased cells and protein level, but the glucose and lactate concentrations are normal. Serologic tests for a variety of viruses and other organisms should be routinely ordered. Viral cultures of the CSF are usually positive. Polymerase chain reaction should be used whenever available since it may give the diagnosis early in the course.

The EEG shows multifocal delta waves, and is useful in monitoring the course of the disease. Visual and brainstem auditory evoked potentials and somatosensory evoked potentials may show delayed latencies.

In AHL, the EEG is more likely to show focal epileptiform activity. Brain biopsy may be necessary to establish the diagnosis. The characteristic findings include vessel necrosis with fiber impregnation and ring ball hemorrhages. Perivascular and inflammation edema and demyelination are also seen. White matter U fibers and gray matter are not significantly involved.

The value of steroids is still being debated. However, if there is evidence of edema, it is recommended that steroids be given, if the edema is severe and generalized. Intravenous dexamethosone should be prescribed initially at 100 mg. Otherwise, methylprednisolone should be given for the first 5 days, followed by oral dosages thereafter, and then discontinuing the daily medication and continuing with alternate-day therapy thereafter. Antacids and an H_2 blocker should be prescribed.

WHIPPLE DISEASE

This rare disease, caused by the bacterium *Topheryma whippeli*, will occasionally affect the nervous system and may alter consciousness. It is often experienced by middle-aged men, causing systemic evidence of weight loss, fever, anemia, steatorrhea, abdominal pain and distention, arthralgias, lymphadenopathy, and hyperpigmentation.[133] Nervous system manifestations are much rarer than systemic ones and, when present, may show varying combinations of excessive sleepiness, mental confusion, supranuclear ophthalmoplegia, ataxia, seizures, myoclonus, and unusual movement of the eyes and jaw, termed oculomasticatory myorrhythmia.[134] The diagnosis may be made by a biopsy of the jejunal mucosa, where macrophages filled with periodic acid–Schiff (PAS)-positive histiocytes are found. The PAS-positive histiocytes have also been identified in the CSF and at autopsy in the periventricular regions, in the hypothalamic nuclei, or scattered diffusely in the brain. Electron microscopy of suspected tissue, such as blood, pleural effusion, etc., demonstrates distinctive bacilliform bodies (Whipple's bacilli), whose presence can now be confirmed by PCR.[135] Scanning of the brain by MRI may reveal multiple lesions in the white or gray matter or at the gray-white matter junctions, especially after gadolinium enhancement.[136]

Treatment with tetracycline or penicillin may be effective, but there is a tendency for the disorder to recur after treatment has stopped.

REFERENCES

1. Scheld WM, Whitley RJ, Durack DT: Approach to the patient with central nervous system infection, in *Infections of the Central Nervous System*. New York, Raven Press, 1991, chap 1.
2. Tyler KL, Martin JB: *Infectious Diseases of the Central Nervous System*. Philadelphia, FA Davis, 1993.
3. Hacke W (ed): *NeuroCritical Care*. Berlin, Springer-Verlag, 1994.
4. Zimmerman SJ, Moses E, Sofat N, et al: Evaluation of a visual rapid membrane enzyme immunoassay for the detection of herpes simplex virus antigen. *J Clin Microbiol* 29:842–845, 1991.
5. Westmoreland BF: The EEG in cerebral inflammatory processes, in Niedermeyer E, Lopes da Silva F (eds): *Electroencephalography: Basic Principles, Clinical Applications and Related Fields*. Baltimore, Urban & Schwarzenberg, 1987, pp 259–273.
6. Romer FK: Difficulties in the diagnosis of bacterial meningitis: evaluation of antibiotic pretreatment and causes of admission to hospital. *Lancet* 2(8033):345–347, 1977.
7. Pfister H-W, Dirnagl U, Haberl R, Anneser F, Kodel U, Mehraein P, Feiden W, Einhaupl KM: Changes of intracranial pressure in a rat meningitis model, in Hoff JT, Betz AL (eds): *Intracranial Pressure*, vol 7. Berlin, Springer-Verlag, 1989, pp 781–783.
8. American College of Chest Physicians/Society of Critical Care Medicine Consensus Conference: Definitions for sepsis and organ failure and guidelines for the use of innovative therapies in sepsis. *Crit Care Med* 20(6):864–874, 1992.
9. Glauser MP, Zanetti G, Baumgartner J-D, et al: Septic shock: pathogenesis. *Lancet* 338:732–736, 1991.
10. Cowloy HC, Heney D, Gearing AJH, Hemingway I, Webster NR: Increased circulating adhesion molecule concentrations in patients with the systemic inflammatory response syndrome: a prospective cohort study. *Crit Care Med* 22(4):651–657, 1994.
11. Palmer RMJ, Ferrige AG, Moncada S: Nitric oxide release accounts for the biological activity of endothelium-derived relaxing factor. *Nature* 327:524–526, 1987.
12. Dhainaut J-FA, Tenaillon A, Le Tulzo Y, Schlemmer B, et al: Platelet-activating factor receptor antagonist BN 52021 in the treatment of severe

sepsis: a randomized double-blind, placebo-controlled, multicenter clinical trial. *Crit Care Med* 22(11):1720–1728, 1994.

13. Yamashima T, Kashihara K, Ikeda K, Kubota T, Yamamoto S: Three phases of cerebral arteriopathy in meningitis: vasospasm and vasodilation followed by organic stenosis. *Neurosurgery* 16:546–553, 1985.

14. Paulson OB, Brodersen P, Hansen EL, Kristensen HS: Regional cerebral blood flow, cerebral metabolic rate of oxygen and cerebrospinal fluid acid-base variables in patients with acute meningitis and with acute encephalitis. *Acta Med Scand* 196:191–198, 1974.

15. Pfister H-W, Koedel U, Haberi RL, et al: Microvascular changes during the early phase of experimental bacterial meningitis. *J Cereb Blood Flow Metab* 10:914–922, 1990.

16. Tauber MG: Brain edema, intracranial pressure and cerebral blood flow in bacterial meningitis. *Pediatr Infect Dis J* 8:915–917, 1989.

17. Ashwal S, Stringer W, Tomasi L, Schneider S, Thompson J, Perkin R: Cerebral blood flow and carbon dioxide reactivity in children with bacterial meningitis. *J Pediatr* 117:523–530, 1990.

18. Ashwal S, Tomasi L, Schneider S, Perkin R, Thompson J: Bacterial meningitis in children: pathophysiology and treatment. *Neurology* 42:739–748, 1992.

19. Quagliariello VJ, Long WK, Scheld WM: Morphologic alterations of blood-brain barrier with experimental meningitis in the rat: temporal sequence and role of encapsulation. *J Clin Invest* 77:1084–1095, 1986.

20. Horwitz SJ, Boxerbaum B, O'Bell J: Cerebral herniation in bacterial meningitis in childhood. *Ann Neurol* 7:524–528, 1980.

21. Williams CPS, Swanson AG, Chapman JT: Brain swelling with acute purulent meningitis. *Pediatrics* 34:220–227, 1964.

22a. Tauber MG, Borschberg U, Sande MA: Influence of granulocytes on brain edema, intracranial pressure, and cerebrospinal fluid concentrations of lactate and protein in experimental meningitis. *J Infect Dis* 157:456–464, 1988.

22b. Tauber MG, Khayam-Bashi H, Sande MA: Effects of ampicillin and corticosteroids on brain water content, cerebrospinal fluid pressure, and cerebrospinal fluid lactate levels in experimental pneumococcal meningitis. *J Infect Dis* 151:528–534, 1985.

23. Tureen JH, Stella FB, Clyman RI, Maury F, Sande MA: Effect of indomethacin on brain water content, cerebrospinal fluid white blood cell response and prostaglandin E_2 levels in cerebrospinal fluid in experimental pneumococcal meningitis in rabbits. *Pediatr Infect Dis J* 6(suppl):1151–1153, 1987.

24. Stovring J, Snyder RD: Computed tomography in childhood bacterial meningitis. *J Pediatr* 96:820–823, 1980.

25. Cabral DA, Flodmark O, Farrell K. Speert DP: Prospective study of computed tomography in acute bacterial meningitis. *J Pediatr* 111:201–205, 1987.

26. Tureen J: Cerebral blood flow and metabolism in experimental meningitis. *Pediat Infect Dis J* 8(12):917–918, 1989.

27. Syrogiannopoulos GA, Nelson JD, McCracken JH Jr: Subdural collections of fluid in acute bacterial meningitis: a review of 136 cases. *Pediatr Infect Dis J* 5:343–352, 1986.

28. Academy of Pediatrics Committee on Infectious Diseases: Dexamethasone therapy for bacterial meningitis in infants and children. *Pediatrics* 86:130–133, 1990.

29. Lebel MH, Freij BJ, Syrogiannopoulos GA, et al: Dexamethasone therapy for bacterial meningitis. *N Engl J Med* 319:964–971, 1988.

30. Odio CM, Faingezicht I, Paris M, et al: The beneficial effects of early dexamethasone administration in infants and children with bacterial meningitis. *N Engl J Med* 324:1525–1531, 1991.

31. Lebel MH, Hoyt J, Wagner DC: Magnetic resonance imaging and dexamethasone therapy for bacterial meningitis. *Am J Dis Child* 143:301–306, 1989.

32. Kline MW, Kaplan SL: Computed tomography in bacterial meningitis of childhood. *Pediatr Infect Dis J* 7:855–857, 1988.

33. Dodge PR, Swartz MN: Bacterial meningitis: a review of selected aspects. II. Special neurologic problems, post meningitis complications and clinicopathological correlations. *N Engl J Med* 272:954–960, 1954.

34. Goiten KJ, Tamir I: Cerebral perfusion pressure in central nervous system infections of infancy and childhood. *J Pediatr* 103:40–43, 1983.

35. Gaussorgues P, Guerin C, Boyer F, et al: Intracranial hypertension in comatose bacterial meningitis. *Presse Med* 16:1420–1423, 1987.

36. Rebaud P, Berthier JC, Hartemann E, Floret D: Intracranial pressure in childhood central nervous

system infections. *Intensive Care Med* 14:522–525, 1988.

37. Dodge PR, Swartz MN: Bacterial meningitis: a review of selected aspects. *New Engl J Med* 272:1003–1010, 1965.

38. Minns RA, Engleman HM, Stirling H: Cerebrospinal fluid pressure in pyogenic meningitis. *Arch Dis Child* 64:814–820, 1989.

39. McMenamin JB, Volpe JJ: Bacterial meningitis in infancy: effects on intracranial pressure and cerebral blood flow velocity. *Neurology* 34:500-504, 1984.

40. Lou HC: The "lost autoregulation hypothesis" and brain lesions in the newborn—an update. *Brain Dev* 10:143–146, 1988.

41. Tureen JH, Dworkin RJ, Kennedy SL, Sachdeva M, Sande MA: Loss of cerebrovascular autoregulation in experimental meningitis in rabbits. *J Clin Invest* 85:577–581, 1990.

42. Jordan KJ: Continuous EEG and evoked potential monitoring in the neuroscience intensive care unit. *J Clin Neurophysiol* 10:445, 1993.

43. Young GB, Jordan KG, Doig GS: An assessment of nonconvulsive seizures in the intensive care unit using continuous EEG monitoring: an investigation of variables associated with mortality. *Neurology* 47:83–89, 1996.

44. Altafullah I, Asaikar S, Torres F: Status epilepticus: clinical experience with two special devices for continuous cerebral monitoring. *Acta Neurol Scand* 84:374, 1991.

45. Archer BD: Computed tomography before lumbar puncture in acute meningitis: a review of the risks and benefits. *Can Med Assoc J* 148(6):961–965, 1993.

46. Friedland IR, Paris MM, Rinderknecht S, McCracken GH: Cranial computed tomographic scans have little impact on management of bacterial meningitis. *AJDC* 146:1484–1487, 1992.

47. Durand ML, Calderwood SB, Weber DJ, Miller SI, Southwick FS, Caviness VS, Swartz MN: Acute bacterial meningitis in adults. A review of 493 episodes. *N Engl J Med* 328:21–28, 1993.

48. Meyding-Lamade U, Hanley DF, Skolkenberg B: Herpesvirus encephalitis, in Hacke W (ed): *Neuro-Critical Care.* Springer-Verlag, Berlin, 1994, pp 455–467.

49. Overturf GD: Pyogenic bacterial infections of the CNS. *Neurol Clin* 4(1):69–90, 1986.

50. Ramirez-Ronda CH, Johnson MT, Thorley JD, Goodman EL, Blankenship R, Gould K, Sanford JP: Clinical presentation, diagnosis, outcome and management criteria for partially treated meningitis in adults. *15th ICAAC* Abstract 119, 1975.

51. McGee ZA, Baringer JR: Acute meningitis, in Mandell GL, Douglas RG, Bennett JE (eds): *Principles and Practice of Infectious Diseases,* 3rd ed. New York, Churchill Livingston, 1990, pp 741–755.

52. Del Rio MD, Chrane D, Shelton S, McCracken GM, Nelson JD: Ceftriaxone versus ampicillin and chloramphenicol treatment of bacterial meningitis in children. *Lancet* 1241–1244, 1983.

53. Bortolussi R, Wort AJ, Casey S: The latex agglutination test versus counter immuno-electrophoresis for rapid diagnosis of bacterial meningitis. *Can Med Assoc J* 127:489–493, 1982.

54. Kaplan SL: Antigen detection in cerebrospinal fluid—pros and cons. *Am J Med* 75(suppl 2B):109–118, 1983.

55. Bhisitkul DM, Hogan AE, Tanz RR: The role of bacterial antigen detection tests in the diagnosis of bacterial meningitis. *Pediatr Emerg Care* 10:67–71, 1994.

56. Ni H, Knight AI, Cartwright K, Palmer WH, McFadden J: Polymerase chain reaction for diagnosis of meningococcal meningitis. *Lancet* 340:1432–34, 1992.

57. Tunkel AR, Scheld WM: Acute bacterial meningitis. *Lancet* 346:1675–1680, 1995.

58. Levine S, Harris AA, Sokalski SJ: Bacterial meningitis, in Vinken PJ, Bruyn GW, Klawans HL (eds): *Handbook of Clinical Neurology,* vol 33. Amsterdam, North Holland, 1978, pp 1–19.

59. Karandanis D, Shulman JA: Recent survey of infectious meningitis in adults: review of laboratory findings in bacterial, tuberculous, and aseptic meningitis. *South Med J* 69:449–57, 1976.

60. Skoldenberg B: Herpes simplex encephalitis. *Scand J Infect Dis* 78(suppl):40–46, 1991.

61. Whitley RJ, Lakeman F: Herpes simplex virus infections of the central nervous system: therapeutic and diagnostic considerations. *Clin Infect Dis* 20:441–420, 1995.

62. Aszkenasy OM, George RC, Begg NT: Pneumococcal bacteraemia and meningitis in England and Wales. *Commun Dis Rep* 5:R45–49, 1995.

63. Tunkel AR, Wispelwey B, Scheld WM: Bacterial meningitis: recent advances in pathophysiology and treatment. *Ann Intern Med* 112:610–623, 1990.

64. McCracken G, Lebel M: Dexamethasone therapy for bacterial meningitis in infants and children (editorial). *Am J Dis Child* 143:287–289, 1989.

65. Pomeroy S, Holmes S, Dodge P, et al: Seizures and other neurologic sequelae of bacterial meningitis in children. *N Engl J Med* 323(24):1651–1657, 1990.

66. Dagbjartsson A, Ludvigsson P: Bacterial meningitis: diagnosis and initial antibiotic therapy, in *Intensive Care*. Pediatric Clinics of North America, vol 34. Philadelphia, WB Saunders, 1987, 219–230.

67. Klein J, Feigin R, McCracken G: Report of the task force on diagnosis and management of meningitis. *Pediatrics* 78(5):969–980, 1986.

68. Baker R, Seguin J, Leslie N, et al: Fever and petechiae in children. *Pediatrics* 84(6):1051–1055, 1989.

69. Moffet H: Rash syndromes, in *Pediatric Infectious Diseases—A Problem-Oriented Approach*, 3rd ed. Philadelphia, JB Lippincott 1989, pp 307–341.

70. Benson CA, Harris AA, Levin S: Acute bacterial meningitis: general aspects, in Vinken PJ, Bruyn GW, Klawans HL (eds): *Handbook of Clinical Neurology*, vol 52. Amsterdam, North Holland Publishing, 1988, pp 1–19.

71. McGravey A: A dilated unreactive pupil in acute bacterial meningitis: ocular nerve inflammation versus herniation. *Pediatr Emerg Care* 5(3):187–188, 1989.

72. Kline M: Review of recurrent bacterial meningitis. *Pediatr Infect Dis* 8(9):630–634, 1989.

73. Schlech WF, Ward JI, Band JD, et al: Bacterial meningitis in the United States, 1978 through 1981. The National Bacterial Meningitis Surveillance Study. *JAMA* 253:1949–1954, 1985.

74. Bonadio W, Bonadio J: Significance of polymorphonuclear leukocytes in CSF of bacteremic children. *Pediatr Emerg Care* 4(3):180–182, 1988.

75. Moffet H: Neurologic syndromes, in *Pediatric Infectious Diseases—A Problem-Oriented Approach*, 3rd ed. Philadelphia, JB Lippincott, 1989, pp 197–264.

76. Pfister H-W, Roos KL: Bacterial meningitis, in Hacke W (ed): *NeuroCritical Care*. Berlin, Springer-Verlag, 1994, p 387.

77. Kennedy PG, Adams JH, Graham DI, Clements GB. A clinico-pathological study of herpes simplex encephalitis. *Neuropathol Appl Neurobiol* 14:395, 1988.

78. Keller TL, Halperin JJ, Whitman M: PCR detection of *Borrelia burgdorferi* DNA in cerebrospinal fluid of Lyme neuroborreliosis patients. *Neurology* 42:32–42, 1992.

79. Kaplan S: Current management of common bacterial meningitides. *Pediatr Rev* 7(3):77–87, 1985.

80. Goldman AP, Kerr SJ, Butt W, et al: Extracorporeal support for intractable cardiorespiratory failure due to meningococcal disease. *Lancet* 349:466, 1997.

81. Madagame ET, Havens PL, Bresnahan JM, Babel KL, Splaingard ML: Survival and functional outcome of children requiring mechanical ventilation during therapy for acute bacterial meningitis. *Crit Care Med* 23:1279–1283, 1995.

82. Contant Jr CF, Robertson CS, Crouch J, et al: Intracranial pressure waveform indices in transient and refractory intracranial hypertension. *J Neurosci Methods* 57:15–25, 1995.

83. Rosner MJ, Coley IC: Cerebral perfusion pressure: a hemodynamic mechanism of mannitol and the postmannitol hemogram. *Neurosurgery* 21:147–156, 1987.

84. Snedeker JD, Kaplan SL, Dodge PR, Holmes SJ, Feigin RD: Subdural effusion and its relationship with neurologic sequelae of bacterial meningitis in infancy: a prospective study. *Pediatrics* 86:163–170, 1990.

85. Santambrogio S, Marinotti R, Sardella F, Parra F, Randazzo A: Is there a real treatment for stroke? Clinical and statistical comparison of different treatments in 300 patients. *Stroke* 9:130–132, 1978.

86. Spetzler RF, Nehlf DG: Cerebral protection against ischemia, in Wood JH (ed): *Cerebral Blood Flow: Physiologic and Clinical Aspects*. New York, McGraw-Hill, 1987, pp 658–659.

87. Haring HP, Berek K, Kampfl A, Pfausler B, Schmutzhard E: Is heparin really indicated in bacterial meningitis? *Arch Neurol* 51:13, 1994.

88. Pfister H-W, Borasio GD, Dirnagl U, Bauer M, Einhaupl KM: Cerebrovascular complications of bacterial meningitis in adults. *Neurology* 42:1497–1504, 1992.

89. Schmutzhard E, Willett J, Langmayr J, Rumpl E, Prugger M, Gerstenbrand F: Hypophysenabszess und cerebrale Arteritis bei todlich verlaufender Pneumokokken-meningitis. *Nervenarzt* 58:176–179, 1987.

90. Haring HP, Rotzer KH, Reindl H, et al: Time course of cerebral blood flow velocity in central nervous system infections: a transcranial Doppler sonography study. *Arch Neurol* 50:98–101, 1993.

91. Des Prez RM, Heim CR: Mycobacterium tuberculosis, in Mandell GL, Douglas RG, Bennett JE

(eds): *Principles and Practice of Infectious Diseases*, 3rd ed. New York, Churchill Livingstone, 1990, pp 1877–1906.

92. Parsons M: *Turberculous Meningitis, Tuberculomas and Spinal Tuberculosis. A Handbook for Clinicians*, 2nd ed. Oxford, Oxford University Press, 1988.

93. Wood M, Anderson M: Neurological infections, in *Major Problems in Neurology*, vol. 16. Philadelphia, WB Saunders, 1988.

94. Selwyn PA, Hartel D, Lewis VA, Schoenbaum EE, Vermund SH, Klein RS, Walter AT, Friedland GH. A prospective study of the risk of tuberculosis among intravenous drug abusers with immunodeficiency virus infection. *N Engl J Med* 320:545–550, 1989.

95. Edlin BR, Tokars JI, Grieco MH, Crawford JT, Williams J, Sordillo EM, Ong KR, Kilburn JO, Dooley SW, Castro KG, Jarvis WR, Holmberg SD: An outbreak of multidrug-resistance tuberculosis among hospitalized patients with the acquired immunodeficiency syndrome. *N Engl J Med* 326:1514–21, 1992.

96. Telzak EE, Sepkowitz K, Alpert P, Mannheimer S, Medard F, El-Sadr W, Blum S, Gagliardi A, Salomon N, Turett G: Multidrug-resistant tuberculosis in patients without HIV infection. *N Engl J Med* 333:907–11, 1995.

97. Schmutzhard E, Roelcke U: Tuberculous meningitis and central nervous system tuberculosis, in Hacke W (ed): *NeuroCritical Care*. Berlin, Springer Verlag, 1994, pp 398–406.

98. Shankar P, Manjunath N, Mohan KK, Prasad K, Behari M, Ahiya GK: Rapid diagnosis of tuberculous meningitis by polymerase chain reaction. *Lancet* 1:5–7, 1991.

99. Lin JJ, Harn HJ: Application of the polymerase chain reaction to monitor *Mycobacterium tuberculosis* DNA in the CSF of patients with tuberculous meningitis after antibiotic treatment. *J Neurol, Neurosurg Psych* 59:175–177, 1995.

100. Kox LFF, Kuijer S, Kolk AHJ: Early diagnosis of tuberculous meningitis by polymerase chain reaction. *Neurology* 45:2228–2232, 1995.

101. Bullock MR, van Dellen JR: The role of cerebrospinal fluid shunting in tuberculous meningitis. *Surg Neurol* 18:274–277, 1982.

102. Offenbacher H, Fazekas F, Schmidt R, Kleinert R, Payer F, Kleinert G, Lechner H: MR in tuberculous meningoencephalitis: report of four cases and review of the neuroimaging literature. *J Neurol* 238:340–344, 1991.

103. Fallon RJ, Kennedy DH: Treatment and prognosis in tuberculous meningitis. *J Infection* 3(suppl):39–44, 1981.

104. Fitzsimons JM: Tuberculous meningitis: a follow-up study on 198 cases. *Tubercle* 44:87–102, 1963.

105. Villanueva PA: Brain abscess and empyema, in Hacke W (ed): *NeuroCritical Care*, Berlin, Springer-Verlag, 1994, Chap. 38.

106. Britt RH: Brain abscess, in Wilkins RH, Rengachary SS (eds): *Neurosurgery*. New York, McGraw-Hill, 1985, pp 1928–1956.

107. Shahzadi S, Lozano AM, Bernstein M, Guha A, Tasker RR: Stereotactic management of bacterial brain abscesses. *Can J Neurol Sci* 23:34–39, 1996.

108. Bannister G, Williams B, Smith S: Treatment of subdural empyema. *J Neurosurg* 55:82–88, 1981.

109. Koskiniemi M: CNS manifestations associated with *Mycoplasma pneumoniae infections*: summary of cases at the University of Helsinki and review. *Clin Infect Dis* 17(1):S52–7, 1993.

110. Hindmarsh T, Lindkvist M, Olding-Stenkvist E, Skoldenberg B: Accuracy of computed tomography in the diagnosis of herpes simplex encephalitis. *Acta Radiol* 209:192–196, 1986.

111. Sartor K: Viral infections, in Sartor K (ed): *MR Imaging of the Skull and Brain*. Springer-Verlag, Berlin, 1991, pp 645–648.

112. Upton A, Gumpert J: Electroencephalography in diagnosis of herpes-simplex encephalitis. *Lancet* 1:650–6542,l 1970.

113. Smith JB, Westmoreland BF, Reagan TJ, Sandok BA: A distinctive clinical EEG profile in herpes simplex encephalitis. *Mayo Clin Proc* 5:469–474, 1975.

114. Nahmias AJ, Witley RJ, Visintine AN, et al: Herpes simplex virus encephalitis: laboratory evaluations and their diagnostic significance. *J Infect Dis* 145:829–836, 1982.

115. Rowley A, Whitley RJ, Lakeman FD, Wolinsky SM: Rapid detection of herpes-simplex-virus DNA in cerebrospinal fluid of patients with herpes simplex encephalitis. *Lancet* 335:440–441, 1990.

116. Aurelius E, Johansson B, Skoldenberg B, et al: Rapid diagnosis of herpes simplex encephalitis by nested polymerase chain reaction assay of cerebrospinal fluid. *Lancet* 337:189–192, 1991.

117. Fox JD, Brink NS, Zuckerman MA, Neild P, Gazzard BG, Tedder RS, Miller RF: Detection of herpesvirus DNA by nested polymerase chain reaction in cerebrospinal fluid of human immuno-

deficiency virus-infected persons with neurologic disease: a prospective evaluation. *J Infect Dis* 172(4):1087–90, 1995.

118. Shoji H, Honda Y, Murai I, Sato Y, Oizumi K, Hondo R: Detection of varicella-zoster virus DNA by polymerase chain reaction in cerebrospinal fluid of patients with herpes zoster meningitis. *J Neurol* 239(2):69–70, 1992.

119. Tiecks F, Pfister HOW, Ray CG: Other viral infections, in Hacke W (ed): *NeuroCritical Care*, Berlin, Springer-Verlag 1994, Chap. 45.

120. Whitley RJ, Arthropod-borne encephalitides, in Scheld WM, Whitley RJ, Durack DT (eds): *Infections of the Central Nervous System*. New York, Raven Press, 1991, pp 87–111.

121. Whitley RJ, Middlebrooks M: Rabies, in Scheld WM, Whitley RJ, Durack DT (eds): *Infections of the Central Nervous System*. New York, Raven Press, 1991.

122. Enzensberger W and Royal III W: HIV infection and associated opportunistic infections, in Hacke W (ed): *NeuroCritical Care*. Berlin, Springer-Verlag, Chap. 47, 1994, pp 500–511.

123. Rosenblum ML, Levy RM, Bredesen DE (eds): *AIDS and the Nervous System*. New York, Raven Press, 1988.

124. Clifford DB, Buller RS, Mohammed S, et al: Use of polymerase chain reaction to demonstrate cytomegalovirus DNA in CSF of patients with human immunodeficiency virus infection. *Neurology* 43:75–79, 1993.

125. Luft BJ, Remington JS. Toxoplasmic encephalitis. *J Infect Dis* 157:1–6, 1987.

126. Zuger A, Louie E, Holzman RS, Simberkoff MS, Rahal JJ: Cryptococcal disease in patients with the acquired immunodeficiency syndrome. *Ann Intern Med* 104:234–240, 1986.

127. Schmidt S, Reiter-Owona I, Hotz M, et al: An unusual case of central nervous system cryptococcosis. *Clin Neurol Neurosurg* 97:23–27, 1995.

128. Berger JR, Kaszovitz B, Post JD, Dickinson G: Progressive multifocal leukoencephalitis associated with human immunodeficiency virus infection. *Ann Intern Med* 107:78–87, 1987.

129. Weber T, Turner RW, Frye S, et al: Progressive multifocal leukoencephalopathy diagnosed by amplification of JC virus-specific SNA from cerebrospinal fluid. *AIDS* 8:49–57, 1994.

130. Fassbinder W, Challah S, Brynger H: The long-term renal allograft recipient. *Transplant Proc* 19:3754–3757, 1987.

131. Storch-Hagenlocher B, Griffin DE: Acute disseminated encephalomyelitis (parainfectious and postvaccinal encephalitis), in Hacke W (ed): *NeuroCritical Care*. Berlin, Springer-Verlag 1994, pp 493–499.

132. Marks WA, Bodensteiner JB, Bobele GB, Hamza J, Wilson DA: Parainflammatory leukoencephalomyelitis: clinical and magnetic resonance imaging findings. *J Child Neurol* 3:205–213, 1988.

133. Adams RD, Victor M, Ropper AH: *Principles of Neurology*, 6th ed. New York, McGraw-Hill, 1997, p 1135.

134. Schwartz MA, Selhorst JB, Ochs AL, et al: Oculomasticatory myorhythmia: a unique movement disorder occurring in Whipple's disease. *Ann Neurol* 20:677, 1986.

135. Dobbins WO: The diagnosis of Whipple's disease (editorial comment). *N Eng J Med* 332:363, 1995.

136. Erdem E, Carlier R, Devalle A, et al: Gadolinium-enhanced MRI in cerebral Whipple's disease. *Neuroradiology* 35:581, 1993.

137. Fishman RA: *Cerebrospinal Fluid in Diseases of the Nervous System*, 2nd ed. Philadelphia, WB Saunders, 1992.

138. Nelson J: *Pocketbook of Pediatric Antimicrobial Therapy, 1991–1992*, 9th ed. Baltimore, Williams and Wilkins, 1991, pp 16–17, 66–80.

139. Pichichero ME: Occult bacteremia in children: what are the odds? *Emerg Med Rep* 12(1):1–10, 1991.

140. Rao KV: Renal transplantation: complications and results in the second decade. *Transplant Proc* 19:3758–3759, 1987.

141. Bolton CF, Young GB: *Neurological Complications of Renal Disease*. Boston, Butterworth, 1990, p 211.

142. Moffet H: Fever and shock syndromes, in *Pediatric Infectious Diseases—A Problem-Oriented Approach*, 3rd ed. Philadelphia, JB Lippincott, 1989, pp 265–306.

143. Caugant DA, Hoiby EA, Froholm LO, Brandtzaeg P: Polymerase chain reaction for case ascertainment of meningococcal meningitis: application to the cerebrospinal fluids collected in the course of the Norwegian meningococcal serogroup B protection trial. *Scan J Infect Dis* 28:149–153, 1996.

144. Williams AL: Infectious diseases, in Williams AL, Haughton VM (eds): *Cranial Computed Tomography. A Comprehensive Text*. St. Louis, CV Mosby, 1987, pp 269–270.

145. Talan D, Hoffman J, Yoshikawa T, et al: Role of empiric parental antibiotics prior to lumbar puncture in suspected bacterial meningitis: state of the art. *Rev Infect Dis* 10(2):365–376, 1988.

146. Whitley RJ, Cobbs CG, Alford CA Jr, et al: Diseases that mimic herpes simplex encephalitis: diagnosis, presentation and outcome. *JAMA* 262:234–239, 1989.

147. Bolton CF: Infection, in Bolton CF, Young GB (eds): *Baillières Clinical Neurology, Critical Care*, vol 5, no 3. London, WB Saunders, 1996, pp 600–616.

Chapter 12

OTHER INFLAMMATORY DISORDERS

G. Bryan Young

This chapter is concerned with inflammatory disorders that affect the brain, other than direct central nervous system (CNS) infections, post-infectious encephalitides, and hemorrhagic leuko-encephalitis, which are addressed in Chap. 8. The following will be discussed:

1. Encephalopathy secondary to systemic inflammation;

2. Toxic encephalopathy;

3. Vasculitis and collagen vascular syndromes:
   Systemic lupus erythematosus,
   Systemic necrotizing vasculitis,
   Angiitis of the CNS,
   Sjögren syndrome,
   Wegener's granulomatosis,
   Temporal (giant-cell) arteritis,
   Takayasu's arteritis,
   Scleroderma,
   Rheumatoid arthritis,
   Behçet disease;

4. Other inflammatory, noninfectious disorders:
   Multiple sclerosis,
   Sarcoidosis;

5. Bacterial endocarditis.

SEPSIS-ASSOCIATED ENCEPHALOPATHY

Definition

"Sepsis" refers to the systemic manifestations of infection. Systemic inflammatory response syndrome (SIRS) consists of the same systemic manifestations, but infection is not essential. All the systemic features of sepsis can occur without infection, e.g., with burns, pancreatitis, or trauma (see Fig. 12-1). An operational definition of SIRS, based on a consensus committee of the American College of Chest Physicians and the Society of Critical Care Medicine, requires two or more of the following criteria: (1) body temperature $>38°C$ or $<36°C$; (2) heart rate >90 beats per minute; (3) tachypnea (respiratory rate >20 breaths per minute or $Pa_{CO_2} < 32\,mmHg$); and (4) alterations in white blood count concentrations ($>12,000$ or <4000 cells per cubic millimeter).[1]

The encephalopathy associated with systemic inflammation is a diffuse disturbance in cerebral function. As a *diagnosis of exclusion*, there should be no clinical evidence of meningitis, macroscopic intracranial abscess, or empyema. Further, the encephalopathy should not be due to a process that is unrelated to the systemic inflammatory

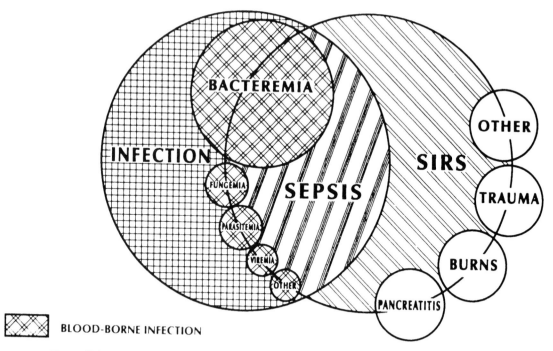

BLOOD-BORNE INFECTION

Figure 12-1
The interrelationships among SIRS, sepsis, and infection. (From American College of Chest Physicians/Society of Critical Care Medicine,[193] with permission.)

response itself, e.g., head trauma, fat embolism, or adverse reactions to medications or sedatives.

Incidence

At least a half-million patients develop sepsis yearly in the United States.[2] Of inpatients with positive blood cultures, the author of this chapter found that over 70 percent had some evidence of brain dysfunction.[3] Forty-six percent of these were in the intensive care unit (ICU), with the rest on the wards.

Diagnosis of Septic Encephalopathy

Septic encephalopathy is a diagnosis of exclusion. Table 12-1 lists various conditions that cause fever and altered mental status. While these are known to all physicians, a broad differential diagnosis is advisable upon the initial assessment. Many of the conditions are life-threatening,

treatable conditions that are easily ruled in or out, providing that they are considered in the first place.

Clinical Features

The principal neurologic findings relate to an altered mental state.[3] Mildly encephalopathic patients demonstrate a fluctuating confusional state and inappropriate behavior. Inattention and writing errors (including spelling, writing full sentences, orientation of writing on the page) are common. More severely affected patients show delirium, an agitated confusional state, or coma.

The most common motor sign is paratonic rigidity or *gegenhalten*, a resistance to passive movement of limbs that is velocity-dependent: the resistance that is felt with movements at normal rate disappears when the limb is moved slowly.[3] Asterixis, multifocal myoclonus, seizures, and

Table 12-1

Causes of fever in encephalopathic patients

Infections	*Immunologic reactions*
Central nervous system	Drug fever
Bacterial: meningitis, cerebritis, brain abscess,	Acetylsalicylic acid poisoning
subdural/epidural empyema	Connective tissue disease
Viral: encephalitis	Postinfectious syndromes
Other: spirochetal, rickettsial, protozoal,	Heat stroke
helminthic, etc.	
	Metabolic conditions
Intracranial thrombophlebitis	Acute adrenal insufficiency
Bacterial endocarditis (meningitis, mycotic aneurysm,	Thyroid storm (porphyria)
abscesses)	Porphyria
Systemic inflammation	*Reye syndrome in children*
Infection of organs	Toxic encephalopathy (adults)
Inflammation, with or without infection (e.g., burns,	
pancreatitis)	*Neoplasms*
	Systemic malignancy with organ failure
Vascular accidents	Brain tumors affecting thermoregulation
CNS: vertebrobasilar stroke, intracranial hemorrhage	
	Hematologic causes
Trauma	Hemolysis (e.g., sickle cell anemia)
Cerebral injury	Leukemia
Fat embolism, other	
	Increased muscular activity
	Seizures
	Malignant neuroleptic syndrome

tremor are relatively infrequent. The cranial nerve functions are spared.

Clinical or laboratory evidence of peripheral nerve dysfunction, termed critical illness polyneuropathy, is also found in 70 percent of encephalopathic patients at the author's hospital.[3] The neuropathy is axonal in type and takes many months to resolve. It is later in onset than the encephalopathy and is much slower to recover than the brain dysfunction.[4] Clinically, one finds decreased movement and the loss of deep tendon reflexes. Motor function is usually more affected than sensation, so that the patient may grimace without other movement when a nailbed is squeezed. In severe cases, the polyneuropathy may affect the phrenic nerves, creating problems in weaning the patient from the ventilator.[5]

Laboratory Features

The electroencephalogram (EEG) serves as the most sensitive test for sepsis-associated encephalopathy.[6] It may show mild, diffuse, reversible slowing in bacteremia, even if the neurologic examination is normal. The severity of the EEG abnormality parallels the mental status impairment. As the encephalopathy worsens, mild slowing in the theta (>4 to <8 Hz) range is followed by diffuse delta (<4 Hz) waves, then generalized triphasic waves, and, finally, by suppression or a generalized burst-suppression (alternating diffuse reductions in voltage with bursts of higher voltage waves) pattern (Figs. 12-2 and 12-3). Mortality is directly related to the severity of the EEG abnormality (Fig. 12-4)

Computed tomography (CT) brain scans are normal.[7] Cerebrospinal fluid (CSF) analysis shows

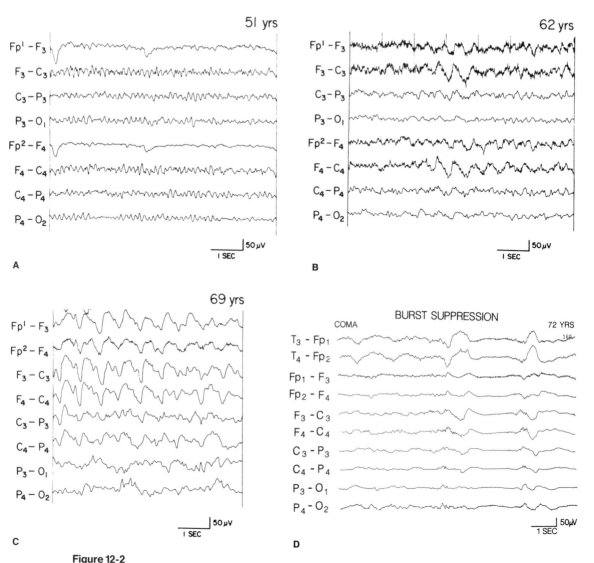

Figure 12-2

Parts A to D illustrate progressively more abnormal EEGs in patients with encephalopathy associated with bacteremia. A. Generalized slowing in the theta (5 to 7 Hz) range; B. excessive generalized delta (<4 Hz) activity; C. triphasic waves; and D. burst-suppression pattern.

only a mild elevation of protein concentration in some, but not all, of the patients and normal cell counts and glucose concentrations, even in patients with brain microabscesses at autopsy.[2,6]

This author and coworkers have not found a significant correlation of severity of encephalopathy with any specific bacteria, but there is a trend

for patients in whom multiple bacteria was recovered from blood cultures and in whom *Candida albicans* is present to have more severe brain dysfunction and a higher mortality rate.[2]

The following biochemical tests show a proportional change with the severity of the encephalopathy: serum urea, creatinine, bilirubin, and

Figure 12-3

The bar histogram shows the correlation of EEG abnormalities with the encephalopathic grade. "Nonencephalopathic" (NE) patients successfully passed a bedside battery of tests of mental funciton. "Mildly encephalopathic" (ME) patients were able to complete the battery of tests but qualified as encephalopathic. "Severely encephalopathic" (SE) patients could not even attempt the battery of tests because of delirium, stupor, or coma. (From Young et al,[3] with permission.)

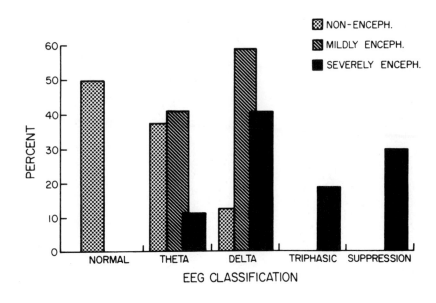

Figure 12-4

The mortality of each EEG abnormality is related to the encephalopathic grade: 0 percent with normal (N), 19 percent with theta, 36 percent with delta, 50 percent with triphasic waves (TWS), and 67 percent with suppression or burst-suppression (Supp). (From Young et al,[6] with permission.)

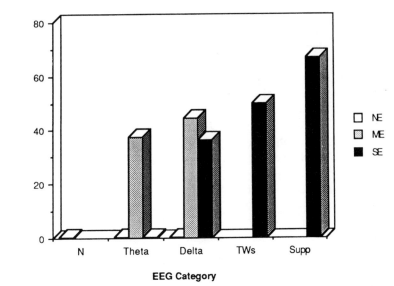

alkaline phosphatase. The degree of renal impairment is, however, rarely sufficient to account for the brain dysfunction.[2] Hepatic failure, on the other hand, is difficult to assess clinically or to quantify biochemically. As in hepatic failure, encephalopathic patients with sepsis have greater elevation of aromatic amino acids and lower concentrations of branched chain amino acids in plasma than do nonencephalopathic patients.[8] With sepsis, this may reflect altered metabolism of amino acids in both muscle and liver.

Pathology and Pathogenesis

The pathogenesis of altered brain dysfunction in the presence of systemic inflammation is not known

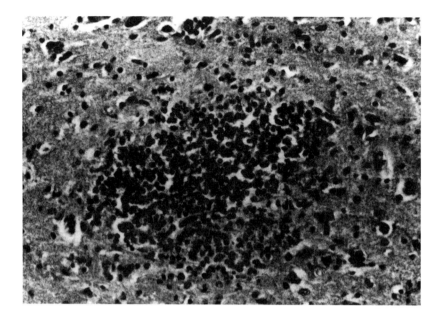

Figure 12-5
A microabscess in the cerebral cortex of a patient dying following a severely encephalopathic illness. (From Jackson et al,[7] with permission.)

with certainty. In advanced cases, it is likely multifactorial, given the variety of pathologic findings. The early fully reversible cases are not associated with structural change and are probably "metabolic" in nature, but of an unknown type. Other mechanisms, in addition to the metabolic disturbances, operate in more advanced cases.

In fatal cases, watershed brain infarctions from sustained hypotension are encountered rarely; however, the brain may show microscopic abnormalities. Eight of 12 of the author's patients with postmortem examinations had disseminated microabscesses (Fig. 12-5). The cerebral cortex is the most common involved site, but deep structures and even the spinal cord may be affected.[6] Some patients who had a protracted septic illness have astrocytic proliferation in the cortex, but the Alzheimer type 2 astrocytes of chronic hepatic encephalopathy are rarely, if ever, encountered.

Other less common lesions include multiple microscopic infarctions, brain purpura, and central pontine myelinolysis.[6]

The main pathogenetic candidates will be reviewed. A number of proposed mechanisms are summarized in Fig. 12-6 and discussed below. They are not mutually exclusive; in specific cases, some may be more relevant than others.

1. Microvascular Disorder The blood-brain barrier, which rigidly maintains a homeostatic environment in the normal brain, becomes leaky in a dynamic, patchy manner within the first few hours of endotoxemia in animal models (Fig. 12-7).[9] In addition, the differential flux of chemicals across the blood-brain barrier is altered; e.g., in sepsis, aromatic amino acids are more readily transported than branched-chain amino acids from blood to brain.[10] Reduced cerebral blood flow and increased cerebrovascular resistance are found in human cases of septic encephalopathy.[11] Microthrombosis may also occur.[12] Most, if not all, of these phenomena likely relate to the production of cytokines (e.g., tumor necrosis factor and interleukins-1 and 2) and their effects on nitric oxide (NO) production.[13–15] Inhibition of NO production leads to impairment of the microcirculation of the brain and other organs by causing vasoconstriction.[16,17] Free radical production may also alter capillary permeability.[18]

2. Amino Acids and Neurotransmitter Imbalance Cases of sepsis in humans and animal models (see above) both show an increased ratio of aromatic to branched-chain amino acids.[19] This may lead to a disturbance

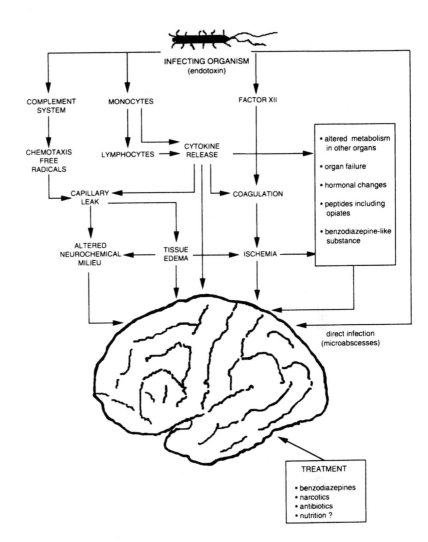

Figure 12-6
Composite figure illustrating different potential mechanisms for sepsis-associated encephalopathy. (From Bolton et al,[4] with permission.)

in neurotransmitter balance, with a reduction of concentrations of norepinephrine, dopamine, and serotonin, and an increase in the "false neuro-transmitter," octopamine.[16]

3. Brain Microabscesses Microabscesses (Fig. 12-5) probably arise from transvascular migration of micro-organisms and inflammatory cells. Chemokines, a recently discovered class of proinflammatory cytokines, could promote entry of inflammatory cells into the brain in sepsis and other inflammatory conditions.[20]

The role of microabscesses in the pathogenesis of septic encephalopathy is uncertain.[6] They are not detected in life, but their presence is inferred when retinal microabscesses are found (a rarity in the author's experience).[21] However, there is no reliable method of detecting them during life. Based on the surrounding histopathologic reaction in the brain, they are probably not all agonal. They are not universally present and are therefore not essential for sepsis associated encephalopathy. They may play a contributory role in some cases of prolonged, severe septic illness in patients in ICUs. Given the multifocal nature of the cortically originating seizures in advanced sepsis, it is possible that microabscesses contribute to this uncommon complication.[7]

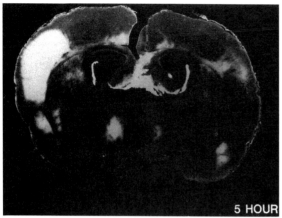

Figure 12-7
Patchy increases in blood-brain barrier (white staining of brain from horseradish peroxidase) 5 h after the injection of Escherichia coli *toxin in the rat. (From Du Moulin et al,[9] with permission.)*

4. Failure of Other Organs   Hepatic or renal failure may, in themselves, cause an encephalopathy. Since septic encephalopathy often precedes multiorgan failure, this secondary mechanism would not explain the *early* encephalopathy of sepsis. Multiorgan failure probably plays a contributory role in producing brain dysfunction in advanced sepsis, however.

5. Other Potential Mechanisms   A number of factors remain relatively unexplored, such as the role of gamma-aminobutyric acid (GABA), altered function or concentration of GABA receptors in the brain, increased systemic production of a benzodiazepine-like substance, and quinolinic acid.[22–25]

Iatrogenically induced encephalopathy always needs to be considered, as many drugs have delayed clearance in sepsis. Nutritional administration may cause variations in serum osmolality and reduced serum phosphate concentration.[26]

Management
First, one must establish the diagnosis by excluding other conditions. It is especially important to perform a lumbar puncture on obtunded patients with SIRS to rule out meningitis.

Seizures (uncommon) should be treated with standard antiepileptic medications such as phenytoin.

Patients with sepsis usually die due to the severity of the systemic illness or from failure of organs other than the brain.[2] Clinicians and nurses must be watchful for early encephalopathy, as it can be a presenting feature of sepsis. Prompt, specific treatment of the septic illness (appropriate antimicrobial therapy, drainage of abscesses, etc.) with prevention of multiorgan failure will save lives, as mortality is directly related to the severity of sepsis and the number of failed organs.[27]

The administration of a mixture of amino acids with high concentrations of branched-chain amino acids successfully reversed septic encephalopathy in five patients studied.[28] This short-term improvement is gratifying, but it is improbable that this will serve as definitive therapy, especially in advanced cases with multiorgan failure.

Potential future therapies may prevent or lessen the severity of sepsis by affecting cytokine or free radical production, the expression of cell adhesion molecules, or nitric oxide generation.[29]

TOXIC ENCEPHALOPATHY

Case report
A 71-year-old man was in his usual health when he developed a cough with grayish sputum for which he took an oral antibiotic without improvement. He remained active for nearly 3 weeks when nausea, vomiting, polyuria, and polydipsia abruptly ensued. He became confused, and then poorly responsive within 2 days.

On admission, he was afebrile; his blood pressure was 130/70 and heart rate was regular at 65 beats per minute. He appeared flushed and acutely ill. He opened his eyes to voice and said, "Leave me alone!" when his name was called. He would not obey commands and slept when not stimulated. There was mild neck stiffness to forward flexion. Cranial nerve reflexes were normal. Tone and deep tendon reflexes were normal.

His complete blood count (CBC), platelets, serum electrolytes, lactate, and urea were normal. Serum glucose was 12.2 mmol/L and serum osmolality was elevated at 317 mosmol/L. Capillary blood gases revealed the following: pH 7.46, P_{O_2} 80 mmHg, P_{CO_2} 34 mmHg, HCO_3 24 mmol/L. The urine showed 1 + glucose, protein, and ketones, and occasional white blood cells on microscopy. Specific gravity was 1.023. Screening for nitrites and drugs was negative. Liver function tests were normal. The CSF showed no cells, increased glucose at 10.7 mmol/L, and slightly increased protein concentration at 135 g/L. Initial CT of the head, chest film and electrocardiogram (ECG) were unremarkable.

Because of the patient's declining alertness and the need for airway management, endotracheal intubation with ventilatory support in the ICU was undertaken. Acyclovir and cefotaxime were administered.

The next day, he was deeply comatose, with no response to stimulation. Both plantar responses were extensor. Cranial nerve reflexes remained intact. The EEG showed a burst-suppression pattern with triphasic waves within bursts and no electrographic reactivity.

He developed systolic hypertension and his temperature rose to 39°C. Generalized tonic-clonic and multifocal clonic seizures ensued; these were confirmed on EEG. These were refractory to phenytoin, benzodiazepines, and phenobarbital; thiopental was required to stop the seizures. Inotropes were needed to raise the blood pressure.

By the next morning, he met the criteria for brain death; the CT scan showed marked cerebral edema. There was no brain perfusion on a radionuclide flow study.

Postmortem examination revealed a swollen, soft brain with bilateral uncal and tonsillar herniation. Meninges and blood vessels were normal. On microscopic examination, there were no microabscesses, inflammation, or microglial nodules. Scattered ischemic neurons were found in the hippocampus, basal ganglia,

cerebellum, and the gray matter of cervical, thoracic, and lumbar portions of the spinal cord.

In this patient, a respiratory infection was followed by a subacute confusional state progressing fairly quickly to stupor, then coma; multifocal seizures followed by fatal cerebral edema. In sepsis-associated encephalopathy, the brain dysfunction parallels the severity of the systemic illness. Here, the encephalopathy was out of proportion to systemic disease. There was no evidence of a primary CNS infection.

The author proposes that the above patient had "toxic encephalopathy," a term coined by Lyon and colleagues.[30] The term is restricted to a syndrome of a profound, diffuse encephalopathy with cerebral edema that is associated with, or following, systemic infection or inflammation. (Some have used the term to refer to encephalopathy from intoxication with exogenous chemicals or related to inborn errors of metabolism.)[31] The encephalopathy in the above patient probably had a microvascular component, but the mechanism remains uncertain. The cerebral edema is reminiscent of that described for Reye syndrome, a disorder, peculiar to childhood, that consists of severe cerebral edema, fatty change in the liver, and hypoglycemia.[32] Adult versions occur rarely.[33] Unlike patients with Reye syndrome, the above patient, and others known to the author, did not have hepatic disease clinically or pathologically.

Hemorrhagic shock and encephalopathy is another postinfectious illness in children that can be associated with severe brain edema.[34,35] A less malignant postinfectious syndrome in children was recently described.[36] The onset is acute—several days after an acute infection—with coma and abnormal (mainly extrapyramidal) movements. The EEG shows generalized slowing but rarely epileptiform activity; the CSF is normal. Neuroimaging is either normal or shows mild cerebral edema. The motor deficits clear quickly, but cognitive function returns more gradually; some patients are left with residual intellectual deficits.

VASCULITIS AND COLLAGEN VASCULAR SYNDROMES

These autoimmune diseases comprise a number of clinical disorders characterized by the production of an immune response (loss of immunologic tolerance) against tissues of the body. The immune response consists principally of autoantibodies, immune complexes, and cytotoxic (T-cell) lymphocytic activation. Immune complexes may be deposited in the walls of blood vessels or in tissues where they activate complement, and induce inflammation and lysosomal enzyme-mediated tissue or blood vessel damage. Antibodies against tissue antigens can directly alter tissue function. In cell-mediated responses, lymphocytes react with tissue antigens, releasing cytokines. Mononuclear cells attracted to the site release lysosomal enzymes or take part in granuloma formation.

Overall, autoimmune diseases affect women much more commonly than men. The peak incidence is in postpubertal and young adult life. There is a relationship of certain autoimmune disorders with HLA-D (human histocompatability leukocyte antigen) and MHC II (major histocompatibility complex) markers on chromosome 6. The role of sex hormones in the initiation of autoimmunity is unclear, but estrogen hydroxylation is increased in a number of autoimmune diseases and androgens are oxidized in greater amounts in systemic lupus erythematosus than in normal individuals.[37]

In the following discussion of specific disease entities, the neurologic complications associated with impairment of consciousness or cognitive functioning are emphasized. Peripheral nervous complications and systemic, nonneurologic manifestations are treated well in standard textbooks of internal medicine (such as *Harrison's Principles of Internal Medicine*) and reviews of rheumatic disorders.

SYSTEMIC LUPUS ERYTHEMATOSUS

Systemic lupus erythematosus (SLE) is a common autoimmune disease in which autoantibodies develop to a number of tissues.[38]

Central nervous system complications occur at some time in about 50 percent of patients and constitute one of the major causes of death.[39,40] Of 288 hospital admissions for SLE, 48 (17 percent) were for nervous system complications.[41] If one includes psychiatric complications, often organic in nature, the figure is somewhat higher. In another 22 (8 percent), nervous system complications contributed to the need for hospitalization. Occasionally, the nervous system is the first clinical target of SLE. Sometimes, the disease is confined to the CNS for years before other parts of the body are affected; the CNS may remain the most affected among various organs.[42]

Clinical Features

Central nervous system complications include: acute confusional state (including acute organic psychosis), stupor or coma, seizures, focal or multifocal dysfunction (including strokes), movement disorders (e.g., chorea or hemiballismus), aseptic meningitis, headaches, and myelopathy.[41,43–45] Cranial nerve lesions include papilledema, ocular movement abnormalities (e.g., third nerve or abducens palsy, unilateral internuclear ophthalmoplegia), nystagmus, tinnitus and vertigo, and trigeminal sensory loss. Peripheral neuropathy is variable; often, it is a predominantly distal polyneuropathy, but mononeuritis multiplex and isolated mononeuropathy and nerve root lesions are described.[46]

Alteration of consciousness or behavior, ranging from confusion to coma, occurred in 8 of 54 (15 percent) cases in the series of Bennahum and Messner[47] and in 35 of the 288 (12 percent) admissions for SLE in the series of Futrell et al.[41] Delirium occurred in 3 (7 percent) of the 43 SLE patients in the series of Miguel et al.[48] Abrupt impairment in alertness or cognitive functioning, including the acute confusional state and psychosis, and generalized seizures are usually unaccompanied by structural lesions. These complications are often fully reversible, while focal deficits, more commonly associated with strokes, are less likely to resolve completely.[49]

Major behavioral or psychiatric changes that have been reported include depression, confusion, decreased alertness, suicide attempts, confusion, hallucinations, paranoia, and schizophreniform psychosis, usually without other focal neurologic findings. Reactive depression is common.[47] Serious underlying systemic infections were present in 5 of 19 patients with normal alertness and 9 of 16 with decreased alertness, of whom 6 died.[47] Thus, screening for systemic infection is important with acutely altered behavior in SLE patients.

Stroke occurs in 14 to 15 percent of acutely hospitalized lupus patients.[41] Impairment of function depends on the sites of involvement, the temporal relationship of various lesions (maximal deficits are apparent if the strokes are closely clustered in time) and complications, such as seizures or mass effect from hemorrhage or edema. Sixty-four percent of patients have multiple infarcts, usually under 3 cm in diameter. Statistically significant associations with stroke include cardiac valvular abnormalities (Libman-Sachs endocarditis), antiphospholipid antibodies, spontaneous abortion, and systemic coagulopathy. Hemorrhages, either intraparenchymal or subarachnoid, occur less commonly. They are usually due to arteritis but sometimes relate to severe thrombocytopenia or to cerebral venous thrombosis.[41]

In the series of Futrell et al,[41] 8 percent of hospitalized SLE patients had seizures; of these, 22 patients had generalized convulsions and 5 had focally originating seizures. These were not always directly related to the SLE: 2 were idiopathic, 1 was posttraumatic, 4 had azotemia, 9 had sepsis, and several had strokes.

Some patients may also have myalgias and fever that can mimic other diseases, such as infections. Often, SLE, including CNS involvement, has a relapsing-remitting course.

Pathology and Pathogenesis

The neurologic complications of SLE are likely to be due to multiple mechanisms that differ in different patients.[50]

Johnson and Richardson found microvascular ischemic lesions in the brains of 80 percent of 24

SLE patients at autopsy.[46] These were usually small cortical infarcts, multifocal white matter changes, or hemorrhages. Large vessel strokes occur, but are less common than small infarcts. Strokes are often associated with antiphospholipid antibodies; patients may present with transient ischemic attacks, completed strokes, a generalized brain dysfunction, seizures, or full-blown disseminated intravascular coagulation.[51,52]

Immune-complex vascular disease with activation of inflammatory mediators may play a role in some patients with strokes, but *vasculitis*, with inflammatory cells within the vessel walls, was found in only 10 percent of patients.[46] Other pathologic studies have revealed a similar low frequency of vasculitis.[53,54] Vascular changes found include hyalinization of vessel walls, endothelial proliferation, and thromboses in small (<100 μm) arteries and capillaries.

Even in patients with clinical CNS dysfunction, the brain may be structurally normal. Alternative mechanisms must therefore apply in these cases.

Antineuronal antibodies are proposed to cause dysfunction without structural change, but their role has yet to be defined.[55,56] Antiribosomal P protein antibodies may cause defective ribosomal synthesis of proteins for enzymes or cell structure.[57] These autoantibodies, found in over 90 percent of SLE patients with psychosis, could affect the brain if they are produced within the CNS or, with systemic production, if there is a defect in the blood-brain barrier.[58,59] A 5- to 30-fold increase in anti-P antibodies occurs during the active phase of psychosis in lupus.[60] Lymphocytotoxic antibodies are commonly present in SLE. These may cross-react with brain cells and correlate with neuropsychiatric complications of SLE.[61] However, the specificity of antilymphocytic antibodies for brain cells has been questioned, and some series do not show any difference in the frequency of antilymphocytic antibodies in SLE patients compared with those without neuropsychiatric manifestations.[62,63]

In many cases, the CNS is indirectly affected, e.g., by septic illness, metabolic disturbances from organ failure, or by treatment side effects. In the series of Futrell et al,[41] of 16 SLE patients with decreased alertness, 11 (69 percent) had severe infections as the probable underlying cause. These included bacteremia, pneumonia (bacterial or fungal), candidemia, septicemia with fungal brain abscesses, and pelvic infection. The author of this chapter has observed brain microinfarcts in "septic encephalopathy"; this mechanism may be more common than lupus-related vasculitis. This has important implications for prompt investigation and therapy. Other potential immunologic mechanisms include aberrant MHC T-cell response and cytokine-induced brain inflammation.[64] Deficiency of Clq may predispose to more severe disease.[65]

Psychiatric disturbances are probably usually organic in nature, in that they correlate with clinical evidence of CNS dysfunction, duration of SLE and enlarged ventricles on the CT scan. Corticosteroids are rarely the cause.[41]

Investigations

The American Rheumatism Association consensus criteria for the diagnosis of SLE are often inadequate for the diagnosis of cerebral lupus. In the differential diagnosis, it is important to determine the underlying mechanism for the brain dysfunction. It is especially important to rule out underlying infectious illness.

All SLE patients with focal, multifocal, or diffuse CNS dysfunction should have antiphospholipid antibody screening and echocardiograms, especially transesophageal echocardiography (TEE). Even this latter may miss the small vegetations on heart valves that constitute Libman-Sachs or nonbacterial thrombotic endocarditis. Hospitalized patients with encephalopathic lupus should be also be carefully investigated for underlying infection or SIRS.

The EEG is helpful in ruling out nonconvulsive status epilepticus, but is otherwise both insensitive and nonspecific.

Neuroimaging is often helpful and may reveal strokes, hemorrhages, or abscesses. Structural neuroimaging with magnetic resonance imaging (MRI) is superior to CT scanning in detecting lesions.[66,67] Lesions may enhance with gadolinium; these may disappear with immunosuppressive treatment, suggesting that they do not result in tissue damage.[68] Commonly detected lesions in the white matter are not specific for lupus, however.

Functional neuroimaging with single photon emission computed tomography (SPECT) is promising in showing areas of regional hypoperfusion (linked to reduced metabolic activity), sometimes without obvious structural changes.[69,70] Positron emission tomography (PET) and functional MRI have similar potential, but are not as readily available as SPECT.

Cerebrospinal fluid evaluation is rarely diagnostic. It should probably be carried out in the patient with suspect sepsis. Even in those with fungal brain lesions, the CSF was unhelpful. Occasionally, a pleocytosis, with under cells 200 per cubic millimeter, may be found, but elevation of protein concentration without pleocytosis is more common and may relate to strokes, peripheral neuropathy, or brain infections, or without any of these, i.e., related to the effects of lupus on the brain. Increased CSF immunoglobulins and positive oligoclonal banding have been reported in about half the patients with clinical CNS involvement.[71] Low CSF glucose concentration is found in about 8 percent of patients; occasionally, this can be protracted.[72,73]

Treatment

Management of CNS lupus should be as specific as possible. Having stated this, symptomatic therapy, e.g., antiepileptic drugs for seizures or antidepressants, is often necessary as well.

Early detection and treatment of SIRS, especially sepsis, can reduce morbidity and mortality.[74]

Patients with strokes in association with positive antiphospholipid antibodies are usually anticoagulated with coumadin. When anticoagulants are used for cardiogenic emboli in lupus, the recommended international normalized ratio (INR) is 2.5 to 4.0; often, lifelong treatment is necessary.[75] Controlled trials are lacking, but the above approach seems wise. It is unclear whether lupus patients with positive antiphospholipid antibodies, but without definite strokes (e.g., encephalopathic patients, and some patients with seizures or migraine-like headaches, or transverse myelitis), should be treated with anticoagulants.

Bona fide immune-mediated CNS dysfunction is an indication for immunosuppressive treatment. It is, however, difficult to know how aggressive to be with subtle or mild cognitive or behavioral abnormalities. Corticosteroids are the mainstay; cyclophosphamide and azathioprine are helpful adjuncts.[76,77] In resistant cases, methotrexate or cyclosporine may be worth considering. Plasma exchange or intravenous immunoglobulin administration may be dramatically helpful in certain patients.[78] The use of monoclonal antibodies is under study. Other strategies, such β-interferon, may be useful in patients with T-cell-mediated neuronal damage.[64] In the future, more targeted therapies may rely on the results of specific immunologic investigations.

SYSTEMIC NECROTIZING VASCULITIS

Classification

The term systemic necrotizing vasculitis encompasses polyarteritis nodosa, allergic angiitis and granulomatosis (Churg-Strauss syndrome), and the overlap syndrome. These entities will be discussed together. The CNS is reported to be involved in anywhere between 8 and 53 percent of cases.[79–82]

Necrotizing vasculitis in association with hepatitis B antigenemia is one of the most common forms of the disease in modern times. Polyarteritis nodosa (PAN) is a necrotizing arteritis affecting small and medium-sized arteries. Men are affected twice as commonly as women. Arteries are affected segmentally, often with aneurysm formation. Although the pulmonary arteries are spared, the kidneys, the heart, the gastrointestinal tract, and the skin are commonly involved.

Allergic and granulomatous angiitis differ from PAN in the following aspects: in the former, pulmonary vessels are commonly affected; veins and venules are affected as well as arteries; intra- and extra-vascular granulomas occur; eosinophilic

tissue infiltrates are found; and severe asthma and peripheral eosinophilia are common.

The overlap syndrome has features of both PAN and allergic granulomatous vasculitis, but it does not fit well into either syndrome.

Clinical Features

Brain involvement commonly presents as a generalized encephalopathy with fluctuating alertness, confusion, visual hallucinations, disorientation, and focal or secondary generalized convulsions.[83] Seizures occur only with acute disease. Although focal signs are found, they are often overshadowed by the diffuse disturbance in cerebral function.[82]

Discrete focal symptoms usually present as a stroke syndrome, sometimes accompanied by accelerated hypertension. Any vascular territory, including the vertebrobasilar system, can be affected. Multiple strokes give a multifocal or diffuse picture.

Some patients with global features have meningeal involvement accompanied by diffuse headaches. Patients may show focal or generalized cognitive deficits; memory impairment is common.

Peripheral nerve involvement is more common than CNS disease in PAN, usually as either mononeuritis multiplex or a symmetric sensorimotor or sensory polyneuropathy.[84]

Investigations

Neuroimaging commonly shows focal or multifocal areas of infarction, or, less commonly, intraparenchymal hemorrhage. Because of the small size of the involved vessels, vasculitis is usually not apparent on angiograms.

Management

Combined treatment with corticosteroids and immunosuppressive drugs give an overall survival of 80 percent.[84] Earlier series of untreated patients showed a 5-year survival rate of only 15 percent; half the patients died within 3 months of diagnosis.[85] The use of immunosuppressives has been associated with prompt reversal of the acute encephalopathy and seizures. Plasmapheresis shows promise, especially in the acute phase of the illness, before starting immunosuppressive agents.[86]

ANGIITIS OF THE CENTRAL NERVOUS SYSTEM

Primary or isolated (granulomatous) angiitis of the central nervous system (PACNS), without other organ or systemic involvement, is a rare (perhaps underrecognized) and variable disorder, characterized by ischemic strokes and intracranial hemorrhages.[87] Both sexes are equally affected; the disorder occurs mainly in individuals over 50 years of age. The diagnosis is one of exclusion of strokes from secondary vasculitides of the CNS and other causes[88] (Table 12-2).

Clinical Features

There are many ways that PACNS can present, including multifocal ischemic strokes, single or multiple intraparenchymal brain hemorrhages, or as a subarachnoid hemorrhage.[89] Disorders of alertness or cognition vary in association with the sites and time course of CNS involvement. Decreased alertness, rarely, can be a presenting feature, before other neurologic signs are found.[90] Some patients present with depression, delirium, or psychosis before frank deterioration in alertness occurs.[91] Worsenings occur often in a multifocal or

Table 12-2

Conditions to exclude in the diagnosis of isolated angiitis of the central nervous system

Acute posterior placoid pigment epitheliopathy and cerebral vasculitis
Antiphospholipid antibody syndrome
Atherosclerotic complications
Arterial dissection with distal emboli or hemorrhage
Behçet disease
Bland or infected (bacterial endocarditis) cardiogenic emboli
Fibromuscular dysplasia and emboli
Infections: herpes zoster with angiitis, HIV complications, bacterial or tuberculous meningitis, meningovascular
    syphilis, rickettsial disease
Malignant hypertension with vasospasm, e.g., with pheochromocytoma
Migraine with vasospasm
Moya-moya disease
Neoplasia, e.g., carcinomatous meningitis, leukemia, lymphoma,
    lymphomatoid granulomatosus/malignant angioendotheliomatosis,
    vascular complications of glioma (surgery or radiotherapy); neoplastic meningitis
Neurofibromatosis: vascular complications
Paradoxical embolism
Pregnancy complications: eclampsia, HELLP[a] syndrome, postpartum angiopathy
Sarcoidosis vasculitis
Sickle cell disease
Systemic vasculitis: SLE, Wegener's granulomatosus, PAN, Churg-Strauss vasculitis, allergic
    granulomatosis, vasculitis with connective tissue disease (e.g., SLE and Sjögren disease), Takayasu's vasculitis,
    Cogan syndrome, hypersensitivity vasculitis group disorders, temporal (giant-cell) arteritis
Thrombotic thrombocytopenic purpura or disseminated intravascular coagulation
Vascular malformation, e.g., aneurysms or arteriovenous malformations with subarachnoid hemorrhage and
    vasospasm
Vasculitis or arterial spasm with drugs, e.g., amphetamines, ephedrine, phenylpropanolamine, cocaine, ergotamine
von Recklinghausen disease with vascular involvement

[a] HELLP = hemolysis, elevated liver enzymes, and low platelets.

stepwise fashion. Headache, often with vomiting, is a common accompaniment or prodrome, with or without intracranial hemorrhage. Seizures, with variable secondary generalization, are common. Intellectual deterioration or focal cognitive deficits, such as aphasia, may occur in some cases. Involvement of cranial nerves includes papilledema, failure of ocular convergence, pupillary abnormalities, monocular visual loss and trigeminal neuropathy.[92] In contrast to many of the conditions in Table 12-2, systemic or constitutional symptoms are usually lacking, but, occasionally, patients have fever and leukocytosis.

When cases with histologic premortem diagnosis are selected, the clinical profile is somewhat more uniform. In this group, patients have had an insidious, chronic illness with diffuse encephalopathic features.[93] Focal deficits from strokes are added later in the course. These cases, however, are likely to be highly selected, as they were diagnostically puzzling, which led to the biopsy. Calabrese and colleagues recently reported a series defined only on the basis of angiography and exclusion of the disorders in Table 12-2.[94] These patients had a more benign course, presenting with an acute, focal event following a monophasic course associated with a relatively benign CSF profile (benign PACNS).

Pathology and Pathogenesis

Most commonly, the leptomeningeal arteries ($<20\,\mu m$) are affected, although intraparenchymal arteries are often involved.[95] Only about one-third of patients have large-artery, e.g., internal carotid or initial segment of the middle cerebral artery, disease.[96–98] Pathologically, the necrotic vessel wall is infiltrated with mononuclear inflammatory cells, multinucleated giant cells, and plasma cells in 80 percent of cases.[87] Vessels may occlude, leading to ischemic infarction; reperfusion of necrotic vessels may produce hemorrhages. The microscopic abnormalities are not, however, diagnostically specific; other vasculitides (giant-cell arteritis and the arteritis associated with sarcoidosis) may have a similar picture. The diagnosis requires clinical and radiologic support.

Investigation

The current key investigation for angiitis is cerebral angiography.[99] This shows a characteristic "beading" or segmental narrowing of the intracranial arteries (Fig. 12-8). Serial angiograms may be needed to see the typical features. Small aneurysms or occlusions of larger arteries may be found occasionally. None of these features is pathognomonic, however. Other disorders (Table 12-2) must be excluded either clinically or by appropriate investigative tests. Unfortunately, the sensitivity of cerebral angiography is not great; nearly 40 percent of patients have normal angiograms.[87]

Magnetic resonance imaging is more sensitive than CT, but neither is specific.[100] Multiple, bilateral supratentorial infarcts are usually found in varied locations. The meninges and cortex may enhance with contrast.

Biopsy of the brain is sometimes performed, but there is some risk to the patient. Also, lesions can be missed, as the disease can skip areas as it is often focal or segmental. One in four biopsies is negative because of this.[87]

Intracranial pressure may be increased and CSF reveals increased protein, red blood cells, and white blood cells, usually lymphocytes in over 90 percent of cases (Case Records of the Massachusetts General Hospital, 1976).[101] (It is normal or near normal in the benign variant described by Calabrese.[94]) Usually the CSF glucose concentration is normal and the IgG index is not elevated. The erythrocyte sedimentation rate (ESR) is only modestly elevated.[92]

Since the diagnosis of PACNS is a diagnosis of exclusion, it is vital to check CSF cultures for bacteria, neoplastic cells, and tuberculosis. Blood cultures, urinalysis and appropriate immunologic screening tests, CBC and platelet count should be carried out to exclude systemic vasculitis. Testing for the human immunodeficiency virus (HIV) and testing for hypercoagulable states, transesophageal echocardiography, and other investigative tests should be performed as required, given the clinical and radiologic picture.

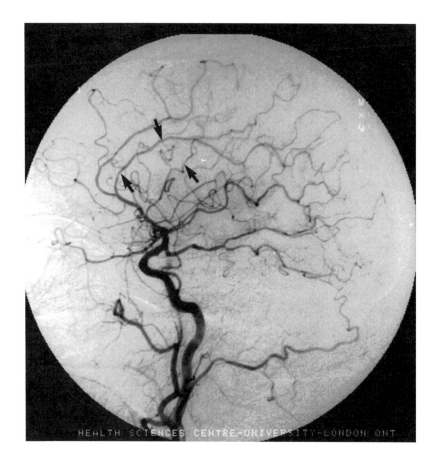

Figure 12-8
Angiogram showing features of vasculitis. The arrows *indicate segmental narrowing in the arteries.*

Treatment

After the exclusion of other diseases and the diagnosis of PACNS is made, the use of corticosteroids and cyclophosphamide is justified for aggressive disease. There have been no controlled trials because of the rarity of the condition. Isolated case reports or small series give some support to the immunosuppressive therapy.[102] Milder cases, e.g., benign PACNS with normal CSF, may respond to corticosteroids and a calcium blocker.[87] Sympathomimetic drugs should be avoided.

Cases of presumed PACNS that fail to respond to immunosuppressive treatment should be carefully re-examined to see if one of the conditions in Table 12-2 applies. Some conditions, e.g., associated systemic or primary CNS lymphoma, may be missed initially.[103]

SJÖGREN SYNDROME

Definition

Sjögren syndrome is an immunologic disorder affecting the exocrine glands, especially the lachrymal and salivary glands, causing dryness of the eyes and mouth (sicca syndrome) and a variety of other autoimmune phenomena, including cutaneous involvement. Middle-aged and older women are the prime targets. Traditionally, Sjögren syndrome has been divided into primary and secondary forms. The primary form occurs without other connective tissue disease, while secondary Sjögren syndrome occurs as part of recognized connective tissue disorders, including rheumatoid arthritis, SLE, or progressive systemic sclerosis. Sjögren syndrome is common, but an epidemiologic survey would be hampered by the lack of standardized diagnostic criteria.[104,105]

Diagnosis

There are no specific rheumatologic criteria. General minimal criteria include the presence of at least two of the following three features: xerostomia (dry mouth), xerophthalmia (dry eyes, confirmed with the Schirmer test) and a positive lachrymal or salivary gland biopsy.[105] Patients should not meet the criteria for systemic lupus erythematosus or mixed connective tissue disease.

The CNS can be involved in Sjögren syndrome.[106] Most often, this is a neuropsychiatric disease with focal or multifocal deficits, seizures, diffuse encephalopathy (usually acute confusional state), or migraine.[107] Occasionally, the disease may mimic multiple sclerosis. Of patients with Sjögren syndrome, 25 to 70 percent may have cognitive dysfunction, often attention-concentration and perceptual speed problems.[108,109] An Alzheimer-like dementia may also occur.[105,110] Patients are often anxious.[109] Focal deficits, e.g., hemiplegia, may onset in a stroke-like fashion, even though angiograms are normal.

Dysfunction of the peripheral nervous system is often more apparent than are CNS complications. These complications include: symmetric sensory polyneuropathy, carpal tunnel syndrome, cranial nerve (especially trigeminal) neuropathies, and a higher-than-expected prevalence of anisocoria.

Pathology and Pathogenesis of Central Nervous System Disease

The most common pathologic finding in patients dying with Sjögren syndrome and CNS involvement is diffuse polymorphous meningitis with microhemorrhages and hemosiderin deposits.[105] Perivascular infiltrates are also found. A cerebral vasculopathy with focal destruction and necrosis of small intrinsic brain vessels has been described in association with focal microinfarcts or, less commonly, microhemorrhages.[105] From preliminary data, it would appear that the CNS complications relate to a multifocal vasculopathy.

Investigations

The MRI shows hyperintense subcortical lesions in 51.3 percent of patients compared with 36.6 percent of controls.[107]

Cerebrospinal fluid shows mild protein elevations; occasionally, oligoclonal banding may be found. Multimodal evoked response testing shows abnormalities in over 80 percent of patients with Sjögren syndrome who have clinical evidence of CNS involvement.[105] Provost and colleagues have shown that in Ro(SS-A) precipitin antibody-positive patients with Sjögren syndrome and SLE, both groups share the following histocompatibility antigens: HLA-DR3, DQ1, DQ2, and DRw52.[105]

Treatment

There is no uniformly agreed-upon treatment modality. Corticosteroids seem to be effective in treating the CNS complications in at least some patients.[105] Other immunosuppressive drugs may also be useful.

WEGENER'S GRANULOMATOSIS

Wegener's granulomatosis is a vasculitis affecting small arterioles, capillaries, and small venules with necrotizing inflammation and granulomata. The upper respiratory tract is involved first, followed, variably, by the lower respiratory tract, kidneys, skin, eyes, and heart. The nervous system is affected in more than half the cases.[111] While the peripheral (including many cranial) nerves are involved more than the CNS, in advanced cases the brain is often affected by hypertensive encephalopathy, cerebral granulomata, ischemic strokes, venous occlusions (from granulomatous extension), or hemorrhage into the brain or subarachnoid space.[111] A generalized encephalopathy, with impairment of consciousness, may also result from multiple system organ failure with advanced systemic disease or infectious complications.[112]

The treatment and prognosis of Wegener's granulomatosis have improved greatly in recent years with more aggressive immunosuppressive therapy using cyclophosphamide.[113]

TEMPORAL (GIANT-CELL) ARTERITIS

Clinical Picture

Temporal arteritis is a disease of the medium-sized arteries of older individuals, most commonly over 65 years.[114] It is a systemic disorder characterized by headache, muscular aches in the shoulder region (polymyalgia rheumatica), and malaise. Other less constant features include low-grade fever, jaw claudication, and mild anemia.

The disorder usually starts in the scalp (most commonly the superficial temporal) arteries. With progression, there may be involvement of the ophthalmic artery and infarction of the optic nerve or retina. Strokes may sometimes occur in a focal or multifocal fashion. The aggregate of these features may produce the picture of a diffuse process with confusion or greater degrees of impaired consciousness.

Investigations

The ESR is usually markedly elevated; the mean being 107 mm in the first hour.[115]

As the disorder can be closely mimicked by a number of other conditions, it is best to obtain a biopsy of the affected scalp artery before committing the patient to a prolonged course of corticosteroids. The sensitivity of superficial temporal artery biopsy is over 90 percent.[116] Flynn and Hellmann recommend taking a 3-cm biopsy of the superficial temporal artery on each side, if there is no clinical involvement of the scalp artery.[116]

Pathology

The artery shows chronic inflammatory changes. The most characteristic feature is loss and fragmentation of parts of the internal elastic lamina in the arterial wall. This is often phagocytosed by multinucleated giant cells. The endothelium proliferates and eventually the artery occludes.

Treatment

Treatment is with prednisone, which should always be successful. The few "refractory" cases turn out to be incorrect diagnoses. The prednisone should be started at 40 to 60 mg per day. The drug dosage can be tapered and therapy switched to alternate days once the disease is under control and the ESR is falling. The ESR can be followed as an index of disease activity and as a guide for the need for continued prednisone therapy.

TAKAYASU'S ARTERITIS

Takayasu's arteritis is a rare disorder that primarily affects young women. It is characterized by granulomatous stenosis or occlusion of the aorta and its major branches.

Clinical Features

Up to 10 percent of affected patients may suffer major strokes, from occlusion of one or both carotid arteries. Seizures and encephalopathy have been reported but are less common than ischemic stroke.[117,118]

Investigation

Angiography that includes the aorta and its branches, including the renal and visceral arteries, is indicated.[119]

Treatment

Treatment involves corticosteroids, using the ESR as a guide for tapering. Most patients require treatment for at least 2 years. If treatment is instituted before disastrous complications occur, the prognosis is reasonably good; the overall 5-year survival rate is 85 percent.[120]

SCLERODERMA

Scleroderma or progressive systemic sclerosis is a disorder of unknown etiology in which endothelial injury is important in the pathogenesis.[121] It is a multisystem disorder affecting the skin and, variably, other organs including the gastrointestinal tract, kidneys, lungs, and heart.

Central nervous manifestations include psychosis in 10 percent of cases.[122] Multifocal deficits may occur over time. Cases of vitamin B_{12} deficiency have resulted from gastrointestinal disease causing malabsorption.[123]

The disease is highly variable and treatment is difficult to evaluate. Corticosteroids are the mainstay of therapy.

RHEUMATOID ARTHRITIS

Rheumatoid arthritis (RA) is an autoimmune disorder, associated with circulating immune complexes, that affects 1 to 2 percent of the population.[124]

Clinical Manifestations

Central nervous system complications are uncommon and may be secondary to rheumatoid nodules, rheumatoid vasculitis, or atlantoaxial subluxation. Impairment of consciousness may occur with multifocal or strategically placed lesions in the ascending reticular activating system (ARAS).[125] With the first two conditions, there may be focal or multifocal deficits or seizures, the latter implying cerebral cortical involvement. Cranial nerve palsies may also occur.

Atlantoaxial subluxation is common in RA. By far the most common CNS complication is compressive myelopathy or drop attacks from intermittent cord compression.[126] Ischemia in the vertebrobasilar system may also occur.[127] This may be due to compression of a vertebral artery by the dens, which can move up or laterally relative to the vertebral column and compress one vertebral artery (see Fig. 12-9).[128] If flow in the opposite vertebral artery is compromised by atherosclerosis or hypoplasia, or is compressed during neck rotation, there may be arrest of circulation in the basilar artery. This may produce transient loss of consciousness preceded or followed by other features of basilar territory ischemia (tetraplegia, diplopia, memory disturbance, and cortical visual disturbance).[129] The author has seen a patient with extensive, fatal infarction in the vertebrobasilar system due compression of one vertebral artery when the other was previously occluded (Fig. 12-10).[127] Anoxic encephalopathy or sudden death may occur with sudden subluxation at the C1–C2 level, with cord compression, respiratory arrest, and quadriplegia.

Management

Rheumatoid vasculitis should be treated as any systemic, immune-mediated vasculitis, i.e., with corticosteroids and immunosuppressants.[130] The role of plasmapheresis is unknown.

Cervical subluxation should be treated conservatively with neck immobilization. Advanced, and life- or cervical cord-threatening subluxation may require surgical fixation.

Symptomatic therapy for seizures or other complications may be necessary.

BEHÇET DISEASE

Behçet disease is a systemic vasculitis that, for diagnosis, requires the presence of aphthous ulcers and any two of the following:[131]

1. genital ulceration,

2. intraocular inflammation (uveitis or retinal vasculitis),

3. defined skin lesions, or

4. a positive skin pathology test.

The disease is relatively common in the Mediterranean and Far East countries (prevalence is 1 in 1000 in Japan), but, it is uncommon in North America and northern Europe. Behçet disease mainly affects young males.

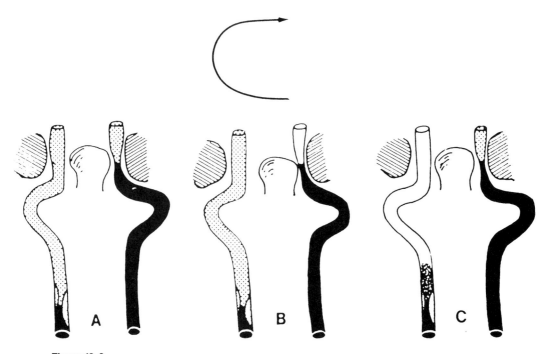

Figure 12-9

Rheumatoid arthritis with basilar invagination. The diagram illustrates the reduced blood flow past an atheromatous stenosis on the left side and past the hourglass constriction between the eccentrically placed odontoid process and the rim of the foramen magnum on the right. A. With the long axis of the head in an anteroposterior position, there are no symptoms. B. Vertigo occurred on rotation of the head to the right side by further restricting vertebral artery blood flow. C. Thrombosis (lower left) of the vertebral artery severely restricted flow to the basilar artery. Infarction could have been precipitated by rotation of the head as in part B. (From Jones and Kaufmann,[127] with permission.)

Clinical Manifestations

Central nervous complications occur in about 18 percent of collected cases.[132] The most common presentation is a meningoencephalitic picture, or acute or subacute brainstem disease.[133–136] These may be associated with impairment of consciousness because of diffuse, discrete lesions of the ARAS or multifocal lesions. Delirium, organic psychoses, and other psychiatric manifestations are frequent and may be the earliest neurologic features.[137] Seizures, focal with variable secondary generalization, ischemic strokes in single or multiple territories, and intracranial venous thrombosis are other mechanisms for impairment of consciousness or cognitive function.[138,139] In a case report from Japan, akinetic mutism was related to bilateral thalamocapsular lesions, presumably infarctions, due to Behçet disease.[140]

The systemic manifestations include the characteristic oral ulcers, either singly or in crops. The larynx or genitals are also affected in some patients. Cutaneous involvement includes folliculitis, erythema nodosum, and an acne-like eruption. Ocular involvement may lead to blindness. Nondeforming arthritis, superficial and deep venous thromboses, and gastrointestinal dysfunction from mucosal ulcerations may occur.

The often relapsing-remitting course and some clinical features may mimic multiple sclerosis.

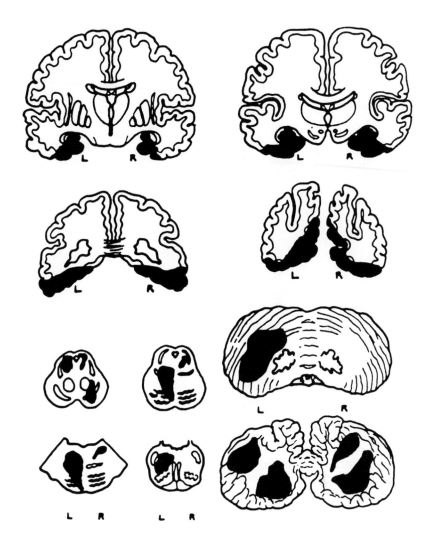

Figure 12-10
Infarction (black areas) in the vertebrobasilar system as a complication of basilar invagination from rheumatoid arthritis; same case as shown in Fig. 12-9. (From Jones and Kaufmann,[127] with permission.)

Pathology and Pathogenesis

The brain reveals chronic meningitis and a vasculitis with lymphocytic infiltration of vessels and perivascular regions.[134] Areas of infarction are common in the brainstem.

The pathogenesis is uncertain, but a vasculitis appears to be operative. The vasculitic changes can often be found in the skin biopsy. There may be a hereditary predisposition; there is an association with HLA-B51 antigen.[141] Although some have speculated about an infectious agent, e.g., a virus, triggering the disease, this has never been proven.[142]

Investigation

The diagnosis is mainly clinical. A skin biopsy may show vasculitic lesions. The CSF is usually abnormal, showing a lymphocytic meningitis with elevated protein concentration and, occasionally, positive oligoclonal banding. The MRI scan is superior to CT in revealing lesions.[143] Fresh lesions typically show high signal intensity on T2-weighted images. Although nonspecific, the lesions are usually different from the periventricular white matter lesions of multiple sclerosis; the MRI may be helpful in the differential diagnosis.

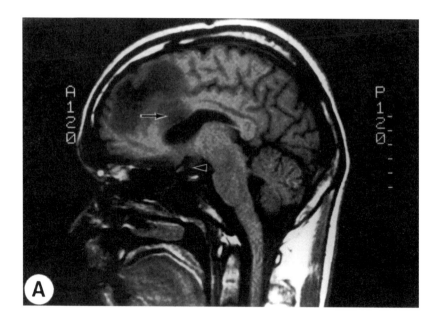

Figure 12-11
An MRI in a case of multiple sclerosis. There are large areas of demyelination, including the deep frontal white matter, the corpus callosum (arrow), *and the optic tracts* (arrow).

Management

Neurologic involvement usually requires treatment with systemic corticosteroids or cytotoxic agents (cyclophosphamide, azathioprine, or chlorambucil). Cyclosporine A or newer immunosuppressives may have a role, but more studies are needed. Symptomatic therapy, e.g., antiepileptic drugs for seizures or anticoagulants for venous thromboses, may be required.

Neurologic involvement, male sex, and earlier age of onset indicate more severe disease, and consequently higher mortality and morbidity. Many patients do well.

MULTIPLE SCLEROSIS

Multiple sclerosis (MS) is a common, immune-mediated demyelinating condition of the CNS.[144–147] The name derives from the fact that lesions are typically multiple, with older lesions consisting of gliotic plaques.

Clinical Features

Impairment of alertness is rarely directly due to MS lesions. Certain fulminant cases, e.g., Marburg's type or "transitional sclerosis" (with acute, large, confluent, inflammatory plaques—see Fig. 12-11), may be associated with impaired consciousness.[148–150] Intermittent impairment of consciousness may relate to epileptic seizures, which occur in a minority of patients.

More commonly, at least in the author's experience, impairment of alertness is an *indirect* complication of MS, usually caused by an underlying infection (most likely urinary tract or respiratory), complications of drugs (either iatrogenic or deliberate overdose), or superimposed renal failure from chronic urinary infections or neurogenic bladder. Occasionally, hypertensive crises may occur as a complication of bladder distention in patients with advanced spinal cord disease—i.e., autonomic hyperreflexia. This can lead to intracranial hemorrhage or to hypertensive encephalopathy. Hypothermia may occur with high spinal cord disease that may prevent appropriate autonomic adjustments to a cold environment (see Chap. 8). There is a single case report of probable hypothalamic dysfunction in which the patient presented with recurrent episodes of altered consciousness, hypothermia, inappropriate antidiuretic hormone secretion and hypoglycemia.[151]

Impairment of cognitive function is common, but may require neuropsychologic testing for its detection. Memory impairment has been documented in a number of studies: learning and remembering verbal and nonverbal material may be impaired, especially during disease exacerbations.[152] The Digit Span test for attention is also often abnormal.[153] Focal deficits in cognition, such as aphasia, are uncommon. Behavioral and affective disturbances are common, but frank dementia with euphoria is found mainly in very advanced disease; such patients are often also quadriplegic with pseudobulbar palsy.

Pathology and Pathogenesis

Acute lesions consist of loss of myelin with relative preservation of axons in plaques. Plaques are typically perivenular and tend to be more common near CSF pathways, i.e., periventricular and surface white matter tracts in the brainstem and spinal cord. With more advanced lesions, an intense astrocytic gliosis and axonal loss ensue. Inflammatory cells, especially T-lymphocytes, are commonly present around veins within plaques.

Disturbed function relates primarily to disturbed axonal conduction of the nerve impulse. The loss of myelin disturbs saltatory conduction in axons. Leakage of current due to the loss of insulation may produce conduction block, so that the axonal conduction totally fails.[154] Incomplete demyelination may allow some nerve impulses to be conducted, but these are conducted more slowly; the axon may not be able to conduct rapid trains of impulses.[155] Such partially demyelinated axons are susceptible to conduction block with even slight elevations (e.g., 0.5°C) of core temperature.[156] This may be due to shortening of the action potential by the elevated temperatures.

Seizures may be due to deafferentation caused by the inflammation of myelinated nerve fibers in the cerebral cortex.

The clinical features related to these physiologic disturbances depend on the regions that are "disconnected" by the demyelinating process. The net effect depends on the accumulated deficits from multiple lesions.

Diagnosis and Investigations

The diagnosis of MS rests on the establishment of CNS white matter lesions that are disseminated in time and space, along with the exclusion of recognized disorders that may mimic this demyelinating disease. A number of "official" sets of diagnostic criteria have been developed, mainly for research purposes.[157–162,194] They suffer from being overly exclusive for clinical purposes; it is estimated that any set of criteria will correctly identify MS in 40 to 87 percent of cases.[163,164] (see Fig. 12-11).

Treatment

After the initial diagnosis, clinicians should resist the tendency to blame all worsenings of the patient's condition on the MS itself. One should carefully screen MS patients with acute worsening in conscious level for the underlying mechanism. It is especially important to exclude underlying systemic infection or inflammation, metabolic or drug-induced disorders, hypothermia, seizures, a depressive illness with superimposed psychomotor retardation, or even a conversion reaction.

Specific therapy should be directed against the pathogenetic mechanism.

Acute MS or exacerbations with significant additional impairment in function are usually treated with intravenously administered high-dose methylprednisolone, which has been shown to be effective in controlled trials.[165,166] The use of other treatments, including copolymer-1, interferons, and other immunosuppressive therapy are undergoing extensive multicenter trials. Recently, six patients with fulminant disease were treated with plasmapheresis; four improved dramatically.[167] Further work is needed to determine if this therapy may have a role with acute fulminant disease.

SARCOIDOSIS

Sarcoidosis is a multisystem granulomatous inflammatory disorder of unknown etiology that is characterized by the presence of noncaseating granulomata in multiple organ systems and by immune dysregulation.

Overall, 5 to 27 percent of patients with sarcoidosis develop neurologic complications, involving either the central or the peripheral nervous system, or both.[168-171] The prevalence of sarcoidosis in the population is 20 to 50 per 100,000.[172]

Clinical Manifestations

The nervous system manifestations reflect the site(s), mechanism, and acuity of the inflammatory disease. Impairment of consciousness may occur with diencephalic involvement, hydrocephalus (either the communicating type with chronic meningitis, or obstructive due to ventricular disease), large parenchymal lesions with herniation, seizures (most commonly secondary generalized convulsive, in 5 to 28 percent of patients), the cumulative effect of parenchymal lesions, or opportunistic systemic or CNS infections secondary to immune deficiency.[171,173] Pituitary involvement may cause metabolic or fluid and electrolyte disorders that may, in turn, cause an encephalopathy. Diabetes insipidus is the most common hormonal disturbance and relates to hypothalamic involvement. Other manifestations of hypothalamic disease include hypersomnolence and hypothermia.[174] Hypercalcemia may also occur with systemic disease; this may cause an encephalopathy (see Chap. 13).[175] Despite vascular involvement, clinical strokes in neurosarcoidosis are rare.[176]

Abnormal mental states are common in sarcoidosis and may be the presenting manifestation: i.e., impaired alertness, psychosis, dementia, or focal features. Delirium may be secondary to diffuse cerebral inflammation.[177]

Additional neurologic problems include optic neuropathy (due to involvement of the optic nerves or chiasm in chronic adhesive meningitis, or infiltration of the nerve or compression by mass lesions), other cranial neuropathies (especially bilateral facial, trigeminal sensory, auditory, vestibular, or vagal neuropathy), peripheral neuropathy (mononeuritis multiplex or polyneuro-pathy), and myelopathy.[176] Patients with meningitis may show meningismus. Brainstem and spinal involvement are rare.

Pathology and Pathogenesis

Chronic granulomatous inflammation is characteristic. The immunopathology involves activation of CD4 lymphocytes that secrete cytokines, including interleukin-2, macrophage chemotactic factor, macrophage colony-stimulating factor, and granulocyte colony-stimulating factor.[178] These stimulate the migration of inflammatory cells that take part in the granulomatous inflammation. The initial trigger is, however, unknown.

Investigations

Scanning by MRI has allowed insight into the site and, to some extent, the nature of the neurologic disease. Infiltration of the diencephalon, optic nerves or chiasm; basal meningitis; ventricular involvement; parenchymal lesions with mass effect, or ischemic lesions, can all be well defined with MRI.

The CSF is usually abnormal, but is not specific. The usual picture is elevation of protein concentration with a mild lymphocytic pleocytosis. Hypoglycorrhachia sometimes occurs. Positive oligoclonal banding is occasionally found.[179]

For systemic disease, gallium scanning is sensitive to inflammatory deposits. A positive gallium scan showing pulmonary involvement may lead to a transbronchial biopsy confirming the presence of noncaseating granulomata. This applies even when the chest film is unremarkable and the patient has no pulmonary symptoms. Biopsy of the lachrymal, salivary, or parotid glands may lead to a histologic diagnosis, if these structures are positive on the gallium scan.

Angiotensin-converting enzyme (ACE) is probably a cytokine produced by macrophages. Its presence in high titer in serum is reasonably specific for sarcoidosis. The combination of elevated serum ACE and a positive gallium scan has high specificity.[180] In the author's experience, elevated ACE concentrations often are not found in CNS sarcoidosis. Thus, the sensitivity may be fairly low.

Anergy to various common antigens, such as *Candida* spp. can be demonstrated. Skin testing with Kviem antigen is seldom performed; a positive result suggests sarcoidosis.[169]

Hypothalamic involvement may be heralded by a modest elevation of the serum prolactin concentration.

Hypercalcemia is sometimes present due to increased production of 1,25-dihydroxyvitamin D, enhanced production from bone, or augmented intestinal absorption of calcium. Increased renal excretion of calcium is commonly found with 24-h collections of urine.

Management

The diagnosis should be specific. Tuberculous meningitis may closely mimic CNS sarcoidosis and must be excluded.

Corticosteroids are the mainstay of therapy, even though controlled trials have not been carried out to demonstrate their effectiveness. Sarcoidosis of the CNS may not respond adequately to corticosteroids alone; immunosuppressive drugs or even radiotherapy may be necessary to check severe disease, especially if the disease is threatening the anterior visual pathways.[181]

The CNS sarcoidosis may persist for months or years without remission. Chronic immunosuppressive therapy is indicated, especially in cases with intra-axial disease or hydrocephalus. Alternate-day prednisone or steroid-sparing immunosuppressive agents, such as azathioprine, are useful treatment modalities.

Symptomatic therapy includes antiepileptic drugs for those with seizures, hormone replacement for some patients with hypothalamic or pituitary disease, and shunting for acute, severe, or steroid-resistant hydrocephalus and raised intracranial pressure. Surgical debulking of large parenchymal lesions may be necessary if there is insufficient response to immunosuppressive therapy. Complications, especially superinfections and steroid-induced osteopenia, should be watched for and treated.

Patients who enter remission need to be counseled and followed regarding the possibility of relapse. An ophthalmologist should conduct follow-up examinations of the patient, as potentially irreversible visual involvement is common.

ENDOCARDITIS

Bacterial endocarditis, either acute or chronic, is accompanied by CNS complications in 20 to 40 percent in most series.[182]

Clinical Features

Table 12-3 lists the CNS complications of bacterial endocarditis that might be accompanied by decreased alertness or altered cognitive functioning. Impaired consciousness, with or without focal signs, in a patient with fever and a murmur should suggest the possibility of endocarditis.

Ocular findings may serve as a clue, especially abnormalities discovered on funduscopy: retinal hemorrhages or Roth spots (see Fig. 3-5) are found in about 25 percent of cases. Acute embolic occlusion of the central retinal artery or defects in the visual pathways are common, but are less specific diagnostically.

Pathogenesis

The various micro-organisms responsible for endocarditis are listed in Table 12-4. Most symptoms are due to emboli that are disrupted from

Table 12-3

Incidence of central nervous system complications with infective endocarditis

Complications	Mean percentage incidence (range)
Embolism	13.4 (6.7–25.9)
Meningitis	7.0 (1.1–15.1)
Septic encephalopathy	6.5 (0.0–8.6)
Hemorrhage	3.6 (0.0–13.9)
Seizure	3.5 (0.00–11.0)
Abscess	1.9 (0.0–8.6)
Mycotic aneurysm	1.5 (0.0–8.6)

Source: From Tunkel and Kaye,[182] with permission.

Table 12-4

Microbiology of infective endocarditis in patients with central nervous system complications

Organism	Cases (n)	CNS complications (n)	Percentage (range)
Staphylococcus aureus	111	62	56 (53–65)
Staphylococci, coagulase-negative	36	10	28 (14–50)
Viridans streptococci	183	48	26 (17–41)
Streptococci, group D	108	31	29 (26–30)
Streptococcus pneumoniae	16	13	81 (75–88)
Other streptococci	45	18	40 (35–57)
Other	74	29	39 (29–47)
Total	**573**	**211**	**37 (33–39)**

Source: From Francioli,[192] with permission.

cardiac vegetations; these lodge in vessels of various sizes.

Strokes, which constitute about two-thirds of the neurologic complications, arise from cardiogenic emboli and may be bland, ischemic lesions or hemorrhagic in nature. Intracranial hemorrhage (intraparenchymal or subarachnoid) may result from rupture of an inflamed, necrotic vessel wall (vasculitis) or from a mycotic aneurysm.

The picture of "septic encephalopathy" (see earlier in this chapter) may relate to a SIRS, but a similar picture may be produced by multifocal microemboli in the cerebral hemispheres, or by meningitis with coma (with ischemia or cerebritis). A similar mechanism probably underlies organic psychosis in these patients.

Meningitis makes up less than 10 percent of neurologic complications of bacterial endocarditis. It is more common with *Streptococcus pneumoniae* or *Staphylococcus aureus* than with endocarditis from other microorganisms.

Single or multiple brain abscesses may uncommonly occur as a result of infected emboli in the brain.

Seizures may result from ischemia to the cortex, infection of the brain, organ failure (e.g., renal failure), reaction to drug therapy (e.g., toxic encephalopathy), and the amounts of penicillin in the presence of renal impairment.

Investigation

In a patient with bacterial endocarditis, the presence of an acute confusional state without focal features should prompt neuroimaging with MRI, or CT if MRI is not available. This often reveals multifocal strokes, regions of cerebritis, or microabscesses. A lumbar puncture is indicated if the patient shows meningismus or is unconscious without showing focal features or mass effect on neuroimaging (a CT or MRI of the head should always be carried out before considering a lumbar puncture in this situation). An EEG will help exclude nonconvulsive seizures as a cause of the confusional state.

Cerebral angiography is advised in the presence of focal or multifocal deficits.[183] Clinically apparent emboli often precede the development of a mycotic aneurysm.[184] The management of mycotic aneurysms is, however, controversial. Some heal with appropriate antibiotic therapy, while others enlarge and rupture. (Also, some arterial ruptures may occur in necrotic vessels that have not expanded in an aneurysmal fashion). Wilson and colleagues recommend serial angiography and CT scans to monitor aneurysms.[185] If the aneurysm enlarges or ruptures, surgery is indicated. The operation involves ligating the parent vessel, then excising the aneurysm and the adjacent vessel wall. An arterial bypass is sometimes used to prevent infarction of the brain tissue supplied by the artery. Such surgical therapy applies especially to aneurysms distal to the first bifurcation of the major artery. Aneurysms proximal to the first bifurcation of the anterior, middle, or posterior cerebral arteries are more hazardous to excise as there is a great risk of a large infarction in that vessel's territory. These sometimes resolve using antibiotic therapy without surgery.[186]

Brain abscesses are usually small and resolve with antibiotic therapy. Occasionally, surgical drainage is necessary for large abscesses with mass effect.[187]

Antiepileptic drugs, e.g., phenytoin, are indicated in patients with seizures.

The roles of heart valve replacement and anticoagulation in infective endocarditis are controversial. There may be a subset of patients who benefit from valve replacement, e.g., those with large aortic valve vegetations due to *Staph. aureus*.[188] Anticoagulation with heparin may have a role in certain cases, but such cases have not been well characterized, nor has anticoagulation been shown to reduce the risk of infected emboli.[189] In two small series, the incidence of intracranial hemorrhages was disproportionately higher in patients receiving anticoagulants than in those without anticoagulation.[190,191]

REFERENCES

1. Bone RC, Balk RA, Cerra FB, et al: Definitions for sepsis and organ failure and the guidelines for the use of innovative therapies in sepsis. The ACCP/ SSP Consensus Conference Committee. American College of Chest Physicians/Society for Critical Care Medicine. *Crit Care Med* 20:864, 1992.

2. *Morbidity and Mortality Weekly Report: Centers for Disease Control.* 39, 1990.

3. Young GB, Bolton CF, Austin TW: The encephalopathy associated with septic illness. *Clin Invest Med* 13:1297, 1990.

4. Bolton CF, Young GB, Zochodne DW: The neurological complications of sepsis. *Ann Neurol* 33:94, 1993.

5. Zochodne DW, Bolton CF, Wells GA, et al: Critical illness polyneuropathy: a complication of sepsis and multiple organ failure. *Brain* 110:819, 1987.

6. Young GB, Bolton CF, Archibald YM, Austin TW, Wells GA: The electroencephalogram in sepsis-associated encephalopathy. *J. Clin. Neurophys* 9:145, 1992.

7. Jackson AC, Gilbert JJ, Young GB, Bolton CF: The encephalopathy of sepsis. *Can J Neurolog Sci* 12:303, 1985.

8. Sprung CL, Cerra FB, Freund HR: Amino acid alterations and encephalopathy in the sepsis syndrome. *Crit Care Med* 19:753, 1991.

9. du Moulin GC Paterson D, Hedley-White J, Broitman SA. *E. coli* peritonitis and bacteremia cause increased blood-brain barrier permeability. *Brain Res* 340:261, 1985.

10. Jeppsson B, Freund HR, Gimmon Z, et al: Blood-brain barrier derangement in sepsis: cause of septic encephalopathy? *Am J Surg* 141:136, 1981.

11. Maekawa T, Fuji Y, Sadamitsu D: Cerebral circulation and metabolism in patients with septic encephalopathy. *Am J Emer Med* 9:139, l981.

12. Glauser MP, Zanetti G, Baumgartner JD, Cohen J: Septic shock: pathogenesis. *Lancet* 338:732, 1991.

13. Belivacqua MP, Pober JS, Majeau GR: Recombinant tumor necrosis factor induces procoagulant activity in cultured human vascular endothelium: characterization and comparison with the actions of interleukin 1. *Proc Natl Acad Sci USA* 83:4533, 1986.

14. Heard SO, Fink MP: Multiple organ failure syndrome—Part 1: epidemiology, prognosis, and pathophysiology. *Intens Care Med* 6:279, 1991.

15. Tracey KJ, Beutler B, Lowry SF, et al: Shock and tissue injury induced by recombinant human cachectin. *Science* 234:470, 1986.

16. Spain DA, Wilson MA, Bar-Natan MF, Garrison RN: Nitric oxide synthetase inhibition aggravates intestinal microvascular vasoconstriction and hypoperfusion of bacteremia. *J Trauma* 36:720, 1994.

17. Kobari M, Fukuuchi Y, Tomita M, et al: Constriction/dilatation of the cerebral microvessels by intravascular endothelin-1 in cats. *J Cereb Blood Flow Metab* 14:64, 1994.

18. Pryor WA: The role of free radical reactions in biological systems, in Pryor WA (ed): *Free Radicals in Biology*, vol 1, New York, Academic Press, 1976, pp 1–43.

19. Freund HR, Muggia-Sullam M, Peiser J, Melamed E: Brain neurotransmitter profile is

deranged during sepsis and septic encephalopathy in the rat. *J Surg Res* 38:267, 1985.

20. Glabinski AR, Tani M, Aras S, et al: Regulation and function of central nervous system chemokines. *Int J Develop Neurosci* 13:153, 1995.

21. Lapresie J, Risvegliato M, Lapresie J, et al: L'éncephalité métatstatique infectieuse. *La Nouvelle Presse Medicale* 9:437, 1980.

22. Schafer DF, Jones EA: Hepatic encephalopathy and the gamma-aminobutyric-acid neurotransmitter system. *Lancet* I:18–20, 1982.

23. Millen KD, Szauter KM, Kaminsky-Russ: "Endogenous" benzodiazepine activity in body fluids of patients with hepalic encephalopathy. *Lancet* 336:81, 1990.

24. Moroni F, Lombardi G, Carlà V, et al: Increase in the content of quinolinic acid in cerebrospinal fliud and frontal cortex of patients with hepatic failure. *J Neurochem* 47:1667, 1986.

25. Anisman H, Zalcman S, Zacharko RM: The impact of stressors on immune and central neurotransmitter activity: bidirectional communication. *Rev Neurosci* 4:147, 1993.

26. Prins JG, Schrijver H, Staghouwer JH: Hyper-alimentation, hypophosphatemia and coma. *Lancet* 1:1253, 1973.

27. Pine RW, Wertz MJ, Lennard ES: Determinants of organ malfunction or death in patients with intra-abdominal sepsis. *Arch Surg* 118:242, 1983.

28. Freund HR, Ryall JA, Fischer JE: Amino acid derangements in patients with sepsis: treatment with branched chain amino acid rich infusions. *Ann Surg* 188:423, 1978.

29. Guillou PJ: Biological variation in the development of sepsis after surgery or trauma. *Lancet* 342:217, 1993.

30. Lyon G, Dodge PR, Adams RD: The acute encephalopathies of obscure origin in infants and children. *Brain* 84:680, 1961.

31. Valk J, van der Knaap MS: Toxic encephalopathy. *Am J Neuroradiol* 13:747, 1992.

32. Reye RDK, Morgan G, Baral J: Encephalopathy and fatty degeneration of the viscera: a disease entity in childhood. *Lancet* 2:749, 1963.

33. Varma RR, Riedel DR, Komorowski RA, et al: Reye's syndrome in nonpediatric age groups. *JAMA* 242:1373, 1979.

34. Levin M, Kay JDS, Gould JD, et al: Haemorrhagic shock and encephalopathy: a new syndrome with a high mortality in young children. *Lancet* 2:64, 1983.

35. Levin M, Pincott JR, Hjelm M, et al: Hemorrhagic shock and encephalopathy: clinical pathologic and biochemical features. *J Pediatr* 114:194, 1989.

36. Sébire G, Devictor D, Hauault G, et al: Coma associated with intense bursts of abnormal movements and long-lasting cognitive disturbances: an acute encephalopathy of obscure origin. *J Pediatr* 121:845, 1992.

37. Lahita RG: The connective tissue diseases and overall influence of gender. *Int J Fertil Menopausal Stud* 41:156, 1996.

38. Tan EM, Cohen AS, Fires JF et al: The 1982 revised criteria for the classification of systemic lupus erythematosus. *Arthritis Rheum* 23:1271, 1982.

39. Bruyn GAW: Controversies in lupus: nervous system involvement. *Ann Rheum Dis* 54:159, 1995.

40. Rubin LA, Urowitz MB, Gladman CL: Mortality in systemic lupus erythematosus. *QJM* 55:87, 1985.

41. Futrell N, Scultz LR, Millikan C: Central nervous system diseases in patients with systemic lupus erythematosus. *Neurology* 42:1649, 1992.

42. Tola MR, Granieri E, Caniatti L, et al: Systemic lupus erythematosus presenting with neurological disorders. *J Neurol* 239:61, 1992.

43. Harris EN, Highes GRV: Cerebral disease in systemic lupus erythematosus. *Springer Emin Immunopathol* 8:251, 1985.

44. Mitsias P, Levine SR: Large cerebral vessel occlusive disease in systemic lupus erythematosus. *Neurology* 44:385, 1994.

45. Sibley JT, Olsynski WP, Decoteau WE, Sundaram MB: The incidence and prognosis of central nervous system disease in systemic lupus erythematosus. *J Rheumatol* 19:47, 1992.

46. Johnson RT, Richardson EP: The neurological manifestation of systemic lupus erythematosus. *Medicine* 47:337, 1968.

47. Bennahum DA, Messner RP: Recent observations on central nervous system lupus erythematosus. *Semin Arthritis Rheum* 4:253, 1975.

48. Miguel EC, Pereira RMR, Pereira CA de B, et al: Psychiatric manifestations of systemic lupus erythematosus: clinical features, symptoms and signs of central nervous system activity in 43 patients. *Medicine* 73:224, 1994.

49. Bluestein HG: Neuropsychiatric manifestations of systemic lupus erythematosus. *N Eng J Med* 317:309, 1987.

50. Denberg JA, Denberg SD, Carbotte RM, Sakic B, Szechtman H: Nervous system lupus: pathogensis

and rationale for therapy. *Scand J Rheumatol* 12:263, 1995.

51. Leach IH, Lennox G, Jaspan T, Lowe J: Antiphospholipid antibody syndrome presenting with complex partial seizures and transient ischemic attacks due to widespread small cerebral arterial thrombosis. *Neuropathol Appl Neurobiol* 15:579, 1989.

52. Tanaka M, Kobayashi S, Tamura N, Hashimoto H, Hirose S: Disseminated intravascular coagulation in a patient with systemic lupus erythematosus with lupus anticoagulant. *Intern Med* 32:513, 1993.

53. Ellis SG, Verity MA: Central nervous system involvement in systemic lupus erythematosus: a review of neuropathologic finding: 57 cases 1955–1977. *Semin Arthritis Rheum* 8:212, 1979.

54. Hanly JG, Walsh NMG, Sangalang V: Brain pathology in systemic lupus erythematosus. *J Rheumatol* 19:732, 1992.

55. Zvaifler NJ, Bluestein HG: The pathogenesis of central nervous system manifestations of systemic lupus erythematosus. *Arthritis Rheum* 25:862, 1982.

56. Futrell N: Connective tissue disease and sarcoidosis of the central nervous system. *Curr Opin Neurol* 7:201, 1994.

57. Elkon K, Weissbach H, Brot N: Central nervous function in systemic lupus erythematosus. *Neurochem Res* 15:401, 1990.

58. Golombek SJ, Graus F, Elkon KB: Autoantibodies in the cerebrospinal fluid of patients with systemic lupus erythematosus. *Arthritis Rheum* 29:109, 1986.

59. Bonfa E, Golombek SJ, Kaufman LD, et al: Association between lupus psychosis and antiribosomal P protein antibodies. *N Eng J Med* 317:265, 1987.

60. Bonfa E, Golombek SJ, Kaufman LD, et al: Association between lupus psychosis and antiribosomal P protein antibodies. *N Eng J Med* 317:265, 1987.

61. Bluestein HG, Williams GW, Steinberg AD: Cerebrospinal fluid antibodies to neuronal cells: association with neuropsychiatric manifestations of systemic lupus erythematosus. *Am J Med* 70:240, 1981.

62. Winfield JB, Brunner CM, Koffler D: Serologic studies in patients with systemic lupus erythematosus and central nervous system dysfunction. *Arthritis Rheum* 21:289, 1978.

63. Long AA, Denburg SD, Carbotte RM, Singal DP, Denburg JA: Serum lymphocytotoxic antibodies and neurocognitive function in systemic lupus erythematosus. *Ann Rheum Dis* 49:249, 1990.

64. Denburg JA, Denburg SD, Carbotte RM, Sakic B, Szechtman HL: Nervous system lupus: pathogenesis and rationale for therapy. *Scand J Rheumatol* 24:263, 1993.

65. Bowness P, Davies KA, Norsworthy PJ, et al: Hereditary Clq deficiency and systemic lupus erythematosus. *QJM* 87:455, 1994.

66. Vermess M, Bernstein RM, Bydder GM, et al: Nuclear magnetic resonance (NMR) imaging of the brain in systemic lupus erythematosus. *J Comput Assist Tomogr* 7:461, 1973.

67. McCune WJ, MacGuire A, Aisen A, Gebarski S: Identification of brain lesions in neuropsychiatric systemic lupus erythematosus by magnetic resonance imaging. *Arthritis Rheum* 31:159, 1988.

68. Miller DH, Buchanan N, Barker G, et al: Gadolinium-enhanced magnetic resonance imaging of the central nervous system in systemic lupus erythematosus. *J Neurol* 239:460, 1992.

69. Nossent JC, Hovestadt A, Schönfeld DHW, Swaak AJG: Single-photon-emission computed tomography of the brain in the evaluation of cerebral lupus. *Arthritis Rheum* 36:1253, 1993.

70. Rubbert A, Marienhagen A, Pirner K, et al: Single-photon emission computed tomography analysis of cerebral blood flow in the evaluation of central nervous system involvement in patients with systemic lupus erythematosus. *Arthritis Rheum* 36:1253, 1993.

71. Winfield JB, Shaw M, Silverman LM, et al: Intrathecal IgG synthesis and blood-brain barrier impairment in patients with systemic lupus erythematosus and central nervous system dysfunction. *Am J Med* 74:837, 1983.

72. Gibson T, Myers AR: Nervous system involvement in SLE. *Ann Rheum Dis* 35:398, 1976.

73. Reinitz E, Hubbard D, Grayzel AJ: Central nervous system systemic lupus erythematosus versus central nervous system infection: low cerebrospinal fluid glucose and pleocytosis in a patient with a prolonged course. *Arthritis Rheum* 25:583, 1982.

74. Young GB, Bolton CF, Austin T: Sepsis-associated encephalopathy. *Clin Invest Med* 13:297, 1990.

75. Derksen RHWM, DeGroot PG, Kater L, Mieuwenhuis HK: Patients with antiphospholipid antibodies and venous thrombosis should receive long term anticoagulant treatment. *Ann Rheum Dis* 52:689, 1993.

76. Redford TW, Small RE: Update on pharmacotherapy of systemic lupus erythematosus. *Am J Health Syst Pharm* 52:2686, 1995.

77. Hay EM: Psychiatric disorder and cognitive impairment in SLE. *Lupus* 3:145, 1994.

78. Corvetta A, Della Bitta R, Gabrielli A, Spaeth PJ, Danieli G: Use of high-dose intravenous immunoglobulin in systemic lupus erythematosus: report of three cases. *Clin Exp Rheumatol* 7:295, 1989.

79. Arkin A: Clinical and pathological study of periarteritis nodosa: report of 5 cases, one historically healed. *Am J Pathol* 6:401, 1930.

80. Ford RG, Siekert RH: Central nervous system manifestations of periarteritis nodosa. *Neurology* 15:114, 1965.

81. Sheehan B, Harriman DGF, Bardshaw JPB: Polyarteritis nodosa with ophthalmologic and neurologic complications. *Arch Ophthalmol* 60:537, 1958.

82. Moore PM, Fauci AS: Neurologic manifestations of systemic vasculitis: a retrospective and prospective study of the clinicopathologic features and responses to therapy in 25 patients. *Am J Med* 71:517, 1981.

83. Prescott JE, Johnson JE, Dice WH: Polyarteritis nodosa presenting as seizures. *Ann Emerg Med* 12:642, 1983.

84. Guillevin L, Jarrouse B, Lok C, et al: Longterm followup after treatment of polyarteritis nodosa and Churg-Strauss angiitis with comparison of steroids, plasma exchange and cyclophosphamide to steroids and plasma exchange: a prospective randomized trial in 71 patients. The Cooperative Study Group for Polyarteritis Nodosa. *J Rheumatol* 18:567, 1991.

85. Frohnert PP, Sheps SG: long -term follow-up study of periarteritis nodosa. *Am J Med* 43:8, 1967.

86. Chalopin JM, Rifle G, Turc JM, et al: Immunologic findings during successful treatment of HBsAg-associated polyarteritis nodosa by plasmapheresis alone. *Br Med J* 1:386, 1980.

87. Calabrese LH: Vasculitis of the central nervous system. *Rheum Dis Clin N Am* 21:1059, 1995.

88. Calabrese LH: Vasculitis of the central nervous system. *Rheum Dis Clin N Am* 21:1059, 1995.

89. Launes J, Iivanainen M, Erkinjuntti T, Vuorialho M: Isolated angiitis of the nervous system. *Acta Neurol Scand* 74:108, 1986.

90. Case Records of the Massachusetts General Hospital: Case 43-1976. *N Eng J Med* 295:944, 1976.

91. Case Records of the Massachusetts General Hospital. Case 41152. *N Eng J Med* 252:634, 1955.

92. Nurick S, Blackwood W, Mair WGP: Giant cell granulomatous angiitis of the central nervous system. *Brain* 95:133, 1972.

93. Vollmer TL, Guarnaccia J, Harrington W, et al: Idiopathic granulomatous angiitis of the central nervous system: Diagnostic challenges. *Arch Neurol* 50:925, 1993.

94. Calabrese LH, Gragg LA, Furan AJ: Benign angiopathy: a distinct subset of angiographically defined primary angiitis of the central nervous system. *J Rheumatol* 30:2046, 1993.

95. Kolondy EH, Rebeiz JJ, Caviness VS, et al: Granulomatous angiitis of the central nervous system. *Arch Neurol* 19:510, 1968.

96. Cupps TR, Moore PM, Fauci AS: Isolated angiitis of the central nervous system. *Am J Med* 74:97, 1983.

97. Huges JT, Brownell B: Granulomatous giant-cell angiitis of the central nervous system. *Neurology* 16:293, 1966.

98. Ozawa T, Sasaki O, Sorimachi T, Tanaka R: Primary angiitis of the central nervous system: report of 2 cases and review of the literature. *Neurology* 36:1783, 1993.

99. Calabrese LH, Duna GF: Evaluation and treatment of central nervous system vasculitis. *Curr Opin Rheumatol* 7:37, 1995.

100. Pierot L, Chiras J, Debussche-Depriester C, et al: Intracerebral stenosing arteriopathies: contribution of three radiological techniques to the diagnosis. *J Neuroradiol* 18:32, 1991.

101. Calabrese LH, Furlan AJ, Gragg LA, et al: Primary angiitis of the central nervous system. Diagnostic criteria and clinical approach. *Cleveland Clin J Med* 59:293, 1992.

102. Cupps TR, Moore PM, Fauci AS: Isolated angiitis of the central nervous system. *Am J Med* 74:97, 1983.

103. Borenstein D, Costa M, Jannotta F, Rizzoli H: Localized isolated angiitis of the central nervous system associated with primary intracerebral lymphoma. *Cancer* 62:375, 1988.

104. Bone R, Fox R, Howell F, Fantozzi R: Sjögren's syndrome: a persistent clinical problem. *Laryngoscope* 95:295, 1985.

105. Provost TT: Sjögren's syndrome: cutaneous, immunologic and nervous system manifestations. *Neurol Clin* 5:405, 1987.

106. Alexander EL: Neurologic disease in Sjögren's syndrome: mononuclear inflammatory vasculopathy affecting central/peripheral nervous system

and muscle. *Rheum Dis Clin North Am* 19:869, 1993.

107. Escudero D, Latorre P, Codina M, Coll-Canti J, Coll J: Central nervous system disease in Sjögren's syndrome. *Ann Med Intern* 146:239, 1995.

108. Selnes OA, Barry G, Malikow KL, Alexander EL: Cognitive dysfunction in primary Sjögren's syndrome. *Neurology* 35(suppl):179, 1985.

109. Mauch E, Völk C, Kratzsch G, et al: Neurological and neuropsychiatric dysfunction in primary Sjögren's syndrome. *Acta Neurol Scand* 89:31, 1994.

110. Alexander EL, Alexander GE: Aseptic meningoencephalitis in primary Sjögren's syndrome *Neurology* 98:155, 1983.

111. Drachman D: Neurological complications of Werener's granulomatosis. *Arch Neurol* 8:145, 1963.

112. Nishino H, Rubino FA, DeRemee RA, et al: Neurologic involvement in Wegener's granulomatosis: an analysis of 324 consecutive cases at the Mayo Clinic. *Ann Neurol* 33:4, 1993.

113. Wolff SM: Wegener's granulomatosis and midline granuloma, in Petersdorf RG, Adams RD, Braumwald E, et al (eds): *Harrison's Principles of Internal Medicine*, 11th ed. New York, McGraw-Hill 1987, pp 1255-1257.

114. Hamilton CR Jr, Shelley WM, Tumulty PA: Giant cell arteritis: including temporal arteritis and polymyalgia rheumatica. *Medicine* 50:1, 1971.

115. Flynn JA, Hellmann DB: Giant cell arteritis and cerebral vasculitis, in Johnson RT, Griffin JW (eds): *Current Therapy in Neurologic Disease*, 5th ed. St. Louis, Mosby, 1997, pp 214-219.

116. Hall S, Persellin S, Lie JT, et al: The therapeutic impact of temporal artery biopsy. *Lancet* II:1217, 1983.

117. Currier RD, DeJong RN, Bole GG: Pulseless disease: central nervous system manifestations. *Neurology* 4:818, 1954.

118. Ross RS, McKusick VA: Aortic arch syndromes: diminished or absent pulses in arteries arising from arch of aorta. *Arch Intern Med* 92:701, 1953.

119. Hall S, Buchbinder R: Takaysu's arteritis. *Rheum Dis Clin North Am* 16:411, 1990.

120. Tshikawa K: Survival and morbidity after diagnosis of occlusive thromboaortopathy (Takayasu's disease). *Am J Cardiol* 47:1026, 1981.

121. Gilliland BC: Progressive systemic sclerosis (diffuse scleroderma), in Petersdorf RG, Adams RD, Braumwald E, et al (eds): *Harrison's Principles of Internal Medicine*, 11th ed. New York, McGraw-Hill 1987, pp 1428-1432.

122. Piper WN, Helwig EB: Progessive systemic sclerosis. *Arch Dermatol* 72:535, 1955.

123. Binder H, Gerstenbrand F: Scleroderma, in Vinken PJ, Bruyn GW (eds): *Handbook of Clinical Neurology*, vol 39, Part II, North Holland, Amsterdam, 1980, pp 355-378.

124. Arnett EC, Edworthy SM, Bloch DA, et al: The American Rheumatism Association 1987 revised criteria for the classification of rheumatoid arthritis. *Arthritis Rheum* 31:315, 1988.

125. Steiner JW, Gelbloom AJ: Intracranial manifestations of two cases of systemic rheumatoid disease. *Arthritis Rheum* 2:537, 1959.

126. Stevens JC, Cartilidge NEF, Saunders M, et al: Atlantoaxial subluxation and cervical myelopathy in rheumatoid arthritis. *QJMed* 40:391, 1971.

127. Jones MW, Kaufmann JCE: Vertebrobasilar artery insufficiency in rheumatoid atlantoaxial subluxation. *J Neurol Neurosurg Psychiatry* 39:122, 1976.

128. Delamarter RB, Bohlman HH: Postmortem osseous and neuropathologic analysis of the rheumatoid cervical spine. *Spine* 19:2267, 1994.

129. Meyding-Lamande U, Rieke K, Krieaer D, et al: Rare diseases mimicking acute vertebrobasilar artery thrombosis. *J Neurol* 242:335, 1995.

130. American College of Rheumatology ad hoc: Committee on Clinical Guidelines: Guidelines for the management of rheumatoid arthritis. *Arthritis Rheum* 39:713, 1996.

131. International Study Group for Behçet's disease: Criteria for diagnosis of Behçet's disease. *Lancet* 1:1078, 1990.

132. Chajek T, Fainaru M: Behçet's disease. Report of 41 cases and a review of the literature. *Medicine* 54:179, 1975.

133. Pallis CA, Fudge BJ: The neurological complications of Behçet's syndrome. *Arch Neurol Psychol* 75:1, 1955.

134. Kawakita H, Nishimura M, Satoh Y, et al: Neurological aspects of Behçet's disease. A case report and clinico-pathological review of the literature in Japan. *J Neurol Sci* 3:417, 1967.

135. Motomura S, Tabura T, Kuriowa Y: A clinical comparative study of multiple sclerosis and neuro-Behçet's disease. *J Neurol Neurosurg Psychiatry* 43:210, 1980.

136. O'Duffy D, Goldstein N: Neurologic involvement in seven patients with Behçet's disease. *Am J Med* 61:170, 1976.

137. Inaba G: Fifteen year's course of Behçet's disease. *Modern Medicine* 43:240, 1980.

138. Pamir MN, Kansu T, Erengi A, et al: Papilledema in Behçet's syndrome. *Arch Neurol* 38:643, 1981.

139. Wadia N, Williams E: Behçet's syndrome with neurological complications. *Brain* 80:39, 1971.

140. Park-Matsumoto Y-C, Ogawa K, Tazawa T, et al: Mutism developing after bilateral thalamo-capsular lesions by neuro-Behçet disease. *Acta Neurol Scand* 91:297, 1993.

141. Welsh KI, Kerr LA: The immunogenetics of Behçet's disease—do they give an indication of the likely mechanisms of the disease?, in Lehner T, Barnes CG (eds): Recent Advances in Behçet's disease. *Int Cong Ser* 103:3, 1986.

142. Lehner T: The role of a disorder of immunoregulation, associated with herpes simpler type 1 in Behçet's disease, in Lehner T, Barnes CG, (eds): Recent Advances in Behçet's disease. *Int Cong Ser* 103:31, 1986.

143. Vidaller A, Carratala J, Moreno R: Magnetic resonance in neuro-Behçet's disease. *Br J Rheumatol* 27:79, 1988.

144. Edland A, Nyland H, Riise T, Larsen JP: Epidemiology of multiple sclerosis in the county of Vestfold, eastern Norway: incidence and prevalence calculations. *Acta Neurol Scand* 93:104, 1996.

145. Van Ooteghem P, D'Hooghe MB, Vlietinck R, Carton H: Prevalence of multiple sclerosis in Flanders, Belgium. *Neuroepidemiology* 13:220, 1994.

146. Beer S, Kesselring J: High prevalence of multiple sclerosis in Switzerland. *Neuroepidemiology* 13:14, 1994.

147. Poser CM: The epidemiology of multiple sclerosis: a general review. *Ann Neurol* 36(suppl 2): S180, 1994.

148. Johnson MD, Lavin P, Whetsell WO Jr: Fulminant monophasic multiple sclerosis, Marburg's type. *J Neurol Neurosurg Psychiatry* 53:918, 1990.

149. Poser S, Luer W, Bruhn H, Frahm J, Bruck Y, Felgenhauer K: Acute demyelinating disease. Classification and non-invasive diagnosis. *Acta Neurol Scand* 86:579, 1992.

150. Niebler G, Harris T, Davis T, Roos K: Fulminant multiple sclerosis. *Am J Neuroradiol* 13:1547, 1992.

151. Ghawche F, Destee A: Hypothermie et sclerose en plaques. Un cas avec trois episodes de hypothermie transitoire. *Rev Neurol* 146:767, 1990.

152. Grant I: Neuropsychological and psychiatric disturbances in multiple sclerosis, in McDonald WI, Silberberg DH, (eds): *Multiple Sclerosis.* London, Butterworth, 1986, pp 134–152.

153. Krupp LB, Sliwinski M, Masur DM, Friedberg F, Coyle PK: Cognitive functioning and depression in patients with chronic fatigue syndrome and multiple sclerosis. *Arch Neurol* 51:705, 1994.

154. McDonald WI, Sears TA: The effects of experimental demyelination on conduction in the central nervous system. *Brain* 93:583, 1970.

155. Slabassi RJ, Namerow NS, Enns NF: Somatosensory response to stimulus trains in patients with multiple sclerosis. *Electroenceph Clin Neurophysiol* 37:23, 1974.

156. Davis FA, Jacobson S: Altered thermal sensitivity in injured and demyelinated nerve: a possible model of temperature effects in multiple sclerosis. *J Neurol Neurosurg Psychiatry* 34:331, 1971.

157. Schumacher GA, Beebe G, Kibler RF, et al: Problems of experimental trials of therapy in multiple sclerosis. *Ann NY Acad Sci* 122:552, 1965.

158. McAlpine D: Course and prognosis, in McAlpine D, Lumsden CE, Acheson ED (eds): *Multiple Sclerosis: A Reappraisal.* Edinburgh, Churchill-Livingstone, 1972, p 55.

159. Bauer HJ: IMAB-Enquette concerning the diagnostic criteria for multiple sclerosis, in Bauer HJ, Poser S, Ritter G (eds): *Progress in Multiple Sclerosis Research.* Berlin, Springer, 1980, p 55.

160. Rose AS, Ellison GW, Myers LW, et al: Criteria for the clinical diagnosis of multiple sclerosis. *Neurology* 26(suppl 20):22, 1976.

161. McDonald WI, Halliday AM: Diagnosis and classification of multiple sclerosis. *Br Med Bull* 33:4, 1977.

162. Poser CM, Paty DW, Scheinberg L, et al: New diagnostic criteria for the multiple sclerosis. *Ann Neurol* 13:227, 1983.

163. Engel T: A clinical-pathoanatomical study of multiple sclerosis diagnosis. *Acta Neurol Scand* 78:39, 1988.

164. Izquierdo G, Hauw JJ, Lyon-Caen O, et al: Value of multiple sclerosis diagnostic criteria. Seventy autopsy confirmed cases. *Arch Neurol* 42:848, 1985.

165. Abbruzzese G, Gandolfo C, Loeb C: Bolus methylpredisolone versus ACTH in the treatment of multiple sclerosis. *Ital J Neurol* 4:169, 1983.

166. Thompson AJ, Kennard C, Swash M, et al: Relative efficacy of intravenous methylprednisolone and ACTH in the treatment of acute relapse in MS. *Neurology* 39:238, 1989.

167. Rodriguez M, Karnes WE, Bartleson JD, Pineda AA: Plasmapheresis in acute episodes of fulminant CNS inflammatory demyelination. *Neurology* 43:1100, 1993.

168. Scott TF: Neurosarcoidosis: Progress and clinical aspects. *Neurology* 43:8, 1993.

169. Stern BJ, Krumholtz A, Johns C, Scott P, Nissim J: Sarcoidosis and its neurologic manifestations. *Arch Neurol* 42:909, 1985.

170. Manz HJ: Pathobiology of neurosarcoidosis and clinicopathologic correlation. *Can J Neurol Sci* 10:50, 1983.

171. Douglas AC, Maloney AFJ: Sarcoidosis of the central nervous system. *J Neurol Neurosurg Psychiatry* 36:1024, 1973.

172. Lieberman J: *Sarcoidosis.* Orlando, Grune and Stratton 1985, p 26.

173. Wiederholt WC, Saiekert RG: Neurological manifestations of sarcoidosis. *Neurology* 15:1147, 1965.

174. Jefferson M: Sarcoidosis of the nervous system. *Brain* 80:540, 1937.

175. Lehrer GM: Neuropsychiatric manifestations of hypercalcemia. *Arch Neurol Psychiatry* 81:709, 1959.

176. Heck AW, Phillips LH II: Sarcoidosis and the nervous system. *Neurol Clin* 7:641, 1989.

177. Ho SU, Berenberg RA, Kim KS, et al: Sarcoid encephalopathy with diffuse inflammation and focal hydrocephalus shown by sequential CT. *Neurology*, 29:1161, 1979.

178. Thomas PD, Hunninghake GW: Current concepts of the pathogenesis of sarcoidosis. *Ann Rev Respir Dis* 135:747, 1987.

179. Kinnman J, Link H: Intrathecal production of oligoclonal IgM and IgG in CNS sarcoidosis. *Acta Neurol Scand* 69:97, 1989.

180. Nosal A, Schleissner LA, Mishkin FS, Lieberman J: Angiotensin-I-converting enzyme and gallium scan in noninvasive evaluation of sarcoidosis. *Ann Intern Med* 90:328, 1979.

181. Bejar JM, Kerby GR, Ziegler DK, Festoff BW: Treatment of central nervous system sarcoidosis with radiotherapy. *Ann Neurol* 18:253, 1985.

182. Tunkel AR, Kaye D: Neurologic complications of infective endocarditis. *Neurol Clin* 11:419, 1993.

183. Frazee JG, Cahan LD, Winter J: Bacterial intracranial aneurysms. *J Neurosurg* 53:633, 1980.

184. Moskowitz MA, Rosenbaum AE, Tyler HR: Angiographically monitored resolution of cerebral mycotic aneurysms. *Neurology* 24:1103, 1974.

185. Wilson WR, Guiliani ER, Danielson GK, et al: Management of complications of infective endocarditis. *Mayo Clin Proc* 57:162, 1982.

186. Brust JCM, Dickinson PCT, Hughes JEO, Holtzman RNN: The diagnosis and treatment of cerebral microaneurysms. *Ann Neurol* 27:238, 1990.

187. Fredericka DN: Endocarditis and brain abscess due to *Bacteroides oralis. J Infect Dis* 145:918, 1982.

188. Wong D, Chandrarathna AN, Wishnow RM, et al: Clinical implications of large vegetations in infectious endocarditis. *Arch Intern Med* 143:1874.

189. Paschalis C, Puglsey W, John R, Harrison MJG: Rate of cerebral embolic events in relation to antibiotic and anticoagulant therapy in patients with bacterial endocarditis. *Eur Neurol* 30:87, 1990.

190. Pruitt AA, Rubin RH, Karchmer AW, Duncan GW: Neurologic complications of bacterial endocarditis. *Medicine* 57:329, 1978.

191. Delahaye JP, Poncet P, Malquarti V, et al: Cerebrovascular events in infective endocarditis: role of anticoagulation. *Eur Heart J* 11:1074, 1990.

192. Francioli P: Central nervous system complications in infective endocarditis, in Sheld WM, Durack D, Whitley R (eds): *Infections of the Central Nervous System.* New York, Raven Press 1998, p 528.

193. Members of the American College of Chest Physicians/Society of Critical Care Medicine Consensus Conference Committee: American College of Chest Physicians/Society of Critical Care Medicine Consensus Conference: Definitions for sepsis and organ failure and guidelines for innovative therapies in sepsis. *Crit Care Med* 20:864, 1992.

194. Allison RS, Millar JHD: Prevalence and familial incidence of disseminated sclerosis: a report to the Northern Ireland authority on the results of a three-year survey. *Ulster Med* 23(suppl 2):1, 1954.

Part 4

METABOLIC, NUTRITIONAL, AND TOXIC ENCEPHALOPATHIES

Chapter 13

METABOLIC ENCEPHALOPATHIES

G. Bryan Young
Debra A. DeRubeis

As long as the brain is at rest the man enjoys his reason, but the depravement of the brain arises from phlegm and bile, either of which you recognize in this manner: those who are mad from phlegm are quiet, and do not cry out or make noise; but those with bile are vociferous, malignant, and will not be quiet, but are always doing something improper.

Hippocrates[1]

Metabolic encephalopathies are chemical disorders that adversely affect brain function and are not primarily due to structural lesions. For the purposes of this chapter, metabolic disorders are considered to be endogenous conditions. Similar brain dysfunction secondary to drugs or toxins is considered separately in Chap. 16. Brain dysfunction consists of alterations in either alertness or cognitive function. Therefore, the ascending reticular activating system or the thalamocortical complex is affected. Bilateral structural disease of the cerebral hemispheres, e.g., nonconvulsive status epilepticus or multifocal lesions of ischemic, neoplastic, hemorrhagic, or inflammatory nature, may occasionally produce a similar picture. However, these are usually not difficult to rule out clinically or with appropriate investigations.

The clinical features that are characteristic of metabolic encephalopathies are described in Chap. 3. In summary, the pupils, ocular movements, and respirations are relatively spared in most metabolic encephalopathies (the few exceptions are discussed in Chap. 3). As a corollary, when a patient is deeply comatose, yet the above-mentioned functions are spared, one should consider a metabolic or toxic etiology. Certain motor features, especially asterixis, tremor, and multifocal myoclonus, are highly suggestive of a metabolic or toxic encephalopathy.

A simplistic analogy is that of a patient undergoing an anesthetic.[2] Although this "model" has some deficiencies, the following apply:

1. There is a graded response of the brain dysfunction to anesthetic dose or duration, similar to the severity of the metabolic disturbance in the body.

2. The electroencephalogram (EEG) response is initially linear, with increasing slowing and simplicity of rhythms with increasing anesthetic dose/severity of metabolic derangement (see Fig. 13-1).

3. The linearity breaks down with higher anesthetic concentrations, and the EEG develops a discontinuous or generalized burst-suppression pattern (sometimes this may evolve into triphasic waves, or suppression).

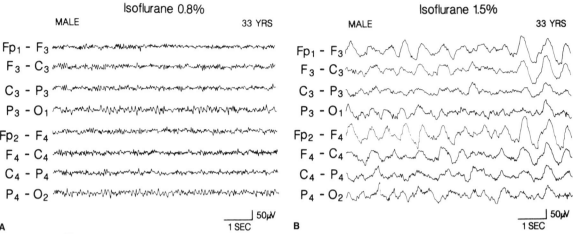

Figure 13-1

The EEG changes of a patient undergoing general anesthesia with halothane. Note the progressive rhythmic slowing and simplification of rhythmic patterns with increasing anesthetic dose. A. This shows only mild slowing of rhythms posteriorly (channels 4 and 8) and faster frequencies anteriorly (channels 1, 2, 5, and 6) at a concentration of 0.8% isoflurane. B. This shows high voltage rhythmic slow waves at 1.5% isoflurane. (From Young et al,[2] with permission.)

4.   The clinical and EEG changes are reversible with removal of the anesthetic or metabolic derangement (see Table 13-1).

The neurophysiologic events are not well defined, and are probably not uniform among different metabolic encephalopathies. However, based on the EEG effects, it appears that synaptic function is affected early in such disorders. It has been shown that for most metabolic encephalopathies and for anesthetics, neuronal energy failure either does not occur or is a very late event. Polysynaptic pathways and complex interactions of various cortical regions are likely affected first, as higher mental functions are the first to be compromised. Thus, cognitive functions such as memory, judgement, attention, and concentration are universally affected as early features. In those conditions that can progress to neuronal death, a final common pathway (discussed in Chap. 15) likely applies.

The biochemical aspects of disorders of brain metabolism are likely to be further clarified with evolving technologies, including molecular biologic techniques, positron emission tomography (PET),

and nuclear magnetic resonance spectroscopy (NMRS) with ^{13}C-labeled isotopes.[3] Increased insights into energy metabolism, substrate utilization, and metabolic pathways should be forthcoming.

The metabolic encephalopathies discussed in this chapter are listed in Table 13-2. Temperature-related encephalopathies, anoxia, nutritional disorders, and toxicology are discussed separately in Chaps. 8, 14, 15, and 16, respectively.

MINERAL, ELECTROLYTE, AND CARBON DIOXIDE DISORDERS

HYPONATREMIA

Definition and Clinical Significance

Hyponatremia, defined as a serum sodium concentration of less than 135 mmol/L, has an incidence of about 1 percent and a prevalence of about 3 percent in inpatients in general hospitals.[4] Hyponatremia constitutes the most common electrolyte disturbance and is associated with a number of diseases.

Table 13-1

Metabolic encephalopathies related to the anesthetic model

Etiology	Additional features	Reversibility of burst-suppression or suppression
Anoxia	Epileptiform activity; alpha/theta coma[a] usually unfavorable	Not reversible; with advanced anoxia (periodicity and epileptiform activity are also unfavorable)[b]
Drug intoxication	Some may produce epileptiform activity; a mixture of beta + theta/delta suggestive of barbiturate or benzodiazepine overdose	Completely reversible
Hepatic failure	Triphasic waves[c]	Not reversible (older literature); ?potentially reversible if liver function improves or with detoxification
Reye syndrome	14 and 6 positive spikes in 50% (controversial significance)	Probably not reversible (dependent on damage from brain swelling and/or hypoglycemia)
Uremic encephalopathy	Triphasic waves[c] or epileptiform activity in some; photic sensitivity	Probably reversible
Septic encephalopathy	Triphasic waves[c] in some	Potentially reversible if patient survives multiple organ failure
Dialytic encephalopathy	Epileptiform activity (gen spike and wave)	Not reversible in advanced cases
Porphyria	Focal features, e.g., spikes, suppression occasionally seen—usually transient	Largely reversible; EEG may be slow to improve
Hypothyroidism	Low amplitude	Should resolve, except in cretinism
Wernicke's encephalopathy	May show sharp and slow wave complexes; periods of suppression in very advanced cases	EEG may improve; many patients with severe amnesia and ataxia
Addison disease	Majority are normal; others show diffuse slowing	Resolves, especially with corticosteroids
Hypercalcemia	May have triphasic waves or FIRDA[d]	Rare, resolves
Hypoglycemia	May show epileptiform activity; periodic complexes	Partly reversible
Hypothermia	Temperature dependent: no change till < 30°C	Burst-suppression at 20–22°C; suppression with $T < 18°C$ completely reversible

[a] Burst-suppression pattern after cardiac arrest is associated with a 96 percent mortality rate; recordings should be done >24 h postarrest and repeated to help establish prognosis.[454]

[b] Alpha or theta coma patterns differ from the patterns for those frequencies seen normally in that they are more widespread, often more prominent frontally, and are unreactive to stimulation.[450–453] The particular frequencies cover a wider spectrum (e.g. 6 to 12 Hz) rather than the narrow frequency band seen normally. Such patterns have been described in anoxic-ischemic encephalopathy, brainstem lesions, and drug intoxications, expecially with barbiturates. The author has also seen it with hydrogen sulfide intoxication. In the intoxications, the prognosis is favorable. In anoxic-ischemic encephalopathy or brainstem lesions, these patterns are usually, but not invariably, associated with a poor prognosis for recovery of full conscious awareness. The alpha-theta pattern coma is unstable and usually changes to more definitive prognostic pattern in 5 to 6 days from coma onset.

[c] Note: triphasic waves were originally thought to be specific for hepatic encephalopathy.[446] However, they can occur in a variety of metabolic encephalopathies, septic encephalopathies, and neurodegenerative conditions.[447,448] In the context of an acute alteration in alertness, however, they are highly suggestive of a metabolic encephalopathy. In the author's experience, hepatic or renal failure or septic encephalopathy are the most common underlying etiologies in this situation.[449]

[d] FIRDA = frontal intermittent rhythmic delta activity.

Source: Reproduced from Young et al,[2] with permission.

Table 13-2
Classification of metabolic encephalopathies (as discussed in text)

Fluid and electrolyte disorders	Endocrinopathies (continued)
Hyponatremia	Acute adrenal failure
Hypernatremia	Pituitary apoplexy
Hypocalcemia	*Vital organ failure*
Hypercalcemia	Hepatic encephalopathy
Hypomagnesemia	Acute hepatic failure
Hypermagnesemia	Chronic hepatic failure
Hypophosphatemia	Uremia
Hypocapnia	Acute renal failure
Hypercapnia	Chronic renal failure
	Complications of treatment
Endocrinopathies	Pancreatic encephalopathy
Thyroid disorders	*Hereditary metabolic disorders*
Myxedema (hypothyroidism)	Porphyria
Hyperthyroidism	Mitochondrial disorders
Hashimoto's thyroiditis	MELAS
Hypoglycemia	Leigh disease
Hyperglycemia	

Classification

Hyponatremia reflects water balance, which determines the osmolality of the plasma, and is classified into four groups, isovolemic, hypovolemic, hypervolemic, and iso-osmolar (see Table 13-3).

Most cases of hyponatremia are associated with hypo-osmolality of the blood or a relative excess of solvent to solute. This is associated with the kidneys not excreting a dilute urine and can be due to (1) inappropriate secretion of antidiuretic hormone (ADH), which can relate to a number of disorders; (2) insufficient glomerular filtrate reaching distal parts of the nephron, either related to decreased glomerular filtration rate or to increased proximal tubular reabsorption of fluid and sodium; or (3) defective sodium transport in the diluting parts of the nephron, or excessive water reabsorption.

Hypo-osmolar hyponatremia can be divided according to volume status. Hypovolemic hyponatremia may be caused by loss of fluid or blood through the gastrointestinal tract, urinary tract (often with secretion of atrial natriuretic factor or loss of aldosterone effect), and skin, or blood loss from various sites, or from third space sequestration (e.g., ascites with hypoproteinemia may be associated with a contraction of the vascular volume). This stimulates the secretion of ADH as volume replacement has precedence over osmolality. Normo- or hypervolemic hyponatremia is usually related to inappropriate secretion of antidiuretic hormone, or drugs that cause this effect.

Artifactual hyponatremia is associated with normal osmolality. It may be caused by hyperlipidemia, hyperglycemia, or certain intoxications. In hyperlipidemia, lipids occupy volume in the plasma as if they formed a compartment. If this compartment is excluded, the osmolality or serum sodium of the remaining component is normal.

Clinical Features

Hyponatremia itself, if symptomatic, causes a metabolic encephalopathy consisting of inappropriate behavior, confusion, headache, speech problems, lethargy, vomiting, tremor, weakness, malaise, and seizures.[5] The latter are usually generalized convulsions. Muscle twitches and cramps may occur. The patient is much more likely to be

Table 13-3

Hyponatremia

Hypovolemic hyponatremia
(combined sodium and water deficiency)

A. Extrarenal losses: gastrointestinal, skin, third space sequestration (e.g., ascites), skin (sweating, burns)
B. Renal losses
    1. Renal disease: chronic renal failure, salt-wasting tubular disease
    2. Diuretic excess
    3. Osmotic diuresis: diabetes mellitus, iatrogenic (e.g., mannitol)
    4. Mineralocorticoid deficiency: Addison disease, hypoadrenalism

Isovolemic hyponatremia
(no significant expansion of extracellular compartment)

A. Nausea, pain, emotion: temporary impairment of water diuresis
B. Psychogenic polydipsia
C. Endocrine (glucocorticoid deficiency, hypothyroidism)
D. SIADH
E. Drugs
    1. Drugs that potentiate ADH action: clofibrate, NSAIDs,[a] ADH analogues, cyclophosphamide
    2. Drugs that stimulate ADH release: vincristine, carbamazepine, narcotics, barbiturates
    3. Drugs that potentiate ADH action and stimulate release: thiazide diuretics, chlorpromazine, ADH analogues
F. Essential: "sick cell syndrome"

Hypervolemic hyponatremia
(expansion of extracellular compartment: edema)

A. Hepatic failure
B. Cardiac failure
C. Nephrotic syndrome

Without plasma hypo-osmolality

A. Osmotic: hyperglycemia, mannitol
B. Artifactual: hyperlipidemia, hyperproteinemia

[a] NSAIDs = nonsteroidal anti-inflammatory drugs.
Source: Modified from Levinski NG, Fluids and electrolytes, in Braunwald E, Isselbacher KJ, Petersdorf RG, Wilson JD, Martin JB, Fauci AS (eds): *Harrison's Principles of Internal Medicine*, 11th ed. New York, McGraw-Hill, 1987, p 199.

symptomatic if the hyponatremia develops acutely or subacutely and if the serum sodium concentration is less than 125 mmol/L. In some chronic cases, the mental changes may be due to the underlying condition, e.g., hypothyroidism, rather than the hyponatremia.

Occasionally, patients may present with focal findings, such as hemiparesis, monoparesis, or ataxia. This may reflect an underlying lesion; the signs may disappear when the hyponatremia is corrected. Cranial nerves are usually not affected.

Risk factors for development of symptomatic hyponatremia include: age over 75 years (and the use of certain drugs, e.g., thiazide diuretics in this age group), female sex, below average body weight,

the rate and extent of fall of serum sodium concentration, and the presence of underlying serious illnesses.[6,7]

Pathophysiology

A decrease in the osmolality of the plasma creates an osmotic gradient between the blood compartment and the cells of the body, including those of the brain. Unless the brain decreases its osmolality, there will be a shift of water across the cell membranes, causing the cells to swell.

The brain *can* adjust to hyponatremia, thereby maintaining intracellular volume, by reducing its osmolality.[7] Powerful mechanisms allow for "regulatory volume decrease" in acute hypo-osmolality.[8] Efflux of potassium and chloride ions out of neurons and glia begins between 3 and 24 h from the introduction of hyponatremia.[8] This is followed by efflux organic osmolites. Creatine and N-acetylaspartate begin to exude after about 2 days. This is followed by expulsion of taurine, glutamate, glutamine, aspartate, gamma-aminobutyric acid (GABA) and myoinositol. The transduction of cellular signals that allow these responses to cell swelling are still not fully identified. Current theory is that volume or stretch sensors may involve the cytoskeleton that has connections with the cell membrane and membrane channels.[8] Thus, the opening of specific stretch-sensitive ion channels can occur fairly quickly.

If hyponatremia develops quickly, the brain does not have time to adjust by reducing its idiogenic osmoles. With acute brain swelling, compensation for the increased volume can be accommodated only by up 30 to 50 mL (Fig. 3-17). After this, the swelling causes an increase in intracranial pressure (ICP). Such swelling can be severe enough to lead to raised intracranial pressure, reduced cerebral perfusion pressure, and brain ischemia. Herniation and respiratory arrest may occur with massive swelling.[9]

The ionic composition of the brain is altered and changes in neurotransmitter function follow. Acute hyponatremia with hypo-osmolality causes partial depolarization of nerve cells, related to the extrusion of potassium, and reduces the threshold for the generation of action potentials and seizures.

The main effects of acute hyponatremia, however, appear to relate to cellular swelling. In rabbits, the neurologic effects of acute hyponatremia begin to resolve only when the brain, and therefore cellular, volume is returned to normal.[10]

Pathology

Four patterns of pathologic outcomes and associated lesions have been described with acute hyponatremia[11]:

- Group A: severe cerebral edema with respiratory arrest, cerebral edema, and tentorial

herniation. This syndrome has been noted in the early postoperative period in young, previously healthy women.[12] The liberal use of intravenous fluids and narcotic analgesics, which can increase retention of water, and repeated vomiting may be relevant contributors. Some patients had the unusual simultaneous combination of diabetes mellitus and insipidus, presumably a late complication of severe brain swelling.[13] Death or permanent disability is the outcome in the majority of patients. This appears to be a rare scenario,[14] but a potentially reversible one if recognized early and treated vigorously.

- Group B: elevation of serum sodium concentration by greater than 25 mmol/L (25 meq/L) during the first 48 h of therapy results in demyelinating lesions with cerebral ischemia. Recovery can occur, but neurologic sequelae are common.

- Group C: respiratory arrest, central diabetes insipidus, hyperglycemia, or spontaneous overcorrection of low serum sodium leads to diffuse demyelinating lesions. Pituitary dysfunction and oculomotor nerve damage are common. There have been no reported survivors.

- Group D: appropriate therapy prior to respiratory arrest leads to a normal brain. Pontine and extrapontine lesions occur only in patients with severe systemic illnesses, such as liver disease, alcoholism, Hodgkin disease, or other malignancy, burns or sepsis.[15]

Management

The management of hyponatremia depends on the underlying cause and the neurologic complications exhibited by the patient. The patient's hyponatremia should be classified into a broad category of hypovolemic, normovolemic, hypervolemic, or normo-osmolar. Then, the specific underlying disorder should be determined using clinical and laboratory means as described in standard medical texts.

Correction of the underlying disorder usually corrects the hyponatremia. Asymptomatic patients with hypotonic hyponatremia who are hypovolemic or normovolemic are treated with fluid restriction to 1.0 L/day and will correct at a maximum rate of 1.5 mmol/L per day.[11]

The management of acutely symptomatic patients is controversial. However, those with seizures probably require more active treatment than water restriction alone.[16,17] In these extreme and rare circumstances, prompt therapy of hypertonic saline with a loop diuretic should be administered such that the correction is no faster than 0.5 to 1.0 mmol/L per hour or 20 mmol/L in the first day. Electrolytes need to be checked hourly, with prompt reporting facilities.

If possible, it is best not to correct the serum sodium too quickly or to normal values. It is important to give just enough treatment to get the serum sodium concentration in the range of 125–130 mmol/L and not to strive for prompt normalization of serum electrolytes. This latter might put the patient at greater risk for central nervous system (CNS) demyelination than the rapidity of sodium elevation.[16] In both chronically and acutely ill humans, rapid correction can result in pontine and extrapontine myelinolysis. However, there is considerable variation in susceptibility.[18] Retrospective studies have led to the recommendation that myelinolysis can be avoided by limiting the rate of rise to less than 12 mmol/L in the first 24 h or 25 mmol/L in the first 48 h.[19] However, even with these guidelines, some patients develop demyelination.[18] Karp and Laureno[18] suggest striving for less than 10 meq/L for the first 24 h and less than 21 meq/L over the first 48 h. Studies on acutely hyponatremic animals showed that an increase of more than 12 mmol/L per day may produce central pontine myelinolysis (CPM) if this rate is continued for 2 to 3 days.[20]

The matter is still shrouded with controversy. Water restriction, if too vigorous, may be associated with complications. In an experimental study, Ayus and colleagues found that if the sodium rose to normonatremic values within 24 h with water restriction, there were scattered brain lesions, including neuronal necrosis and myelin damage, but not the typical features of CPM.[21] Treatment of hypovolemic shock may be necessary and may force a more rapid rise in osmolality than

planned. The use of half-normal saline might be considered in this circumstance.

Central Pontine Myelinolysis

This was first described by Adams and colleagues in three alcoholic, malnourished patients.[22] Since then, it has been described in the central region of the basis pontis, as well as in extrapontine sites.[23] The incidence is estimated to be 0.17 to 0.28 percent of general autopsy patients.[23,24] All cases have developed in systemically ill, hospitalized patients. Most have been in adults between 30 and 70 years of age, but cases have been described in children as young as 3 years.[25]

Clinical Picture and Investigations

Almost all patients have impairment of consciousness, ranging from confusion to coma, in the early phase.[18] The onset may be subacute, over several days. These features may be preceded by convulsive seizures, vomiting, clumsiness, or mental changes including hallucinations, restlessness, confusion, and obtundation.[5] Mental changes may reflect extrapontine involvement. Corticospinal and corticobulbar signs (pseudobulbar palsy) may be found in noncomatose patients; this usually relates to the classic lesion in the basis pontis.[26] The upper limbs are commonly more involved than the lower. Less commonly, bilateral sixth nerve palsies, dystonia, or rigidity may occur. If the tegmentum of the brainstem is involved, the pupils may be dilated, unreactive, or hyporeactive. Lesions of the descending sympathetic tracts result in bilateral miosis. Occasionally, conjugate gaze palsy or ocular bobbing is found.[18] Large pontine lesions produce a complete "locked-in syndrome" (see Chap. 2). If the lesion is small and centered in the midpons, it may not produce any clinical symptoms.

Imaging studies reveal radiolucent lesions on computed tomography (CT) scans and areas of increased signal on T2-weighted magnetic resonance imaging (MRI) scans (see Fig. 13-2). Brainstem auditory evoked responses may show

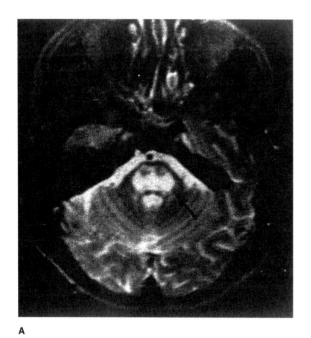

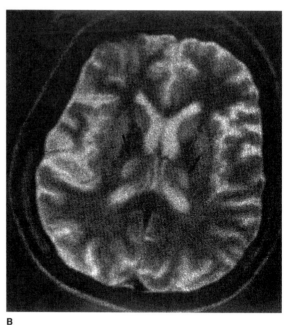

A

B

Figure 13-2

Central and extrapontine myelinolysis. A. This shows large, symmetric areas of increased signal in the basis pontis (arrow) *on a T2-weighted MRI scan. B. This shows thalamic lesions* (arrows) *in extrapontine myelinolysis. (From Karp and Laureno,[18] with permission.)*

evidence of a pontine lesion while the imaging tests are still normal.[27]

Pathogenesis

Early reports emphasized the association of CPM with alcoholism, dehydration, or serious systemic illnesses.[22,23] Indeed, this appears to be the case; other cases have occurred in patients with liver disease, sepsis, burns, or underlying malignancies. Within the past 20 years, it has been recognized that, in most cases, CPM occurred following fairly prompt correction of hyponatremia at rates greater than 20 to 30 mmol/L over 3 days or more than 12 mmol/L per day.[18] Further support came from experimental work in which lesions identical to CPM were induced in animals made hyponatremic with dextrose and water plus ADH, and then given hypertonic saline.[28,29]

McKee and colleagues[24] showed that central

pontine myelinolysis can occur in burns patients who terminally developed hypernatremia, having been normonatremic and normo-osmolar earlier in their course. Thus, it would appear that it is a sudden rise in serum sodium concentration or osmolality that is important and that risk is not restricted to the hyponatremic population.

Several hypotheses have been advanced to explain the demyelination. Norenberg proposed osmotic damage to the capillary endothelium, exposing the brain to myelinotoxic factors in the plasma and/or vasogenic edema.[30] Plasminogen in the plasma could become activated, forming plasmin that would, in turn, hydrolyze the myelin. It has been suggested that the edema itself may cause demyelination.[31] This led to further speculation that white matter tracts in the pons were compressed within the grid-like arrangement of fibers.[32]

Norenberg[30] also proposed that patients with systemic illness may not be able to increase cellular idiogenic osmoles to match the changing osmolality of the plasma during the treatment of hyponatremia.

Pathology

In the original cases described by Adams et al,[22] the lesions occupied the center of the basis pontis and consisted of myelin loss but with sparing of axons and neurons. There was little inflammation. Extrapontine lesions occur in about 10 percent of cases and involve various structures, including the internal capsule, thalamus, cerebellum, lower layers of the cerebral cortex (myelinated nerve fibers within these structures), and adjacent white matter.[33]

Management and Outcome

To prevent CPM, it is best that rapid correction of hyponatremia should be avoided provided that the patient is not in an extreme situation, e.g., severe hyponatremia with convulsions. Sterns et al[19] recommend that serum sodium level be corrected at a rate no faster than 12 mmol/L per day, primarily by water restriction and discontinuation of thiazide diuretics.

Central pontine myelinolysis can be diagnosed clinically, but it is probably best to perform an MRI scan to define the lesions and to differentiate CPM from basilar artery occlusion. Evoked responses and EEG are abnormal, but do not significantly contribute to management.

There is no specific effective therapy for CPM. Supportive care, including intubation and early tracheostomy, is often necessary.

Corticosteroids do not help.[18] Improvement may occur, usually beginning in the first weeks of the illness; most patients are left with significant residua and some show no improvement.[18,34]

HYPERNATREMIA

Definition

Hypernatremia is defined as a rise in serum sodium concentration above 145 mmol/L. Hypernatremia results from a deficit of solvent (water) relative to solute (sodium), and indicates a general hypertonicity of body fluids. Hypernatremia can be divided into acute and chronic categories. Only acute hypernatremia has established primary effects on the CNS. It is difficult-to-impossible to separate chronic hypernatremia from its associated diseases; the latter are usually more likely than the hypernatremia to affect neurologic function.

Pathophysiology

Thirst and the secretion of ADH are two powerful homeostatic mechanisms that normally maintain osmolality of the blood and, by osmotic equilibrium, all the body fluids. Thirst is the most powerful mechanism. Hypernatremia may occur in the face of excessive loss of free water, decreased water intake with immobility, or impaired consciousness that impairs satisfaction of the strong thirst drive. With an increase in serum osmolality, water shifts from the intracellular to the extracellular compartment. Therefore, net rises in serum sodium or osmolality reflect large losses of body water.

Table 13-4 lists the main causes of hypernatremia. Patients who suffer hypothalamic damage and coma are at risk for hypernatremia. Some conscious individuals with hypothalamic damage to their osmoreceptors may not be sensitive to hypernatremia. Hypernatremia from ADH deficiency or excessive mineralocorticoid activity produces only modest elevation of serum sodium. The former may cause significant hypernatremia only if the patient cannot satisfy thirst needs. Conscious individuals drink 15 L of water or more per day to compensate for renal losses. Insensible losses of water from skin and lungs may reach several liters per day in cases of extreme heat, fever, burns, or hyperventilation. Patients who lose both sodium and water usually have contraction of blood volume. Water losses exceed those of sodium in sweating and osmotic diuresis, so hypernatremia is the rule. Exceptionally, hypernatremia results from excessive sodium administration. This has happened inadvertently with infant formula preparations and in the preparation

Table 13-4
Causes of hypernatremia

A. Water loss	B. Water loss with sodium loss
1. Extrarenal	1. Extrarenal
a. Skin: insensible perspiration	a. Skin: sweat
b. Lungs	2. Renal
2. Renal	a. Osmotic diuresis
a. Diabetes insipidus (CNS or nephrogenic)	C. Sodium gain
3. Hypothalamic dysfunction	a. Excessive sodium administration
	b. Adrenal hyperfunction (hyperaldosteronism, Cushing syndrome)

Source: Modified from Levinski NG, Fluids and electrolytes, in Braunwald E, Isselbacher KJ, Petersdorf RG, Wilson JD, Martin JB, Fauci AS (eds): *Harrison's Principles of Internal Medicine*, 11th ed. New York, McGraw-Hill, 1987, pp 198–208.

of hemodialysis solutions, or with excessive administration of hypertonic saline solutions to comatose patients. Occasionally, vigorous correction of metabolic acidosis by the administration of sodium bicarbonate is responsible.[45]

Central Nervous System Complications of Hypernatremia

Acute and subacute hypernatremia with neurologic manifestations occur predominantly in very young infants and the elderly. However, it may occur at any age, especially in the presence of a net loss of water, iatrogenic or self-induced salt loading, and obtundation or inability to express needs or to satisfy thirst.

Neurologic signs and symptoms relate to loss of volume of cells in the CNS, as brain cell membranes are highly permeable to water, allowing shifts to follow osmotic gradients. Potent homeostatic mechanisms prevent cell shrinkage by allowing "regulatory volume increases" of neurons and glia, even in the face of acute hyperosmolality.[35] Within minutes, activation of a "cotransporter" causes an influx of sodium, potassium, and chloride ions into cells.[35] About 10 h later, there is an increase in organic osmolites, especially myoinositol, glutamate, glutamine, and taurine.[35] Myoinositol makes up much of the compensatory increase in osmolality through increased production of a sodium-dependent cotransporter messenger RNA (mRNA).[35] The increase in organic compounds

offsets some of the electrolyte imbalance that can alter neuronal functioning, e.g., seizures.[35]

From the above, it follows that because the brain adjusts its idiogenic osmoles to maintain cellular volume, only very acute hypernatremia causes a loss of brain volume and neurologic complications, including lethargy, delirium, stupor, or coma.[36] Encephalopathic patients show increased muscular tone, probably paratonic rigidity. Brain shrinkage may be accompanied by tearing of bridging veins running from the cerebral cortex to the superior sagittal sinus, creating subdural hematomas.[37] Capillary and venous congestion and bleeding, with multiple microscopic hemorrhages, and macroscopic subcortical intracerebral and subarachnoid hemorrhages have been described.[39] Furthermore, venous thrombosis, including the superior sagittal sinus, has also been described in the context of acute hypernatremia.[39]

Rarely, CPM can occur with the acute development of hypernatremia, in the context of severe systemic illness (see "Hyponatremia" above).[40]

Seizures mainly occur during the rehydration phase of patients with chronic hypernatremia, presumably due to acute osmotic swelling of cells following the administration of fluids that are lower in osmolality than the patient's sera and brain.[41] Patients with elevated serum urea, or acidosis are especially at risk for seizures during rehydration.[41] Seizures are sometimes related to the above-mentioned vascular complications.[42,43]

Table 13-6
Causes of hypercalcemia

1. Disruption of normal bone-extracellular fluid equilibrium
   a. Metastatic tumor
   b. Multiple myeloma
   c. Lymphoma
   d. Hyperthyroidism
   e. Immobilization in a young individual or those with underlying disease, e.g., Paget disease
2. Exessive parathyroid hormone
   a. Primary hyperparathyroidism
   b. Non parathyroid-tumor producing parathormone-like substance, e.g., lung, breast, kidney, etc
   c. Lithium therapy
   d. Familial hypocalciuric hypercalcemia
3. Excess vitamin D
   a. Hypervitaminosis D
   b. Sarcoidosis (increased formation of 1,25-dihydrolecalciferol)
   c. Idiopathic hypercalcemia of childhood
4. Other
   a. Adrenal insufficiency
   b. Thiazide administration
   c. Milk-alkali syndrome
   d. Hypervitaminosis A

concentration of calcium and associated medical conditions. Mental status abnormalities commonly occur with serum calcium concentrations above 14 mg/dL (3.2 mmol/L; meq/L) and consist of behavioral changes (ranging from personality changes to severe organic psychosis) and confusion, progressing to lethargy, stupor, and coma, with clinical features of a diffuse or bihemispheric encephalopathy.[54] Convulsions occasionally occur. Severe hypercalcemia with impaired consciousness is more common in cancer patients than in those with hyperparathyroidism. Ocular palsies, including internuclear ophthalmoplegia, and muscular wasting, weakness and areflexia have been associated with hyperparathyroidism.[55] The association is not necessarily cause-and-effect, but, in one study, a patient with this constellation improved with removal of the parathyroid adenoma and another had hemorrhagic lesions in the anterior horns of the spinal cord, as has been described with experimental animals with iatrogenic hyperparathyroidism.[55]

Commonly associated problems include marked dehydration, abdominal pains, renal calculi, and metabolic bone disease. Renal insufficiency (either prerenal, renal, or obstructive uropathy) may add to the acute picture.

Laboratory Features

Ionized calcium is the physiologically active component of extravascular calcium. Calcium is largely protein bound, but the concentration of the ionized unbound portion is 1.16 to 1.32 mmol/L. In hypoproteinemia, it is important to correct for serum albumin concentration or to obtain an ionized calcium concentration.

Management

Severe, life-threatening hypercalcemia should be diagnosed from a combination of the clinical and laboratory features. It is important to sort out the underlying cause and to treat it, if possible.[56] The decision to treat should be based on the patient's

Diagnosis

Serum electrolyte determination establishes the presence of hypernatremia. The cause should be apparent from the clinical setting.

The EEG changes are nonspecific, consisting of diffuse slowing that reverses after uncomplicated correction. Interictal epileptiform discharges are not seen in acute or chronic hypernatremia in the absence of vascular complications.[44]

Management

Calculations of water deficit should be based on total body water, which equals about 60 percent of body weight in nonobese patients. If there is an associated volume deficit, i.e., combined water and sodium loss, replacement should begin with normal or 0.9 saline solution. Volume deficits must be replaced first.[45] Only profound acidosis, with pH less than 7.15, should be treated with sodium bicarbonate.[46] If the neurologic syndrome of acute hypertonicity predominates, replacement should start with half-normal or 0.45% saline. It is best to avoid decreases of plasma osmolality of greater than 2 mosmol/L per hour.[45] Pure glucose solutions should be avoided, as the brain will not have time to adjust to the resultant shift of water into the intracellular compartment. This will likely result in coma, convulsions, and acute brain swelling from cytogenic edema. Such complications are much more likely if the hypernatremia has been established for some time (e.g., days to weeks). Serum electrolytes should be monitored every 2 to 4 h during acute therapy.

Along with the above measures, the underlying disease process should be sought and treated. Excessive losses of water should be corrected. This often involves changes of medication and correction of hyperthermia.

HYPOCALCEMIA

Calcium exists in the plasma in three forms: an ionized or unbound portion (normally 50 percent of total), a protein-bound fraction (40 percent) and a chelated component (10 percent). The ionized portion is physiologically active and homeostatically regulated.[47]

Hypocalcemia is defined as a serum calcium concentration of <8.15 mg/dL (2.12 mmol/L). About 10 percent of patients in intensive care units (ICUs) have hypocalcemia, following correction for serum albumin levels and ionized calcium concentrations.[48] A considerably smaller proportion is symptomatic.

Pathogenesis

The ionized portion can be altered by a change in pH; for example, with acidosis, the protein binding is lessened and the percentage free fraction is increased. Conversely, in respiratory alkalosis, the protein binding is increased and the free fraction is less, sometimes producing tetany.

Calcium homeostasis is regulated by secretion of parathyroid hormone (PTH). The parathyroid glands are sensitive to the plasma concentration of ionized calcium; secretion is prompt if the calcium concentration falls. The PTH causes increased reabsorption of calcium from the kidney and gastrointestinal tract, as well as increased mobilization of calcium from bone. A component of this is the PTH-mediated renal conversion of 25- to 1,25-hydroxyvitamin D. A deficiency of either PTH or vitamin D can produce hypocalcemia. Parathyroid hormone secretion is inhibited by severe hypo- or hypermagnesemia. Table 13-5 provides a classification of the major causes of hypocalcemia, with emphasis on patients in ICUs.

Extracellular calcium ions have a stabilizing effect on the neuronal membrane. When reduced in concentration, the membrane is hyperexcitable because of this membrane effect and the decrease in calcium-mediated potassium conductance.

Intracellularly, calcium is required for the activity of many enzymes and in the maintenance of the integrity of cells.[49] In hypoparathyroidism, the concentration of intracellular calcium is reduced by 10 percent in the cerebral cortex, but by about 35 percent in the white matter.[49]

Table 13-5

Causes of hypocalcemia

Category	Specific cause	Mechanism
Hypoparathyroidism	Postsurgical	Reduced PTH secretion
	Autoimmune disease	Reduced PTH secretion
	Infiltrative (e.g., cancer, hemochromatosis, sarcoid)	Reduced PTH secretion
	Irradiation	Reduced PTH secretion
	Severe hypomagnesemia	Inhibits PTH secretion
Vitamin D deficiency	Inadequate intake	Decreased formation of 25 or
	Severe liver or kidney disease	1,25-hydroxyvitamin D
Acute complexing or sequestration of calcium	Acute pancreatitis	Sequestration of ionized calcium
	Rhabdomyolysis	in an acute situation
	Massive tumor lysis	(PTH secretion cannot
	Phosphate infusion	compensate)
	Toxic shock syndrome	
	Acute severe illness	
	Alkalosis	
Increased osteoblastic activity	Hungry bone disease	Postparathyroidectomy
	Osteoblastic metastases	Prostate or breast cancer
Drugs		
Anticalcemic	Biphosphonates	
	Plicamycin	
	Calcitonin	
	Gallium nitrate	
	Phosphate	
Antineoplastic agents	Asparaginase	
	Doxorubicin	
	Cytosine arabinoside	
	WR2721	
	Cisplatin	
Others	Ketoconazole	
	Pentamidine	
	Foscarnet	

Abbreviation: PTH = parathyroid hormone.

Clinical Features

Although the threshold for neurologic symptoms is not well defined, life-threatening complications frequently develop when the ionized portion falls to less than 2 mg/dL (0.5 mmol/L).

Seizures, usually of the generalized convulsive type, are the main complication of acute, severe hypocalcemia.[50] They are more likely to occur in patients with pre-existing seizure disorders. Mental changes include depression, agitation, hallucinations, and psychosis, but these are nonspecific. Tetany with carpopedal spasm may occur, along with muscle spasms and cramps, paresthesiae, and weakness.

The most important clinical signs are those of neuromuscular irritability: increased deep tendon reflexes and positive Chvostek's and Trousseau's signs. Pseudotumor cerebri with papilledema may complicate hypoparathyroidism.

Many of the classic clinical signs and symptoms of hypocalcemia may be absent or blunted in the ICU because of the use of drugs with paralyzing, sedating, and antiepileptic properties.

Laboratory Tests

Most hospital and private laboratories report the total serum calcium concentration; this comprises the protein-bound, free ionized, and complexed forms. The normal total serum calcium concentration is 8.5 to 10.5 mg/dL (2.12 to 2.62 mmol/L). The concentration of calcium varies with the serum albumin; as a rule of thumb, for each 1.0 g/L decrease in albumin, the serum calcium drops by 0.8 mg/dL (0.02 mmol/L). The normal ionized serum calcium is 4.1 to 5.1 mg/dL (1.02 to 1.27 mmol/L). One can estimate the ionized calcium under most conditions on regular wards. However, in many ICU situations, e.g., rapid chelation by blood transfusions, rhabdomyolysis, or pancreatitis, the extent of protein binding varies unpredictably; it is important to measure the ionized serum calcium.

Management

All patients with signs or symptoms of hypocalcemia should be treated. Patients with seizures and impaired consciousness require emergency treatment. Etiology-specific therapy is ideal.

Emergency management of hypocalcemia involves the prompt administration of calcium gluconate. This is given as 10 to 20 mL of 10% calcium gluconate, containing 93 mg of elemental calcium, administered intravenously over 10 min. A more rapid infusion may cause cardiac irregularity. A continuous infusion can follow: an infusion of 15 mg/kg will raise the serum calcium by 2 to 3 mg/dL; 11 ampoules are required to achieve this for a 70-kg man.[51]

Chronic management requires correction of the underlying cause. In the case of hypoparathyroidism, lifetime supplementation is necessary. The mainstay of treatment is vitamin D. Orally administered, elemental calcium supplements, e.g., 1 to 1.5 g/day of elemental calcium in the form of calcium carbonate, citrate, lactate, gluconate, or glubionate, are usually required as well. In malabsorption syndromes, there may be malabsorption and deficiency of vitamin D itself. Large doses of vitamin D may be required, leading to a risk of vitamin D intoxication.

Hypocalcemia due to magnesium deficiency does not respond to calcium supplementation alone, but does recover following magnesium replacement. As a corollary, it is generally wise to measure the serum magnesium whenever hypocalcemia is found, and to correct any deficiency.

HYPERCALCEMIA

Definition

A significant increase in serum calcium conce_____ tion, sufficient to cause alteration of central ne_____ function, is fairly common in certain popul_____ e.g., 5 percent of patients with cancer. Hyp_____ mia has a prevalence of 0.5 percent of hos_____ patients.[52]

Pathogenesis

Table 13-6 gives a list of causes of hyp_____ Severe hypercalcemia is most comm_____ malignancy or hyperparathyroidisr_____ (less frequently) by sarcoidosis, mil_____ drome, and adrenal insufficiency. In_____ the main mechanisms are the _____ parathyroid-related peptide by th_____ malignant bone destruction itself.[5]

Calcium plays a vital role in _____ release and in the activation_____ processes that result from neurc_____ well as in electrical stabiliza_____ membranes. A high extracellul_____ calcium decreases membran_____ reduces its excitability.

Early generalized weak_____ relate to reduced neuromusc_____

Clinical Features

The severity of neurologi_____ value and the acuity c_____

anticipated quality of life and personal preferences, and the diagnosis and prognosis of the underlying cause (often cancer). Hypercalcemia secondary to parathyroid adenoma, however, can be cured with surgery.

Once a decision to treat has been made, it is usually best not to rapidly correct the hypercalcemia. The first step is to correct dehydration or effect volume replacement with intravenous saline. Usually, potassium supplements are also needed. Subsequent specific treatment involves the correction of hypercalcemia over the next 24 to 48 h.

A loop diuretic and further infusion of saline, after intravascular volume is adequate, enhance renal clearance of calcium. An intravenous biphosphonate drug (e.g., pamidronate or clodronate) is currently considered to be the drug of choice.[57] Plicamycin (mithramycin), which inhibits bone resorption, is often effective, but has significant dose and dose-duration toxic effects on the liver, bone marrow, coagulation system, and kidneys. Gallium nitrate can be used as an alternative to plicamycin. Corticosteroids and calcitonin usually have modest or transient effect, at best, in controlling the hypercalcemia of malignancy.[58,59] Calcitonin can help acutely while waiting for the effects of the biphosphonate. Corticosteroids may be effective in myeloma, lymphoma, sarcoidosis and vitamin D intoxication. Peritoneal dialysis or hemodialysis have been used to treat hypercalcemia from secondary hyperparathyroidism in patients with chronic renal failure.[60]

To prevent recurrence of the hypercalcemia, the malignant process needs to be controlled. Acute primary hyperparathyroidism requires surgical removal of the offending gland. Oral phosphate treatment is effective in many patients, but tolerated by few.

HYPOMAGNESEMIA

Definition

In hypomagnesemia, the serum magnesium concentration is less than 2.0 mg/dL (0.8 mmol/L; 1.33 meq/L).[61] Neurologic features are usually only present with a serum concentration of less than 1.2 mg/L (0.5 mmol/L; 0.8 meq/L). Since only 10 percent of magnesium is extracellular, the estimate of total body magnesium deficiency may be grossly inaccurate. A low serum concentration usually reflects a severe body deficit in magnesium, but the serum magnesium may be normal despite a general body deficiency. Magnesium concentrations are higher in the cerebrospinal fluid (CSF) than in the plasma, due to active secretion by the choroid plexus.[62]

Prevalence and Significance

Since magnesium is present in abundance in most foods, its deficiency in normal individuals is rare. In hospitals, however, the estimated percentage of patients with low body amounts of magnesium ranges from 4 to 47 percent.[63–65] The prevalence is highest in acute care, especially intensive care, settings.

Magnesium is absorbed from the small bowel. Most of the body's magnesium is intracellular and chelated to adenosine triphosphate (ATP), adenosine diphosphate (ADP), proteins, RNA, DNA, and citrate. Only 5 to 10 percent of the intracellular magnesium is free or ionized. In the plasma, 60 percent is free or unbound. The kidney is responsible for maintaining the serum concentration of magnesium within a narrow range. Phosphate depletion can produce hypomagnesemia through an uncertain renal mechanism. Intracellular Mg is maintained at the expense of extracellular Mg and bone reservoirs.[66]

Etiology and Pathogenesis

The most common causes of hypomagnesemia are protein-calorie malnutrition, malabsorption, diabetic ketoacidosis, sepsis, diuretic use, alcohol abuse, hyperaldosteronism, and hypocalcemia.[67] In addition, certain drugs, such as loop diuretics, aminoglycosides, cisplatin, and cyclosporin, may lower the body's magnesium stores. There may also be an inborn error of metabolism in some affected infants.[62] Some of these causes may act synergistically to create an acute deficiency syndrome: in alcoholics, pre-existing magnesium depletion, catecholamine-induced Mg redistribution, and respiratory alkalosis (causing a shift of Mg intracellularly) may coincide to precipitate seizures and other features of the alcohol-withdrawal syndrome.[61]

The main effects of low magnesium are membrane effects. Low intracellular magnesium can modify current flow through calcium, potassium, and chloride channels.[68] Magnesium ions also reversibly occlude the ion channels governed by the N-methyl-D-aspartate receptor, one of the main excitatory receptors in the brain. Thus, some ionic currents may be affected. Magnesium, however, likely plays a more important role in relation to receptor sites, because of its association with second messenger systems.[69] Magnesium is involved in many enzyme systems: those for intermediary metabolism, biosynthesis of nucleic acids, proteins and lipids and most enzymes that require ATP.[62]

Serum magnesium is maintained within a narrow range by the kidneys and small intestine, and concentrations in the CSF and brain are well regulated. It requires extremely severe malnutrition to significantly lower brain magnesium concentration, sufficient to interfere with enzymatic function.[62]

Some of the manifestations of hypomagnesemia may be due to low extracellular concentrations of ionized calcium. This may explain the hyperexcitability found in some patients. In others, the features may be due to the membrane effects of hypomagnesemia itself.[70]

Clinical Picture

Neurologic manifestations are similar to those of hypocalcemia, including hyperexcitability, muscle cramps, tetany (with positive Chvostek's and Trousseau's signs), hyperreflexia, and seizures. Other clinical features that have been described include vertigo, nystagmus, and dysphagia, athetoid movements, and focal signs such as hemiparesis and aphasia.[71–73] An acute organic brain syndrome with psychiatric manifestations may develop.

In children, problems are found mainly in the neonate and early infancy. Causes include decreased intestinal or renal absorption of magnesium, neonatal hepatitis and maternal conditions (vomiting, diabetes mellitus, diuretics, and excessive lactation). Seizures, tetany, irritability and impaired consciousness are the main clinical features.

Serious cardiac complications including arrythmias and congestive heart failure, which are refractory to standard therapy, are due to magnesium deficiency.[74]

Laboratory Investigations

Besides the serum magnesium concentration, there are other methods of estimating the deficiency of magnesium. A simple physiologic test is the measurement of magnesium excretion in a 24 h urine collection.[75] If the value exceeds 24 mg in 24 h, there is evidence of renal magnesium wasting. If 12 mg or less are excreted, magnesium deficiency is highly likely.

The measurement of magnesium in erythrocytes or leukocytes offers a more accurate assessment of the total body deficit in magnesium.[76] This test is not commonly available, however.

Treatment

Parenteral magnesium is needed when convulsions occur. In such symptomatic magnesium deficiency, the average body deficit is 12 to 24 mg/kg body weight.[77] This should be replaced by magnesium sulfate as a 50 percent solution, given in divided doses. About 50 percent will be lost in the urine. It can be given intravenously or intramuscularly for a total dose of 8 to 12 g of magnesium sulfate or 0.8 to 1.2 g of elemental magnesium. Caution should be exercised in the presence of renal failure since magnesium toxicity may develop acutely. In any case, the serum magnesium and deep tendon reflexes should be closely monitored. Calcium should be available as a treatment in the event of hypermagnesemia. Since hypocalcemia often accompanies hypomagnesemia, calcium supplementation is usually needed. Potassium supplements are also often needed in magnesium deficiency.[78] Prophylaxis by adding 100 to 200 mg magnesium per day to parenteral nutrition helps to prevent hypomagnesemia in the intensive care setting. A diet rich in magnesium will allow more gradual replacement of magnesium stores. Correction of risk factors (alcoholism, hypophosphatemia, or uncontrolled diabetes mellitus) may prevent excessive urinary losses.

HYPERMAGNESEMIA

Definition and Prevalence

Normal serum magnesium concentration ranges from 1.3 to 2.1 meq/L (0.8 to 1.3 mmol/L; 2 to 3 mg/dL); values over 2.1 meq/L therefore constitute hypermagnesemia, although clinical symptoms begin at 4 meq/L. It is almost certainly underrecognized. A survey in a hospital in Oklahoma, Virginia revealed elevated serum magnesium in 59 of 1033 samples (5.7 percent).[79] Of these, physicians had requested serum magnesium determination in only 7 (12 percent).

Pathogenesis

Clinically significant hypermagnesemia occurs mainly in the context of renal failure and magnesium administration. The latter may be administered as a cathartic or as an antihypertensive, e.g., as treatment for pre-eclampsia or eclampsia.[80] Hypermagnesemia has been reported in cases of abuse of laxatives and/or antacids.[81]

Magnesium excess reduces the metabolic rate of glucose utilization in both the gray and the white matter of the rat spinal cord.[82]

Magnesium may effect neuromuscular and parasympathetic cholinergic transmission.[83]

Clinical Features

Oral ingestion may cause gastrointestinal irritation and diarrhea. Hypotension may occur; this is usually mild, but can be marked if hypovolemia is also present.[84]

Although hypermagnesemia causes CNS depression, the loss of deep tendon reflexes usually precedes the mental status changes, and occurs at 5 to 6 meq/L. At 8 to 10 meq/L, CNS depression develops. Indeed, neuromuscular paralysis may precede the clinical recognition of encephalopathy. Lethargy and confusion are, however, common early manifestations.[85] Besides coma, neuromuscular paralysis (including cranial nerve-innervated and respiratory muscles), and areflexia, high serum levels, e.g., more than 9 meq/L, may also cause parasympathetic paralysis.[83] At times, this may mimic a brainstem stroke.

One should be suspicious of hypermagnesemia in any patient with renal failure who develops encephalopathy with weakness and areflexia, with or without palsy of cranial nerve-innervated muscles.

Laboratory Features

Serum magnesium determination is essential. However, since magnesium is mainly intracellular, it gives only a rough estimate of the total body burden of magnesium.

Slowing of the EEG is found with serum magnesium concentrations above 15 meq/L.[86] Electromyography (EMG) may show a presynaptic defect in neuromuscular transmission: compound muscle action potential amplitudes are reduced; there is a decremental amplitude of response to muscle nerve stimulation at low rates and marked amplitude increase following brief exercise or high stimulation rates.[87]

Treatment

Since the effects of magnesium on the neuromuscular junction are the most life-threatening, and since these are antagonized by calcium, treatment of magnesium intoxication includes calcium gluconate administration. This is usually given as 10 mL of a 10% solution and can be repeated, as necessary, to overcome neuromuscular blockade. Hemodialysis may be necessary to lower the serum magnesium concentration in very symptomatic patients, especially in the presence of renal failure.

Supportive care, especially concerning ventilatory function in the ICU, may be necessary.

Blood pressure support, especially with optimization of blood volume, may be necessary if the patient is hypotensive.

HYPOPHOSPHATEMIA

Definition and Significance

Hypophosphatemia is defined as a serum phosphate concentration of <2.5 mg/dL (<0.83 mmol/L). "Severe hypophosphatemia" (Table 13-7), during which symptoms relevant to the serum phosphate concentration appear, is reserved for a serum phosphate of <1.5 mg/dL (0.5 mmol/L).[88]

Pathophysiology

Like magnesium and potassium, phosphate is mainly intracellular, and a low serum phosphate may or may not reflect a total body deficiency. Most bound phosphate is attached to calcium in bone. Phosphate is extremely important in cellular energy and enzymatic processes.[89] Intracellular phosphate exists mainly as organic phosphate compounds such as creatine phosphate and adenosine mono-, di-, or triphosphate. In red blood cells, phosphate is involved in 2,3-diphosphoglycerate (2,3-DPG), which is involved in the energy metabolism of the erythrocyte. In hypoxia, phosphate stimulates anerobic metabolism by

Table 13-7
Causes of severe hypophosphatemia

Chronic alcoholism and alcoholic withdrawal
Dietary deficiency and phosphate-binding antacids
Severe thermal burns
Recovery from diabetic ketoacidosis
Hyperalimentation
Nutritional recovery syndrome
Marked respiratory alkalosis
Therapeutic hyperthermia
Neuroleptic malignant syndrome
Recovery from exhaustive exercise
Renal transplantation
Acute renal failure
Shock occurring with replacement by high volumes of
    glucose solutions

---

activating phosphofructokinase, an enzyme that controls the rate of glycolysis.[90]

Hypophosphatemia may arise from loss of total body phosphate, e.g., in the urine in diabetic ketoacidosis, poor absorption or inadequate phosphate in feeds (oral hyperalimentation), shifts from serum into cells (treatment of diabetic ketoacidosis, administration of high volumes of glucose-containing fluids, hyperventilation), and in alcoholism, with or without alcohol withdrawal (possibly due to increased phosphaturia).[91–93]

The nadir of serum phosphate concentration is within 24 h in diabetic ketoacidosis, between 2 and 4 days in acutely hospitalized alcoholics, and often after 10 days of hyperalimentation.[91]

All levels of the nervous system can be clinically affected in hypophosphatemia. The cause of CNS dysfunction in hypophosphatemia is uncertain. It may relate to inadequate oxygenation of tissues due to 2,3-DPG dysfunction of red blood cells. Associated hyperventilation, e.g, in hyperammonemia, hypoxemia, or with decreased 2,3-DPG may cause reduced cerebral blood flow and further compromise cerebral energy metabolism. Altered neurotransmitter function has been found in an animal model, but uncertainty exists as the animal may have been hypotensive.[88,94]

In clinical practice, there are often coexisting disorders that may also cause an encephalopathy, e.g., alcoholism with infections, pancreatitis, hypomagnesemia, and hepatic failure. It may be difficult to know which are the main factors causing the impaired consciousness. The fact that apparently isolated severe hypophosphatemia can cause encephalopathy especially if there is cellular depletion of phoshate, is an argument for replacement therapy.[91]

Clinical Features

Patients with hypophosphatemia may demonstrate an acute confusional state with irritability and apprehension, variable motor abnormalities including athetosis, ballismus, myoclonus, ataxia, asterixis, weakness or paralysis with areflexia (peripheral), or a Guillain-Barré-like syndrome. Lethargy, distal paresthesiae, dysarthria, and abnormal respiratory patterns may be early features.[95]

A syndrome of impaired eye movements, confusion, and ataxia, closely resembling Wernicke's encephalopathy, has been noted.[96] This can be a diagnostic problem in treating alcoholics or the nutritionally deprived. Hypophosphatemia should be considered in patients with the clinical picture of Wernicke's encephalopathy who fail to respond to thiamine. Leigh syndrome may also be mimicked in infants. Other cranial nerve palsies may resemble botulism.

Reversible coma can occur, with or without seizures. The author and colleagues have also seen hypophosphatemia mimic brain death in a trauma patient who received large amounts of glucose solutions.[97] The cranial nerve areflexia and paralysis of movements were reversed by phosphate administration.

Management

It is wise to consider hypophosphatemia (as well as hypomagnesemia) when patients at risk (i.e., patients with malnutrition who are being fed, patients on hyperalimentation, and hospitalized alcoholics) show altered consciousness or awareness, with or without the other neurologic complications mentioned above. Long-term enteral or parenteral infusions that do not contain phosphate, calcium, or glucose may be especially problematic.[95,98]

While replacing phosphate, it is best to temporarily stop the hyperalimentation program, or to reduce calorie supplementation, until the neurologic, symptoms clear. This is often essential for prompt recovery; phosphate supplementation alone may not affect the clinical condition for as some time.[95]

In most cases, it is unclear whether hypophosphatemia reflects a total body deficiency of phosphorus. In previously healthy patients who become acutely ill, it is unlikely that there is a phosphate deficiency. In the nutritionally deprived, however, it is likely that there is such a deficit. In milder cases, the need for phosphate supplementation can be determined by history; review of

medications, nutrition and therapy; blood gases; and urinary phosphorus and creatinine levels (calculation of fractional excretion of phosphate).

If supplements are needed and the patient is able to take fluids orally, it is safest to give milk, which contains 0.9 mg of phosphorus per millimeter. Other oral phosphate solutions are available. Parenteral administration of 9 mmol of phosphorus in 77 mM NaCl solution over 12 h, to provide 4 mg/kg body weight over this time, has been implemented.[99] Magnesium supplementation should also be considered, as magnesium deficiency will contribute to further excessive losses of phosphate in the urine.[88]

Complications of phosphate administration include hyperphosphatemia, hypocalcemia, hyperkalemia (if potassium salts of phosphate are used), metabolic acidosis, and volume excess with intravenous solutions. Oral treatments may cause diarrhea. It is thus important to monitor the serum phosphate, and other electrolytes and calcium, during therapy.

HYPOCAPNIA

Hypocapnia is the lowering of the arterial carbon dioxide concentration to less than 35 mmHg. This almost always relates to increased ventilation.

Arterial carbon dioxide concentration (Pa_{CO_2}) is closely linked to cerebral blood flow (CBE). As the carbon dioxide concentration falls, so does CBF. Hyperventilation to a Pa_{CO_2} of 22 mmHg will reduce CBF by 40 percent.[100]

Clinical Features

Hyperventilation may be associated either with a metabolic acidosis or a respiratory alkalosis. Hyperventilation is never sufficient, by itself, to cause coma. Coma may, however, relate to other disease processes. These are listed in Table 13-8.

HYPERCAPNIA

Hypercapnia is defined as a carbon dioxide (CO_2) concentration in the arterial blood (Pa_{CO_2}) of more than 60 mmHg. Only marked elevations of Pa_{CO_2} affect brain metabolism and function.

Table 13-8

Hyperventilation

Metabolic acidosis	Respiratory alkalosis
Uremia	Cardiopulmonary problems (see family doctor for OK to travel)
Diabetic ketoacidosis	Psychogenic
Lactic acidosis including sepsis	Hepatic failure
Salicylate poisoning	Salicylate poisoning (early)
Other poisons: ammonium chloride, paraldehyde, ethylene glycol, methanol	Sepsis (early)

Pathophysiology

Like most tissues, the cells of the brain are freely permeable to CO_2, but not to ions, including hydrogen (H^+) and bicarbonate (HCO_3^-). Since the CO_2 in the blood freely diffuses into the extracellular fluid of the brain and thence into neurons and glia, any changes in Pa_{CO_2} have an immediate impact on the acid-base balance of those cells, as shown by the Henderson-Hasselbach equation:

$$pH = pKa + \frac{\log[HCO_3^-]}{\log[H_2CO_3]}$$

Hypoventilation is usually associated with hypoxemia, but if oxygen is supplemented in a patient with an insensitive respiratory center, the Pa_{CO_2} can rise to high concentrations without hypoxemia. This can produce an encephalopathy.

Carbon dioxide narcosis is associated with an increase in CBF, but there is no change in the cerebral metabolic consumption of oxygen, ATP, ADP, or energy charge potential (a net measure of high-energy phosphate activity in cells).[101,102] However, at very high Pa_{CO_2} concentrations, there is a reduction of phosphocreatine (PCr) in the brain.[103] This fall in PCr is associated with a rise in the lactate/pyruvate ratio.[104] Both the PCr fall and the lactate/pyruvate rise are likely to be due to intracellular acidosis from the effect of increased carbonic acid on enzyme systems.[104] Additional metabolic changes include increased glucose-6-phosphate and fructose-6-phosphate, and decreases in tricarboxylic acid (TCA) cycle and amino acid pools.[105] There is a state of substrate depletion for the TCA cycle with carbohydrate metabolism that is compensated for by increased amino acid oxidation.[106] This leads to increased intracellular ammonia and, hence, glutamine concentration.[106] It is speculated that this may alter normal neuronal function.[106] Despite all the above biochemical discussion, the exact mechanism of CO_2 narcosis is not known.

These changes occur acutely; there is likely to be greater intracellular buffering of the effects of chronic respiratory acidosis.

Clinical Features

There is usually a background of chronic pulmonary problems with acute decompensation. Neuromuscular disorders may also lead to ventilatory failure. The precipitant may be an intercurrent illness, or a sedative or narcotic drug that suppresses the ventilatory drive.

Early symptoms of CO_2 toxicity include diffuse headache, followed by impairment of conscious level, through impaired attention, to coma.[107] There may be considerable fluctuations in the degree of obtundation. Brainstem reflexes are spared, but pupils may be miotic. Exceptionally, with the combination of hypoxemia and hypercarbia, an early herniation syndrome may produce pupillary nonreactivity, sometimes unilaterally.[108] Coarse tremor, asterixis, and multifocal myoclonus are very common. Paratonic rigidity and extensor plantar responses are also frequently found. Chronic hypercarbia may be associated with papilledema due to the increase in intracranial blood volume because of arterial dilatation and increased brain blood flow.

Investigations

The principal investigation is the performance of arterial or capillary blood gas determination. This usually reveals hypercarbia with Pa_{CO_2}, usually over 70 mmHg and often over 90 mmHg. Oxygenation of the arterial blood is usually reduced, because of the hypoventilation.

Cerebrospinal fluid is under increased pressure. The EEG shows diffuse slowing.

Differential Diagnosis

The differential diagnosis includes other forms of metabolic or toxic encephalopathies that may be associated with CO_2 retention: e.g., hypothyroidism and drug intoxication (especially opiates, benzodiazepines, and barbiturates).

Papilledema may cause one to consider a primary intracranial process, such as a frontal lobe tumor or obstruction to CSF pathways.

Myoclonus may cause one to consider nonconvulsive status epilepticus or uremia.

Treatment

The treatment of CO_2 narcosis is forced ventilation and correction of the underlying precipitant/cause.

ENDOCRINOPATHIES

THYROID DISORDERS

Function of Thyroid Hormones

The principal thyroid hormones include thyroxine (T_4) and 3,3',5'-triiodothyronine (T_3). The biologically active hormone is T_3, with T_4 serving as a prohormone with large plasma reserve. Both T_4 and T_3 readily diffuse into cells; T_4 is converted to T_3, and T_3 binds to a specific nuclear receptor protein. This complex then interacts with DNA to stimulate or inhibit transcription of specific mRNAs. The mRNAs then direct the synthesis of certain proteins. Besides nuclear receptors, receptor sites have been described in mitochondria, ribosomes, and plasma membrane. These may mediate posttranscriptional, pretranslational, and posttranslational phenomena. Thyroid hormone regulates cellular protein metabolism by affecting transcription, RNA stabilization, or both, at the level of the nucleus. Thyroid hormones also appear to act at the level of the mitochondrion to influence oxidative metabolism. There are probably other actions at the cell membrane that may affect certain conductances, e.g., by increasing sodium-potassium ATPase activity. The latter may account for the physiologic effect of thyroid hormone on cellular respiratory function.

The net effect is the result of the combined interaction of T_3 and other factors in determining gene expression in various tissues. The effects in various tissues differ. For example, while protein synthesis is stimulated in some tissues, net protein catabolism occurs in skeletal muscle. In the CNS, thyroid hormone is important embryologically in the proliferation of axons and the development of dendrites; enzymes involved in the synthesis of myelin and energy generation are decreased in activity. In the mature brain, thyroid hormone plays a role in the metabolic activity of the brain and in alertness, memory, learning, responsiveness to external and internal stimuli (e.g., hunger), and in the regulation of normal emotional tone and reproductive activity.

The secretion of T_4 is controlled by the hypothalamic-pituitary axis in a negative feedback system. Falling serum concentrations of derived T_3 stimulate the pituitary thryotopic cells to produce more thyroid-stimulating hormone (TSH).

MYXEDEMA (HYPOTHYROIDISM)

Clinical Significance and Classification

Most cases are primary hypothyroidism; hypothyrotropic hypothyroidism, related to pituitary or hypothalamic dysfunction, is rare.

The frequency of hypothyroidism increases with advancing age, although cretinism or congenital hypothyroidism affects 1 in 5000 neonates.

Pathogenesis

Hypothyroidism can be classified as primary when the thyroid gland fails or there is hypothyrotropic hypothyroidism related to pituitary insufficiency. Most cases of coma related to myxedema are due to acute decompensation in patients with hypothyroidism. The decompensation often relates to stresses, with development of neurologic or cardiovascular collapse.

There is reduced beta-adrenergic response in hypothyroidism, related to downregulation of beta receptors and second messenger activation. Alpha-adrenergic responses remain intact. This explains the bradycardia and cool, vasoconstricted skin. Thermogenesis is also impaired and there is central hypothermia.

The reduced metabolic activity and beta-adrenergic insufficiency put the myxedematous patient at risk. At times of stress, the heart may not be able to increase its output adequately. Gluconeogenesis and reduced insulin resistance may result in hypoglycemia. Drug clearances are reduced, allowing a greater cumulative effect. Also, impaired free water clearance and increased antidiuretic hormone levels commonly result in hyponatremia.

Clinical Features

History   Most patients are elderly and commonly manifest mental slowing or frank dementia. Alternatively, presentations include a confusional state with disorientation, impaired attention, drowsiness, or agitation and delusions. The development of late-life psychosis should prompt a search for hypothyroidism. Frontal or occipital headaches and abnormal gait are common. Seizures may occur, related to hyponatremia, in at least some patients.

The adult patient may have preceding increasing fatiguability and somnolence, cold intolerance, constipation, menorrhagia, reduced hearing, hair loss, and a hoarse voice. The background history may help, e.g., previous thyroid disease, especially with replacement therapy by surgical removal or radioactive destruction of part of the thyroid gland.

The onset of impaired consciousness or coma is usually acute or subacute, and is often precipitated by one of the following:

1.   Serious intercurrent infection, urinary tract sepsis, or pneumonia.

2.   Cold exposure or hypothermia.

3.   Certain medications that increase the metabolism of T_4 and T_3: phenytoin, rifampin, amiodarone, and lithium. Drugs with sedative effects, such as narcotics, may precipitate coma in severely hypothyroid patients.

4.   Hypoglycemia.

5.   Serious acute illnesses: stroke, congestive heart failure, gastrointestinal bleeding, acute infection such as pneumonia.

6.   Withdrawal from thyroid replacement therapy.

Examination

The most common acute emergency room presentations of a neurologic nature are[109]:

1.   "Mom won't wake up." An older patient, usually female, is found unarousable after a period of declining function.

2.   Unexplained carbon dioxide retention or hypothermia with impaired consciousness, sometimes due to an underlying stressor, e.g. pneumonia.

In patients with decreased alertness, the cranial nerve reflexes are spared. In the noncomatose patient, there is often evidence of cognitive dysfunction, ataxia, nystagmus, or muscle spasms. Deep tendon reflexes characteristically show a prolonged relaxation phase.

On general examination, key features are hypoventilation, hypothermia, sinus bradycardia, and hypotension. Bradycardia would be very unusual in patients with other disorders with either hypotension or systemic infection. The skin is pale, cool, doughy, and puffy. There is often periorbital swelling. The tongue may be enlarged. Signs of pericardial effusion may be found. The patient typically hypoventilates.

The features of hypothyroidism in children depend on the age at which the insufficiency occurs. The neonate shows prolongation of physiologic jaundice, a hoarse cry, constipation, somnolence, and poor feeding. In the older child, hypothyroid manifestations are a cross between those of the neonate and the adult.

Investigations

Specific tests of thyroid function include TSH and serum-free T_4. These tests are rarely available on an emergency basis. If myxedema coma is strongly suspected, treatment should be initiated immediately after blood for tests is drawn (see Table 13-9).

The Pa_{CO_2} is increased and Pa_{O_2} is reduced.

Hyponatremia, related to the syndrome of inappropriate antidiuretic hormone secretion (SIADH), is frequent.

Hypoglycemia is less common and may relate to cortisol deficiency. The latter may relate to Schmidt syndrome associated with autoimmune adrenal insufficiency. Hypoglycemia should also raise the possibility of panhypopituitarism.

Table 13-9

Blood tests in hypothyroidism

Test result	Primary hypothyroidism	Hypothyrotropic hypothyroidism
Serum TSH	Increased	Decreased
Free T_4	Decreased	Decreased
Free T_3	Decreased	Decreased
Pa_{CO_2}	Increased	Increased
Pa_{O_2}	Decreased	Decreased
Serum CK	Increased	Increased
Serum glucose	Possibly decreased	Decreased
Serum Na	Decreased	Decreased
Hemoglobin	Decreased	Decreased

Creatine kinase (CK) serum concentrations, related to the skeletal muscle coenzyme with variable contributions from the myocardial fraction, are often increased. Rarely, myoglobinuria related to rhabdomyolysis may be found.

Anemia is common. Serum cholesterol may be elevated.

A pericardial effusion may be found clinically or on chest film. The cardiac silhouette is often enlarged in primary hypothyroidism, but may be reduced in size in hypothyrotropic hypothyroidism.

Differential Diagnosis

Myxedema may mimic any of the following: hypothermia, carbon dioxide narcosis, hyponatremia or other causes of SIADH, hypoglycemia, depression from medication, severe emotional depression, chronic nephritis, nephrotic syndrome, or carbon dioxide retention.

Treatment

Myxedema coma is a medical emergency and prompt replacement therapy is necessary to reduce mortality. After a clinical diagnosis, it is best to proceed promptly with treatment, before the test results are back. Even if there are other possibilities, it is better to treat for hypothyroidism than to wait.[110] The optimum dose of T_4 is not known. Recommended intravenous doses vary from 100 to 1000 μg. The latter dose is probably excessive and places the patient at risk for myocardial infarction or other complications; 100 to 400 μg is probably a better dose.

Cook and Boyle argue that hypothyroidism, especially myxedema coma, should be treated with T_3 rather than with T_4.[111] Reasons include the following: (1) Metabolic studies suggest that T_3 is more active than T_4 at the cellular level.[112] (2) In myxedema, the conversion of T_4 to T_3 is slowed.[113] (3) Transport of T_3 across the blood-brain barrier is superior to that of T_4.[114] However, the cardiovascular risks of such treatment with T_3 are likely to be greater than for T_4 in the elderly and in those with ischemic heart disease; carefully titrated T_3 or T_4 may be advisable in such patients.

Additional investigative and therapeutic considerations include the following:

1. Administration of glucose in hypoglycemic patients.

2. The patient should be screened for underlying infection.

3. Hypotension can be treated with volume replacement and/or with dopamine.

4. Hypothermia is treated by covering the patient with additional blankets.

5. Tamponade from pericardial infusion demands prompt pericardiocentesis.

6. Glucorticoid administration for myxedema coma is controversial. There appears to be no difference in survival between those given steroids compared with those not given steroids, although such supplementation is still recommended in endocrinology texts. If they are used, corticosteroids should not be given in large doses, as they impair the conversion of T_4 to T_3. If hypothyrotropic hypothyroidism is suspected, pretreatment with corticosteroids is essential in order to prevent crisis of acute adrenal insufficiency.

Prognosis

Factors associated with a poor prognosis include: body temperature less than 93°F, hypothermia not responding after 3 days of therapy, bradycardia with heart rate of less than 44 beats per minute, and hypotension or associated sepsis or myocardial infarction.[115]

HYPERTHYROIDISM (THYROID STORM)

"Thyroid storm" contains the accentuated features of thyrotoxicosis but also refers to an acute decompensation involving central nervous, cardiovascular, thermoregulatory, and gastrointestinal-hepatic systems. It is important to recognize as there is still a high associated mortality.[116]

The syndrome has been shown, at least in some cases, to be associated with elevated free (unbound) plasma concentrations of T_3 and T_4.[117,118] However, the cerebral metabolic rate for consumption of oxygen is not increased, nor do mitochondria undergo changes found in many tissues. There appears to be an increased adrenergic sensitivity in the brain.[119] It is unlikely that this accounts for all the manifestations as adrenergic blockers do not correct all the CNS manifestations of hyperthyroidism.[119] Since there are neuronal receptors for T_4 and T_3, it is probable that thyroid hormones have a direct neuronal effect.[120]

Clinical Features

Table 13-10 lists the diagnostic criteria for thyroid storm. Milder encephalopathies consist of impaired concentration and attention, and impaired recent memory as well as impaired performance on the Paired Associates Learning Task.[121] With further progression of the encephalopathy, delirium or organic psychosis with agitation, confusion, delusions, and hallucinations may occur. Then impairment of consciousness supervenes, sometimes due to, or punctuated by, generalized convulsive seizures.

The abnormal mental status findings in conscious patients are typically superimposed on other typical neurologic features of hyperthyroidism, including postural-action tremor and brisk deep tendon reflexes. Patients with superimposed thyroid myopathy may be weak. There is no evidence that "Basedow's paraplegia" is due to a myelopathy. It is more likely that the weakness relates to a myopathy and that the upgoing plantar responses reflect a metabolic encephalopathy, along with the physiologically brisk deep tendon reflexes.[122] An infiltrative ophthalmopathy produces ophthalmoplegia in Graves disease. Movement disorders, including chorea, have been described.

Investigative Tests

Thyroid function tests reveal an elevated free T_4 and free T_3 with suppression of TSH.

The EEGs are abnormal in most encephalopathic patients, showing acceleration of the occipital rhythm frequency.[123] Beta waves (≥ 13 Hz activity) may also be accentuated. Paroxysmal bursts, including grand mal seizures, have been

Table 13-10
Diagnostic criteria for thyroid storm

Central nervous system effects		Cardiovascular (continued)	
Absent	0	130–139	20
Mild: agitation	10	≥140	25
Moderate		Congestive heart failure	
Delirium	20	Absent	0
Psychosis	20	Mild: pedal edema	5
Extreme lethargy	20	Moderate: bibasilar crackles	10
Severe		Severe: pulmonary edema	15
Seizure	30	Atrial fibrillation	
Coma	30	Absent	0
		Present	10
Thermoregulatory dysfunction			
Temperature		*Gastrointestinal-hepatic dysfunction*	
99–99.9°F	5	Absent	0
100–100.9°F	10	Moderate	
101–101.9°F	15	Diarrhea	10
102–102.9°F	20	Nausea/vomiting	10
103–103.9°F	25	Abdominal pain	10
>104°F	30	Severe	
		Unexplained jaundice	20
Cardiovascular		*Precipitant history*	
Tachycardia: beats/min		Negative	0
90–109	5	Positive	10
110–119	10		
120–129	15		

Points are assigned to the highest weighted description in each category and the results tallied. When it is not possible to distinguish the effects of an intercurrent illness from those of severe thyrotoxicosis, the points are awarded to favor thyroid storm and empiric therapy. An aggregate score of ≥ 45 is highly suggestive of thyroid storm; 25–44 for impeding storm, and <25 makes thyroid storm unlikely.
Source: From Burch and Wartofsky.[455]

reported.[124] Sleep may be disturbed, with prolonged sleep latency and prolonged periods of rapid-eye-movement (REM) sleep. With more marked encephalopathy, diffuse slowing occurs, sometimes with superimposed bursts of faster frequencies.[125] Triphasic waves may appear.[126]

Therapy

Therapy is aimed at reducing the secretion and effects of thyroid hormone, treating systemic decompensation, and at the precipitating event for the thyroid storm. The first three should be done in concert from the beginning.

Correcting the hormonal-metabolic abnormality is fundamental. None of the neurologic or systemic effects will resolve until this is done. This includes epileptic seizures, which are often refractory to antiepileptic drugs until the hyperthyroidism is under control.[124] Blocking the synthesis of thyroid hormone is usually attempted through the use of the antithyroid drugs, propylthiouracil (PTU) or methimazole (MMI). The PTU is given in a loading dose of 600 to 1000 mg, followed by 200 to 250 mg every 4 h. It is not available parenterally, so it is given orally, per nasogastric tube or via retention enema. The MMI is usually given as 20 mg every 4 h. The drug of choice is PTU as it also prevents the peripheral conversion of T_4 to T_3, while MMI does not. Other agents that prevent this conversion include corticosteroids, propranolol, and ipodate. Inorganic iodine helps reduce T_4 release from the thyroid gland and should be added to the therapeutic regime as the thyroid gland may store up to 2 months worth of hormone.

Peripheral effects of hyperthyroidism can be antagonized by beta-adrenergic blockers, usually propranolol; verapamil, a calcium channel blocker, has been used effectively to slow the heart rate. Esmolol, an ultra-short-acting beta blocker can also be used, and this allows a more rapid titration of dosage for desired effect. These have fewer side effects than guanethidine, a catecholamine release inhibitor. Reserpine, which depletes peripheral catecholamines, has also been used. (Caution should be exercised in treating patients suffering from congestive heart failure with such drugs.) Plasmapheresis or charcoal hemoperfusion to remove circulating hormone have also been used successfully in extreme cases.[127,128]

Systemic support includes correcting hyperthermia with acetaminophen, ice packs, and cooling blankets. (Salicylates should be avoided as they can cause dissociation of thyroid hormone from serum binding sites.) Dehydration, congestive heart failure, and psychotic behavior require standard treatment. In most cases, it is wise to prevent relative adrenal insufficiency by giving corticosteroids. These drugs improve survival, probably by a number of actions. Hypoglycemia should be prevented by the administration of 5 to 10% glucose solution. Vitamin supplements should be added.

Precipitating events include surgery, labor and delivery, withdrawal of antithyroid drugs, especially thionamindes, and recent use of radioiodine therapy. In mild cases of thyrotoxicosis, these measures should be approached cautiously to avoid worsening or recurrence of thyrotoxicosis until the patient is under control.

Definitive therapy, e.g., surgery, should follow to control the thyroid condition, and to prevent recurrence.

ENCEPHALOPATHY IN HASHIMOTO'S THYROIDITIS

An encephalopathy has been described in cases of Hashimoto's thyroiditis that is not explainable by hypothyroidism or the toxic effects of excessively released thyroid hormone.[129,130]

Clinical Features

The encephalopathy has a subacute onset and relapsing course. Confusion, memory impairment, psychosis, tremor, ataxia, altered consciousness, myoclonus, and seizures are common. Some develop a stroke-like picture with focal signs and symptoms. There are several reports of nonconvulsive or myoclonic status epilepticus in association with Hashimoto's thyroiditis.[131] A reversible afferent pupillary defect was noted in 2 of 7 patients in one series.[132]

Patients were usually clinically euthyroid at the time of the encephalopathy.

Investigations

The MRI scans may show multiple white matter lesions although CT scans and cerebral angiograms are often unremarkable. These may be immediately subcortical. The CSF protein is often elevated, sometimes showing oligoclonal banding and increased gamma globulin concentration. The EEGs are varied: diffuse, bifrontal, or multifocal rhythmic slowing in the delta or theta range; and generalized triphasic or periodic sharp waves.[132] Epileptiform activity may occur in the presence of seizures.

A number of immunologic abnormalities have been found, including suppressor T-cell abnormalities and immune complex formation. Patients with Hashimoto's thyroiditis often have extrathyroid autoantibodies and may have other coexistent autoimmune diseases, including rheumatoid arthritis, pernicious anemia, and myasthenia gravis.[133]

Hashimoto's thyroiditis is characterized by increased antithyroid cytoplasmic antibody, antithyroglobulin, or antithyroid microsomal titers. Ultrasound of the thyroid may be abnormal.

Pathogenesis

It would appear the syndrome of Hashimoto's encephalopathy has nothing to do directly with the effects of the thyroid hormone. It has been proposed that the brain dysfunction relates to an autoimmune encephalitis or vasculitis from immune complex disease.[130,134] The following features are supportive: the response of the encephalopathy to corticosteroid therapy, the coexistence with other autoimmune diseases such as Sjögren syndrome and primary biliary cirrhosis,[131] and the immune reaction in the CSF (see above) that correlates with the severity of the encephalopathy.[135–137]

Grawche et al[131] suggest that thyroid-releasing hormone (TRH) is responsible for the encephalopathy, as some cases have not resolved until thyroid-stimulating hormone is in the normal range. Thyroid-releasing hormone acts as a neurotransmitter and may affect a number of extrahypothalamic systems.[138] However, there is no evidence for elevated TRH levels; TSH elevation may occur without TRH increase.

Management

It is important to have a high index of suspicion as the clinical features and many of the laboratory features are not specific. Shaw and coworkers[130] found that patients responded well to corticosteroid or other immunosuppressive therapy.

HYPOGLYCEMIA

The human brain is almost entirely dependent on glucose as its energy source. Normally, about 31 μmol of glucose are utilized per 100 grams of brain tissue per minute.[139] The utilization of glucose, however, varies widely in different brain regions, e.g., the neocortical metabolic rates are higher than the cerebellar cortex and subcortical white matter.[140] As with oxygen, the metabolic rates of regions increase when they are engaged in processing or other activity. In addition to energy metabolism, glucose is involved in the synthesis of acetylcholine, amino acids, proteins, and lipids in the brain.[141]

In hypoglycemia, dysfunction is first manifest in regions of higher order activity as a reversible alteration. With greater severity, lower centers are

affected, with cranial nerve nuclei being among the last; and neuronal death may occur at various sites (see below).

Definition

Hypoglycemia has been defined as a serum glucose concentration of less than 2.5 mmol/L (40 mg/dL).[142,143]

Epidemiology

A classification of causes of hypoglycemia and a list of drugs associated with hypoglycemia are given in Tables 13-11 and 13-12.

The etiologies vary from center to center, but the largest group, comprising 37 to 88 percent in different series,[159,286] consists of diabetics on insulin.

In the era of tighter control of serum glucose in diabetic patients, hypoglycemic reactions are common. In a study of 34 continuously monitored insulin-dependent diabetic children, 6 had asymptomatic hypoglycemia in sleep and 5 had symptomatic episodes while awake.[144] Longer term studies indicate symptomatic hypoglycemia affects over

Table 13-11
Etiologic classification of hypoglycemia

Postprandial
    Glucose-induced
    Fructose, galactose, leucine-induced (pediatric patients)

Fasting hypoglycemia
    Hepatic disease
    Excess insulin from tumor (insulinoma)
    Deficiency of growth hormone, cortisol
    Renal failure
    Sepsis
    Alcoholism
    Drugs (see Table 13-12)
    Exogenous insulin
    Malnutrition
    Heart failure
    Tumors that secrete IGF_1 (insulin-like growth factors)
        Sarcomas
        Mesotheliomas
        Hepatomas

Table 13-12

Drugs (other than insulin) reported to cause hypoglycemia

Acetaminophen	Manganese
Acetylsalicyclic acid	Monoamine oxidase
Amphetamine	inhibitors
Chloramphenicol	Onion extract
Dextropropoxyphene	Orphenidrine
Dicumarol	Oxytetracycline
Dispyramide	Pentamidine
Ethylenediaminetetra-acetate	Phenothiazines
Halofenate	Phenylbutazone
Haloperidol	Quinine
Hypoglycin	Sulfa drugs
Kerola (herb)	

Source: Modified from Lee,[205] with permission.

90 percent of insulin-dependent diabetic patients.[145] Seventeen percent of these reactions were severe enough to require glucagon injections. It has been estimated that 3 to 5 percent of insulin-requiring diabetics die from hypoglycemic reactions, although this seems quite high from this author's experience.[146] When one considers that, overall, the prevalence of insulin-dependent diabetes mellitus in North America is between 0.2 and 0.4 percent of the population, significant hypoglycemia is a common clinical problem.[147]

Pathophysiology and Pathology of Hypoglycemic Encephalopathy

Mild, reversible hypoglycemia alters general cognitive performance and the processing of information without altering functions of receptors and lower order processing. McCrimmon and colleagues performed an experiment on normal volunteers with a paradigm that tightly controlled serum glucose within either normal or hypoglycemic (2.5 mmol/L) ranges in a manner that the subjects did not know whether or not they were receiving insulin at the time.[148] They found that acuity and stereopsis were not affected, but the following were compromised during hypoglycemia: general cognitive tests (Digit Symbol and Trail Making B Tests) and visual processing tests

(inspection time, and test requiring detection of movement and changes of direction and contrast). These tests all require higher order processing, with visual processing discriminative tests requiring communication of visual centers with those for working memory.[149] The pathophysiology of these reversible disturbances in mental functioning is not known.

Hypoglycemia itself can cause neuronal death. Severe hypoglycemic reactions are commonly accompanied by generalized convulsive seizures or by status epilepticus which may contribute to neuronal death. Status epilepticus may damage the brain by excitotoxic mechanisms but also by systemic effects: hypoxemia, hyperthermia, and, ultimately, circulatory failure (see Chap. 17).

Brierley and colleagues[156] produced hypoglycemia with insulin in monkeys. Electroencephalography and somatosensory evoked responses become abolished after 2 to 5 h of profound hypoglycemia. After abolition of somatosensory evoked responses for 49 to 92 min in adult monkeys, dead neurons were found diffusely in the neocortex, the hippocampus, the caudate, and the putamen. Hypoglycemia that is of intermediate severity, uncomplicated by status epilepticus, may occasionally lead to selective hippocampal damage in humans.[150]

In hypoglycemic coma, extracellular calcium concentration falls profoundly and intracellular calcium rises before energy stores are depleted.[151] It is presumed that neuronal death is calcium-mediated, with activation of free radicals and various autodestructive enzymes.[152] In hypoglycemia, aspartate is released from neuronal metabolic pools into the extracellular space; this exceeds the release of glutamate that is released more in seizures and ischemic insult.[153] Quinolinic acid, another endogenous neurotoxin in the brain, is also increased in the brain in profound hypoglycemia.[154] In contrast to anoxic-ischemic encephalopathy, there is probably minimal lactate production; this may account for the lack of increase in vascular permeability in hypoglycemic compared with anoxic-ischemic encephalopathy.[155] These factors may explain some of the topographic differences in the neuropathology and

Figure 13-3

Cerebral cortex, 1 week after ischemia of 6 min duration (left panel, ISCH), *hypoglycemia with isoelectric encephalographic activity for 60 min* (middle panel, HG), *and 2 h of status epilepticus* (right panel, EP). *There is selective neuronal necrosis of the middle cortical laminae in ischemic encephalopathy and of the superficial laminae in hypoglycemia. Status epilepticus produces selective neuronal necrosis restricted to the lower portion of lamina 3 and the upper portion of lamina 4, where the thalamocortical afferents terminate. Necrotic neurons are rendered dark and punctate because of intense acidophilia. Cortical laminae are indicated on the right.* (From Auer and Siesjö,[154] with permission.)

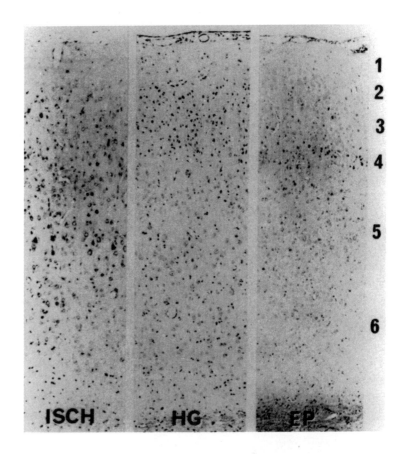

anoxic-ischemic encephalopathy. With hypoglycemia, energy failure is usually late and incomplete; cerebral blood flow and oxygen supply are maintained. Because of the shortage of glucose, lactic acidosis does not occur unless glucose is replaced and seizure activity continues. Cerebral blood flow is well maintained. For these reasons, hypoglycemic-induced brain damage develops only with longer episodes and is usually less severe than with ischemia.

The pattern of brain damage in hypoglycemia differs from that found in anoxia-ischemia and as a result of seizures (see Figs. 13-3 and 13-4). Hypoglycemia affects the cerebral cortex and basal ganglia more diffusely, and the thalamus and cerebellum are much less damaged than in anoxia-ischemia[156–158] (see Fig. 13-5). Long-duration hypoglycemia causes neuronal death in superficial neocortical layers in contrast with ischemia that affects the middle cortical region, and status epilepticus which first affects layer 4.[154] Hypoglycemia tends to affect the medial subiculum and the crest of the dentate gyrus, and dentate granule cells in the hippocampus.

Clinical Features

Although the principal CNS effects of hypoglycemia are of primary interest, sympathetic autonomic responses to hypoglycemia related to epinephrine release provide important clues to the diagnosis of early hypoglycemia. They include cold perspiration, tachycardia, palpitations, and associated anxiety. These signs are prevented by beta-adrenergic blocking agents, such as propranolol.

Central nervous system manifestations of hypoglycemia can be divided into the following

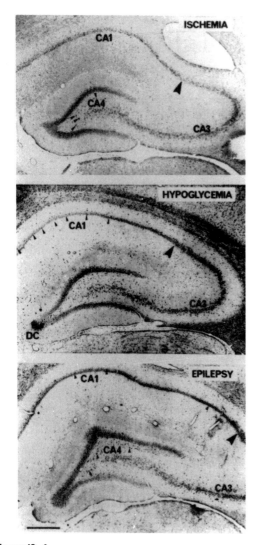

Figure 13-4

Hippocampus, 1 week after 8 min of cerebral ischemia (upper panel), 30 min of hypoglycemia with isoelectric *encephalographic activity (middle panel), and 2 h of status epilepticus (lower panel). Ischemia causes dense selective neuronal necrosis uniformly affecting the CA1 pyramidal cells, but hypoglycemic damage shows a gradient, affecting medial CA1 cells more than lateral ones. Involvement of the dentate crest (DC) is prominent only in hypoglycemia. Epilepsy is not distinguishable from mild ischemia. The border between CA1 and CA3 is indicated in each photomicrograph (large arrowhead)* and necrotic neurons are delineated *(small arrowheads). (Acid fuschin/cresyl violet; bar= 50 μm). (From Auer and Siesjö,[154] with permission.)*

groups: confusion or delirium, stupor or coma, motor manifestations, seizures and focal deficits.

Confusion and altered behavior represent the mildest form of acute hypoglycemic encephalopathy. Prior to this, patients may complain of feeling hungry or of headache. Decreased attention and concentration, and impaired orientation and memory are typical. Behavior can be bizarre, suggesting an acute psychiatric illness or drunkenness. Mental symptoms are often associated with agitation, sweating, tachycardia, tremor, palpitations, dizziness, and other signs and symptoms of increased epinephrine release. Mild changes are associated with generalized slowing on the EEG.

Seizures are usually of the generalized convulsive type, commonly as status epilepticus, with EEG spikes indicating a cortical origin. Multifocal seizures evolving to generalized convulsions occasionally occur.[159–161]

Focal neurologic signs, especially hemiplegia and aphasia, constitute less than 3 percent of the neurologic complications.[159] However, because hypoglycemia is common, this complication is occasionally encountered. The lateralized signs may occur without reduced consciousness and may solve promptly with glucose administration.[162] Thus, hypoglycemia should be considered in the early differential diagnosis of a "stroke" syndrome. These episodes, when investigated, are not related to arterial stenosis or vasospasm. Transient hemiplegias have been documented in children; postmortem examinations in adults do not reveal infarction. Further, the hemiplegia may alternate sides with different attacks. Although focal findings have been attributed to "selective vulnerability," the mechanism remains unclear.

Recurrent attacks of choreiform or athetoid movements may also accompany hypoglycemia and also resolve promptly with intravenous glucose administration.[163] These may due to administration of exogenous insulin or to an insulinoma.

In differential diagnosis, hypoglycemia should be considered in unexplained seizures, especially generalized convulsive, episodic confusion (especially early morning or at a certain time interval after meals), transient ischemic attacks, transient movement disorders, unexplained stupor

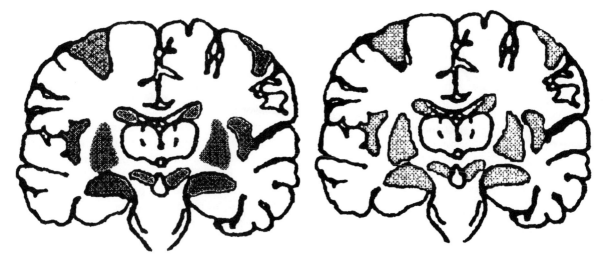

Figure 13-5

Topography of MRI changes in patients with persistent vegetative state after severe hypoglycemia. The changes (shaded areas) *depicted in the basal ganglia, cerebral cortex, substantia nigra, and hippocampus probably reflect neuronal death, glial proliferation, paramagnetic substance deposition, and/or lipid accumulation. The left figure in T1-weighted and the right figure is T2-weighted. (From Fujioka et al,*[158] *with permission.)*

or coma, acutely altered behavior, or acute confusion. The probability of hypoglycemia is increased if the patient is taking insulin or other glucose-lowering medication, or with alcoholism, dumping syndrome, liver disease, or if the person shows increased sympathetic nervous activity.

Severely damaged individuals may remain in a persistent vegetative state, permanent coma, or may die of complications.

Case report

A 30-year-old woman was admitted to hospital with generalized convulsive seizures.

She had a 15-year history of insulin-dependent diabetes mellitus and routinely took 22 units of insulin suspension isophane (NPH) and 17 units of regular insulin in the morning, and 12 units of NPH and 7 units of regular insulin in the evening. She also had a history of bulimia.

Prior to being discovered alone in her apartment with generalized convulsions, she was last seen 20 h earlier when she had an argument with her boyfriend.

Six milligrams of diazepam, administered intravenously, abolished the seizures, but she remained comatose with intact brainstem reflexes and no response to stimulation. Deep tendon reflexes were brisk and both plantar responses were extensor. Her temperature was 39.7°C; heart rate was 150 beats per minute with sinus rhythm on monitored electrocardiograph (ECG); blood pressure was 100/62. The general examination was unremarkable.

The initial serum glucose concentration was 1.0 mmol/L. Drug screen was negative for ethanol, benzodiazepines, tricyclics, and barbiturates. Blood gases revealed a metabolic acidosis with pH 7.21 and no anion gap. The white blood count was 19.0×10^9 cells per liter. A CT scan of the brain showed mild, diffuse cerebral edema. Cerebrospinal fluid was unremarkable, except for mild depression of glucose in keeping with hypoglycemia. The EEG showed relative suppression of voltage in the left hemisphere, and left-hemisphere periodic lateralized epileptiform discharges at a rate of one every 2 s.

Glucose infusions were sufficient to ensure euglycemia and she received a loading dose and a daily maintenance dose of phenytoin. Brainstem reflexes remained intact.

With EEG monitoring, her EEG did not show seizures, but a progressive decline in voltage. By the next day, the EEG showed a complete suppression and the N20 component of the somatosensory evoked response with median nerve stimulation at the wrist was absent bilaterally.

She regained spontaneous eye opening after 1 week, but remained in a persistent vegetative state until her death 20 days after admission.

At postmortem, her cerebral cortex showed widespread loss of neurons in all cell layers.

This case exemplifies the worst complication of severe, protracted hypoglycemia, namely extensive neuronal death. The patient presumably took an overdose injection of insulin. The protracted hypoglycemia and the superimposed status epilepticus may have acted synergistically to produce neuronal damage, which may have been amplified by hyperthermia. Although clinical evolutionary changes occurred after admission, it is unlikely that the process could have been reversed by the time she reached medical attention.

Management of Hypoglycemia

Management can be divided into prevention of further events, the treatment of the acute hypoglycemic episode, management of complications, and investigation and definitive treatment of specific causes.

In diabetics, prevention of severe hypoglycemic reactions consists of education of patients and relatives, and selection of specific therapy for specific patients with estimation of the degree of metabolic control necessary. Education includes knowledge of the warning symptoms and signs of hypoglycemia, the effects of specific foods and exercise on serum glucose concentration, and routine measurement of serum glucose concentration. Instruction of the family in first aid for hypoglycemia and the advisability of a Medic-Alert bracelet are important additions. Patients who are at the greatest risk for hypoglycemia should be treated less aggressively with insulin or hypoglycemic agents. Such patients include those with pituitary, adrenal, and autonomic insufficiency; end-stage hepatic or renal failure; psychiatric disturbances, or conditions requiring high doses of beta blockers. Relative caution also needs to be exercised for patients who live alone and cannot measure their serum glucose or who cannot be educated in self-care measures for diabetics.

Acute, severe hypoglycemia requires vigorous and sustained treatment, especially with insulin or oral hypoglycemic drug overdose. A bolus of 25 to 50 g of a 50% solution should be given, followed by a steady, intravenous infusion sufficient to provide a normal serum glucose. Serum glucose should be monitored at least hourly. Using a glucometer, it should possible to monitor the blood glucose level at least every 30 min. In cases of insulin overdose, the glucose infusion may need to be considerable, e.g., a 30% concentration. This should be continued until the patient is conscious and able to eat a meal. This is very important, as the glycogen stores need to be replenished to prevent further serious hypoglycemia. One should not assume that a 5% glucose infusion at 2 mL/min is sufficient to maintain the serum glucose in the normal range or to prevent hypoglycemia; monitoring is an essential component of management.

The cause of the hypoglycemia should always be sought. This is obvious in most cases, but when a cause is not found, vigorous investigation is necessary. It is helpful to freeze and store plasma for possible later analysis.

Insulinomas are best treated surgically. Medical treatment with diazoxide can help prevent further hypoglycemic attacks until the surgery is performed.

Idiopathic postprandial hypoglycemia and alimentary hypoglycemia are best treated by dietary management, e.g., small, frequent meals.

Table 13-13

Nonketotic hyperglycemia: some predisposing conditions

1. Serious systemic illness
   a. Unobserved dehydration
   b. Fundamental metabolic change
   c. Surgery or anesthesia[456,457]
2. Combination of transient reduction in carbohydrate tolerance with increased carbohydrate intake, e.g., burns, drug therapy (corticosteroids, phenytoin) plus parenteral hyperalimentation
3. Inhibition of fat mobilization in ketosis-susceptible patients, e.g., propranolol therapy
4. Inadequate insulin dosage

Source: Revised from Uribarri and Carroll[185] and Arieff and Carroll.[168b]

HYPERGLYCEMIA

Definition and Classification

Hyperglycemia, the elevation of serum glucose above 140 mg/L (7.8 mmol/L), can occur in two main contexts: diabetic ketoacidosis (DKA) and nonketotic hyperglycemia (NKH). Hyperglycemia is rarely associated with impaired consciousness if serum glucose values are under 300 mg/dL (16.7 mmol/L) in DKA or 600 mg/dL (33 mmol/L) in hyperosmolality from NKH.

Hyperglycemia can arise from an increase in the intake of exogenous glucose, or from gluconeogenesis or glycolysis. Lack of insulin or insulin resistance fosters hyperglycemia by preventing glucose entry into cells. This, in turn, leads to an alteration in hormone balance that worsens regulation of carbohydrate metabolism.

Causes and Clinical Features

Hyperglycemia with impaired consciousness can occur spontaneously or in the context of a serious systemic metabolic stress such as burns, infections, pancreatitis, corticosteroid or other drug therapy, or dialysis. In some of the latter cases, the systemic stressor may contribute to the encephalopathy. (A list of predisposing conditions for NKH is given in Table 13-13.)

Focal signs of CNS dysfunction occur commonly in NKH. The latter include hemiplegia, aphasia, and even brainstem signs. Movement disorders, including dystonic posturing, can occur. Seizures, usually focal and usually, but not invariably, associated with a clear sensorium, are common. Focal tonic seizures, movement-induced or kinesigenic seizures, and epilepsia partialis continua have been reported.[164–166] The author's group have observed nystagmus retractorius associated with coma and periodic lateralized epileptiform discharges on EEG (see Fig. 13-6).[167]

The author has also studied a patient who had more elaborate hallucinations and cognitive dysfunction with seizures, and an increase in regional blood flow on single photon emission computed tomography (SPECT) (Fig. 13-7). Others have also reported seizures arising from the posterior cerebrum in KNH.[168a]

Premonitory symptoms include polyuria, polydipsia, increased thirst, malaise, lethargy, and weakness. Abdominal pain is frequent; its pathogenesis is obscure.

Alteration in mental status is more common and more marked in NKH than DKA.

Physical examination reveals evidence of dehydration and blood volume contraction. Mucous membranes are dry; there is decreased tissue turgor. There is orthostatic hypotension with flat jugular veins; tachycardia may be present. Patients with DKA usually show tachypnea with hyperventilation (Kussmaul's respiration) related to the metabolic acidosis. Acetone gives the breath a fruity odor. Hyperventilation and the acetone breath are absent in NKH.

Laboratory Investigation

Serum glucose is elevated, usually >350 mg/dL (19 mmol/L) in patients with impaired consciousness. There is usually glucosuria.[168b]

Patients with DKA show an elevation of acetone and ketone bodies (acetoacetic acid and β-hydroxybutyric acid). If there is systemic ischemia, the conversion of acetate to acetoacetate is impaired and the ketone bodies are mainly

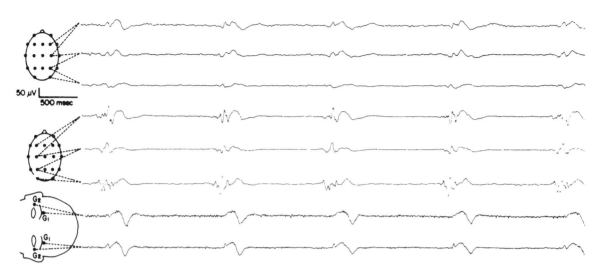

Figure 13-6

Periodic lateralized epileptiform discharges (PLEDs) in the left hemisphere appearing 150 ms before eye movement artifact. There is cross firing to the right hemisphere. (From Young et al,[457] with permission.)

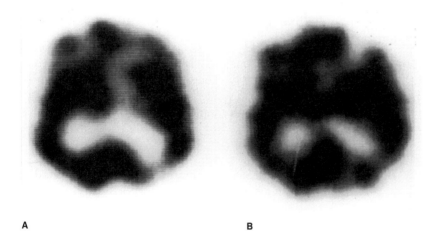

A   B

Figure 13-7

Single photon emission computed tomographic scan. A. This shows decreased perfusion in the left posterior head while the patient was acutely symptomatic during nonketotic hyperglycemia. B. Several months later, when the patient was asymptomatic, the focal defect was no longer apparent.

β-hydroxybutyric acid. Since some laboratory kits screen only for acetoacetic acid in testing for ketone bodies, false negatives may occur. There is an increase in anion gap; serum bicarbonate is usually suppressed to 10 mmol/L or less. In DKA, the presence of a metabolic acidosis with ventilatory compensation to some degree is confirmed on blood gas evaluation. Rarely, vomiting (with loss of hydrochloric acid) may reduce the anion gap acidosis; protracted vomiting could even produce a metabolic alkalosis.

Patients with NKH form a heterogeneous group with severe hyperglycemia, hyperosmolality, and little ketone production. With time, the serum glucose falls spontaneously, due to glucose loss from glucosuria, glucose metabolism, and fluid shifts from the intracellular compartment.

Hemoglobin, hematocrit, serum urea, and plasma proteins are commonly elevated in NKH, reflecting blood volume contraction. Serum sodium is usually decreased and serum potassium concentration may be normal, increased, or decreased.

Pathophysiology of Altered Mental Status in Hyperglycemia

Impairment of consciousness correlates with the degree and rapidity of the hyperosmolality in patients and animals (Fig. 13-8). Fulop and colleagues[169] and Arieff and Carroll found a close correlation between plasma osmolality and altered mental status.[168b] Cellular dehydration or volume loss has been proposed as the main mechanism. The electrical activity of the reticular formation is affected by the altered osmolality.[170] The abrupt development of plasma hyperosmolality may be the main factor, rather than hyperglycemia, per se. Indeed, patients with longstanding, severe hyperglycemia (serum glucose concentrations between 45.8 and 92 mmol/L),

Figure 13-8

The relationship between depression of consciousness and plasma osmolality in 70 patients with diabetic ketoacidosis. Note that there is considerable overlap among groups. (From Arieff and Carroll,[168b] with permission.)

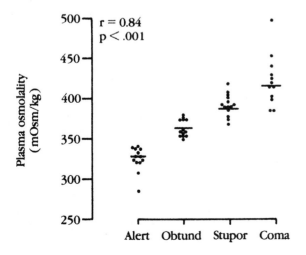

hyponatremia, and renal impairment do not show mental impairment.[171]

Acetoacetate, but not β-hydroxybutyric acid, in high concentrations in DKA produces impaired consciousness and decreased cerebral oxygen utilization.[172,173] Systemic metabolic acidosis, in itself, probably does not produce coma.[174] There is no significant correlation with the level of consciousness and the pH of either the plasma or CSF in patients with nonketotic hyperosmolar coma.[168b] Infusions of acid have not been associated with coma, except in one report (Walther cited in Ref. 185). Furthermore, coma is not a feature of the metabolic acidosis in renal tubular acidosis or diarrhea.

Seizures in NKH, but not DKA, may relate to a decrease in the brain concentration of GABA, due to defective production of this substance by mitochondria.[175] The decrease in neuronal inhibition from GABA deficiency favors excitation and seizures.

There is preliminary evidence of altered monoamine activity in the CNS in hyperglycemia.[176] Serotonin turnover is increased in DKA; reductions in metabolism of noradrenalin, dopamine and serotonin are also noted. Insulin administration also alters monoamine activity. The significance of these observations needs further exploration.

Cerebral Edema

In severe, acute hyperglycemia there is a dehydration of the brain. Within 4 h, there is a homeostatic adjustment of brain intracellular osmolality to match that of the plasma.[177] The increase in osmolality relates to increases in intracellular potassium, chloride, amino acids, myoinositol and sorbitol, and "idiogenic" osmoles (Fig. 13-9). Some expansion of the extracellular space may occur with an increase in blood-brain barrier permeability during the hyperglycemic phase.

Cerebral edema with raised intracranial pressure occasionally occurs during or following the treatment of hyperglycemia.[178,179] It occurs in some patients with DKA, but is very rare in

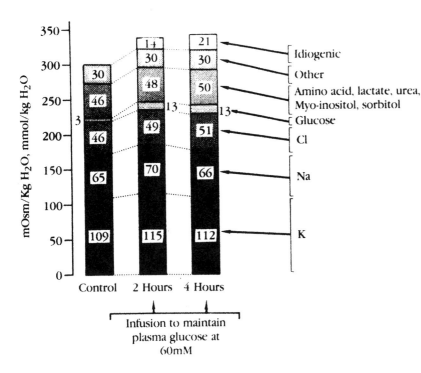

Figure 13-9

Brain composition of osmoles in normal rabbits and those rendered hyperglycemic for 2 to 4 h with plasma glucose maintained at about 60 mmol/ L (1080 mg/dL). After 4 h of hyperglycemia, there is an increase of 21 mosmol/kg of solute in the brain. This solute is commonly referred to as "idiogenic osmoles." (From Arieff et al,[177] with permission.)

those with NKH.[180–182] This sometimes fatal complication almost certainly relates to a shift of fluid from the plasma into the intracellular compartment, with resulting cellular edema.[183] Thus, the correction of sustained hyperglycemia should be gradual. Monitoring of the level of consciousness with a high index of suspicion is important. Clinical changes should prompt a CT or MRI scan to look for edema. The judicious use of mannitol for patients at risk of herniation may be life-saving.

Treatment

The restoration of blood volume is extremely important; the administration of normal saline should take priority, especially if the patient is severely dehydrated.[184] There is a risk of suddenly dropping the serum osmolality due to dilution with large volumes of saline, but the risks of not correcting hypovolemic hypotension and vascular instability are of greater importance.

Some authors recommend the administration of more water than salt by alternating half-normal saline with normal saline.[185] This may be unwise if large volumes are needed. Recently, however, three cases of severe hyperosmolar coma with hyperglycemia occurred in the context of pulmonary edema.[186] A solute-free fluid, intravenous sterile water, was successful treatment in each case. Glucose administration should be avoided.

Insulin administration is necessary to stop the gluconeogenesis and glycolysis that have been contributing to the vicious cycle of hyperglycemia and, in the case of DKA, ketone body production.

Potassium deficiency is the rule in hyperglycemia. This may relate to the increase in aldosterone activity related to the hypovolemia, solvent drag during cellular dehydration, and other causes. Potassium replacement can be started at about 10 mmol/h, then adjusted according to urine output and to requirement.

To prevent cerebral edema and raised ICP, it is usually sufficient to stop giving insulin in the acute situation before the serum glucose is lowered to 250 mg/dL (14 mmol/L).[168b,168c]

ACUTE ADRENAL FAILURE (ADRENAL CRISIS)

Definition

Adrenal crisis is a life-threatening event consisting of acute adrenocortical failure with insufficiency of secretion of adrenal hormones.

Pathophysiology

Adrenocorticotropic hormone (ACTH) release from the hypothalamic-pituitary axis directs cortisol secretion by the adrenal gland. Cortisol, in turn, inhibits the hypothalamic center that secretes corticotropin-releasing factor (CRF), which is responsible for ACTH release. The CRF secretion is increased at times of stress and varies with the diurnal cycle. Cortisol plays a role in the metabolism of proteins, amino acids, lipids, and nucleic acids, usually opposing, or performing the opposite action of, insulin. Cortisol stimulates gluconeogenesis, glucagon secretion (with elevation of serum glucose), protein catabolism, and hepatic enzyme activity. It inhibits delayed immunity and lymphocyte activity.

Aldosterone, locally regulated by the adrenal-renal axis, maintains extracellular (including intravascular) volume by increasing sodium retention by the kidney, and regulates plasma potassium concentration by increasing its secretion into the urine.

Adrenocortical deficiency can be *primary* (Addison disease), with reduced glucocorticoid and mineralocorticoid activity, or *secondary* to pituitary failure, with diminishing cortisol but usually not aldosterone secretion.

Primary adrenal failure is usually an autoimmune disorder; this may be combined with other endocrinopathies, usually with hypofunction. Other causes include: tuberculosis, fungal infections, acquired immunodeficiency syndrome (AIDS), adrenoleukodystrophy, metastatic carcinoma, adrenal hemorrhage, and meningococcemia.

Secondary adrenal failure is often related to prolonged use of exogenous corticosteroids with inadequate replacement at time of crisis, adrenal suppression from excess endogenous steroid production, and disorders of the hypothalamic pituitary axis.

In severe stress, the adrenals cannot keep up the metabolic needs, creating a crisis and circulatory collapse. This can indirectly affect brain function by diminishing perfusion, or by causing the development of hypoglycemia or electrolyte imbalance.

The CNS may be *directly* affected by adrenal insufficiency. Baethman and Van Harreveld found that after adrenalectomy, water, sodium and potassium accumulated in both the intra- and extracellular compartments of the brain, causing increased volume.[187] They proposed that the metabolic failure or altered energy-dependent, blood-brain barrier transport mechanisms were responsible. Associated hyponatremia may aggravate the encephalopathy with or without brain swelling (see "Hyponatremia" above).

Clinical Features

Cognitive disturbances, especially problems with attention and concentration, apathy, lethargy, depression, and fatigue are common.[188] Frank collapse or fainting may occur with hypotension in acute adrenal crisis; less commonly, high output cardiac failure is seen.[189] Complications related to associated hyponatremia or hypoglycemia may produce an acute encephalopathy. Addison disease may occasionally present with cerebral edema, along with papilledema and impairment of consciousness.[190] This may be fatal if unrecognized and undertreated.[191]

Acute primary adrenal failure can be the result of acute adrenal dysfunction or an exacerbation of chronic adrenal insufficiency. In the latter condition, the patient often shows signs of hyperpigmentation.

Laboratory Features

Electrolyte disorders are found in half the patients with chronic adrenal insufficiency. With mineralocorticoid deficiency (primary adrenal failure), hyponatremia, hyperkalemia, and dehydration are characteristic. With glucocorticoid deficiency, a picture similar to the SIADH is commonly found. Hypercalcemia (uncertain mechanism) occasionally occurs.[192]

In acute adrenal crisis, serum cortisol is low (less than 20 µg/dL). A formal ACTH stimulation test shows reduced or absent cortisol rise in primary adrenal failure.

Therapy

Treatment should begin as soon as diagnostic blood samples are taken, without waiting for results. Hydrocortisone, 100 mg, should be given intravenously every 6 h. Hypovolemia or shock should be treated with volume replacement while monitoring central venous pressure. Glucocorticoid therapy is then tapered to maintenance as soon as the clinical situation permits. Chronic adrenal insufficiency can then be managed with glucocorticoids and a mineralocorticoid supplement if the adrenal failure is primary, or with a glucocorticoid, plus other hormone supplementation as required, in secondary adrenal insufficiency. Table 13-14 gives the relative glucocorticoid and mineralocorticoid activity of available preparations.

Associated life-threatening cerebral edema with raised ICP can be treated successfully with hyperventilation and mannitol.[190]

PITUITARY APOPLEXY

Definition

Pituitary apoplexy refers to a clinical syndrome related to abrupt hemorrhage, infarction, or necrosis of a pituitary adenoma or, less commonly, a normal pituitary gland.[193] Although the condition is rare, it is a true emergency; failure to recognize the acute entity and to manage it appropriately carries a serious risk of mortality. Acute problems arise from sudden deficiency of pituitary hormones, especially the failure of adrenal function. Occasionally, compression of the hypothalamus may produce impaired consciousness. Significant morbidity may arise, especially from compression of the optic apparatus.

Epidemiology

Pituitary apoplexy probably complicates about 1 percent of pituitary adenomas.[194,195] There are no data on hemorrhage or necrosis of the normal

Table 13-14
Relative potency of commonly used corticosteroids

Steroid	Glucocorticoid potency	Equivalent dose (mg) of glucocorticoid	Mineralocorticoid activity
Short-acting			
Cortisol	1	20	1
Cortisone	0.8	25	0.8
Prednisone	4	5	0.8
Methylprednisolone	5	4	0.5
Intermediate-acting			
Triamcinolone	5	4	0
Long-acting			
Dexamethasone	39	0.5	0
Aldosterone	0–1	—	400

Source: From Werbel SS, Ober KP, Acute adrenal insufficiency, in Ober KP (ed): *Endocrinol Metab Clin N Am* 22:303, 1993, based on data from Axelrod L, Glucocorticoid therapy. *Medicine* 55:39, 1976 and Koller, *Adrenal Insufficiency*, in *Clinical Endocrinology*. New York, John Wiley, 1986, pp 208–235.

pituitary gland. Some authors have found that pituitary apoplexy shows a male predominance, probably because women are more likely to present earlier with endocrine abnormalities, especially amenorrhea and galactorrhea, which leads to earlier detection of the adenoma.[196] Any age may be affected.

Clinical Features

Patients present with a violent frontal, retro-orbital, or diffuse headache, vomiting, signs of meningeal irritation and nuchal rigidity to forward flexion, or impaired consciousness, thus mimicking subarachnoid hemorrhage.[197] Impaired consciousness may relate to acute compression of the hypothalamus by the expanding suprasellar mass, or it may occur later, being related to endocrinologic and metabolic complications. Ophthalmoplegias are common, related to compression of cranial nerves III, IV, and/or VI in the cavernous sinus (Fig. 15-9). Ptosis and pupillary defects may occur with third nerve compression. The mass commonly expands upwards, acutely compressing the region of the optic chiasm, tracts, or posterior optic nerves, resulting in various patterns of acute loss of vision. The latter most commonly include bitemporal hemianopsia, but can result in complete bilateral blindness with absent pupillary reflexes.

The patient may develop acute secondary adrenal insufficiency (see "Acute adrenal failure").

This may occur on the background of previous endocrine dysfunction related to an unrecognized pituitary tumor, e.g., amenorrhea. Some predisposing factors that have been observed (not in controlled series) include: hypertension, diabetes mellitus, pregnancy, radiotherapy to the pituitary, anticoagulation, and open heart surgery.

Differential Diagnosis

Among the main diagnoses to be excluded are aneurysmal subarachnoid hemorrhage and bacterial meningitis. Many clinical and CSF findings can be similar. Bilateral third nerve palsies favor pituitary apoplexy. Radiologic studies are helpful, in

that most patients with pituitary apoplexy have evidence of enlarged pituitary fossae, or a sellar or suprasellar mass that is not entirely vascular, related to the pre-existing adenoma.

Meningitis rarely has such an acute onset as pituitary apoplexy and would not produce visual failure, ophthalmoplegia, ptosis, and pupillary nonreactivity acutely.

Pathophysiology

The mechanism for pituitary apoplexy is uncertain. The vascular hypothesis proposes that the tumor outgrows the blood supply, leading to necrosis and possible hemorrhage.[198] This does not adequately explain the apoplexy arising in small adenomas, however. A large tumor may compress the pituitary stalk as it enlarges, thus causing ischemia and then hemorrhage into the infarcted tumor and gland. Predisposing factors for stroke, including diabetes and hypertension, may support a primary vascular etiology. Cholesterol emboli in some necrotic tumors have been reported. It is unclear what causes infarction or hemorrhage of normal pituitary glands, unless the gland suffers a "stroke" like other neural structures.

Hemorrhage or necrotic tissue may disrupt the arachnoid membrane overlying the pituitary fossa, producing meningeal irritation or pressure on the surrounding optic apparatus or hypothalamus.

Stresses such as trauma and angiography occasionally appear to precipitate hemorrhage into an adenoma.[199]

Laboratory Features

Plain skull films often show bony changes in the sella from a pituitary adenoma. The CT scan typically shows a large pituitary mass that may or not be hemorrhagic. Extension into the suprasellar cistern is very common. Cerebral angiograms show lateral displacement of the intracavernous portion of the carotid artery.

Cerebrospinal fluid usually shows an elevated protein concentration. Evidence of recent hemorrhage (red blood cells or xanthochromia) may be present. Some patients show a pleocytosis of granulocytes, but glucose values are usually normal.

Endocrine tests usually reveal various deficiencies of anterior pituitary hormones (gonadotropic, thyroid, or adrenal hormones). Some hormones, e.g., prolactin, may be elevated from the underlying pituitary tumor. The SIADH may be present.

Management

It is important to provide substitution of corticosteroid function (e.g., hydrocortisone, 100 mg, intravenously immediately, then subsequent steroid coverage) and correction of fluid and electrolyte imbalance. Most patients can be managed medically and do not require surgery acutely, but most have transsphenoidal surgery later for the pituitary adenoma. The use of steroids and possibly bromocriptine (for large prolactinomas) may allow some time for the clinical condition to improve.[200]

Surgery is probably indicated if vision is seriously or progressively compromised due to compression of the optic apparatus, or if consciousness is affected due to compression of the hypothalamus. Most neurosurgeons prefer the transsphenoidal technique.[201] A suprasellar approach is probably necessary for large suprasellar extensions or hematomas with optic nerve or hypothalamic compression. A conservative, support and watch approach is reasonable for the others in most cases.[202] It is possible, however, that early decompressive surgery may allow a quicker and more complete recovery of pituitary and other functions.[203]

Outcome

Consciousness usually returns, along with full cognitive function, unless cerebral infarction occurs. Ocular palsies resolve or improve in the majority patients with this complication, even without surgical decompression.[197] Those with visual field deficits or monocular visual impairment often have residual visual impairment and later develop optic atrophy. Similarly, motor deficits may endure. Subarachnoid bleeding may be complicated by vasospasm and cerebral infarction.

Panhypopituitarism persists in most patients. Diabetes insipidus is usually transient. Pituitary adenomas may recur.

VITAL ORGAN FAILURE

HEPATIC ENCEPHALOPATHY

Definition and Classification

Hepatic failure and its associated encephalopathy can be classified into two distinct clinical entities: acute and chronic. Acute hepatic failure is characterized by encephalopathy and coagulopathy within 6 months of the onset of acute liver disease.[204] A subcategory, "fulminant hepatic failure," usually refers to the development of cerebral dysfunction within 8 weeks of the initial development of the liver disorder.[205] Chronic liver disease evolves over a longer time (greater than 8 weeks), with a fluctuating course or relapses. It is related to a combination of hepatocellular failure and portal-systemic shunting in which blood is diverted from the hepatic portal to the systemic circulation.

The evolutionary time course of onset is dependent on the etiology. One week or less is suggestive of a toxic cause, while acute hepatic failure of more than 4 weeks duration is characteristic of viral hepatitis.

Incidence and Significance of Acute and Chronic Hepatic Encephalopathy

Acute liver failure affects over 2000 persons in the United States per year. All such patients are encephalopathic. The mortality is nearly 80 percent.[205]

There are no reliable data on the incidence or prevalence of chronic hepatic encephalopathy. In North America and Europe, chronic liver failure is mainly related to alcoholism. In the United States and Germany, the prevalence of alcohol dependence-abuse is about 13 percent of the population.[206,207] Only 1.3 percent of men and 0.9 percent of women met the DSM-III (*Diagnostic and Statistical Manual of Mental Disorders*) definition of alcoholism, however.[207] About 10 percent of alcoholics develop cirrhosis.[208] About one-third of cirrhotics have portal-caval shunts and would be at least *susceptible* to develop episodes of encephalopathy or chronic hepatic encephalopathy.[209] This yields a conservative risk of about 1 in 3000 of the population.

Acute Hepatic Failure

A classification of the causes of acute liver failure is given in Table 13-15.

Acute viral hepatitis accounts for 70 percent of cases of acute hepatic failure. Types A though E have been incriminated. Type A occurs in epidemics and is spread from person to person by fecal-oral contamination. Type B, usually spread by the parenteral route, e.g., the sharing of intravenous needles, typically causes a more severe

Table 13-15
Some principal causes of acute liver failure

Cause	Agent responsible
Viral hepatitis	Hepatitis A, B, C, D, and E
	Herpes simplex virus
Drug-induced liver injury	Acetaminophen
	Idiosyncratic reactions
Toxins	Carbon tetrachloride
	Amanita phalloides
	Phosphorus
Vascular events	Ischemia
	Veno-occlusive disease
	Heatstroke
	Malignant hyperthermia
Miscellaneous	Wilson disease
	Acute fatty liver of pregnancy
	Reye syndrome
	Lymphoma
	Status epilepticus in children (rare) (Decell et al[210])

Source: From Lee,[205] with permission.

hepatitis. Type C rarely causes severe hepatitis alone, but does so in coinfections with Type B. Fulminant type D hepatitis is peculiar to drug abusers. Type E may cause fulminant hepatitis in pregnant women. Other viruses, e.g., the Epstein-Barr virus and herpesvirus 1, 2, and 6, may occasionally cause acute liver failure.

Fluorinated hydrocarbons (trichloroethylene and tetrachloroethane) may cause acute hepatic and renal damage, especially among glue sniffers and those exposed to cleaning solvents. *Amanita phalloides*, the death-cap mushroom, may cause acute hepatic failure preceded by muscarinic cholinergic side effects. Acetaminophen toxicity, especially when combined with ethyl alcohol, may produce severe hepatic damage associated with extremely high serum transaminase concentrations. (Acetylcysteine is an effective antidote.) Repeat anesthetic exposure to halothane anesthetic may cause acute hepatic necrosis. Idiosyncratic reactions to certain drugs (e.g., isoniazid, valproate, phenytoin, carbamazepine, or the drug combinations of trimethoprim-sulfamethoxazole or amoxicillin-clavulanic acid) may cause acute liver damage.

Ischemic hepatic necrosis may accompany heart failure or other causes of severe, systemic hypotension. Rarely, fulminant hepatic failure may follow status epilepticus, possibly as a complication of hypoxia and ischemia.[210] An interaction between various antiepileptic drugs and chemicals produced in status epilepticus may lead to increased free radical production that could be hepatotoxic. Venous congestion, as in the Budd-Chiari syndrome, or sinusoidal obstruction by metastatic carcinoma or amyloidosis may also lead to acute liver failure.

In persons under 20 years of age, acute hepatic damage should raise consideration of Wilson disease. A clue is the very high serum bilirubin concentration (i.e., >500 µmol/L). This relates partly to the liver disease and partly to hemolysis.[204]

Fulminant hepatic failure is a rare complication of status epilepticus in children. It is associated with cerebral edema and is usually, but not invariably, fatal.[211–213]

Hepatic Encephalopathy with Chronic Liver Disease

Chronic hepatic encephalopathy in North America is most commonly related to chronic alcoholism, but it may follow any condition which acutely damages the liver and disturbs its architecture to allow portal-systemic shunting of blood.

The encephalopathy related to long-standing liver disease is due to a combination of hepatocellular insufficiency and the shunting of blood from the portal to the systemic circulation, bypassing the liver. Chronic liver disease causes a wide spectrum of impaired cognitive functioning; patients are susceptible to recurrent, sudden deterioration with stupor or coma.

Neuropathology of Hepatic Encephalopathy

The classic paper describing changes in the brain in patients with liver failure was published by Adams and Foley in 1953.[214] Abnormalities were found only in those patients who had suffered at least one episode of hepatic coma; others with alcoholic liver disease did not show abnormalities on light microscopic studies of the brain.

The characteristic change is the increase in number and size of cells that resemble enlarged protoplasmic astrocytes, Alzheimer type II astrocytes (see Fig. 13-10), in numerous CNS gray matter structures: the cerebral cortex (especially layers 5 and 6), the putamen, globus pallidus, caudate, amygdala, subthalamic nucleus, red nucleus, substantia nigra, midbrain tectum, pontine nuclei, cerebellar nuclei and Purkinje cell layer, and the inferior olive. Other regions, such as the hypothalamus, the midline thalamic nuclei, and motor nuclei, are spared. Some, but not all patients dying with hepatic encephalopathy show evidence of neuronal death and replacement gliosis in deeper neocortical layers.

Electron microscopy combined with studies of animals with portal-caval anastomoses gives insight into the development of astrocytic

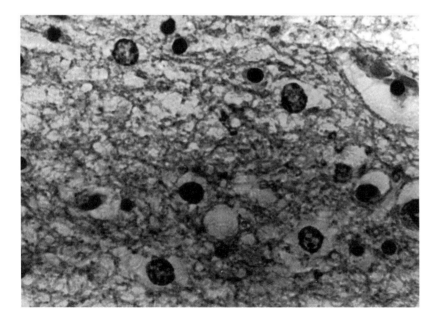

Figure 13-10

A hematoxylin and eosin preparation showing Alzheimer type II astrocytes (the cells with large pale nuclei and inconspicuous cytoplasm) in a patient with chronic hepatic encephalopathy. Note the enlarged nucleus, the margination of the chromatin, and the prominent nucleolus. Such cells can be produced in experimental animals with portocaval shunts or with intoxication with ammonia. Alzheimer type II cells are highly characteristic but are not specific to hepatic disease and/or hyperammonemia. They have been described in conditions of other metabolic stresses. The early changes are reversible.

change.[215] The initial, reversible phase is one of astrocytic swelling associated with dilated endoplasmic reticulum in all parts of the cytoplasm. Glial filaments then disappear from pericapillary end feet which were dilated. This is followed by a reactive phase with increased number of ribosomes and mitochondria, and increases cytoplasmic glycogen stores. The preceding features suggest a marked increase in metabolic activity in astrocytes. However, some dystrophic changes are also found. The matrix of the mitochondrial cristae is often altered. Subsequent degenerative phenomena include the loss of myelinated axons in the caudate-putamen and the dentate nucleus of the cerebellum.

Acquired hepatocerebral degeneration is a subcategory of hepatic encephalopathy that is distinct clinically and neuropathologically. A larger proportion of such patients suffered postnecrotic (coarsely nodular hepatitic) rather than alcoholic cirrhosis. In addition to the above-described changes of hepatic encephalopathy, the following features were noted by Victor et al[216]: pseudolaminar necrosis of the cerebral cortex, especially in the parietal and occipital lobes; thinning of the cerebral cortex in other regions; necrosis or neuronal loss in the lenticular nuclei in some patients; consistent cerebellar changes including reduction of Purkinje cells and proliferation of Bergmann astrocytes; and degeneration in subcortical white matter, and polymicrocavitation in both gray matter and white matter, in severely affected patients. The spinal cord showed posterior and/or lateral column degeneration in 3 of 9 cases. It is unclear if these changes were due to hepatic failure itself. For example, neuronal loss might have been produced by hypotensive episodes and the cerebellar findings may relate to alcohol-nutritional factors (see Chaps. 14 and 15).

An unusual case of acute necrotizing encephalopathy in a patient with postnecrotic liver cirrhosis was described by Mizuguchi and colleagues.[217] Symmetric, sharply demarcated regions of necrosis with marked surrounding edema were present in the deep central gray matter structures of the cerebral hemispheres extending into the gray matter of the rostral brainstem. The mammillary bodies were spared. The lesions were not due to Wernicke's encephalopathy, but more closely resembled those of Leigh disease. Mizuguchi et al proposed that a breakdown in the blood-brain barrier and the metabolic derangements of hepatic insufficiency produced this picture. It is possible, however, that an "inborn error of metabolism" was unmasked by stressors. This could not be proven.

Pathophysiology of Hepatic Encephalopathy

Biochemical Factors The putative endogenous toxin producing hepatic encephalopathy should meet several criteria: (1) It should be present in the blood, brain or CSF during the encephalopathy. (2) Administration of the toxin to experimental animals should produce coma by altering the neurochemistry of the brain, affecting metabolic or synaptic function. (3) Correction or reduction of the concentration of the substance should reverse the encephalopathy. (4) The toxin should be able to cross the blood-brain barrier or to alter the permeability of the blood-brain barrier. (5) The toxin should normally be present in the portal blood (going to the liver via the portal venous system).[218]

The detailed biochemical mechanisms have not been firmly established or entirely explained. Hypothetical mechanisms and toxic chemicals include: increased benzodiazepine receptor activity, ammonia, abnormalities of neurotransmission, mercaptans, short-chain fatty acids, and manganese intoxication. These will be discussed in turn:

1. *Benzodiazepine receptors and endogenous benzodiazepines*: Hepatic encephalopathy resembles encephalopathies produced by drugs that potentiate GABA neurotransmission.[219] Activation of $GABA_A$ receptors increases chloride conductance in neurons, causing hyperpolarization and, hence, inhibition. Neurons from animals with hepatic encephalopathy show increased sensitivity to benzodiazepines and other GABA facilitators. These neurons are also more sensitive to, or are excited by, benzodiazepine receptor antagonists at concentrations that do not affect normal neurons, suggesting tonic benzodiazepine or

GABA-mediated inhibition in hepatic encephalopathy.[220,221] Also, GABA and endogenous benzodiazepine-like chemicals, or endozepines that bind to benzodiazepine receptors, are elevated in the CSF in animals with experimental hepatic encephalopathy.[222,223] The source is uncertain, but the liver fails to reduce circulating systemic concentrations of such toxins. Since at least some of these, but not GABA itself, can cross the blood-brain barrier, they could alter brain function.[224] Manifestations of hepatic encephalopathy can be ameliorated by benzodiazepine antagonists, both in humans and experimental animals with hepatic encephalopathy.[225] However, such benefit is not universal, consistent, or of sustained duration, even with continuous infusions (see below). Randomized controlled trials are needed.

In addition, the antiepileptic drug Vigabatrin (gamma-vinyl GABA) increases brain GABA levels by inhibiting the GABA-degrading enzyme, GABA transaminase, but this rarely produces an encephalopathy.

2. *Ammonia*: Arguments that favor a role for ammonia include those listed below.

a. There is a correlation of the severity of the encephalopathy with arterial serum ammonia concentration.[226]

b. The metabolic by-products of ammonia detoxification by the brain, glutamine and α-ketoglutaramate, are increased in the CSF in hepatic encephalopathy.[227]

c. Ammonia intoxication can produce an encephalopathy in animals and humans with deficiencies in certain enzymes of the urea cycle. This resembles hepatic encephalopathy, including cerebral edema. Hyperammonemia in childhood may result from defects in urea cycle enzymes. Acquired hyperammonemia may result from ingestion of ammonium compounds or may develop in patients who have had surgical anastomosis of a ureter to the bowel or to a breakdown of a bladder repair. Urea-splitting enzymes from bacteria in the gut may then lead to hyperammonemia. One such patient, with a severe, protracted hyperammonemic encephalopathy, had characteristic Alzheimer type II astrocytes in the basal ganglia at autopsy.[228]

d. Morphologic, changes similar to the Alzheimer type II change (see "Neuropathology" above) occur in protoplasmic astrocytes exposed to ammonia in tissue culture.[229] With chronic exposure to ammonia, there was reduction in ATP production and in isoproterenol-stimulated cyclic AMP production, as well as an increase in benzodiazepine receptors. Other chemicals, including octanoic acid and phenol, play a synergistic role with ammonia in producing these changes.

e. Serum ammonia: brain dysfunction correlates only in a rough way with the serum ammonia concentration. However, there is a good correlation of encephalopathic grade with the concentrations of glutamine and α-ketoglutaramate which are formed in the detoxification of ammonia.[230]

Ammonia, mainly in the form of ammonium ions, has a number of biochemical actions. In the acute phase of encephalopathy, ammonium ions impair the inhibitory postsynaptic potentials (IPSPs) that normally follow action potentials.[231] This relates to a shift in the equilibrium potential for IPSPs toward the usual resting membrane potential for the neuron, which is, in turn, due to impairment of chloride extrusion.[232]

On the excitatory side, ammonium ions prevent the action of glutamate on alpha-amino-3-hydroxy-5-methyl propionic acid (AMPA) receptors.[233] Further, ammonium ions depolarize neurons, probably by reducing the intracellular concentration of potassium. Ammonium ions themselves can pass through ion channels, causing depolarizations. Brain serotonin turnover is increased.[234] Ammonia leads to increased extracellular glutamate that may result in down regulation of N-methyl-D-asparate (NMDA) receptors.

In an experimental model of acute hepatic encephalopathy, using the hepatotoxin thioacetamide, messenger RNA (mRNA) for the glutamate-cycle enzymes was assayed: mRNA for glutamic acid dehydrogenase was decreased; mRNA for glutaminase and glutamine synthetase were increased; and glutamic acid decarboxylase mRNA was unaffected.[235] Thomas et al postulate that these changes reflect increased glial metabolism related to fixing ammonia, increased neuronal

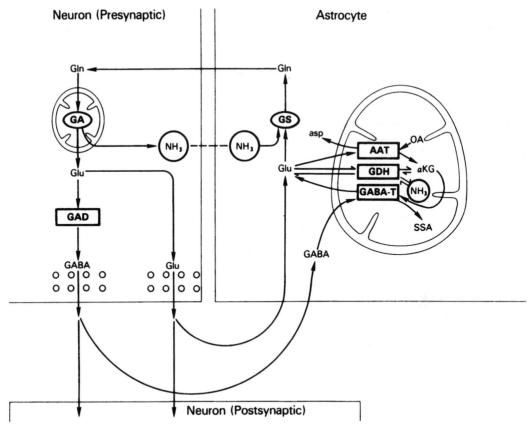

Figure 13-11

Diagram of some important enzyme reactions in a model of the glutamate/GABA system in the brain. Glutamate (Glu) is converted to glutamine (Gln) by glutamine synthetase (GS) in astrocytes; the glutamate is then transported to neurons. Glutaminase (GA) generates more glutamate in neurons; glutamate can be released as a neurotransmitter or is converted into gamma-aminobutyric acid (GABA) by glutamic acid decarboxylase (GAD). The malate-aspartate shuttle (not shown) provides energy for the astrocyte. An important enzyme for this system is aspartate aminotransferase (AAT). The mitochondria of neurons and glia are represented by double-membrane ellipses. Other abbreviations: aKG, alpha-ketoglutarate; asp, aspartate; GABA-T, GABA transaminase; GDH, glutamic acid dehydrogenase; NH3, ammonia; OA, oxaloacetate; SSA, succinic semialdehyde. (From Thomas et al,[235] with permission.)

activity in the deamination of glutamine to form glutamate as a neurotransmitter, and decreased availability of glutamate in astrocytes to produce energy via the malate-aspartate shuttle (see Fig. 13-11).

3. *Biogenic amines and neurotransmitters*: Liver disease is associated with a relative increase of plasma concentrations of straight-chain and aromatic amino acids (e.g., tryptophan, tyrosine, and phenylalanine) compared with branched-chain amino acids (valine, leucine, and isoleucine).[236] Histamine is also increased in the hypothalamus and histidine generally in the brain.[237] It is argued that this leads to an alteration in neurotransmitters in the brain. In support of this is the finding of increased concentrations of octopamine, which is

derived from shunting of phenylalanine into alternative metabolic pathways. It is proposed that octopamine functions as a "false neurotransmitter," i.e., it is taken up by neurons, where it takes the place of more active, specific catecholaminergic neurotransmitters. However, even large doses of octopamine injected into the cisterna magna failed to produce encephalopathy in experimental animals.[238]

The effects of hepatic failure on brain glutamate and aspartate, the principal excitatory neurotransmitters synthesized and regionally active in the cortex, are complex. Sera and CSF from patients dying of hepatic failure inhibit the reuptake of glutamate and aspartate into hippocampal neurons.[239] Also, stimulated release of glutamate leads to elevated levels in the cortex of experimental rats with portacaval shunting, likely due to reduced reuptake.[240] This might allow these neurotransmitters to be active at receptor sites for longer periods of time. However, the synthesis and release of glutamate are reduced.[241] This would diminish the activity of receptor sites. Pathophysiologically, these effects could account, at least in part, for initial excitatory phenomena (e.g., delirium) and then reduced excitation (e.g., stupor).

The hypothesis of decreased CNS dopaminergic activity led to trials of levodopa therapy, which were largely unsuccessful. Similarly, infusions containing high ratios of branched-to-unbranched and aromatic amino acids have met with variable and conflicting results in experimental animals and humans (see "Management" below).[242]

Tryptamine is increased in the CSF of patients with chronic hepatic encephalopathy. A postmortem study of patients with cirrhosis revealed decreased tryptamine binding sites in various brain regions.[243] This may reflect increased tryptamine turnover and a down regulation of receptor sites.

Putative neurotransmitters found to be increased in the brain in hepatic encephalopathy include: serotonin, norepinephrine, GABA, and the neurotransmitter metabolites asparagine, glutamine, homovanillic acid, normetanephrine,

5-hydroxyindoleacetic acid, and indoleacetic acid.[244]

The density of receptors for the excitatory amino acids, glutamate and aspartate, are decreased in an experimental model of hepatic encephalopathy by using galactosamine.[245] Conversely, the receptors for GABA and glycine, as well as for benzodiazepines, are increased. Thus, there appears to be a shift towards increased inhibition from the neurotransmitter perspective.

Cholecystokinin, a putative neuromodulator released locally in the brain, may produce excitatory effects.

4. *Mercaptans*: These organic thioalcohols contain sulfhydral rather than hydroxyl groups and inhibit urea cycle enzymes, contributing to hyperammonemia.[246] They also depress mitochondrial respiration in liver and brain; some have direct membrane effects.[247] Methanethiol, the most abundant mercaptan in the body, may contribute to the encephalopathy by acting synergistically with ammonia or fatty acids to produce an encephalopathy.[248] However, there does not seem to be a simple concentration-dependent effect for methanethiol and encephalopathic severity.[248]

5. *Lipids*: Coma has been produced by the intraperitoneal injection of short- and medium-chain fatty acids. Free fatty acids are increased in the plasma of patients with hepatic coma.[249] Impairment may occur via a variety of mechanisms. Cellular redox potentials in mitochondria are decreased. The enzymes involved in urea and glutamate synthesis are inhibited and sodium-potassium ATPase activity is reduced. A synergistic role with ammonia in producing impairment of brain function is possible. These mechanisms may be especially important in the pathogenesis of the encephalopathy and hepatic dysfunction in Reye syndrome.

Ketone production by the liver is decreased, as reflected in decreased plasma hydroxybutyrate.

6. *Phenols*: Phenols, increased in the plasma in hepatic encephalopathy, can depress various brain and hepatic enzymes.

7. *Manganese*: Manganese (Mn) concentration is increased in the blood and brain (striatum,

substantia nigra, and globus pallidus) in patients with liver failure.[250,251] Manganese produces the increase in the reversible T1-weighted increase in globus pallidus signal on MRI; semiquantitative scores of T1-weighted signal hyperintensity on MRI correlate with serum Mn concentration.[250,252]

There are some similarities between Mn neurotoxicity and hepatic encephalopathy: sleep disorders, depression of mood, and irritability. Extrapyramidal features, including dystonia and parkinsonian-like syndrome, are more typical of Mn intoxication, but these may also develop in chronic hepatic encephalopathy.[253,254] Both parkinsonism and hepatic encephalopathy may respond to levodopa. The similarities between hepatic and Mn-induced encephalopathy are limited, however. Attention and concentration are more profoundly affected in hepatic encephalopathy. Although tremor is not typical of Mn-induced encephalopathy, it is of parkinsonism. Manganese toxicity is more likely to be associated with dystonic posturing than is hepatic encephalopathy.[255]

The mechanism for Mn neurotoxicity is not known, but in excess amounts it is a known cellular toxicant that can impair transport systems, mitochondrial and other enzyme activities, and membrane receptor function.[256,257] There is experimental evidence that Mn leads directly or indirectly to mitochondrial damage in the striatum.[258] With toxicity, Mn accumulates in the basal ganglia and is associated with a decrease in dopamine concentration in the pallidum.[259] This, in turn, may relate to increased activity of monoamine oxidase, as well as displacement of dopamine from presynaptic storage sites.[260,261] There are also decreased D2 receptor binding sites in the striatum in the pallidum in patients with chronic hepatic failure.[262]

Manganese gains access to the body through diet and intestinal absorption. It is normally concentrated in the liver and actively excreted in the bile. Thus, it accumulates in the body in hepatic failure. Trivalent Mn (Mn^{3+}), the most toxic form, is produced in the liver and transported linked to transferrin in the plasma. The Mn^{3+}-transferrin complex crosses the blood-brain barrier where it is taken up by neurons. Manganese also gains access to ventricular fluid through the choroid plexus.

The Mn hypothesis is new and is worthy of being addressed. The mechanisms for its accumulation and its neuropathogenic role need to be clarified. (Is it a cause or just a marker of hepatic encephalopathy?) It seems reasonable to suggest that Mn may play a role in the extrapyramidal manifestations of hepatic encephalopathy, but it is unlikely that Mn accounts for the mental status changes.[263]

8. *Copper*: increased accumulation of copper has recently been found in the pallidum of patients dying with chronic liver disease. This suggests similarities with Wilson disease, but the role of copper in acquired hepatolenticular degeneration, if any, has not been clarified.[264]

9. *Free radicals*: Free radical damage has been proposed for some cases of fulminant hepatic failure. Free radical production is increased following the induction of mixed-function oxidase by certain drugs (e.g., phenobarbital, phenytoin, and carbamazepine), after ischemia with reperfusion injury and during hyperthermia, leading to increased xanthine oxidase activity.[265-269] These factors may operate in isolation or together, e.g., in status epilepticus, to cause oxidative hepatic membrane damage by superoxide radicals.[212]

Other Factors

1. *Cerebral edema and blood-brain barrier permeability*: Cerebral edema is more likely with acute than chronic liver disease. It is found in over 80 percent of patients dying of acute liver failure.[270] The cerebral edema of acute hepatic failure relates both to loss of "cell membrane integrity" with cell swelling (cytotoxic edema) and to increased permeability of the blood-brain barrier (vasogenic edema).[271-273] The mechanism for the two types of edema is uncertain.[274] Accumulation of toxic metabolites, such as glutamine, alteration of sodium-potassium ATPase, and disturbed ionic gradients in astrocytes, have been suggested.[275,276] The resultant increase in ICP could compromise

cerebral perfusion pressure, producing ischemia.[275]

Following hepatectomy, there is increased permeability to certain substances that are normally excluded from the brain in animals. Even without producing cerebral edema, altered barrier function could alter the chemical milieu of the brain, including the balance of neurotransmitters.

2. *Blood, oxygen and glucose supplies*: Cerebral blood flow and metabolic consumption of glucose and oxygen are decreased in both acute and chronic liver failure.[277] This is, however, secondary to decreased demand; energy charge potential, related to high-energy phosphate stores, is well maintained.[278]

Hypoxemia may result from pulmonary shunts as a complication of cirrhosis.[279] This, compounded by a decrease in the affinity of hemoglobin for oxygen and a shift of the oxygen-hemoglobin dissociation curve to the right, could reduce the oxygen supply to the brain.

Hypoglycemia may occur in severe liver disease with decreased gluconeogenesis. In Reye syndrome, this is associated with mitochondrial failure.[280]

3. *Acid-base and electrolyte abnormalities*: Respiratory alkalosis and hypokalemia are common in hepatic encephalopathy; sometimes metabolic alkalosis and, occasionally, a metabolic acidosis are superimposed.

4. *Multiple organ failure syndrome*: Features include peripheral vasodilatation with hypotension, pulmonary edema, acute renal tubular necrosis, and disseminated intravascular coagulation (DIC). This complication is associated with disturbed microvascular circulation resulting from endothelial injury, the release of actin from dying hepatocytes, and delayed clearance of vasoactive substances.[281,282]

Synergism

Various mechanisms likely *act together* to impair brain function in most cases of hepatic encephalopathy. Synergism for encephalopathy has been demonstrated experimentally for the following

chemicals: ammonia, mercaptans, fatty acids, phenols, hypoglycemia, and hypoxemia.[230]

Precipitants of Hepatic Encephalopathy in Patients with Chronic Hepatic Disease

Increased ammonia production can produce an encephalopathy; causes include increased protein in the diet, constipation, azotemia, and gastrointestinal hemorrhage. The latter may aggravate the illness by producing hypovolemic shock.

Drugs, especially sedatives, tranquilizers and narcotics, may precipitate encephalopathy in patients with badly diseased livers. Diuretics—producing hypovolemia, electrolyte imbalance, and increased renal ammonia production—can contribute to the encephalopathy. Hypoxemia or impaired organ perfusion from hypovolemic or septic shock may augment the metabolic derangements and precipitate frank encephalopathy.

Infections, such as pneumonia, or other conditions associated with the systemic inflammatory response syndrome (SIRS), produce a large number of metabolic abnormalities that add to those of hepatic failure (see Chaps. 11 and 12).

Clinical Features of Hepatic Encephalopathy

Fulminant Hepatic Failure Delirium with delusions and hyperkinesis occur commonly in fulminant hepatic failure and may precede icterus. Typically, the agitated confusional state (stages I and II) is followed within hours, by stupor with preserved arousal (stage III), and then by coma (stage IV). Mania has been described in children with the acute phase. Mortality is directly related to the encephalopathic grade. Patients with cerebral edema (about 80 percent of those with stage IV coma) frequently show a widened pulse pressure and bradycardia (Cushing response), decortication, decerebration, and herniation (see Chap. 4).

Portal-Systemic (Chronic) Hepatic Encephalopathy Abnormalities on neuropsychologic tests precede the clinical syndrome. Initial deficits are in visuospatial and perceptuomotor tasks. The Reitan Trail-making B, digit symbol and block design of the Wechsler Adult Intelligence Scale (WAIS), digit copying, and Purdue pegboard and tactual performance tests are the most affected.[283] Concentration and attention are affected later.

With portal-systemic encephalopathy, the progression from stages I to IV is more gradual, and potentially reversible, than with acute hepatic failure. The course is variable, with relapses and remissions or bouts of recurring stupor. Patients commonly show decreased spontaneity, a fixed stare, apathy and slowness, or unusual brevity of response. Occasionally an organic psychosis with hypomania, depression, or a paranoid schizophrenic-like state prevails. Delirium, an agitated confusional state with disorientation, sometimes occurs, but a quiet confusional state, with impaired concentration and attention, and progressive obtundation, is more common. Hypersomnia and reversal of the normal sleep-wake cycle are common. Reversible cortical blindness has been described. With recurrent bouts of hepatic encephalopathy, patients can become demented.

Hyperventilation and respiratory alkalosis, probably due to stimulation of the respiratory center by peptides from the gut, are almost universal. Hyperthermia is a near-terminal event, unless it is due to a complication such as infection.

Asterixis (see Chap. 3) is common; it is mainly sought in the upper limbs, but also frequently affects the head and neck, or lower limbs, tongue; or jaw. Although asterixis was originally thought to be peculiar to hepatic encephalopathy, it is now recognized as a nonspecific feature associated with a variety of metabolic encephalopathies as well as with structural midbrain or parietal lesions. An intention or postural-action tremor occasionally appears. Frontal lobe signs (e.g., sucking, and grasp and palmomental reflexes) are common. Extrapyramidal features, including parkinsonian rigidity, sometimes occur. *Gegenhalten*, or paratonic rigidity, is almost universal. Dysarthria occurs in stage II; this can deteriorate to an unintelligible speech. Some patients have an ataxic gait. With deep coma, "false localizing signs" may

appear. These include hemiparesis, ocular bobbing, skew deviation, dysconjugate eye movements, or tonic downward deviation of the eyes.[284,285] These can fluctuate or last minutes, hours, or days. They should prompt neuroimaging to search for structural lesions (e.g., intracranial hemorrhage, or central pontine myelinolysis). However, peripheral ocular palsies and pupillary abnormalities (apart from mild miosis) do not occur. Early coma may also be accompanied by limb spasticity, sustained ankle clonus, and extensor plantar responses.[286] These disappear in deep coma. Decerebrate posturing in deep coma has been described. Multifocal myoclonus occurs late and is not as common in hepatic as in renal failure. Convulsive seizures are found only in advanced encephalopathy or with complications such as hypoglycemia.

The diagnosis of hepatic encephalopathy is helped by the almost universally present jaundice and stigmata of liver disease, including spider levi, fetor hepaticus, enlarged or shrunken liver, signs of portal hypertension, parotid enlargement, clubbing, and palmar erythema.

The differential diagnosis includes psychiatric disturbances, Wernicke's encephalopathy, Wilson disease, drug or alcohol intoxication, or withdrawal for mild or incipient hepatic encephalopathy. Bilateral subdural hematomas may produce altered mental status and gait disturbance without lateralizing signs.[287] A metabolic encephalopathy from *other* causes, such as hyponatremia, should be excluded. In deeper obtundation, hemiparesis may mimic a structural lesion. The signs mentioned above suggest intrinsic brainstem disease, especially if combined with decerebrate posturing. However, pupillary and oculovestibular reflexes would not be preserved in brainstem compromise from herniation. These features and preservation of individual cranial nerve functions would be atypical in brainstem ischemic or infiltrative lesions.

Investigative Tests

Biochemistry The most sensitive and specific confirmatory test of hepatic encephalopathy is elevated CSF glutamine concentration.[288,289] However, this is not commonly available, and lumbar puncture is hazardous if there is an associated coagulopathy. The diagnosis of hepatic encephalopathy is strengthened by the demonstration of abnormal liver function tests. These reflect the acuity and severity of the problem, as well as providing information that is helpful in management. With acute hepatocellular damage, there is marked elevation of serum transaminase values. Serum bilirubin and alkaline phosphatase concentrations are increased. As mentioned above, a respiratory alkalosis accompanies hepatic encephalopathy. Serum glucose should be monitored; hypoglycemia relates to defective gluconeogenesis as well as elevated serum insulin levels from inadequate uptake of insulin by the failing liver. Serum glucose is often depressed in acute liver failure and in Reye syndrome, but seldom in chronic hepatic encephalopathy. Hypokalemia and hyponatremia are common.

Oliguric renal failure occurs with the hepatorenal syndrome, related to intrarenal shunting of blood. This complication occurs in half the patients with acute hepatic failure, producing abnormal renal function tests and contributing to electrolyte abnormalities.

Hematology Severe coagulopathy is common. This relates, in part, to the defective synthesis of coagulation factors II, V, VII, IX, and X, causing elevation of the prothrombin time [or international normalized ratio (INR)] and partial thromboplastin time. Antithrombin III is decreased, platelet counts are usually less than 100,000 per cubic millimeters, and platelet function is altered.

Electroencephalogram The EEG shows the progression of abnormalities often seen in other metabolic encephalopathies (see Chap. 3). Mild cases are associated with intermittent or persistent diffuse theta waves ($>4 < 8$ Hz frequencies). With further progression, triphasic waves or frontally predominant intermittent, high-amplitude, rhythmic delta waves (<4 Hz frequencies) are seen.[290] These subside and are followed by diffuse, persistent arrhythmic delta waves and then by

Table 13-16

Electroencephalographic grading of hepatic encephalopathy

	Grade of encephalopathy			
	0	1	2	3/4
Mean dominant Frequency (Hz)	>6.4	>6.4	<6.4	<6.4
Theta (%)	<35	>35		
Delta (%)	—	—	<70	>70

Source: From van der Rijt et al.[291]

suppression with progressive deepening of coma. Epileptiform discharges, spikes or seizures, either multifocal or diffuse, occur in acute, rapidly progressive or very advanced, (usually) ultimately fatal chronic hepatic encephalopathy.

Quantitative EEG (QEEG) is probably more sensitive than standard, visually read recordings, although great care is necessary to obtain valid samples during maximal alertness. Using the mean dominant frequency and power spectra of the theta and delta bands, it is possible to separate patients with grade I encephalopathy from patients with grade II encephalopathy, but the differentiation between grade II and grade I is greatest (Table 13-16).[291] Of 34 clinically nonencephalopathic patients, 12 were found to have latent encephalopathy using QEEG. The compressed spectral array affords an opportunity to objectively examine the trends of voltage and frequencies over time; several hours of reading can be shown on the same page or screen.[292] Not surprisingly, prognosis is related to the severity of the EEG abnormality.[293]

Event-Related Potentials The P300, a late cortical response to an "oddball stimulus," that differs qualitatively from a series of similar auditory stimuli, is characteristically abnormal in even mild encephalopathies.[294] This response is probably the most useful in detecting an early encephalopathy, especially if a baseline normal response had been obtained earlier.

Visual evoked responses, with flash or pattern stimuli, have been in found to be abnormal in hepatic encephalopathy in a minority of clinically nonencephalopathic patients with liver disease.[295,296] However, similar abnormalities have been attributed to the effects of alcohol on the brain in alcoholics.[297]

Auditory brainstem evoked responses are characteristically normal. These and somatosensory evoked responses, although occasionally abnormal, offer little help in the diagnosis and management of patients with suspected encephalopathy.[298,299]

Neuroimaging In chronic hepatic encephalopathy, CT scans show widened sulci over the frontal lobes, and a narrowed third ventricle, even in patients without any history of alcoholism.[300] Neuroimaging tests, CT or MRI, may also demonstrate cerebral edema, especially in patients with stages III and IV fulminant hepatic encephalopathy, and exclude other structural lesions, such as subdural hematomas.[301] Wijdicks et al developed a grading system (see Table 13-17) for determining the severity of brain edema (Fig. 13-12). This correlates with the clinical severity of coma ICP. This could prove helpful in signaling

Table 13-17

Computed tomography grading of cerebral edema in acute hepatic encephalopathy

Feature	Score
Visibility of cortical sulci	
Three CT scan slices of upper cerebral area (L/R)	6
Visibility of white matter	
Internal capsule (L/R)	2
Centrum semiovale (L/R)	2
Vertex (L/R)	2
Visibility of basal cisterns	
Sylvian fissure (horizontal-vertical, L/R)	4
Frontal interhemispheric fissure	1
Quadrigeminal cistern	1
Paired suprasellar cisterna (L/R)	2
Ambient cistern (L/R)	2
Maximal total	22

Abbreviation: CT = computed tomographic; L/R = left and right cerebral hemispheres.

the likelihood of raised ICP and the need for prompt therapy to lower ICP. However, like the ICP rise, CT-verified brain edema is a late development in the evolution of fulfilmant hepatic encephalopathy.[302]

The globus pallidus shows an increase in the signal on the T1-weighted MRI in most patients with cirrhosis (Fig. 13-13).[303] The intensity of the globus pallidus does not correlate with the severity of the hepatic encephalopathy among patients with cirrhosis.[304] This increase is reversible following normalization of the biochemical derangements or after successful liver transplantation.[305,306]

Management

Acute and Chronic Hepatic Failure with Encephalopathy Patients with acute hepatic failure should be cared for in an ICU setting. In patients with residual liver function, careful medical management, designed to reduce and treat complications, will often produce useful survival. Severely affected patients survive only with liver transplantation.

The level of consciousness should be carefully monitored, and any worsening should be investigated.[307] In conscious patients, the mental status, including tests of constructional praxis (drawing a house or arranging sticks to form a five-pointed star), orientation, attention, and handwriting, should be checked several times daily. Sedative drugs should be avoided.

Since patients are prone to infections, systemic inflammatory response syndrome, hypoglycemia, coagulopathy, and pulmonary and peripheral shunting, close surveillance is necessary.[308] Charting of temperature, pulse, intake and output, daily weights, and chest examination should be performed. Serum urea, glucose, bilirubin, electrolytes, hemoglobin, and white cell and platelet count should be checked daily. Ten percent glucose should be administered as necessary for hypoglycemia. Serum electrolytes must be appropriately monitored and managed. If platelets drop below 50,000 per cubic millimeter, platelet transfusion may be necessary. Fresh-frozen plasma is warranted only for active bleeding problems. Since

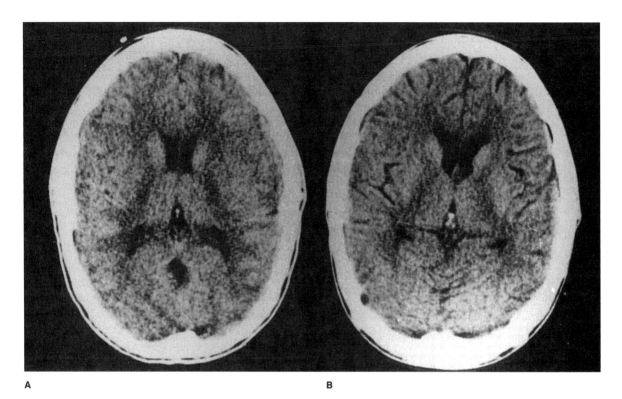

A   B

Figure 13-12
A. *Serial tomographic scan of the brain in a patient with fulminant hepatic failure and signs of cerebral edema (virtual absence of cortical sulci and sylvian fissures).* B. *Follow-up scan shows reappearance of sulci and fissures after treatment of increased ICP. (From Wijdicks et al,[301] with permission.)*

infection is a common, life-threatening complication, surveillance and prompt therapy are essential.

For patients with chronic liver disease, it is essential to aggressively determine and treat/eliminate the precipitant (see above). Sepsis and gastrointestinal bleeding may not be obvious and require careful investigation and treatment.

As well as possible, the patient should be monitored for cerebral edema and raised ICP.[309] Coagulopathy often makes most invasive methods of continuously monitoring ICP hazardous, but the epidural monitor may be an effective compromise.[310] Monitoring of ICP should be considered for patients with grade 3 or 4 hepatic encephalopathy who are at high risk for cerebral edema. Monitoring is especially useful in the pre- and postoperative period in patients with acute

liver failure who are undergoing liver transplantation.[311] If invasive monitoring is not feasible, transcranial Doppler monitoring of cerebral blood flow may be useful.[312] Increased velocity is an indication of advanced edema and raised ICP. A CT scan of the head is recommended to exclude intracranial hemorrhages and as an approximate evaluation of brain edema.

Elevation of the head of the bed by 45° has been recommended in the management of raised ICP. However, this is hazardous, as elevations of greater than 20° reduce cerebral perfusion pressure.[313]

Mannitol administration is useful for cerebral edema and increased ICP, at least for those in stage III encephalopathy.[301] Treatment consists of 100 to 200 mL of 20% mannitol, administered by

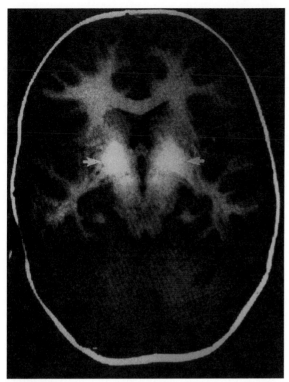

Figure 13-13

Brain T1-weighted MRI scan showing symmetric hyperintense lesions of the globus pallidus in a child with postnecrotic cirrhosis. (From Ballauff et al,[458] with permission.)

rapid infusion; this can be repeated. Tachyphylaxis, or rapidly developing tolerance, occurs with mannitol; therefore, it is a temporary measure. Dexamethazone is not effective in hepatic encephalopathy.[314] Although hyperventilation may reduce raised ICP, it further reduces brain perfusion. It was not helpful in a trial for ICP management in acute liver failure.[315] Pentobarbital coma or thiopental may help control ICP in desperate situations when mannitol is no longer effective or not possible because of renal impairment, e.g., to buy time before liver transplantation. Anesthetic barbiturates eliminate much of the clinical evaluation of coma, but such patients are in deep coma in any case. Hypotension must be prevented. The prevention/treatment of massively raised ICP should take precedence

over concerns regarding drug clearance in this situation.

General management for both acute and chronic hepatic failure includes reducing ammonia production from the gastrointestinal tract by bowel clearance with enemas, lactulose or lactilol, and antimicrobials. Lactulose and lactilol probably work by promoting the fixation of nitrogen by colonic bacteria, thus increasing nitrogen excretion in the stool.[316] Lactulose alone is often sufficient in patients with portal-systemic encephalopathy and decompensation. Enemas are used in the comatose patient. Antimicrobials, e.g., neomycin, tetracycline, vancomycin, or metronidazole, are often given to help reduce ammonia production in the gut by bacteria. These agents also have been proposed as measures to prevent superinfections in cases of fulminant liver failure. A prospective, randomized controlled trial using selective parenteral and enteral antimicrobials in fulminant liver failure proved no more effective for survival rates than placebo, however.[317]

Calorie intake should be maintained with carbohydrate to prevent protein catabolism and ammonia production; dietary protein should be stopped initially and glucose given (drinks, and gastric, or intravenous infusions) at 1600 calories per day. Prothrombin times should be checked and additional vitamin K administered if necessary. Fresh-frozen plasma may be necessary in the face of active bleeding and a hepatic-related coagulopathy that is unresponsive to vitamin K. Potassium supplements and B-complex vitamins should be provided for hypokalemia.

The use of infusions of branched-chain amino acids, levodopa, or bromocriptine or flumazenil may benefit some patients in the short term. Naylor and colleagues performed a careful meta-analysis on five randomized controlled trials that used branched-chain amino acids in hepatic encephalopathy.[318–323] The studies all had short follow-up times (<2 weeks) and were too heterogeneous to judge comparative survival rates. Statistical evidence favored improvement in mental status with this therapy, however. Another review by Erikson and Conn also found no evidence of improved survival.[324] There is need for a large, controlled trial with adequate duration of follow-up before the net effectiveness of this therapy, especially survival, can be determined. The practical benefit of branched-chain amino acids remains to be proven.

Flumazenil was found to have an inconsistent beneficial effect in a series of seven children with encephalopathy secondary to fulminant hepatic failure: only one patient transiently improved in level of consciousness.[325] A definitive randomized controlled study is needed to evaluate the role of flumazenil.

Occasionally, the occlusion of portal-caval anastomoses or esophageal varices is beneficial, the latter to stop gastrointestinal bleeding as well as to reduce shunting of blood past the liver.

Liver transplantation is appropriate for selected patients with acute hepatic failure.[326] Rates of recovery allowing hospital discharge are now over 70 percent.[327] O'Grady and colleagues at King's College in London, England recently prepared guidelines for liver transplantation in acute hepatic failure (see Table 13-18).[328] This has been

Table 13-18

Criteria for consideration of liver transplantation in acute liver failure

Acetaminophen toxicity
   pH <7.3 (regardless of coma grade)
   or
   Prothrombin time >100 s and serum creatinine >3.4 mg/dL (300 μmol/L) in patients with grade III or IV encephalopathy

All other causes
   Prothrombin time >100 s (regardless of coma grade) or any three of the following (regardless of coma grade):
      Age <10 years but >40 years
      Liver failure caused by non-A, non-B hepatitis, halothane-induced hepatitis, or idiosyncratic drug reactions
      Duration of jaundice before the onset of encephalopathy >7 days
      Prothrombin time >50 s
      Serum bilirubin >300 μmol/L (17.5 mg/dL)

Source: From O'Grady et al,[328] with permission.

an important milestone. Clinicians often recommend transplantation too late, after severe brain damage from cerebral edema or a series of life-threatening complications (especially sepsis or multiple organ failure) has developed. Therefore, it is wise to put the patient on the list for hepatic transplantation as soon as the prognosis is less than 70 percent; delays are usually more than 2 days. In general, as long as there is not marked cerebral edema, liver transplantation has a good chance of success.

Charcoal hemoperfusion and administration of prostaglandin E_1 have not improved outcomes over standard care in controlled trials.[328,329] Despite some experimental support for improvement in hepatocellular regeneration, a controlled trial of insulin and glucagon proved unsuccessful in the treatment of fulminant hepatic failure.[330]

Other procedures such as hepatocyte transplantation and bioartificial liver devices are promising. Intrasplenic hepatocellular transplantation in portacaval shunted rats improves locomotor activity.[331] Extracorporeal hybrid bioartificial livers with porcine hepatocytes and charcoal filters can carry or "bridge" patients until a transplant is possible. Patients tolerate the procedure well and show an improvement in level of consciousness, ICP, cerebral perfusion pressure, and plasma biochemistry, as detailed in a preliminary report.[332]

UREMIA

Uremia can affect brain function either directly, through the effects of retained uremic toxins, or indirectly, through complications of renal failure or its treatment.[333] These are discussed under the headings "Acute Uremic Encephalopathy," "Chronic Renal Failure," and "Complications of Dialysis." Complications of renal transplantation are discussed in Chapter 21.

Uremic Encephalopathy

Uremia is defined as the clinical syndrome related to profound loss of renal function. Uremic encephalopathy can be divided into acute renal failure (ARF) or chronic renal failure (CRF) varieties.

These differ in more than acuity, as there are a number of metabolic and endocrine disturbances and compensatory adjustments that take time to evolve completely to their full manifestations in chronic renal failure. Some may ameliorate and others may contribute to adverse effects of kidney failure on the CNS.

Uremia is prevalent: there are over 100,000 patients undergoing treatment for chronic renal failure in the United States.

Acute Uremic Encephalopathy

Etiology Acute renal failure can be divided into prerenal (circulatory failure), postrenal (obstructions to outflow), and specific renal causes.[334] At least 40 percent of ARF cases occur in an acute medical setting.[335] Most cases are due to renal ischemia with either systemic hypotension or local ischemia related to aortic disease. Nephrotoxic medical materials, such as aminoglycosides and radiographic contrast agents, are more common causes than the organic solvents, heavy metals, and glycols of the past. Massive release of myoglobin into the circulation (crush injuries, ischemia to muscle, alcoholism, and malignant neuroleptic and malignant hyperthermia syndromes), massive hemolysis, and complications of pregnancy may produce acute tubular necrosis.

The pathophysiology of the brain dysfunction is discussed in the section on "Chronic Renal Failure."

Clinical Features

There are few specific features that differentiate uremic encephalopathy from other metabolic encephalopathies. However, the following combination suggests uremia, after the exclusion of exogenous agents: (1) an encephalopathy with hyperventilation from a metabolic acidosis; and (2) excitability, including prominent myoclonus or seizures.

As with other metabolic encephalopathies, early changes include lethargy, irritability, problems with concentration and attention, disorientation, omissions in speech, and sleep disturb-ances.[336] Patients are usually subdued, but delirium, or an agitated confusional state, may be found. There may be periods of profanity, euphoria, depression, or catatonic stupor.[337] Coma from acute uremia is found when the patient is *in extremis.*[338]

Cranial nerves are usually intact, although fundi may reflect arterial hypertension. Seizures, usually in the form of generalized convulsions and often multiple, occur in the oliguric phase.[336] Focal seizures may occur, but are not usually consistently from the same site, unless they relate to an associated structural lesion. Patients may feel weak and demonstrate multifocal myoclonus that is so prominent that the muscles appear to be fasciculating.[339] Action myoclonus has been described.[340] Tetany may also be found. Focal signs such as hemiparesis are not rare, but subside with dialysis and may switch sides with recurrent episodes.

Investigative Tests Specific medical tests are discussed in the "Management" section.

The EEG reflects the level of consciousness: slowing of frequencies occurs in parallel with the severity of the encephalopathy.[341] Generalized epileptiform discharges occur in about 25 percent of children with acute uremia, but these are rare in adults.[342]

Differential Diagnosis The main differential diagnosis is accelerated hypertension with hypertensive encephalopathy. The latter is usually associated with papilledema, which is rare and unexpected in uremic encephalopathy. Elevated CSF protein is more characteristic of hypertensive than uremic encephalopathy.

Other conditions that may cause both encephalopathy and systemic acidosis include exogenous toxins, such as methanol, ethylene glycol, salicylates, and paraldehyde. These, along with laboratory work, are discussed in Chap. 16. Diabetic ketoacidosis, anoxia, sepsis with circulatory failure, and lactic acidosis should not pose diagnostic difficulty (see earlier in this Chapter).

Penicillin intoxication (huge doses) may cause an encephalopathy with seizures, as well as acute renal failure. In children, lead intoxication enters the differential diagnosis.[343] Papilledema and other evidence of raised ICP are commonly present in childhood lead intoxication with impaired consciousness. There may be a "lead line" in the gingivae and radiologic bony abnormalities.[344]

Management The first step is to determine the category and specific cause of ARF, especially to detect and treat reversible causes. Pre- and post-renal causes, precipitants (myoglobin, hemoglobin, and urate crystals) and nephrotoxic drugs should be sought first. These require the specific management steps contained in general medical texts.

Fluid intake needs to be adjusted with respect to the cause of ARF, but usually needs to be restricted depending on urinary output. Steps should be taken to reduce catabolism by increasing carbohydrate intake. Serum potassium needs to be closely monitored, as life-threatening hyperkalemia is a constant risk. Complications such as congestive heart failure, acute hypertension, fluid and electrolyte imbalance, and infections need to be looked for, prevented, and managed promptly if they occur.

Not all patients require dialysis; some can be managed conservatively with correction of the underlying cause and expectant observation. Absolute indications for dialysis include: development of CNS complications, resistant hypertension, fluid overload, severe acidosis, and uremic pericarditis.

Other management, including antiepileptic drug therapy, is discussed under "Chronic Renal Failure."

Chronic Renal Failure

Pathogenesis The specific neurotoxin of uremia has not been identified. It is unlikely that a single retained chemical species will account for uremic encephalopathy for all patients. Instead, there is likely a synergism, similar to that described for hepatic encephalopathy, in which a combination of factors has been proposed to produce the syndrome.

It seems reasonable to expect the uremic neurotoxin to meet the criteria developed by Massry.[345]

1. The substance must be identifiable, and its chemical structure known.

2. The substance should be elevated in the blood of uremic patients. Furthermore, a linear, positive relationship should be shown between the degree of encephalopathy and the blood concentration of the chemical.

3. The substance should be capable of causing the encephalopathy when given to experimental animals in doses that produce blood concentrations similar to those observed in symptomatic human patients. There should be a correlation of the plasma/tissue concentrations with the severity of encephalopathy.

4. Removal of the substance from the blood of affected humans and experimental animals should improve the cerebral function.

The following chemicals and hormones have been proposed to play a role in producing the uremic syndrome: urea, creatinine, guanidine and related compounds, uric and oxalic acids, phenols, aromatic acids, indican, amines, amino acid imbalance (and resultant neurotransmitter imbalance), myoinositol, middle molecules (2000 to 5000-Da molecules—mainly consisting of peptides), parathormone (with altered calcium metabolism), and aluminum. These are reviewed in the monographs by Bolton and Young[346a] and Arieff and Griggs.[346b] The chemicals that come closest to meeting the listed criteria are elevated parathyroid hormone and possibly aluminum intoxication.[347]

It has been hypothesized that the uremic toxin(s) alter the brain function in the following way:[346a]

1. altered neurotransmitter and synaptic function;

2. enzyme inhibition;

3. altered sodium-potassium pump mechanism—mainly based on increased sensitivity;

4. interference with a number of intracellular processes including transcription from

DNA to mRNA, phosphodiesterase and phosphoinositide (second messenger) functions, phosphate transfer in various enzymes, and microtubular function.

Clinical Features The neurologic features in CRF do not differ in kind from those of ARF. In CRF, they are less florid or fulminant; they are also considerably ameliorated by treatment, such as dialysis. Lethargy and fatiguability, problems concentrating, slowness in thinking and impaired memory function are common with CRF, whether or not patients are on regular dialysis programs.[348,349] Headaches, sleep disturbances, dysarthric speech and abnormal hormonal, including sexual, functions occur *parri passu* with these issues.

The following motor phenomena are common manifestations of uremic encephalopathy: tremor, myoclonus, asterixis, paratonic rigidity, and primitive reflexes (rooting, grasp, and snout). Tremor is a coarse, irregular postural-action tremor, best seen on supporting the limbs against gravity or on reaching for something. Myoclonus may be multifocal or synchronous in uremia.[350] Asterixis is the brief relaxation in a part of the body that is being actively supported by muscular contraction. It relates to sudden relaxation of muscle. Paratonic rigidity is the resistance to passive movement of a limb. It is distinct from extrapyramidal rigidity in that paratonic rigidity is velocity dependent, tending to disappear when the limb is moved slowly. Interestingly, tone in uremia tends to remain increased, even when the patient is comatose.[351]

Cerebral seizures are encountered occasionally, usually as generalized convulsions. Seizures may occur as a near-terminal event, preceded by coma, in very advanced, untreated uremia.[352] They are uncommon in hemodialyzed patients, unless they occur near the start of therapy or if a complication arises, e.g., stroke or metabolic upset, such as a sudden change in acid-base or electrolyte composition, or hypocalcemia.[353] Focal seizures do occur, but are not often repeated in a stereotypic fashion unless there is an underlying structural lesion.

Uremic meningitis may complicate chronic uremic encephalopathy. Consciousness is not seriously compromised, but patients exhibit nuchal rigidity and a positive Kernig's sign.[354]

Investigations Routine EEG may be normal with mild encephalopathy, but often shows intermittent bursts of low voltage theta (>4, <8 Hz rhythmic waves). With more severe encephalopathy, the EEG shows slowing of frequencies and an increase in amplitude. The occipital rhythm may show progressive slowing in serial EEGs. Bursts of rhythmic delta (<4 Hz waves) are common, especially upon arousal from sleep.[355] Triphasic waves may be superimposed on background slowing (see Chap. 3). A photomyogenic response (muscle twitches of the face coincident with light flashes) or photoparoxysmal response (generalized epileptiform discharges in response to photic stimulation) may be found. Bursts of irregular generalized spike and wave may also occur spontaneously during the recording.

Frequency changes can be detected more readily with quantitative methods using the strategies developed by Teschan, Bourne, and their respective colleagues.[356,357] This can be a sensitive method for determining the optimal effectiveness of dialysis strategies.[357] Event-related potentials, especially middle latency auditory evoked responses, can be used in a similar fashion to show improvement with dialysis (Fig. 13-14).

Management Every effort should be made to correct reversible causes of renal failure and to maximize the function of the kidneys with conservative means. Dietary restrictions of fluid, potassium, sodium, phosphate, and, ultimately, protein are usually necessary.

When CNS symptoms persist or develop after correction of reversible factors and institution of conservative therapy, dialysis is necessary. Peritoneal dialysis and hemodialysis reverse many of the neurologic and systemic complications of uremia, but many are incompletely corrected. Patients on dialysis often feel chronically ill, with reduced stamina and problems concentrating or maintaining attention, they have memory problems and sleep

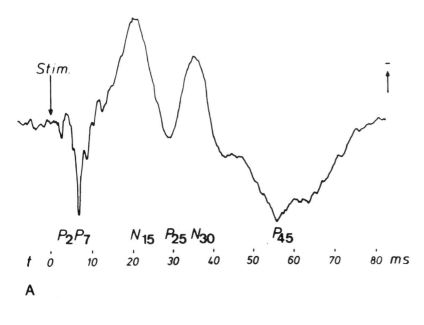

A

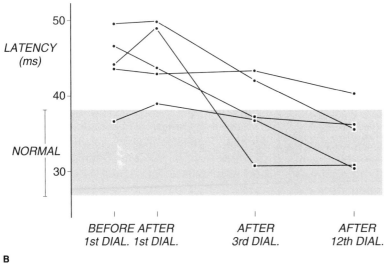

B

Figure 13-14

A. This shows early auditory evoked response components: 2048 responses were averaged. Stim = stimulus; t = time. Note the N30 peak. B. This shows latencies of the N30 component during initiation of regular hemodialysis treatment (DIAL.) in five patients with chronic renal failure. (Reprinted with permission from Knoll A, Harbort U, Schulte K, Zimpel F: Quantitative survey of uremic brain dysfunction by auditory evoked potentials, in Courjon J, Mauguiere F, Revol M (eds): Advances in Neurology, vol 32: Clinical Applications of Evoked Potentials in Neurology. New York, Raven Press, 1982, pp 227–232.)

disorders. Some may continue to have seizures. Peripheral neuropathy may persist. In addition, a host of systemic problems, including chronic anemia, secondary hyperparathyroidism, osteopenia, malnutrition, hypertension, immunologic deficiency, bleeding diatheses, and pruritis, may persist.

Many of these are completely reversed by successful renal transplantation.[358] Some problems related to immunosuppression are discussed in Chap. 21.

Complications of Dialysis Therapy

Adverse effects from dialysis, especially hemodialysis, occur in every renal unit. These include: dialysis dementia, dysequilibrium syndrome, subdural hematoma, and vitamin deficiencies. These will be discussed in turn.

Dialysis Dementia

This is a clinical syndrome initially described in clusters of patients on chronic hemodialysis, although a similar syndrome may occur in patients on peritoneal dialysis.[359] The cause appears to be an accumulation of aluminum in the brain. The condition is progressive and fatal unless recognized and treated vigorously. The condition is often associated with a fracturing osteodystrophy and a severe, refractory, microcytic anemia.

Clinical Features The essential components are an initial nonfluent speech disturbance (aphasia plus dysarthria), involuntary motor phenomena (especially myoclonus and seizures), gait disturbance (apraxia or ataxia), and mental changes.[346a] The latter consist initially of apathy and behavioral changes, combined with speech and writing errors. The mental changes can blend with the features described above as part of the uremic syndrome, but a striking behavioral *change* in a patient with CRF should raise the possibility of dialysis dementia. Confusional states appearing transiently shortly after dialysis are a typical early feature. These last longer with further dialysis treatments until they are persistent. Memory failure, poor attention, disorientation, psychotic behavior, apraxia, and dyscalculia have been described. Eventually, the patient becomes bedridden, incontinent and stuporous.

Investigations The EEG can be helpful diagnostically and in assessing therapy. Typically, patients have frequent "projected" bursts of rhythmic delta activity, triphasic waves, or irregular generalized epileptiform discharges, despite an adequate, e.g., thrice weekly, dialysis program. Serum aluminum levels are helpful but often not definitive. Although serum aluminum levels of <50 µg/L are unlikely to be associated with dialysis dementia, occasional cases may have low levels. Bone aluminum measurements and the desferoxamine infusion test are further refinements.[346a]

Pathogenesis There is good epidemiologic evidence that aluminum accumulation in the brain is the main cause of dialysis dementia. Early outbreaks occurred in centers that had high levels of aluminum in their dialysate.[360] Elimination of the aluminum essentially eliminated epidemics of this syndrome. Sporadic cases since then have been related to the absorption of aluminum from the gastrointestinal tract (e.g., from the use of aluminum-containing phosphate binders). In dialysis dementia the burden of aluminum in the brain is clearly elevated above that found in any other condition.[361]

Aluminum is neurotoxic and interferes with a number of intracellular and membrane effects when present in toxic amounts.[346a]

The mechanism by which aluminum gains access to the brain in patients with CRF is not entirely clear. Uremic patients accumulate aluminum from dietary sources, dialysis and medicines, but it is unlikely that the brain accumulation relates only to the body burden. Many normal individuals have considerably higher exposure to aluminum. In addition, there appears to be either a defect in the blood-brain barrier function or an active uptake that accounts for the brain accumulation and neurotoxicity. The role of parathyroid hormone in facilitating transport of aluminum into the brain may be an important factor.[362]

Management A high index of suspicion and vigilance for dialysis dementia in the uremic population is vital. With first symptoms of the condition, the patient should be withdrawn from all sources of aluminum or (especially in dialysate, or aluminum-containing antacids). Desferoxamine, a chelating agent for aluminum, can be given safely on an intermittent or long-term basis.[346a] This can help in arresting the progression of the disorder and may reverse many of the features, although sometimes not completely.[346a]

Symptomatic therapy with antiepileptic drugs such as phenytoin or valproate, may be necessary. Although benzodiazepines may have a transiently beneficial effect on the clinical features, their long-term usefulness has not been shown.

Dialysis Dysequilibrium

Dialysis dysequilibrium is a syndrome with a close temporal relation to hemodialysis treatment. The condition is more likely during or after the initial dialysis treatment in patients with chronic renal failure. The very young and very old may be more susceptible.[363] The condition is reversible, but serious complications, including death or damage from seizures can occur in severe cases.[364,365]

Pathophysiology Dialysis dysequilibrium syndrome is thought to be related to an osmotic mismatch between the plasma and brain, with relatively lower osmolality in the blood because of the dialysis process. (The brain had increased its idiogenic osmoles because of the uremic state.) There is then a net shift of water into the brain which causes cellular edema.[366] This has been substantiated by densitometric measurements by CT scanning of uremic patients undergoing dialysis.[367] Pappius et al have shown that the concentration gradient is not maintained: it is maximal at 30 to 60 min from the onset of hemodialysis, but then equilibration occurs over the next 1 to 3 h.[368] More recently, Arieff and colleagues have shown that an intracellular acidosis occurs in the brain, in association with dialysis dysequilibrium.[369] The relative roles of osmotic and pH changes in producing the neuronal dysfunction are unclear.

Clinical Features Mild forms consist of headache, nausea, vomiting, restlessness or drowsiness, and muscle cramps. Moderate features include disorientation, somnolence, asterixis, and myoclonus. Severe cases develop an acute organic psychosis, coma, or generalized convulsions. These features start either during or immediately following the dialysis treatment.

Investigations The EEGs in acutely symptomatic patients show bursts of slow-frequency waves, with higher voltage and slowing with increasing severity of the encephalopathy.[370] These occur against a background that is either normal, mildly slowed, or markedly dysrhythmic. Generalized epileptiform activity may be found in those with seizures. The EEG returns to normal with resolution of the encephalopathy. Quantitative methods may be more sensitive in detecting early changes during dialysis, but it is difficult to control for normal drowsiness.[371] The CSF becomes acidotic during attacks.[372]

Management Dialysis dysequilibrium is due to a rapid osmotic shift of water into the brain. This can be largely prevented by using slower blood flow rates in dialysis[369] and/or by increasing the osmolality of the dialysate by the addition of urea, sodium, mannitol, or glycerol.[363,371,373] Glycerol has some theoretical advantages, as it prevents the intracellular acidosis noted by Arieff and colleagues.[371] The substitution of bicarbonate for acetate in the dialysate has also been recommended. The use of peritoneal dialysis or hemofiltration in place of dialysis are other preventive strategies.[372]

Subdural Hematoma Subdural hematomas occur in 1 to 3.3 percent of patients on hemodialysis and associated anticoagulant therapy.[374,375] Subdural hematomas can occur at any age in uremia. The shift to older individuals for nontraumatic subdural hematomas, found in the normal population, does not apply to uremic patients. Rotter and Roettger found nontraumatic subdural hematomas at autopsy in 2.7 percent of routinely hemodialyzed uremic patients.[376] The hematomas were large in only 1 of 9 cases; most had fresh bleeding with evidence of older hemorrhage. The iatrogenic and intrinsic uremic coagulopathies probably combine to predispose to subdural hemorrhage.

Clinically, patients are likely to present with headache, associated with tenderness of the head to percussion. The patient may show decreased alertness and cognition, and may seem depressed. These are insidious and common features in the uremic population and can easily be overlooked. Focal signs may predominate in some patients. Hemiparesis or a language disturbance may occur, but could be misinterpreted. Gait apraxia is common in older patients with subdural hematoma.[377] Patients walk as if they are "glued to the floor," especially at the

134. Mauriac L, Roger P, et al: Thyroiditis de Hashimoto et encéphalopathie. *Rev Franç Endocrinol Clin* 23:147, 1982.

135. Shein M, Apter A, Dickerman Z, Tyano S, Gadoth N: Encephalopathy in compensated Hashimoto thyroiditis: a clinical expression of autoimmune cerebral vascultis. *Brain Dev* 8:60, 1986.

136. Claussman C, Offner C, Chevalier Y, Sella F, Collard M: Encephalopathie et thyroidite de Hashimoto. *Rev Neurol* 150:166, 1994.

137. Takahashi S, Mitamura R, Itoh Y, Suzuki N, Okuno A: Hashimoto encephalopathy: etiologic considerations. *Pediatr Neurol* 11:328, 1994.

138. Latinville D, Bernardi O, Cougoule JP, et al: Thyroidite d'Hashimoto et encéphalopathie myoclonique. Hypotheses pathogeniques. *Rev Neurol* 141:55, 1985.

139. Sokoloff L: The metabolism of the central nervous system in vivo, in Field J, Magoun HW (eds): *Handbook of Physiology-Neurophysiology*, vol 3. Washington, American Physiological Society, 1960, pp 1843–1864.

140. Sokoloff L: Local energy metabolism: its relationships to functional activity and blood flow, in Purves MJ, Elliott P (eds): *Cerebral Vascular Smooth Muscle and its Control*. Ciba Foundation Symposium 56. Amsterdam, Elsevier/Excerpta Medica/North Holland, 1978, pp 171–197.

141. Stone WE, Tews JK, Whisler KE, et al: Incorporation of carbon from glucose into cerebral amino acids, proteins and lipids, and alterations during recovery from hypoglycemia. *J Neurochem* 19:321, 1972.

142. Koh THHG, Aynsley-Greene A, Tarbit M, Eyre JA: Neural dysfunction during hypoglycemia. *Arch Dis Child* 63:1353, 1988.

143. Surtees R, Leonard JV: Acute metabolic encephalopathy: a review of causes, mechanisms and treatment. *J Inher Metab Dis* 12(suppl 1):42, 1989.

144. Winter RJ: Profiles of metabolic control in diabetic children—frequency of asymptomatic nocturnal hypoglycemia. *Metabolism* 30:666, 1981.

145. Basdevant A, Costagliola D, Lanöe JL, et al: The risk of diabetic control: a comparison of hospital versus general practice supervision. *Diabetiologia* 22:309, 1982.

146. Paz-Guevara AT, Hsu TH, White P: Juvenile diabetes mellitus after 40 years. *Diabetes* 2:569, 1981.

147. Olefsky JM: Diabetes mellitus, in Wyngaarden JB, Smith LH (eds): *Cecil Textbook of Medicine*, 18th ed. Philadelphia, WB Saunders, 1988, pp 1361–1362.

148. McCrimmon RJ, Deary IJ, Huntly BIP, MacLeod KJ, Frier BM: Visual information processing during controlled hypoglycemia in humans. *Brain* 119:1277, 1996.

149. Deary IJ, Hunter R, Langan SJ, Goodwin GM: Inspection time, psychometric intelligence and clinical estimates of cognitive ability in presenile Alzheimer's disease and Korsakoff's psychosis. *Brain* 114:2543, 1991.

150. Boeve BF, Bell DG, Noseworthy JH: Bilateral temporal lobe MRI changes in uncomplicated hypoglycemic coma. *Can J Neurol Sci* 22:56, 1995.

151. Siesjö BK: Hypoglycemia, brain metabolism, and brain damage. *Diabetes/Metabolism Rev* 4:113, 1988.

152. Siesjö BK: Calcium-mediated processes in neuronal degeneration. *Ann NY Acad Sci* 47:140, 1994.

153. Sandberg M, Butcher SP, Hagberg H: Extra cellular overflow, of neuroactive amino acids during severe insulin-induced hypoglycemia: in vivo dialysis of the rat hippocampus. *J Neurochem* 47:178–184, 1986.

154. Auer RN, Siesjö BK: Biological differences between ischemia, hypoglycemia and epilepsy. *Ann Neurol* 24:699–707, 1988.

155. Öztas B, Kücük M, Sandalci U: Effect of insulin-induced hypoglycemia on blood-brain barrier permeability. *Exp Neurol* 87:129, 1985.

156. Brierley JB, Brown AW, Meldrum BS: The nature and time course of the neuronal alterations resulting from oligemia and hypoglycaemia in the brain of *Macaca mulata*. *Brain Res* 25:483, 1971.

157. Kalimo H, Olsson Y: Effects of severe hypoglycemia on the human brain. Neuropathological case reports. *Acta Neurol Scand* 62:345, 1980.

158. Fujioka M, Okuchi K, Hiramatsu K-I, et al: Specific changes in human brain after hypoglycemic injury. *Stroke* 28:584, 1997.

159. Malouf R, Brust JCM: Hypoglycemia: causes, neurological manifestations and outcome. *Ann Neurol* 17:421, 1985.

160. Reiher J, Rivest J, Grand'Maison F, Leduc CP: Periodic lateralized epileptiform discharges with transitional rhythmic discharges: association with seizures. *Electroenceph Clin Neurophysiol* 78:12, 1991.

161. Hepburn DA, Deary IJ, Frier BM, et al: Hypoglycemia convulsions cause serious musculoskeletal injuries in patients with IDDM. *Diab Care* 12:32, 1989.

162. Wallis WE, Donaldson I, Scott RS, Wilson J: Hypoglycemia masquerading as cerebrovascular disease (hypoglycemic hemiplegia). *Ann Neurol* 18:510, 1985.

163. Shaw C, Haas L, Miller D, Delahunt J: A case report of paroxysmal dystonic choreoathetosis due to hypoglycaemia induced by an insulinoma. *J Neurol Neurosurg Psychiatry* 61:194, 1996.

164. Venna N, Sabin TD: Tonic focal seizures in non-ketotic hyperglycemia of diabetes mellitus. *Arch Neurol* 38:512, 1981.

165. Hennis A, Corbin D, Fraser H: Focal seizures and non-ketotic hyperglycemia. *J Neurol Neurosurg Psychiatry* 55:195, 1992.

166. Duncan MB, Jabbari B, Rosenberg ML: Gaze-evoked seizures in nonketotic hyperglycemia. *Epilepsia* 32:221, 1991.

167. Young GB, Brown JD, Bolton CF: Periodic lateralized epileptiform discharges (PLEDs) and nystagmus retractorius. *Ann Neurol* 2:61, 1977.

168a. Harden CL, Rosenbaum DH, Daras M: Hyperglycemia presenting with occipital seizures. *Epilepsia* 32:215, 1991.

168b. Arieff AI, Carroll HJ: Cerebral edema and depression of sensorium in nonketotic hyperosmolar coma. *Diabetes* 23:525, 1974.

168c. Arieff AI, Kleeman CR: Studies on the mechanisms of cerebral edema in diabetic comas: effects of hyperglycemia and rapid lowering of plasma glucose in normal rabbits. *J Clin Invest* 52:571, 1973.

169. Fulop M, et al: Ketotic hyperosmolar coma. *Lancet* 2:635, 1973.

170. Tachibana Y, Yasuhara A: Hyperosmolar syndrome and diffuse CNS dysfunction with clinical implications. *Funct Neurol* 1:140, 1986.

171. Popli S, Leehey DJ, Daugirdas JT, et al: Asymptomatic, nonketotic, severe hyperglycemia with hyponatremia. *Arch Intern Med* 150:1962, 1990.

172. Schneider R, Droller H: The relative importance of ketosis and acidosis in the production of diabetic coma. *Q J Exp Physiol* 28:3223, 1938.

173. Kety SS, et al: The blood flow and oxygen consumption of the human brain in diabetic ketoacidosis and coma. *J Clin Invest* 27:500, 1948.

174. Posner JB, Plum F: Spinal fluid pH and neurologic symptoms in systemic acidosis. *N Eng J Med* 277:605, 1967.

175. Guisado R, Arieff AI: Neurologic manifestations of diabetic comas: correlation with biochemical alterations in the brain. *Metabolism* 24:665, 1975.

176. Rowland NE, Bellush LL: Diabetes mellitus: stress, neurochemistry and behavior. *Neurosci Biobehav Rev* 13:199, 1989.

177. Arieff AI, Kleeman CR, Keushkerian A, et al: Studies on the mechanisms of cerebral edema in diabetic comas: effect of hyperglycemia and rapid lowering of plasma glucose in normal rabbits. *J Clin Invest* 52:571, 1973.

178. Clements RS Jr, Blumenthal AS, Morrison JI, Winegrad AI: Increased cerebrospinal pressure during treatment of diabetic ketoacidosis. *Lancet* II:671, 1971.

179. Hoffman WH, Steinhart CM, Gammal TE, et al: Cranial CT in children and adolescents with diabetic ketoacidosis. *Am J Neuroradiol* 9:733, 1988.

180. Prockop LD: Hyperglycemia: effects on the nervous system, in Vinken PJ, Bruyn GW (eds): *Handbook of Clinical Neurology*, vol 27, part 1, New York, Elsevier, 1976, pp 79–98.

181. Hammond P, Wallis S: Cerebral oedema in diabetic ketoacidosis. *BMJ* 305:203, 1992.

182. Lebovitz HE: Diabetic ketoacidosis. *Lancet* 345:767, 1995.

183. Fein IA, Rackow EC, Sprung CL, Grodman R: Relation of colloid osmostic pressure to arterial hypoxemia and cerebral edema during crystalloid volume loading of patients with diabetic ketoacidosis. *Ann Intern Med* 96:570, 1982.

184. Soni A, Rao SV, Bajaj R, Treser G: Extreme hyperglycemia and hyperosmolality. *Diabetes Care* 13:181, 1990.

185. Uribarri J, Carrol HJ: Neurologic manifestations of diabetic coma, in Arieff AI, Griggs RC (eds): *Metabolic Brain Dysfunction in Systemic Disorders*. Boston, Little, Brown, 1992, pp 107–127.

186. Worthley LI: Hyperosmolar coma treated with intravenous sterile water. *Arch Intern Med* 146:945, 1986.

187. Baethman A, Van Harreveld A: Effect of adrenal insufficiency on water and electrolyte distribution in the brain. *J Neuropath Exp Neurol* 32:394, 1973.

188. Cleghorn RA: Adrenal cortical insufficiency: psychological and neurological observation. *Can Med Assoc J* 65:449, 1951.

189. Dorin RI, Kearns PJ: High output circulatory failure in acute adrenal insufficiency. *Crit Care Med* 16:296, 1988.

190. Geenen C, Tein I, Erlich RM: Addison's disease presenting with cerebral edema. *Can J Neurol Sci* 23:141, 1996.

191. Jefferson A: Clinical association between encephalopathy and papilloedema in Addison's disease. *J Neurol Neurosurg Psychiatry* 19:21, 1956.

192. Burke CW: Adrenocortical insufficiency. *Clin Endocrinol Metab* 14:947, 1985.

193. Kovacs K: Necrosis of the anterior pituitary in humans. *Neuroendocrinology* 4:170, 1969.

194. Mueller-Jensen A, Ludecke D: Clinical aspects of spontaneous necrosis in pituitary tumors (pituitary apoplexy). *J Neurol* 224:267, 1981.

195. Mohr G, Hardy J: Hemorrhage, necrosis, and apoplexy in pituitary adenomas. *Surg Neurol* 18:181, 1982.

196. Brougham M, Heusner AP, Adams RD: Acute degenerative changes in the adenomas of the pituitary body. *J Neurosurg* 7:421, 1950.

197. Vital E, Cevellos R, Vidal J, Ravon R, et al: Twelve cases of pituitary apoplexy. *Arch Intern Med* 152:1893, 1992.

198. Rovit RL, Fein JM: Pituitary apoplexy: a review and reappraisal. *J Neurosurg* 37:280, 1972.

199. Tamasawa N, Kurahashi K, Baba T, et al: Spontaneous remission of acromegaly after pituitary apoplexy following head trauma. *J Endocrinol Invest* 11:429, 1987.

200. Reid RL, Quigley ME, Yen SSC: Pituitary apoplexy. *Arch Neurol* 42:712, 1985.

201. Cardoso ER, Peterson EW: Pituitary apoplexy: a review. *Neurosurgery* 14:363, 1984.

202. Pelkonen R, Kuusisto A, Salmi J, et al: Pituitary function after pituitary apoplexy. *Am J Med* 65:773, 1978.

203. Rolih CA, Ober KP: Pituitary apoplexy, in Ober KP (ed): *Endocrinol Metab Clin N Am* 22:291, 1993.

204. Lee WM: Acute liver failure. *Am J Med* 96:1A–3S, 1994.

205. Lee WM: Acute liver failure. *N Eng J Med* 329:1862, 1993.

206. Regier DA, Farmer ME, Rae DS, et al: Comorbidity of mental disorders with alcohol and other drug abuse. *JAMA* 264:2511, 1990.

207. Bronisch T, Wittchen HU: Lifetime and 6-month prevalence of abuse and dependence of alcohol in the Munich Follow-up Study. *Eur Arch Psychiatry Clin Neurosci* 241:273, 1992.

208. Podolsky DK, Isselbacher KJ: Cirrhosis, in Braunwald E, Isselbacher KJ, Petersdorf RG, Wilson JD, Martin JB, Fauci AS (eds): *Harrison's Principles of Internal Medicine*, 11th ed. New York, McGraw-Hill, 1987.

209. Itai Y, Kurosaki Y, Saida Y, Nitsu M, Kuramoto K: AT and MRI in detection of portosystemic shunts in patients with liver cirrhosis. *J Comput Assist Tomog* 18:768, 1994.

210. Decell MK, Gordon JBN, Silver K, Meagher-Villemure K: Fulminant hepatic failure associated with status epilepticus in children: three cases and a review of potential mechanisms. *Intens Care Med* 20:375, 1994.

211. Smith D, Cullity G, Silberstein D: Fatal hepatic necrosis associated with multiple anticonvulsant therapy. *Aust NZ J Med* 18:575, 1989.

212. Ussery X, Henar E, Black D, Berger S, Whitington P: Acute liver injury after protracted seizures in children. *J Pediatr Dostroenterol Nutr* 9:421, 1989.

213. Decell MK, Gordon JB, Silver K, Neager-Villmure K: Fulminant hepatic failure associated with status epilepticus in children: three cases and a review of potential mechanisms. *Intens Care Med* 20:375, 1994.

214. Adams RD, Foley JM: The neurological disorder associated with liver disease, in Merritt HH, Hare C (eds): *Metabolic and Toxic Diseases of the Nervous System*. Baltimore, Williams and Wilkins, 1953, pp 198–237.

215. Lockwood AH: *Hepatic Encephalopathy*. Boston, Butterworth-Heinemann, 1992.

216. Victor M, Adams RD, Cole M: The acquired (nonWilsonian) type of chronic hepatocerebral degeneration. *Medicine* 44:345, 1965.

217. Mizuguchi M, Tomonaga M, Fukusato T, Sasno M: Acute necrtotizing encephalopathy with widespread edematous lesions of symmetrical distribution. *Acta Neuropathol* 78:108, 1989.

218. Lockwood AH: *Hepatic Encephalopathy*. Boston, Butterworth-Heineman, 1992, p 109.

219. Jones EA, Skolnick P, Gammal SH, Basile AS, Mullen KD: NIH Conference. The gamma-aminobutyric acid A (GABAA) receptor complex and hepatic encephalopathy. Some recent advances. *Ann Intern Med* 110:532, 1989.

220. Gammal SH, Basile AS, Geller D, et al: Reversal of behavioral and electrophysiological abnormalities of an animal model of hepatic encephalopathy by benzodiazepine receptor ligands. *Hepatology* 11:371, 1990.

221. Basile AS, Pannell L, Jaouni T, et al: Brain concentrations of benzodiazepines are elevated in an animal model of hepatic encephalopathy. *Proc Natl Acad Sci USA* 87:5263, 1991.

222. Ferenci P, Covell D, Schafer DF, et al: Metabolism of the inhibitory neurotransmitter gamma-aminobutyric acid in a rabbit model of fulminant hepatic failure. *Hepatology* 3:507, 1983.

223. Olasmaa M, Rothstein JD, Guidotti A, et al: Endogenous benzodiazepine receptor ligands in human and hepatic encephalopathy. *J Neurochem* 55:2015, 1990.

224. Basile AS, Pannell L, Jouni T, et al: Brain concentrations of benzodiazepines are elevated in an animal model of hepatic encephalopathy. *Proc Natl Acad Sci USA* 87:5263, 1990.

225. Basile AS, Jones EA, Skolnik P: The pathogenesis and treatment of hepatic encephalopathy: evidence for the involvement of benzodiazepine receptor ligands. *Pharmacol Rev* 43:27, 1991.

226. Sherlock S: Pathogenesis and management of hepatic coma. *Am J Med* 24:737, 1958.

227. Duffy TE, Vergara F, Plum F: Alpha-ketoglutaramate in hepatic encephalopathy, in Plum F (ed): Brain Dysfunction in Metabolic Disorders. *Res Publ Assoc Nerv Ment Dis* 53:39, 1974.

228. Boogerd W, Zoetulder FA, Moffie D: Hyperammonemic encephalopathy due to suture line breakdown after bladder operation. *Clin Neurol Neurosurg* 92:255, 1990.

229. Norenberg MD: The role of astrocytes in hepatic encephalopathy. *Neurochem Pathol* 6:13, 1987.

230. Zieve L: Pathogenesis of hepatic encephalopathy. *Metab Brain Dis* 2:147, 1987.

231. Raabe W, Gumnit RJ: Disinhibition in cat motor cortex by ammonia. *J Neurophysiol* 38:347, 1875.

232. Lux HD, Loracher C, Neher E: The action of ammonium on postsynaptic inhibition of cat spinal motor neurons. *Brain Res* 11:431, 1970.

233. Szerb JC, Butterworth RF: Effect of ammonium ions on synaptic transmission in the mammalian nervous system. *Prog Neurobiol* 39:135, 1992.

234. Bergeron M, Swain MS, Reader TA, Grondin L, Butterworth RF: Effect of ammonia on brain serotonin metabolism in relation to function in the portacaval shunted rat. *J Neurochem* 55:222, 1990.

235. Thomas JW, Banner C, Whitman J, Mullen KD, Freese E: Changes in glutamate-cycle enzyme mRNA levels in a rat model of hepatic encephalopathy. *Metab Brain Dis* 3:81, 1988.

236. Fischer JE, Baldasarini RJ: False neurotransmitters and hepatic failure. *Lancet* 2:75, 1971.

237. Fogel WA, Andrezejewski W, Maslinski C: Neurotransmitters in hepatic encephalopathy. *Acta Neurobiol* 50:281, 1990.

238. Zieve L, Olsen RL: Can hepatic encephalopathy be caused by a reduction of brain noradrenalin or octopamine. *Gut* 18:688, 1977.

239. Schmidt W, Wolf G, Grüngreiff K, Meier M, Reum T: Hepatic encephalopathy influences high-activity uptake of neurotransmitter glutamate and aspartate into the hippocampal formation. *Metab Brain Dis* 5:19, 1990.

240. Butterworth RF, Le O, Lavoie J, Szerb J: Effect of portacaval anastomosis on electrically stimulated release of glutamate from rat hippocampal slices. *J Neurochem* 56:1481, 1991.

241. Hamberger A, Hequist B, Nyström B: Ammonium ions inhibition of evoked release of endogenous glutamate from hippocampal slices. *J Neurochem* 33:1295, 1979.

242. Lockwood AH. Hepatic encephalopathy: experimental approaches to human metabolic encephalopathy. *CRC Rev Neurobiol* 3:105, 1987.

243. Mousseau DD, Layargues GP, Butterworth RF: Region-sensitive decreases in [^{3}H]tryptamine binding sites in autopsied brain tissue from cirrhotic patients with hepatic encephalopathy. *J Neurochem* 62:621, 1994.

244. Borg J, Warteer JM, Schliengeer JL, Imleeer M, Marescauzz C, Mack G: Neurotransmitter modifications in human cerebrospinal fluid and serum during hepatic encephalopathy. *J Neurol Sci* 57:343, 1982.

245. Baraldi M, Zeeneroli ML: Experimental hepatic encephalopathy. Changes in binding gamma aminobutyric acid. *Science* 216:427, 1982.

246. Der RF, Zieve L: Methanethiol and fatty acids depress urea synthesis by the isolated rat liver. *J Lab Clin Med* 100:585, 1982.

247. Vahlkamp T, Meijer AJ, Wilms J, Chamuleau RAFM: Inhibition of mitochondrial electron transfer in rats by ethanediol and methanethiol. *Clin Sci* 56:147, 1979.

248. Zieve L, Doizaki W, Zieve FJ: Synergism between mercaptans and ammonia or fatty acids in the production of coma: a possible role for mercaptans in the pathogenesis of hepatic coma. *J Lab Clin Med* 83:16, 1974.

249. Moritaux A, Dawson AM: Plasma free fatty acid in liver disease. *Gut* 2:304, 1961.

250. Krieger D, Krieger S, Jansen O, et al: Manganese and chronic hepatic encephalopathy. *Lancet* 346:270, 1995.

251. Mergler D: Manganese: the controversial metal. At what levels can deleterious effects occur? *Can J Neurol Sci* 23:93, 1996.

252. Hauser RA, Zesiewicz TA, Martinez C, Rosemurgy AS, Olanow CW: Blood manganese correlates with brain magnetic resonance imaging changes in patients with liver disease. *Can J Neurol Sci* 23:95, 1996.

253. Calne DB, Chu NS, Hung CC, Lu CS, Olanow CW: Manganism and idiopathic parkinsonism: similarities and differences. *Neurology* 44:1583, 1994.

254. Sherlock S, Summerskill WHJ, White LP, Phear EA: Portal-systemic encephalopathy: neurological complications of liver disease. *Lancet* 267:453, 1954.

255. Barbeau A: Manganese and extrapyramidal disorders. *Neurotoxicology* 5:13, 1984.

256. Aschner M, Aschner JL: Manganese neurotoxicity: cellular effects and blood-brain barrier transport. *Neurosci Behav Rev* 15:333, 1991.

257. Brouillet EP, Shinobu L, McGarvey U, Hochberg F, Beal MF: Manganese injection into the rat striatum produces excitotoxic lesions by impairing energy metabolism. *Exp Neurol* 120:89, 1993.

258. Brouillet EP, Shinobu L, McGarvey U, Hochberg F, Beal MF: Manganese injection into the rat striatum produces excitotoxic lesions by impairing energy metabolism. *Exp Neurol* 120:89, 1993.

259. Bird ED, Anton AH, Bullock B: The effect of manganese intoxication on basal ganglia dopamine concentrations in rhesus monkey. *Neurotoxicology* 5:59, 1984.

260. Subhash MN, Padmashree TS: Effect of manganese on biogenic amine metabolism in regions of the rat brain. *Food Chem Toxicol* 29:579, 1991.

261. Lista A, Abarca J, Ramos C, Daniels AJ: Rat striatal dopamine and tetrahydrobioterin content following intrastriatal injection of magnesium chloride. *Life Sci* 38:2121, 1986.

262. Mousseau DD, Perney P, Pormier Layrargues G, Butterworth RF: Selective loss of pallidal dopamine D2 receptor density in hepatic encephalopathy. *Neurosci Lett* 162:192, 1993.

263. Butterworth RF, Spahr L, Fontaine S, Pormier Layrargues G: Manganese toxicity, dopaminergic dysfunction and hepatic encephalopathy. *Metabol Brain Dis* 10:259, 1995.

264. Pomier Layrargues G, Shapcott D, Spahr L, Butterworth RF: Accumulation of manganese and copper in pallidum of cirrhotic patients: role in the pathogenesis of hepatic encephalopathy. *Metab Brain Dis* 10:353, 1995.

265. Karenlampi S, Tuomi K, Korkalainen TZ, Raunio H: Induction of cytochrome P-450 IAI in mouse hepatoma cells by several chemicals. *Biochem Pharmacol* 38:1517, 1989.

266. McCord J: Oxygen-derived free radicals in postischemic tissue injury. *N Eng J Med* 312:159, 1985.

267. Skibba JL, Stadnicka A, Kalbfleisch JH: Effects of hyperthermia on xanthine oxidase activity and glutathione levels in the perfused rat liver. *J Biochem Toxicol* 4:119, 1989.

268. Pyke S, Lew H, Quintanilha A: Severe depletion of liver glutathione during physical exercise. *Biochem Biophys Res Commun* 139:926, 1986.

269. Roy D, Snodgrass W: Phenytoin metabolic activation: role of cytochrome P450, glutathione, age and sex in rats and mice. *Res Commun Chem Pathol Pharmacol* 59:173, 1988.

270. Ede RJ, Williams R: Hepatic encephalopathy and cerebral edema. *Semin Liver Dis* 6:107, 1989.

271. Traber PG, Dal Canto M, Ganger DR, Blei AT: Electron microscopic evaluation of brain edema in rabbits with galactosamine-induced fulminant hepatic failure: ultrastructure and integrity of the blood-brain barrier. *Hepatology* 7:1272–1277, 1987.

272. McClung HJ, Sloan HR, Powers P, et al: Early changes in the permeability of the blood-brain barrier produced by toxins associated with liver failure. *Pediatr Res* 28:227, 1990.

273. Kato M, Hughes RD, Keays RT, Williams R: Electron microscopic study of brain capillaries in cerebral edema from fulminant hepatic failure. *Hepatology* 15:1060, 1992.

274. Livingstone AS, Potvin M, Goresky CAA, Finlayson MH, Hinchey EJ: Changes in the blood-brain barrier permeability in hepatic coma after hepatectomy in the rat. *Gastroenterology* 73:697, 1977.

275. Blei AT: Cerebral edema and intracranial hypertension in acute liver failure: distinct aspects of the same problem. *Hepatology* 13:376, 1991.

276. Seda HWM, Hughes RD, Gove CD, Williams R: Inhibition of rat brain NA^+-K^+-ATPase activity by serum from patients with fulminant hepatic failure. *Hepatology* 4:74, 1984.

277. Almdal T, Schroeder T, Ranek L: Cerebral blood flow and liver function in patients with encephalopathy due to acute and chronic liver diseases. *Scand J Gastroenterol* 24:299, 1989.

278. Derr RF, Zieve L: Decreased cerebral uptake of oxygen in coma—a consequence of decreased utilization of ATP. *J Neurochem* 21:1555, 1973.

279. Barbe T, Losay J, Grimon G, et al: Pulmonary arteriovenous shunting in children with liver disease. *J Pediatr* 126:571, 1995.

280. DeVivo DC: Reye syndrome. *Neurol Clin* 3:95, 1985.

281. Lee WM, Galbraith RM: The extracellular actin-scavenger system and actin toxicity. *N Eng J Med* 326:1335, 1992.

282. Bihari DJ, Gimson AES, Williams R: Cardiovascular, pulmonary, and renal complications of fulminant hepatic failure. *Semin Liver Dis* 6:119, 1986.

283. Tarter RE, Hegedus AM, Van Thiel DH, et al: Nonalcoholic cirrhosis associated with neuropsychological dysfunction in the absence of overt evidence of hepatic encephalopathy. *Gastroenterology* 86:1421, 1984.

284. Caplan LR, Scheiner D: Dysconjugate gaze in hepatic coma. *Ann Neurol* 8:328, 1980.

285. Rai G, Buxton-Thomas M, Scanlon M: Ocular bobbing in hepatic encephalopathy. *Br J Clin Pract* 30:202, 1976.

286. Plum F, Posner JB: *The Diagnosis of Stupor and Coma*. Philadelphia, FA Davis, 1980, pp 189–190.

287. McLachlan RS, Bolton CF, Coates RK, Barnett JHM: Gait disturbance in chronic subdural hematoma. *Can Med Assoc J* 125:865, 1981.

288. Horani BT, Hamlin BM, Reynolds TB: Cerebrospinal fluid glutamine as a measure of hepatic encephalopathy. *Arch Intern Med* 127:1033, 1971.

289. Gilon E, Szeinberg A, Tauman G, Bodonyi E: Glutamine estimation in cerebrospinal fluid in cases of liver cirrhosis and hepatic coma. *J Clin Lab Med* 53:714, 1959.

290. Brenner RP: The electroencephalogram in altered states of consciousness. *Neurol Clin* 3:615, 1985.

291. Van der Rijt CD, Schalm SW, de Groot GH, de Vlieger M: Objective measurements of hepatic encephalopathy by means of activated EEG analysis. *Electroenceph Clin Neurophysiol* 57:423, 1984.

292. Bickford RG; Fleming JI, Billinger TW: Compression of EEG spectra by isometric power spectral plots. *Electroenceph Clin Neurophysiol* 31:632, 1971.

293. Van der Rijt CD, Schalm SW: Quantitative EEG and survival in liver disease. *Electroenceph Clin Neurophysiol* 61:502, 1985.

294. Davies MG, Rowan MJ, Keeling PWN, Weir DG, Feely J: The auditory P300 event related potential: an objective marker of the encephalopathy of chronic liver disease. *Hepatology* 12:688, 1990.

295. Zeneroli ML, Pinelli G, Gallini G et al: VEP: a diagnostic tool for the assessment of hepatic encephalopathy. *Gut* 25:291, 1984.

296. Levy LJ, Bolton RP, Losaowsky MS: The use of VEP in delineating a state of subclinical encephalopathy. *J Hepatol* 5:211, 1987.

297. Chan YW, McLeod JG, Tuck RP, Walsh JC, Feary PA: Visual evoked response in chronic alcoholics. *J Neurol Neurosurg Psychiatry* 49:945, 1986.

298. Davies MG, Rowan MJ, Feely J: EEG and event related potentials in hepatic encephalopathy. *Metab Brain Dis* 6:175, 1991.

299. Kullman F, Hollerbach S, Holstege A, Scholmerich J: Subclinical hepatic encephalopathy: the diagnostic value of evoked potentials. *J Hepatol* 22:101, 1995.

300. Tarter RE, Hays AL, Sandford SS, et al: Cerebral morphological abnormalities associated with non-alcoholic cirrhosis. Lancet II:893, 1986.

301. Wijdicks EF, Plevak DJ, Rakela J, Wiesner RH: Clinical and radiological features of cerebral edema in fulminant hepatic failure. *Mayo Clin Proc* 70:119, 1995.

302. Munoz SJ, Robinson M, Northrup B, et al: Elevated intracranial pressure and computed tomography of the brain in fulmilant hepatocellular failure. *Hepatology* 13:209, 1993.

303. Herrmann S, Krieger D, Jansen A, et al.: Effect of liver transplantation on hepatic encephalopathy and hyperintense globus pallidus on T1-weighted MRI in liver failure. *Neurology* 45 (Suppl 4):298, 1995.

304. Weissenborn K, Ehrenheim Ch, Hori A, Kubicka S, Manns MP: Pallidal lesions in patients with liver cirrhosis: clinical and MRI evaluation. *Metab Brain Dis* 10:219, 1995.

305. Ballauff A, Engelbrecht V, Voit T: Hyperintense lesions of the globus pallidus on MRI in children with liver disease. *Eur J Pediatr* 153:802, 1994.

306. Barron TF, Devenyl AG, Mamourian AC: Symptomatic manganese neurotoxicity in a patient with chronic liver disease: correlation of clinical symptoms with MRI findings. *Pediatr Neurol* 10:145, 1994.

307. Weissborn K, Marsano L, Diehl AM, Kunze K: Hepatic coma, in Hacke W (ed): *Neuro-Critical Care*. Berlin, Springer-Verlag, 1994, pp 937–950.

308. Atillasoy E, Berk PD: Fulminant hepatic failure: pathophysiology, treatment and survival. *Annu Rev Med* 46:181, 1995.

309. Donovan JP, Shaw BW Jr, Langnas AN, Sorrell MF: Brain water and acute liver failure: the emerging role of intracranial pressure monitoring. *Hepatology* 16:267–268, 1992.

310. Blei AT, Olafsson S, Webster S, Levy R: Complications of intracranial pressure monitoring in fulminant hepatic failure. *Lancet* 341:157, 1993.

311. Keays R, Potter D, O'Grady J, Peachy T, Alexander G, Williams R: Intracranial and cerebral perfusion pressures before, during and immediately after orthotopic liver transplantation for fulminant hepatic failure. *QJM* 79:425, 1991.

312. Sidi A, Mahla ME: Noninvasive monitoring of cerebral perfusion by transcranial Doppler during fulminant hepatic failure and liver transplantation. *Anesth Analg* 80:194, 1995.

313. Davenport A, Will EJ, Davison AM: Effect of posture on intracranial pressure in patients with fulminant heptic and renal failure after acetaminophen self-poisoning. *Crit Care Med* 18:286, 1993.

314. Canalese J, Gimson AES, Davis C, et al: Controlled trail of dexamethazone and mannitol for the cerebral edema of fulminant hepatic failure. *J Hepatol* 2:43, 1986.

315. Ede RJ, Gimson AES, Bihari D, Williams R: Controlled hyperventilation in the prevention of cerebral oedema in fulminant hepatic failure. *J Hepatol* 2:43, 1986.

316. Weber FL Jr, Fresard KM, Lally BR: Nitrogen in fecal bacterial, fiber, and soluble fractions of patients with cirrhosis: Effects of lactulose and neomycin. *J Lab Clin Med* 82:213, 1987.

317. Rolando N, Gimson A, Wade J, et al: Prospective controlled trail of selective parenteral and enteral antimicrobial regimen in fulminant liver failure. *Hepatology* 17:196, 1993.

318. Naylor CD, O'Rourke K, Detsky AS, Baker JP: Parenteral nutrition with branched-chain amino acids in hepatic encephalopathy: a meta-analysis. *Gastroenterology* 97:1033, 1989.

319. Rossi-Fanelli F, Riggio O, Cangiano C, et al: Branched chain amino acids versus lactulose in the treatment of hepatic coma. A controlled study. *Dig Dis Sci* 27:929, 1982.

320. Wahren J, Denis J, Desurmont P, et al: Is intravenous administration of branched chain amino acids effective in the treatment of hepatic encephalopathy? A multicenter study. *Hepatology* 3:475, 1983.

321. Michel H, Pomier-Layrargues G, Aubin JP, et al: Treatment of hepatic encephalopathy by infusion of a modified amino acid solution: results of a controlled study of 47 cirrhotic patients, in Capocaccia L, Fischer JE, Rossi-Fanelli F (eds): *Hepatic Encephalopathy in Chronic Liver Failure*. New York, Plenum Press, 1984, pp 301–310.

322. Fiaccadori F, Ghinelli F, Pedretti G, et al: Branched chain amino acid enriched solutions in the treatment of hepatic encephalopathy: a controlled trial, in Capocaccia L, Fischer JE, Rossi-Fanelli F (eds): *Hepatic Encephalopathy in Chronic Liver Failure*. New York, Plenum Press, 1984, pp 323–333.

323. Cerra FB, Chung NK, Fischer JE, et al: Disease specific amino-acid infusion (F080) in hepatic encephalopathy: a prospective randomized, double-blind controlled trial. *J Parenter Nutr* 9:288, 1985.

324. Erikson LS, Conn HO: Branched-chain amino acids in the management of hepatic encephalopathy: an analysis of variants. *Hepatology* 10:228, 1989.

325. Devictor D, Tahiri C, Lanchier C, et al: Flumazenil in the treatment of hepatic encephalopathy in children with fulminant hepatic failure. *Intens Care Med* 21:253, 1995.

326. Chapman RW, Forman D, Peto R, Smallwood R: Liver transplantation for acute hepatic failure. *Lancet* 335:32, 1990.

327. Lidofsky SD: Fulminant hepatic failure. *Crit Care Clin* 11:415, 1995.

328. O'Grady JG, Gimson AES, O'Brien CJ, et al: Controlled trails of charcoal hemoperfusion and prognostic factors in fulminant hepatic failure. *Gastroenterology* 94:1186, 1988.

329. Sheiner P, Sinclair S, Greig P, et al: Randomized controlled trial of prostaglandin E_1 in the treatment of fulminant hepatic failure. *Hepatology* 16:88A, 1992.

330. Woolf GM, Redeker AG: Treatment of fulminant hepatic failure with insulin and glucagon: a randomized, controlled trial. *Dig Dis Sci* 36:92, 1991.

331. Ribeiro J, Noprdlinger B, Ballet F, et al: Intrasplenic hepatocellular transplantation corrects hepatic encephalopathy in portacaval-shunted rats. *Hepatology* 15:12, 1992.

332. Demetriou AA, Rozga J, Podestas L, et al: Early clinical experience with a hybrid bioartificial liver. *Scand J Gastroenterol* 30(suppl 208):111, 1995.

333. Fraser CL, Arieff AI: Metabolic encephalopathy as a complication of renal failure. *New Horiz* 2:518, 1994.

334. Conger JD, Schrier RW: Acute renal failure: pathogenesis, diagnosis, and management, in Schrier RW (ed): *Renal and Electrolyte Disorders*. Boston, Little, Brown, 1985.

335. Hou SH, et al: Hospital-acquired renal insufficiency: a prospective study. *Am J Med* 74:243, 1983.

336. Locke S, Merrill JP, Tyler HR: Neurologic complications of acute uremia. *Arch Intern Med* 108:519, 1961.

337. Wilson SAK: *Neurology*. London, Edward Arnold, 1940, p 1097.

338. Gowers WR: *A Manual of Diseases of the Nervous System*. Philadelphia, P Blackiston 1888, pp 535–536.

339. Plum F, Posner JB: *The Diagnosis of Stupor and Coma*. Philadelphia, FA Davis, 1980, p 228.

340. Chadwick D, French AT: Uraemic myoclonus: an example of reticular reflex myoclonus? *J Neurol Neurosurg Psychiatry* 42:52, 1979.

341. Cadilhac J, Ribstein NI: The EEG in metabolic disorders. *Word Neurol* 2:296, 1961.

342. Chaptal J, Passouant P, Puech P: Sur la forme hypertensive des glomérulonéphrites de l'enfant. *Arch Fr Pediatr* 11:192, 1954.

343. Bartlop D: Lead poisoning in children. *Postgrad Med* 44:537, 1968.

344. Piomelli S, Rosen JF, Chisholm JJ Jr, et al.: Management of childhood lead poisoning. *J Pediatr* 105:260, 1976.

345. Massry SG: Current status of the role of parathyroid hormone in uremic toxicity. *Contrib Nephrol* 49:1, 1985.

346a. Bolton CF, Young GB: *Neurological Complications of Renal Disease*. Boston, Butterworths, 1990.

346b. Arieff AI, Griggs RC (eds): *Metabolic Brain Dysfunction in Systemic Disorders*. Boston, Little, Brown, 1992.

347. Moe SM, Sprague SM: Uremic encephalopathy. *Clin Nephrol* 12:251, 1994.

348. Tyler HR: Neurologic disorders seen in the uremic patient. *Arch Intern Med* 126:781, 1970.

349. Heilman KM, Moyer RS, Melendez F, et al: A memory defect in uremic encephalopathy. *J Neurol Sci* 26:245, 1975.

350. Stark RJ: Reversible myoclonus with uremia. *Br Med J* 282:1119, 1981.

351. Raskin NH, Fishman RA: Neurologic disorders in renal failure (first of two parts). *N Eng J Med* 294:143, 1976.

352. Glaser GH: Brain dysfunction in uremia, in Plum F (ed): *Brain Dysfunction in Metabolic Disorders*. New York, Raven Press, 1974, 173–199.

353. Tyler HR: Neurologic disorders in renal failure. *Am J Med* 44:734, 1968.

354. Madonick MJ, Berke K, Schiffer I: Pleocytosis and meningeal signs in uremia. *Arch Neurol Psychiatry* 64:431, 1950.

355. Jacob JC, Gloor P, Elwan OH, et al: Electroencephalographic changes in chronic renal failure. *Neurology* 15:419, 1965.

356. Teschan PE: Electroencephalographic and other neurophysiological abnormalities in uremia. *Kidney Int* 7:S210, 1975.

357. Bourne JR, Teschan PE: Computer methods, uremic encephalopathy and adequacy of dialysis. *Kidney Int* 24:496, 1983.

358. Teschan PE, Ginn HE, Bourne JR, Ward JW: Neurobehavioral probes for adequacy of dialysis. *Trans Am Soc Artif Organs* 23:556, 1977.

359. Alfrey AC, Mishell JM, Burks J, et al: Syndrome of dyspraxia and multifocal seizures associated with chronic hemodialysis. *Trans Am Soc Artif Organs* 18:257, 1972.

360. Wing AJ, Brunner FP, Brynger H, et al: Dialysis dementia in Europe. *Lancet* 2:190, 1980.

361. Sideman S, Manor D: The dialysis dementia syndrome and aluminum intoxication. *Nephron* 31:1, 1982.

362. Fraser CL: Neurologic manifestations of the uremic state, in Arieff AI, Griggs RC (eds): *Metabolic Brain Dysfunction in Systemic Disorders*. Boston, Little, Brown, 1992, pp 139–166.

363. Port FK, Johnson WJ, Klass DW: Prevention of dialysis dysequilibrium syndrome by the use of a high sodium concentration in the dialysate. *Kidney Int* 3:327, 1973.

364. Peterson H DeC, Swanson AG: Acute encephalopathy occurring during hemodialysis. *Arch Intern Med* 113:877, 1964.

365. Wakim KG: The pathophysiology of the dialysis dysequilibrium syndrome. *Mayo Clin Proc* 44:406, 1969.

366. Peterson H deC, Swanson AG: Acute encephalopathy occurring during hemodialysis. *Arch Intern Med* 113:877, 1964.

367. LaGreca G, Biasioli S, Chiaramonte S, et al: Studies of brain density in hemodialysis and peritoneal dialysis. *Nephron* 31:146, 1982.

368. Pappius HM, Oh JH, Dossetor JB: The effects of rapid hemodialysis on brain tissues and cerebrospinal fluid of dogs. *Can J Physiol Pharmacol* 45:129, 1966.

369. Arieff AI, Massry SG, Barrientos A, Kleeman CR: Brain, water and electrolyte metabolism in uremia: effects of slow and rapid hemodialysis. *Kidney Int* 4:177, 1973.

370. Kennedy AC, Linton AL, Luke RG, Renfrew S: Electroencephalographic changes during haemodialysis. *Lancet* 1:408, 1963.

371. Arieff AI, Lazarowitz VC, Guisado R: Experimental dialysis dysequilibrium syndrome: prevention with glycerol. *Kidney Int* 14:270, 1978.

372. Arieff AI: Dialysis dysequilibrium syndrome: current concepts on pathogenesis and prevention. *Kidney Int* 45:629, 1994.

373. Gilliland KG, Hegstrom RM: The effect of hemodialysis on cerebrospinal fluid in uremic dogs. *Trans Am Soc Artif Organs* 9:44, 1963.

374. Talalla A, Halbrook H, Barbour BH, et al: Subdural hematoma associated with long-term hemodialysis for chronic renal disease. *JAMA* 212:1847, 1970.

375. Leonard A, Shapiro FL: Subdural hematoma in regularly hemodialyzed patients. *Ann Intern Med* 82:650, 1975.

376. Rotter W, Roettger P: Comparative pathologic-anatomic study of cases of chronic global renal insufficiency with and without preceding dialysis. *Clin Nephrol* 1:257, 1973.

377. McLachlan RS, Bolton CF, Coates RK, Barnett HJM: Gait disturbance in chronic subdural hematoma. *Can Med Assoc J* 125:865, 1981.

378. Lopez RI, Collins GK: Wernicke's encephalopathy: a complication of chronic hemodialysis. *Arch Neurol* 18:248, 1968.

379. Jagadha V, Deck JHN, Halliday WC, Smyth HS: Wernicke's encephalopathy in patients on chronic peritoneal dialysis or hemodialysis. *Ann Neurol* 21:78, 1987.

380. Scharf B, Levy N: Pancreatic encephalopathy, in Vinken PJ, Bruyn GW (eds): *Handbook of Clinical Neurology*, vol 27, part I, New York, Elsevier, 1976, pp 449–458.

381. Estrada RV, Moreno J, Martinez E, et al: Pancreatic encephalopathy. *Acta Neurol Scand* 59:135, 1979.

382. Rothermich NO, Van Haam K: Pancreatic encephalopathy. *J Clin Endocrin* 1:872, 1941.

383. Plum F, Posner JP: *The Diagnosis of Stupor and Coma*, 3rd ed. Philadelphia, FA Davis, 1980, pp 233–234.

384. Boon P, deReuck J, Achten E, de Bleecker J: Pancreatic encephalopathy. A case report and review of the literature. *Clin Neurol Neurosurg* 93:137, 1991.

385. Purtscher O: Noch unbekannte Befunde nach Schädeltrauma. *Versamml Deutschen Ophthamol Gesell* 36:294, 1910.

386. Semlacher EA, Chan-Yan C: Acute pancreatitis presenting with visual disturbance. *Am J Gastroenterol* 88:756, 1993.

387. Jacob HS, Goldstein IM, Shapiro I, et al: Sudden blindness in acute pancreatitis: possible role of complement-induced retinal leukoembolization. *Arch Intern Med* 141:134, 1981.

388. Vogel FS: Central demyelination and focal visceral lesions in a case of acute hemorrhagic pancreatitis. *Arch Path* 52:355, 1951.

389. Bertrand I, Cerbonnet G, Gdet-Guillain J: Contribution a l'étude des encéphalopathies d'origine pancréatique. *Rev Neurol* 98:245, 1958.

390. Delarue J, Chomette G, Monsaingeon A, Pinaudeau Y, Brocheriou C: Encéphalopathie subaguë secondaire à une pancréatite nécrosante hémorrhagique. *Arch Anat Path* 13:45, 1965.

391. Vogel FS: Demyelination induced in living rabbits by means of a lipolytic enzyme preparation. *J Exp Med* 93:297, 1951.

392. Johnson DA, Tong NT: Pancreatic encephalopathy. *South Med J* 70:165, 1977.

393. Bunao RM, Meyer KK: Pancreatitis with encephalomalacia and ascites. *Am J Gastroenterol* 55:145, 1971.

394. Sharf B, Bental E: Pancreatic encephalopathy. *J Neurol Neurosurg Psychiatry* 34:357, 1971.

395. Kincaid MC, Green WR, Knox DL, et al: A clinicopathologic case report of retinopathy of pancreatitis. *Br J Ophthalmol* 66:219, 1982.

396. Craddock PR, Hammerschmidt DE, White JG, et al: Complement (C5a)-induced granulocyte aggregation in vitro. A possible mechanism of complement-mediated leukostasis and leukopenia. *J Clin Invest* 60:260, 1977.

397. Jacob HS, Goldstein IM, Shapiro I, et al: Sudden blindness in acute pancreatitis: possible role of complement-induced retinal leukoembolization. *Arch Intern Med* 141:134, 1981.

398. Hammerschmidt DE, Harris PD, Wayland JH, et al: Intravascular granulocyte aggregation in live

animals. A complement-mediated mechanism of ischemia. *Blood* 52(suppl 1):125, 1978.

399. Dadreiling DA, Blum L, Sanders M: Thrombophlebitis, blood coagulation and pancreatic disease. *Arch Int Med* 96:490, 1955.

400. Tran DD, Cuesta MA, Schneider AJ, Wesdrop RIA: Prevalence and prediction of multiple organ system failure and mortality in acute pancreatitis. *J Crit Care* 8:145, 1993.

401. Gerzof SG: Percutaneous drainage as an option in multiple system organ failure, in Fry DE (ed): *Multiple System Organ Failure.* St. Louis, Mosby, 1992, pp 336–343.

402. Fry DE: Multiple system organ failure, in Fry DE (ed): *Multiple System Organ Failure.* St. Louis, Mosby, 1992, pp 3–14.

403. Hedstrom J, Sainio V, Kemppainen E, et al: Serum complex of trypsin 2 and alpha 1 antitrypsin as a diagnostic marker of acute pancreatitis: a clinical study in consecutive patients. *BMJ* 313:333, 1996.

404. Hermann RE, Knowles RC: Effect of a new trypsin inhibitor in the therapy of experimental pancreatitis. *Surg Form* 13:306, 1962.

405a. Brion S, Aillet J, Graveleau J, Léonardon N: Encéphalopathie pancréatique probable guérie par les antitrypsiques. *Presse Med* 76:9, 1968.

405b. Ettien JT, Webster PD III: The management of acute pancreatitis. *Adv Intern Med* 25:169, 1980.

406. Lee JS, Anvret M: Identification of the most common mutation within the porphobilinogen deaminase gene in Swedish patients with acute intermittent porphyria. *Proc Natl Acad Sci USA* 88:10912, 1991.

407. Stein JA, Tschudy DP: Acute intermittent porphyia. A clinical and biochemical study of 46 patients. *Medicine* 49:1, 1970.

408. Bylesjo I, Forsgren L, Lithner F, Boman K: Epidemiology and clinical characteristics of seizures in patients with acute intermittent porphyria. *Epilepsia* 37:230, 1996.

409. Sorenson HWS, With TK: Persistent pareses after porphyric attacks. *Acta Med Scand* 190:219, 1971.

410. Tefferi A, Colgan JP, Solberg LA: Acute porphyria: diagnosis and management. *Mayo Clin Proc* 69:991, 1994.

411. Greer M. Porphyria, in Vinken PJ, Bruyn GW (eds): *Handbook of Clinical Neurology.* Amsterdam, Elsevier/North Holland, 1976, pp 429–447.

412. Beattie AD, Moore MR, Goldberg A, Ward RL: Acute intermittent porphyria: response of tachycardia and hypertension to propranolol. *BMJ* 3:257, 1973.

413. Nicoll RA: The interaction of porphyrin precursors with GABA receptors in the isolated frog spinal cord. *Life Sci* 19:521, 1976.

414. Loots JM, Becker DM, Meyer BL, et al: The effect of porphyrin precursors on monosynaptic reflex activity in the isolated hemispected frog spinal cord. *J Neural Trans* 36:71, 1975.

415. Becker D, Viljoen D, Kramer S: The inhibition of red cell and brain ATPase by δ-aminolaevulinic acid. *Biochim Biophys Acta* 225:26, 1971.

416. Feldman DS, Levere RD, Lieberman JS, Cardinal R, Watson CJ: Presynaptic neuromuscular inhibition by porphobilinogen and porphobilin. *Proc Nat Acad Sci* 68:383, 1971.

417. Litman DA, Correia MA: L-Tryptophan: a common denominator of biochemical and neurological events of acute hepatic porphyria. *Science* 222:1031, 1983.

418. Hierons R: Changes in the nervous system in acute porphyria. *Brain* 80:176, 1957.

419. Denny-Brown D, Sciara D: Changes in the nervous system in acute porphyria. *Brain* 68:1, 1945.

420. King PH, Bragdon AC: MRI reveals multiple reversible cerebral lesions in an attack of acute intermittent porphyria. *Neurology* 41:1300, 1991.

421. Gibson JB, Goldberg A: The neuropathology of acute porphyria. *J Path Bact* 71:495, 1956.

422. Tschudy DP, Welland FH, Collins A, Hunter G Jr: The effect of carbohydrate feeding on the induction of L-amino-levulinic synthetase. *Metabolism* 13:396, 1964.

423. Hirano M, Pavlakis S: Mitochondrial myopathy, encephalopathy, lactic acidosis and stroke-like episodes (MELAS): current concepts. *J Child Neurol* 9:4, 1994.

424. Sparaco M, Bonilla E, DiMauro S, Powers J: Neuropathology of mitochondrial encephalopathies due to mitochondrial DNA defects. *J Neuropathol Exp Neurol* 52:1, 1993.

425. Love S, Nicoll JAR, Kinrade E: Sequencing and quantitative assessment of mutant and wild-type mitochondrial DNA in paraffin sections from cases of MELAS. *J Pathol* 170:9, 1993.

426. Pavlakis SG, Gould R, Zito J: Stroke in children. *Adv Pediatr* 38:151, 1990.

427. Choi D: Bench to bedside: the glutamate connection. *Science* 258:241, 1992.

428. Ohama E, Ohara S, Ikuta F, et al: Mitochondrial angiopathy in cerebral blood vessels of mito-

chondrial encephalopathy. *Acta Neuropathol* 74:226, 1987.

429. Clark JM, Marks MP, Adalsteinsson E, et al: MELAS: clinical and pathologic correlations with MRI, xenon/CT, and MR spectroscopy. *Neurology* 46:223, 1996.

430. Johns DR, Stein AG, Wityk R: MELAS syndrome masquerading as herpes simplex encephalitis. *Neurology* 43:2471, 1993.

431. Stroh E, Winterkorn J, Jalkh A, Lessell S: MELAS syndrome: a mitochondrially inherited disorder. *Int Ophthalmol Clin* 33:169, 1993.

432. Matthews PM, Tamperi D, Berkovic SF, et al: Magnetic resonance imaging shows specific abnormalities in the MELAS syndrome. *Neurology* 41:1043, 1991.

433. Penn AM, Lee JW, Thuiller P, et al: MELAS syndrome with mitochondrial tRNA (leu) (UUR) mutation L correlation of clinical state, nerve conduction, and muscle 31P magnetic resonance spectroscopy during treatment with nicotinaminde and riboflavin. *Neurology* 42:2147, 1992.

434. Ihara Y, Namba R, Kuroda S, Sato T, Shirabe T: Mitochondrial encephalomyopathy (MELAS): pathological study and successful therapy with coenzyme Q and idebenone. *I Neurol Sci* 90:263, 1989.

435. David RB, Mamunes P, Rosenblum WI: Necrotizing encephalomyelopathy (Leigh), in Vinken PJ, Bruyn GW (eds): *Handbook of Clinical Neurology*, vol. 28, New York, Elsevier/North Holland, 1976, pp 349–363.

436. Reynaud P, Loiseau H, Coquet M, Vital C, Loiseau P: Un cas adulte d'encephalopathie necrosante aubaigue de Leigh. *Rev Neurol* 144:259, 1988.

437. Spranger M, Schwab S, Wiebel M, Becker CM: Das adulte Leigh-Syndrom. Eine seltene Differentialdiagnose einer zentralen. Atemregulationsstorung. *Nervenzart* 66:144, 1995.

438. Monpetit VJA, Andermann F, Carpenter S, et al: Subacute necrotizing encephalopathy—a review and a study of two families. *Brain* 94:1, 1971.

439. Krageloh-Mann I, Grodd W, Schoning M, et al: Proton spectroscopy in five patients with Leigh's disease and mitochondrial enzyme deficiency. *Dev Med Child Neurol* 35:769, 1994.

440. Tatuch Ym, Christodoulou J, Feignebaum A, et al: Heteroplasmic mtDNA mutation (T–G) at 8993 can cause Leigh disease when the percentage of abnormal mtDNA is high. *Am J Hum Genet* 54:385, 1994.

441. Koga Y, Nonaka I, Nokao M, et al: Progressive cytochrome c oxidase deficiency in a case of Leigh's encephalopathy. *J Neurol Sci* 95:63, 1990.

442. Robinson BH, De Meirleir L, Glerum M, et al: Clinical presentation of mitochondrial respiratory chain defects in NADH-coenzyme Q reductase and cytochrome oxidase: clues to the pathogenesis of Leigh disease. *J Pediatr* 110:216, 1987.

443. Hinman LM, Sheu KF, Baker AC, Kim YT, Blass JP: Deficiency of pyruvate dehydrogenase complex (PDHC) in Leigh's disease fibroblasts: an abnormality in lipoamide dehydrogenase affecting PDHC activation. *Neurology* 9:70, 1989.

444. Cavanagh JB: Selective vulnerability in acute energy deprivation syndromes. *Neuropathol Appl Neurobiol* 19:461, 1993.

445. Geyer CA, Sartor KJ, Prensky AJ, et al: Leigh disease (subacute necrotizing encephalopathy) CT and MRI findings. *J Comput Assist Tomogr* 12:40, 1988.

446. Bickford RG, Butt HR: Hepatic coma: the electroencephalographic pattern. *J Clin Invest* 34:790, 1955.

447. Karnaze DS, Bickford RG: Triphasic waves: a reassessment of their significance. *Electroenceph Clin Neurophysiol* 57:193, 1984.

448. Sundaram MBM, Blume WT: Triphasic waves: clinical correlates and morphology. *Can J Neurolog Sci* 14:136, 1987.

449. Young GB, Bolton CF, Austin TW, Archibald Y, Wells GA: The encephalopathy associated with septic illness. *Clin Invest Med* 13:297, 1990.

450. Synek VM: Prognostically important EEG coma patterns in diffuse anoxic and traumatic encephalopathies in adults. *J Clin Neurophysiol* 5:161, 1988.

451. Synek VM, Synek BJL: "Theta pattern coma" a variant on alpha pattern coma. *Clin EEG* 15:116, 1984.

452. Synek VM, Synek BJL: "Theta pattern coma" occurring in younger adults. *Clin EEG* 18:54, 1987.

453. Young GB, Blume WT, Jacono V: Alpha, theta and alpha-theta coma patterns. *Can J Neurolog Sci* 16:248, 1989.

454. Kuroiwa Y, Celesia GG: Clinical significance of periodic EEG patterns. *Arch Neurol* 37:15, 1980.

455. Burch HB, Wartofsky L: Life-threatening thyrotoxicosis: thyroid storm, in Ober KP (ED): *Endocrinol Metab Clin N Am* 22:263, 1993.

456. Maioli M, Arca GM, Ganau A, et al: A case of hyperglycemic hyperosmolar non-ketotic coma

during anesthesia: a possible casue of failed re-awakening. *Diabetes Res* 18:45, 1991.

457. Young GB, Brown JD, Bolton CF, Sibbald WJ: Periodic lateralized epileptiform discharges (PLEDs) and nystagmus retractorius. *Ann Neurol* 2:61, 1977.

458. Ballauff A, Engelbrecht V, Voit T: Hyperintense lesions of the globus pallidus on MRI in children with chronic liver disease. *Eur J Pediatr* 153:802, 1994.

459. Cino M, DelMaestro RF: Generation of hydrogen peroxide by brain mitochondria: the effects of re-oxygenation following postdecapitative ischemia. *Arch Biochem Biophys* 269:623, 1989.

Chapter 14

NUTRITIONAL DEFICIENCY AND IMPAIRED CONSCIOUSNESS

G. Bryan Young

Vitamins are essential to the normal functioning of the brain. Deficiencies can cause impairment of alertness and various cognitive functions. The principal deficiencies are reviewed in this chapter. The specific nutrient deficiencies and their neurochemical effects are known with various degrees of certainty. Furthermore, the conditions may coexist with other disorders so that the adverse effects on consciousness are amplified.

WERNICKE'S ENCEPHALOPATHY

Definition

Wernicke's encephalopathy is an acute disturbance in brain function related to a deficiency of thiamine. The classic features of disturbed mentation, eye movement abnormalities, ataxia, and absent ankle reflexes may not all be present, or additional features, such as hypothermia, may predominate.

Epidemiology and Significance

An autopsy study from a university hospital in Sweden observed Wernicke's encephalopathy in 52 cases (0.74 percent) of 6964 autopsies. Of these, 40 (77 percent) were alcoholics and 12 (23 percent) were nonalcoholics.[1] Males outnumbered

females by 4:1 in the alcoholic population with Wernicke's encephalopathy.[2] Lindboe and Loberg found evidence of acute or previous Wernicke's encephalopathy in 12.5 percent of the alcoholics. A prevalence figure for Wernicke's encephalopathy of 2.8 percent of autopsies was found in Australia; this is close to the figures in large American cities.[3a]

Wernicke's encephalopathy is clinically important for the following reasons: it is common (see data above); it is often undiagnosed in life (only 20 percent of patients had been clinically diagnosed in the autopsy study by Harper et al[3b]); the associated mortality is 10 to 20 percent; it has a high morbidity—80 percent of cases develop Korsakoff's psychosis (see later); the condition is preventable and early cases may be completely reversed with thiamine therapy.[3-6] In developed countries, Wernicke's encephalopathy is seldom considered in even in malnourished nonalcoholics; these individuals are at great risk of inadequate treatment.[7]

Pathogenesis

Wernicke's encephalopathy is primarily related to a deficiency of thiamine. The daily requirements are approximately 1 mg/day or 0.5 mg for each

1000 calories, reflecting the proportional need for thiamine in carbohydrate metabolism. A state of body depletion for thiamine develops after 18 days of a thiamine-free diet.[8]

In developed countries, most cases of Wernicke's encephalopathy occur in alcoholics who replace nutritious food with alcohol. In addition, alcoholics also suffer impaired gastrointestinal absorption of thiamine (as a consequence of alcohol itself).[9] With alcoholic liver disease, activation of thiamine pyrophosphate from thiamine is decreased and the ability of the liver to store thiamine is reduced.[10] Other causes of nutritional deficiency or vomiting that lead to Wernicke's disease include: starvation (prolonged fasting), anorexia nervosa and other psychogenic types of food refusal, hyperemesis gravidarum, gastric carcinoma, complications of gastric surgery for carcinoma or partitioning for morbid obesity, pancreatitis, prolonged administration of intravenous fluids, and thiamine-deficient parenteral nutrition.[11-18] It may also accompany systemic malignancy in children and adults.[19,20] This may relate to inadequate vitamin intake or to incomplete absorption, related to chemotherapy-induced nausea and vomiting. It occasionally occurs in patients on hemodialysis or peritoneal dialysis, when water-soluble thiamine is not adequately replaced.[21] It has also been reported in patients suffering from acquired immunodeficiency syndrome (AIDS).[22] Rarely, Wernicke's encephalopathy may be drug induced; e.g., tolazamide may precipitate Wernicke's encephalopathy in patients with a genetic defect in transketolase activity.[23]

Thiamine is converted into its active form, thiamine pyrophosphate, which acts as a coenzyme for a number of enzymes involved in the pentose phosphate pathway and the tricarboxylic acid cycle (Fig. 14-1).[24] If thiamine pyrophosphate is deficient, affected cells may have abrupt energy failure, and may malfunction or die. Focal accumulation of lactate has also been invoked as a cause of cell death.[25] It has been postulated that glutamate release may cause excitotoxic damage by activation of N-methyl-D-aspartate (NMDA) or alpha-amino-3-hydroxy-5-methyl-4-isoxazole propionic acid (AMPA) receptors, allowing calcium influx into

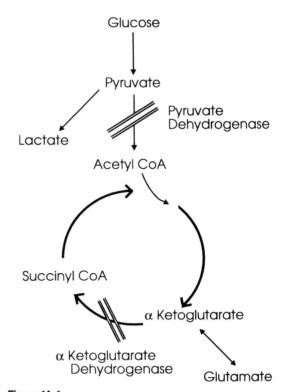

Figure 14-1

Depression of the enzymes pyruvate dehydrogenase and α-ketoglutarate dehydrogenase (parallel lines) in thiamine deficiency leads to increased lactate and glutamate concentrations. The circle represents the Kreb's (citric acid) cycle, only part of which is detailed. (Redrawn from Engel et al,[20] with permission.)

neurons (Fig. 14-1). Evidence for the latter comes from the protective effect of MK 801, an NMDA receptor antagonist, in the pyrithiamine-treated rat model for Wernicke's encephalopathy.[26] Failure of synaptic transmission and impairment of DNA synthesis may occur.[27,28] Deficiency of synthesis of gamma-amino butyric acid (GABA), a neurotransmitter that is involved in inhibition, also occurs as a reversible component of thiamine deficiency.[29] Since magnesium is a cofactor in thiamine-dependent enzyme systems, its deficiency may aggravate features of Wernicke's encephalopathy.[30]

Wernicke disease is associated with increased blood-brain barrier permeability in certain affected regions.[31] This could alter the chemical milieu of the cells in this region and contribute to the encephalopathy.

There may be a genetic susceptibility to develop Wernicke's encephalopathy in the presence of thiamine deficiency. One patient developed Wernicke's encephalopathy after taking tolazamide, an oral hypoglycemic drug.[32] It was thought that this had occurred because the drug increased the patient's glucose metabolism. Fibroblasts from the patient and his relatives showed a lower Michaelis-Menten constant for transketolase compared with diabetic controls.[33] When the enzyme has low affinity for thiamine pyrophosphate, the individual may develop Wernicke's encephalopathy following a sudden influx of glucose into cells.

The cerebellum has a higher rate of thiamine turnover than the cerebral cortex (0.55 µg/g per hour compared with 0.159 µg/g per hour).[34] It has been proposed that an irreversible cerebellar lesion that follows acute, severe thiamine deficiency is due to damage of the climbing fibers that connect the inferior olive with the anterior superior vermis.[35]

Acute Wernicke's encephalopathy is often precipitated by carbohydrate loading in patients with deficient thiamine stores. The mechanism for this is still controversial, but it may be due to acute energy failure, excitotoxic or free radical damage, acute deficiency of transmitters, altered neuronal membrane function, or combinations of these factors. This underlies *the importance of adequate thiamine supplementation in any patient who may be nutritionally deprived or depleted, before carbohydrates are administered.*

Neuropathology and Mechanisms for Clinical Signs

There is a characteristic anatomic distribution of lesions in the central gray structures surrounding the third and fourth ventricles and the cerebral aqueduct. Thus, the medial thalamus, the hypothalamus (always including the mammillary bodies), the periaqueductal gray matter, and the floor of the fourth ventricle (vestibular, abducens, and vagal nuclei) are affected.

The mammillary bodies show more damage of the neuropil than of the neurons (Fig. 14-2), while the reverse is true in the medial dorsal nucleus of the thalamus.[36] Changes in the neuropil include prominent endothelial swelling in capillaries, small hemorrhages, microglial reaction, and accumulations of macrophages with destruction of tissue. The thalamus, on the other hand, shows loss of neurons, pyknosis of neurons, and replacement gliosis without macrophage infiltration or vascular changes. The changes in these two regions progress in parallel; there is not an adequate explanation for their difference. Affected regions frequently become gliotic and atrophic.

The anatomic distribution of the lesions correlates with clinical features (see below). In addition, there may be cerebral cortical dysfunction related to metabolic or neurotransmitter alterations.

Clinical Features

Wernicke's encephalopathy should be suspected in any patient with altered mental status who is at risk for nutritional deficiency. The diagnosis is more often missed in nonalcoholics than in alcoholics.[6]

The classic features include the encephalopathy, ocular abnormalities, and ataxia, although a retrospective survey showed that only 16.5 percent of autopsy-diagnosed patients had all three features.[37]

In more than one-third of patients, an abnormality of mentation is the only abnormality.[37] The nature and degree of the encephalopathy are variable, but the most frequent is an acute, global confusional state.[3] Elements of the acute confusion include: inattention and impaired concentration, reduced level of consciousness with decreased responsiveness, disorientation, deranged perceptual function and memory impairment. There may be an overlap with the features of alcohol withdrawal, such as a delirium with visual hallucinations. Because of the confusional state, extensive assessment of mental status functioning, including memory, is difficult to impossible. Most patients are quiet and readily drift off to sleep when not stimulated. However 1 to 4 percent may be in a

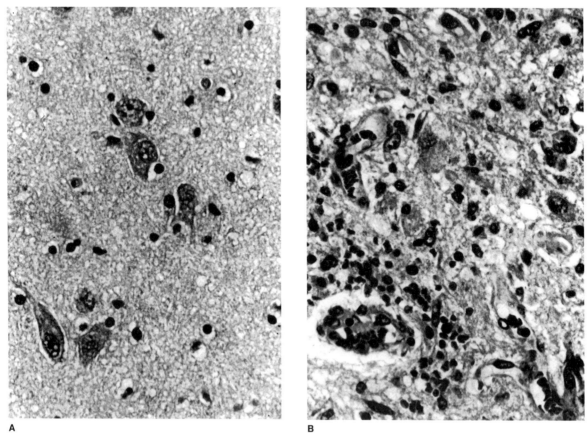

Figure 14-2
A. *This shows the histology of the normal mammillary body (enlarged 98×). Note the neurons and the fine, fibrillary background of the neuropil.* B. *This shows the mammillary body of a patient who died with acute Wernicke's encephalopathy (enlarged 98×). Note the swelling of the endothelium of capillaries, petechial hemorrhages, and chromatolytic change in a minority of neurons* (bottom left).

stupor or in coma.[3,38] The patient who is more alert and attentive may display severe memory dysfunction, even early in the course of the illness. This affects recall of past memories as well as the ability to retain new information.

Ocular abnormalities, due to the periaqueductal and periventricular lesions (or early reversible dysfunction) described above, occur in most patients, led by, in frequency, horizontal nystagmus in 85 percent of cases.[37] This is followed by bilateral abducens palsies (54 percent) and conjugate gaze palsy (45 percent).[37] Bilateral inter-

nuclear ophthalmoplegia, usually associated with multiple sclerosis, has also been described in Wernicke's encephalopathy.[39] In some patients with advanced disease, all ocular movements, including vertical ones, may be lost. Patients typically lose the oculovestibular response to caloric testing; the author of this chapter has found this to be a helpful diagnostic finding. Pupillary reactions are usually preserved, but some patients may have small pupils that are unreactive to light.

Ataxia, related to the above-described lesions of the anterior-superior vermis, affects stance and gait much more than the arms. However, the early marked imbalance has been attributed to a central vestibular disturbance (confirmed by caloric testing).[40]

Hypothermia requires emphasis as an important presenting feature.[41] Hypotension, likely related to involvement of the sympathetic centers in the hypothalamus, may be associated with hypothermia or can occur independently.[42]

The memory loss in patients who later develop Korsakoff syndrome is believed to be due to lesions in the medial dorsal thalamic nuclei that occur during Wernicke's encephalopathy.[3]

Differential Diagnosis

Conditions that produce a reversible syndrome of ocular movement disturbances, such as gaze palsies, ataxia, and mental changes, include: intoxication with phenytoin, barbiturates, or carbamazepine; and high-dose oxifluridine (a chemotherapeutic agent used for rectal carcinoma).[43]

Other conditions that cause abnormal mentation and hypothermia are hypothyroidism; intoxication with alcohol, barbiturates, or neuroleptic agents; brainstem encephalitis; vertebrobasilar territory strokes; central and extrapontine myelinolysis; and hypothermia itself. In addition, hypophosphatemia has been reported to cause an acute confusional state with disorientation and hallucinations, gaze paresis, areflexia, tremor, paresthesiae, and leg paresis.[44,46] Ocular movement abnormalities and somnolence sometimes occur in the Fisher variant of Guillain-Barré syndrome.[45]

Diagnosis

The diagnosis should be suspected with the above constellation of clinical features, or any in isolation, in a patient at risk of nutritional deprivation (see "Pathology and Pathogenesis.") The diagnosis can be confirmed by the measurement of transketolase enzyme and its saturation in red blood cells, as well as by increased plasma pyruvate, but such testing is rarely necessary or available.

The acute lesions of Wernicke's encephalopathy, especially in the mammillary bodies and periaqueductal gray matter, show increased signal on proton density images and enhance with gadolinium magnetic resonance imaging (MRI) scanning (see Fig. 14-3).[46,47] The abnormal signal usually, but not always, decreases with time and the affected structures atrophy.

Figure 14-3

Contrast-enhanced, T-1 weighted MRIs in the transaxial and coronal planes, showing enhancement of the mammillary bodies (white arrows) *and inferior quadrigeminal plate* (black arrow) *in a 35-year-old woman with Wernicke's encephalopathy. (From D'Aprile et al,[46] with permission.)*

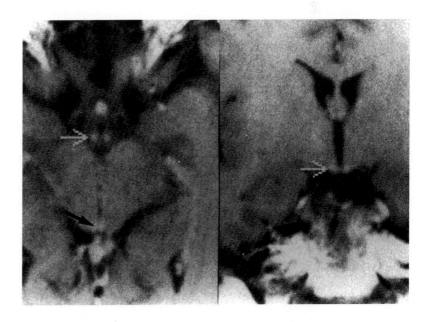

Brainstem auditory evoked response testing reportedly shows a delay in the interpeak latency between waves I and III, indicative of a pontine tegmental abnormality, in 32 percent of patients suffering from Wernicke's encephalopathy.[48] This finding is not specific for Wernicke's encephalopathy, as other brainstem lesions, e.g., multiple sclerosis, brainstem tumor, or stroke, might produce the same abnormality. The abnormality is, however, found in only 6 percent of chronic alcoholics without Wernicke's encephalopathy.[48]

Wernicke's encephalopathy may coexist with other illness, including central pontine myelinolysis, sepsis, and traumatic lesions. One should not be too parsimonious in arriving at a diagnosis, especially in alcoholics and the nutritionally deprived.

Management

Prevention of Wernicke's encephalopathy by the addition of thiamine to alcoholic beverages has been debated. No country seems to have embarked on such a systematic program. It is wise for physicians to treat any nutritionally deprived patient with thiamine, to prevent Wernicke's encephalopathy. Such individuals are at risk upon admission to hospital, where they receive increased calories.

It is a good policy to administer 50 to 100 mg of thiamine either intravenously or intramuscularly, to any patient in coma when the diagnosis is uncertain or questionable.

Wernicke's encephalopathy is a medical emergency. Thiamine, 50 mg, should be promptly administered intramuscularly, along with 50 to 100 mg added to the first liter of intravenous solution. Following this, 50 to 100 mg can be given, either by mouth or parenterally, daily for the first week in hospital. Then, one multivitamin tablet containing thiamine can be given daily for at least several months.

The ocular movements usually normalize within a few minutes to a few hours. Alertness should return at least within a few days and recovery of other functions occurs over several weeks. Gait ataxia may not recover, because of neuronal loss in the anterior superior vermis.

Chronic institutionalization is often necessary for those patients who are left with Korsakoff's psychosis.

Outcome

The outcome can vary between complete recovery and death, and the prognosis is dependent on the early diagnosis and treatment with thiamine supplementation. Patients may be left with an amnestic-confabulatory (Korsakoff's) state or may have varying degrees of memory deficit. However, Korsakoff's psychosis is uncommon in nonalcoholics. This may relate to more severe nutritional deficiency in the alcoholics or to a role of the alcohol itself in contributing to neurotoxicity.[49] Some are left with permanent ataxia of stance and gait, related to degeneration of the anterior-superior vermis of the cerebellum.

MARCHIAFAVA-BIGNAMI DISEASE

Definition and Epidemiology

Marchiafava-Bignami disease consists of a demyelination or necrosis of the corpus callosum, variably associated with similar lesions of the adjacent centrum semiovale and anterior commissure.[50] It is associated with a variable encephalopathy typically occurring in the context of alcoholism and nutritional deficiency. It must be distinguished from other causes if there is central leukomalacia, e.g., trauma, radiation/chemotherapy, necrotizing hemorrhagic leukoencephalopathy, extrapontine myelinolysis, carbon monoxide poisoning, delayed hypoxic change, or Binswanger disease.

Since the clinical syndrome was not specific, the disorder was previously defined by the pathology. Since the advent of computed tomography (CT) and MRI, the disorder can be recognized during life. The true incidence is unknown. It was considered to be rare, based on the infrequency of pathologically proven cases.[51] It had previously been assumed that all cases were fatal, but in recent years survivors have been described.[52–54] Thus, Marchiafava-Bignami disease may be underrecognized, as patients may survive the illness, the clinical features are not specific, and neuroimaging may not have been performed.

Pathology and Pathogenesis

The corpus callosum is the defining site of pathology. The middle portion is consistently involved. If the anterior portion is affected, the disease is most marked in the midline, but involvement is more diffuse or separately affects the lateral parts in the mid and posterior segments. The white matter may be truly demyelinated with sparing of the axis cylinders. Most often, the white matter is also necrotic and cavitated. Reactive gliosis borders the necrotic tissue. New vessel growth into the region is common, if the patient survives long enough.

Other lesions have been described in the anterior commissure, the optic chiasm, posterior columns of the spinal cord, and the superior or middle cerebellar peduncles. The central demyelination may extend into the cerebral hemispheres from the corpus callosum, extending through the centrum semiovale to the subconvolutional white matter. The internal capsule and arcuate "U" fibers are usually spared. Occasionally, the lesions may extend into the posterior commissures.

A recent study showed that the cerebral metabolic rate of glucose was diminished in the frontal-temporal-parietal-occipital association cortices.[55] This was attributed to the disruption of transcollosal cortical-cortical networks. Neuronal loss and/or subcortical lesions may be additional or alternative explanations, however. The loss of cortical neurons in layers 3 and 5 may be due to transsynaptic degeneration, with absence of communication from homologous regions in the other hemisphere. This also remains speculative.

The etiology is unclear. There is a strong association with alcoholism, but this is not essential.[51] Early attention was directed towards a metabolic cause. Although most patients with Marchiafava-Bignami disease are nutritionally deprived, no consistent vitamin or nutrient deficiency has been established. The condition is distinct from central pontine myelinolysis and

does not appear to be a form of extrapontine myelinolysis since no overlap cases have been reported; brainstem lesions are distinct in the two conditions and there is no link of Marchiafava-Bignami disease to osmotic problems, such as hyponatremia, as has been established for central pontine myelinolysis.

Dysfunction of the oligodendroglia has been proposed, because similar lesions have been produced by cyanide intoxication (cyanide is toxic to oligodendroglia). Cyanide interferes with oxidative enzymes, especially those of the mitochondria. Cyanide is also incorporated into cyanocobolamine. Vitamin B_{12} has been proposed as an antagonist of cyanide; therefore it is possible that patients with Marchiafava-Bignami disease were deficient in vitamin B_{12} and at risk when a toxic or metabolic stress occurred.

The edema, likely vasogenic as evidenced by contrast enhancement on neuroimaging (see later), raises the possibility of a vascular or microvascular pathogenesis. However, this remains speculative.

The central portion of the corpus callosum may be vulnerable because it is more active metabolically (there is a higher rate of protein turnover here) than other regions and, therefore, more vulnerable to metabolic stress. Perhaps it is also more vulnerable to osmotic or vascular stresses.

It has recently been discovered that the interleukins tumor necrosis factor-alpha (TNF) and interleukin-1 (IL-1) are expressed in glial cells of the corpus callosum.[56] These can be expressed at times of injury and could contribute to tissue damage in a trauma model. Further, in a rat glioma model, the intravenous infusion of TNF caused breakdown in the blood-brain barrier, with edema and pericapillary halos in the corpus callosum. This was a necrotizing reaction that extended from the tumor.[57] The intravenous injection of TNF without a tumor did not produce this necrotizing brain lesion. These findings raise the possibility that the corpus callosum is predisposed to damage mediated by inflammatory mediators if a physical lesion is present in the brain and there is activation of the cytokine system, either locally in the brain or systemically. In the latter instance, there may be a requirement for the blood-brain barrier to be breached.

As a pathologic-clinical syndrome without a known pathogenesis, it is unclear if there is a single etiology or mechanism. Should any lesion more-or-less confined to the corpus callosum be called Marchiafava-Bignami disease? For the present, it is probably best to keep an open mind and consider this a controversial syndrome in need of clarification.

Clinical Features

As mentioned, the clinical syndrome is variable and not at all specific. This may relate, at least in part, to the coexistence of Marchiafava-Bignami disease with other acute, subacute, and chronic disorders of the nervous system: alcohol withdrawal syndromes, pellagra, Wernicke's encephalopathy, sepsis, volume and electrolyte disturbances, hepatic dysfunction, trauma, pancreatitis, seizures, etc. Despite these confounding factors, acutely ill patients, later discovered on neuroimaging or autopsy to have the lesions of Marchiafava-Bignami disease, present with dysphagia, muteness, and then seizures, stupor, or coma.

A subacute course with rapidly progressive dementia leading to a vegetative state, or to coma and convulsions, is perhaps the most common presentation.[58] Patients are unable to stand in the early stages. There may be relative remissions and exacerbations. Prominent *gegenhalten* or paratonic rigidity (including the neck) is common. Diffuse muscular hypertonia and a grasp reflex are common accompaniments.

About 10 percent of cases have a more protracted course of behavioral change, cognitive deficits (including apraxia and aphasia), gait apraxia, and dysarthria. Reflecting the pathology, the presence of frontal lobe symptoms or signs of callosal disconnection should suggest the diagnosis. More chronically affected patients may develop a syndrome similar to communicating hydrocephalus, with dementia, gait disturbance, and incontinence.

Disease of the corpus callosum typically causes defects involving interhemispheric transfer of information, including bimanual tasks, left-sided praxis, and defects in the transfer of somesthetic sensation.[59] Mutism is common in patients who have just undergone callosotomy; this is reversible in 2 or more weeks. Recently, Balint syndrome (ocular apraxia, paralysis of voluntary gaze, and ataxia of visually guided movements and fluctuating visual inattention) was described, in association with findings of callosal disconnection, in a case of Marchiafava-Bignami disease.[54] Other deficits, including those affecting transfer of visual and auditory information, can be detected with special neuropsychologic techniques.[59,60] With posterior callosal involvement, crossed hemianopsia can occur and also left hemispatial neglect.[61]

Extracallosal damage may account for other findings: dementia, lack of initiative, and psychomotor retardation.[59]

The differential diagnosis is broad and, depending on the time course, includes encephalitis, meningitis, sepsis-associated encephalopathy, pellagra, intoxications, Creutzfeldt-Jakob disease, bilateral strokes or subdural hematomas, metastases, and metabolic encephalopathies or intoxications for the acute and subacute forms. The chronic form can be mimicked by communicating hydrocephalus, Alzheimer disease, or frontal neoplasms.

Laboratory Diagnosis

Scanning by MRI and CT are the most useful diagnostic procedures.[52,62,63] In the acute stage, there is swelling of the corpus callosum, probably due to edema and demyelination. There may be extension into the adjacent hemispheric white matter (see Fig. 14-4). There may be contrast enhancement in this early stage.[62] In the chronic stage, there is characteristically low signal intensity in the central portion of the corpus callosum on T1-weighted imaging.[64] These changes were reported to have been reversible, along with the clinical findings, in one survivor.[54] Atrophy of the same region, with or without cystic change, showing as a hypodensity on T2-weighted images, has also been reported.[65]

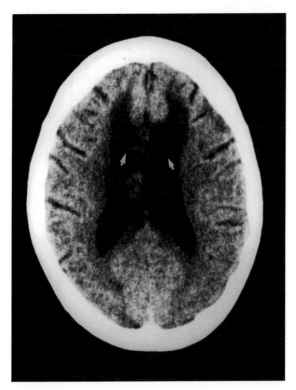

Figure 14-4

A CT scan showing typical features of Marchiafava-Bignami disease. Arrows indicate the posterior border of the swollen, necrotic corpus callosum. The white matter change extends anteriorly into the forceps minor. The patient was a 24-year-old alcoholic man who had preceding sepsis and pancreatitis. He had multifocal seizures and impaired consciousness at the time of the scan. Residual sequelae included a right hemiplegia and paralysis of the left lower limb.

Management

Since the cause is not known, there is no specific treatment. If the disorder is due to metabolic stress from nutritional deficiency and systemic stress, it is important to correct these problems. The following are recommended measures but are not proven to be effective: supplementation with a broad range of B vitamins and fat-soluble vitamins; prompt treatment of sepsis or infections, including coagulopathies; and prevention of marked shifts in electrolyte concentrations, especially sodium.

PELLAGRA ENCEPHALOPATHY

Definition and Epidemiology

Pellagra is a disorder attributed to deficiency of nicotinic acid or niacin (closely related and interconverted compounds that are synthesized from tryptophan), with a clinical syndrome consisting of mental changes, dermatitis, and diarrhea. Primary pellagra, found mainly in alcoholics, is considered to be extremely rare in developed countries but is probably underrecognized.[66,67] Secondary pellagra, related to interference with absorption or metabolism of niacin, is found in patients with malignant carcinoid and in those treated with isoniazid, 6-mercaptopurine, 5-fluorouracil, or puromycin.[68] It may also occur in Hartnup disease, an autosomal recessive disorder with impaired intestinal absorption of tryptophan, and in children who have abnormalities in the synthetic pathway from tryptophan to nicotinic acid or niacin.[69–71]

Clinical Features

The triad of dementia, dermatitis and diarrhea may not always be apparent. The rash is typically erythematous and appears chiefly in sun-exposed regions. There may be an associated glossitis. Of nine autopsy-proven cases of pellagra without other neurologic findings, Serdau and colleagues[66] described an acute confusional state in eight (89 percent). The confusional state fluctuated and was associated with clouding of consciousness. Global memory loss, visual hallucinations, and motor restlessness alternating with apathy or stupor were frequent. Eventually, patients progressed to stupor, then coma before death.

One of the main features was *gegenhalten* or paratonic rigidity, affecting the limbs and less often the trunk. The neck was uncommonly involved. Hypertonus usually appears within a few days of the onset of mental features. Myoclonus, spontaneous or stimulus-induced, and affecting the limbs more commonly than the face, was common, but action and palatal myoclonus were not observed. Ataxia may also be present initially. A mild to moderate motor-sensory polyneuropathy may also occur. With an encephalopathy, the sensory component may be hard to detect. A myelopathy may be present, but is usually masked by the other features.

Pathogenesis and Pathology

Niacin deficiency has been held to be the main cause of pellagra, based on observations of responsiveness when patients were selectively supplemented with this vitamin. Similar patients given thiamine or other vitamins failed to recover. Many cases have an overlap of syndromes with mixed vitamin deficiencies.[72] Still, some patients fail to respond to niacin. It is possible that other vitamin deficiencies also play a role. Victor and colleagues have produced an animal model with identical neuropathology in which pyridoxine was the deficient vitamin.[73] They maintain that the dermatologic and gastrointestinal signs and symptoms relate to deficiency of niacin or its precursor, tryptophan, while the neurologic syndrome relates to riboflavin deficiency. This is still controversial, however, as Jolliffe et al found that supplementation of patients with only thiamine and pyridoxine did not reverse the

encephalopathy, which progressed.[74] The timing of administration of vitamins in human cases is undoubtedly important. There could be a threshold of reversibility in that more severely affected patients may not respond, while others in the early phases of the disease may be completely cured.

Pellagra affects central nervous system neurons in various locations, producing "central chromatolysis" (Fig. 14-5). The cell bodies are distended and the nucleus, often smaller than normal, is displaced to the periphery of the soma. There is loss of Nissl substance in the central portion of the neuronal cell body. Hauw and coworkers noted that, in cases of "pure" pellagra, the brainstem nuclei were predominantly involved.[72] The pontine reticular and cerebellar dentate nuclei were the most severely affected structures. Changes were also frequent in the fifth, sixth, seventh, and vestibular nuclei. In the midbrain, the third nuclei, mesencephalic reticular formations were affected. The cerebral cortex was only mildly affected, usually in the large-cell layers of the frontal lobe and the Betz cells of the motor cortex. The spinal cord, especially the posterior horn cells and cells of Clark's column, may also be affected.

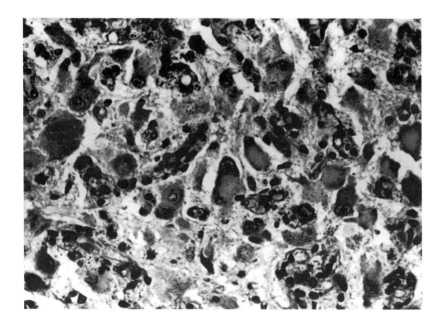

Figure 14-5

Photomicrograph showing chromatolytic neurons in the mammillary body of a patient who died with pellagra. Note the eccentric nuclei and the lack of Nissl substance in the central portions of the neurons.

Such chromatolysis typically results from retrograde changes from the degeneration of cell processes (especially the axon), but, in the case of pellagra, is probably due to a primary cellular deficiency lesion.

Hauw and coworkers found, in their autopsy series of alcoholics, that pellagra is more commonly associated with Marchiafava-Bignami disease than with Wernicke's encephalopathy.[72] These three conditions can exist independently of each other, but the statistically stronger association with Marchiafava-Bignami disease raises the possibility of a common pathogenetic mechanism.

Niacin's role in the nervous system is primarily as a component of nicotinamide adenine dinucleotide (NAD) and nicotinamide adenine dinucleotide-phosphate (NADP), nucleotides that are important in a number of enzymatic reactions. The latter are important in carbohydrate, fatty acid, and glutathione metabolism. A deficiency in niacin causes a reduction in NAD and NADP and the activity of their associated enzymes in the nervous system.

Management

For the prevention of pellagra, it is suggested that patients suspected to be deficient in vitamins be given multivitamins, including niacin. The same advice might be applied to any patient with an unexplained encephalopathy.

For the established case, prompt supplementation with niacin and other vitamins, is advised.

VITAMIN B₁₂ DEFICIENCY

Epidemiology

Neurologic complications developed in about half the 369 patients with vitamin B_{12} deficiency studied at the Columbia-Presbyterian Medical Center and Harlem Hospital in New York by Healton et al.[75] The peak age of onset of neurologic symptoms was between 70 and 80 years, but 40 percent of patients developed symptoms before age 40 years; the range was 17 to 98 years.

Clinical Features

Encephalopathic features have included acute confusion, poor memory, irritability, and impaired judgment and cognition in about 25 percent of patients, while an equivalent number develop psychotic symptoms including depression, auditory or visual hallucinations, paranoid delusions, or mania.[76] Coma, or significant impairment in alertness, is rare and occurs more commonly in infants.[77–80] While a few patients are demented, virtually all patients with abnormal mental status have other neurologic signs as well, e.g., subacute combined degeneration and peripheral nerve involvement.[75] When mental changes occur, they may, however, constitute the most prominent and disabling abnormality.[75]

Retrobulbar neuropathy with central scotomata occurs in about 3 percent of patients with subacute combined degeneration of the spinal cord. Occasionally, retinopathy with venous dilatation and retinal hemorrhages are found. This is mainly a manifestation of severe anemia rather than a direct complication of vitamin B_{12} deficiency itself. Rarely, disorders of ocular movement occur in the context of vitamin B_{12} deficiency, and they respond to its replacement. These include downbeat nystagmus, paralysis of upward gaze, and internuclear ophthalmoplegia.[81–83]

The earliest neurologic symptoms resemble those of a peripheral neuropathy, with paresthesiae, ataxia, and decreased dexterity of the hands, followed by some muscle weakness distally in the lower limbs.[75] The sensory modalities affected are large-fiber or posterior column in type (impaired vibratory and position sense), leaving pain and temperature sensation relatively unaffected. Reflexes may be lost, in association with the peripheral involvement. Impotence in males and bowel and bladder incontinence may occur. With these, however, there are upgoing plantar responses, indicating central involvement.

Neurologic complications usually occur late in the series of symptoms and relate to the severity of the vitamin B_{12} deficiency. Curiously, there is an inverse relationship of the anemia to the neurologic complications that is not entirely explained by folate supplementation.[75]

Nonneurologic symptoms include dyspnea on exertion, lassitude, palpitations, angina, anorexia, diarrhea, and vague generalized complaints.[84] Visual signs comprise premature graying or whitening of the hair, sallow-colored skin, and loss of papillae on the tongue.

Pathology and Pathogenesis

Humans cannot synthesize vitamin B_{12} and must obtain it from organisms that produce it.[85] Only 1 to 3 µg/day are required; it is rare for dietary deficiency to be responsible for vitamin B_{12} deficiency. Much more commonly, the problem is in absorption from the gastrointestinal tract. Pernicious anemia is an autoimmune disease, due either to autoantibodies directed against the parietal cells of the gastric mucosa (that secrete "intrinsic factor" needed for B_{12} absorption in the ileum), the intrinsic, factor itself, or the intrinsic factor binding site on ileal receptors.[86] Disorders of the distal small bowel or tapeworm infestation are less common causes of the failure of vitamin B_{12} to be absorbed in the gut.

Vitamin B_{12} (cobolamin) functions as a co-enzyme in a number of biochemical reactions.[87] In humans, two relevant enzymes are methylmalonyl-CoA-mutase and methionine synthetase. With the latter, there is an interaction with folate, in the form of tetrahydrofolate, to produce methionine that acts as a methyl donor in a number of reactions. Some of the deficiencies that occur with vitamin B_{12} deficiency include defective nucleotide (especially DNA) and lipoid synthesis. The former relates to the production of a megaloblastic anemia and the latter to defective myelin synthesis and/or repair.

The main neuropathic finding is vesicular demyelination in the posterior (fasiculus cuneatus and later gracilis) and lateral columns (corticospinal tracts and ascending cerebellar tracts) of the spinal cord (subacute combined degeneration). Axons undergo irreversible degeneration later. The brain, like the spinal cord, reveals multiple or diffuse areas of demyelination; there is no frank necrosis or glial reaction. Changes are most marked in the corpus callosum and the frontal and parietal white matter. There may be areas of microscopic hemorrhage around blood vessels. There may be some loss of neurons in the cerebral cortex.[88]

Investigations

Measurement of the serum concentration of vitamin B_{12} (cobolamin) reveals a deficiency in most patients with pernicious anemia. The measurement of serum or urinary methylmalonic acid (MMA), however, has greater specificity and sensitivity.[89,90] Elevation of serum MMA is found in pernicious anemia, hypothyroidism, and renal failure; urinary MMA may be affected by diet, however. A Schilling's test will demonstrate the lack of intrinsic factor in patients with pernicious anemia. In the Schilling test, an injection of 1000 µg of vitamin B_{12} is given parenterally, followed by the oral administration of labeled vitamin B_{12}. After the urine collection, the test is repeated with the oral administration of labeled B_{12} along with intrinsic factor. A positive result is the presence of reduced gastrointestinal absorption of B_{12} without intrinsic factor that is corrected by adding the latter. There are, however, some false negatives and false positives depending on how the oral preparation is constituted.[86] Determining the urinary methylmalonic acid is probably a more sensitive method of establishing vitamin B_{12} deficiency.[86] A more sensitive test that avoids confounders that produce false positive and false negative results is the measurement of serum, or both urinary and serum, methylmalonic acid.[86]

Usually, a megaloblastic picture of the peripheral blood is found, but hematologic indices are *normal* in about 30 percent of patients.[91] The "classic" picture includes anemia with oval macrocytes (mean corpuscular volume usually greater than 112 fL), granulocytopenia with multilobulated nuclei, and thrombocytopenia. Bone marrow examination is usually not necessary, but typically shows large erythroid and myeloid precursors with high mitotic activity and delayed nuclear maturity.[86]

Electrophysiologic studies reveal a reduction in motor and sensory conduction velocity on peripheral nerve conduction studies and some fibrillation on needle electromyography.[92,93] Somatosensory evoked potential studes show abnormalities of central and peripheral sensory pathways.[94]

Treatment and Prognosis

The treatment is the parenteral supplementation with vitamin B_{12}. This is usually effective in clearing the encephalopathy. The improvement in subacute combined degeneration depends on the severity and duration of the myelopathy. Overall, about half the patients respond well to such and therapy and make a complete recovery.[75] For pernicious anemia, lifelong replacement therapy with vitamin B_{12} is necessary. There are no known syndromes associated with vitamin B_{12} overdose, so there is no upper limit to dosage. Usually, 1000 μg daily are given intramuscularly for 1 week, then 1000 μg once weekly for 1 month; thereafter, 1000 μg intramuscularly once monthly should suffice.[86,95]

REFERENCES

1. Lindboe CF, Loberg EM: Wernicke's encephalopathy in nonalcoholics. An autopsy study. *J Neurol Sci* 90:125, 1989.
2. Lindboe CF, Loberg EM: The frequency of brain lesion in alcoholics. Comparison in the 5-year periods 1975–1979 and 1983–1987. *J Neurol Sci* 88:107, 1988.
3a. Victor M, Adams RD, Collins GH: *The Wernicke-Korsakoff Syndrome: A Clinical and Pathological Study of 245 Patients, 82 with Post-Mortem Examinations*. Philadelphia, FA Davis, 1971.
3b. Harper C, Gold J, Rodriguez M, Perdices M: The prevalence of the Wernicke-Korsakoff syndrome in Sydney, Australia: a prospective necropsy study. *J Neurol Neurosurg Psychiatry* 52:282, 1989.
4. Torvik A, Lindboe CF, Rogde S: Brain lesions in alcoholics: a neuropathological study with clinical correlations. *J Neurol Sci* 56:233, 1982.
5. Editorial: Wernicke's preventable encephalopathy. *Lancet* 1:1122, 1979.
6. Ebels EJ: Underlying illness in Wernicke's encephalopathy: analysis of possible causes of underdiagnosis. *Eur Neurol* 12:226, 1974.
7. Sands GH: Wernicke's encephalopathy: what we don't teach. *JAMA* 258:2530, 1987.
8. Ziporin ZZ, Nunes WT, Powell RC, Waring PP, Sauberlich HE: Thiamine requirement in the adult human as measured by excretion of thiamine metabolites. *J Nutr* 85:297, 1965.
9. Tomasulo PA, Kater RMH, Iber FL: Impairment of thiamine absorption in alcoholism. *Am J Clin Nutr* 21:1341, 1968.
10. Camilo ME, Morgan MY, Sherlock S: Erythrocyte transketolase in alcoholic liver disease. *Scand J Gastroenterol* 16:273, 1981.
11. Parkin AJ, Blunden J, Rees JE, Hunkin NM: Wernicke-Korsakoff syndrome of nonalcoholic origin. *Brain Cogn* 15:69, 1991.
12. Tan GH, Farnell, Hensrud DD: Acute Wernicke's encephalopathy attributable to pure dietary thiamine deficiency. *Mayo Clin Proc* 69:849, 1994.
13. La Pia S, Agata Spitaleri DL, Vitolo S, et al: Sidrome di Wernicke-Korsakoff post gastrectomia: studio clinico di due casi. *Riv Neurol* 58:121, 1988.
14. Ohkoshi N, Ishii A, Shoji S: Wernicke's encephalopathy induced by hyperemesis gravidarum, associated with bilateral caudate lesions on computed tomography and magnetic resonance imaging. *Eur Neurol* 34:177, 1994.
15. Bruck W, Christensen HJ, Hanefeld F, Friede RL: Wernicke's encephalopathy in a child with acute lymphoblastic leukemia treated with polychemotherapy. *Clin Neuropathol* 10:134, 1991.
16. Abarbanel JM, Beringer VM, Osimani A, Solomon H, Charuzi I: Neurologic complications after gastric restriction surgery for morbid obesity. *Neurology* 37:196, 1987.
17. Bergin PS, Harvey P: Wernicke's encephalopathy and central pontine myelinolysis associated with hyperemesis gravidarum. *BMJ* 305:517, 1992.
18. Doraiswamy PM, Massey EW, Wright K, et al: Wernicke-Korsakoff syndrome caused by psychogenic food refusal: MR findings. *AJNR* 15:594, 1994.
19. Pihko H, Saarinen U, Paetau A: Wernicke encephalopathy—a preventable cause of death: report of 2 children. *Pediatr Neurol* 5:237, 1989.
20. Engel PA, Grunnet M, Jacobs B: Wernicke-Korsakoff syndrome complicating T-cell lymphoma:

unusual or underrecognized? *South Med J* 84:253, 1991.

21. Jagadha V, Deck JH, Halliday WC, Smyth HS: Wernicke's encephalopathy in patients on peritoneal dialysis or hemodialysis. *Ann Neurol* 21:78, 1987.

22. Scwenk J, Gosztonyi G, Thierauf P, Ingleias J, Langer E: Wernicke's encephalopathy in two patients with acquired immune deficiency syndrome. *J Neurol* 237: 445, 1990.

23. Mukherjee AB, Ghazanfari A, Svoronos S, et al: Transketolase abnormality in tolazamide-induced Wernicke's encephalopathy. *Neurology* 36:1508, 1986.

24. McCandless DW, Schenker S, Cook M: Encephalopathy of thiamine deficiency: studies of intracerebral mechanisms. *J Clin Invest* 47:2268, 1968.

25. Kinnersley HW, Peters RA: Brain localization of lactic acidosis in avitaminosis B1 and its relation to the origin of symptoms. *Biochem J* 24:711, 1930.

26. Langlais PT, Mair RG: Protective effects of the glutamate antagonist MK-801 on the pyrithiamine-induced lesions and amino acid changes in the rat brain. *J Neurosci* 10:1664, 1990.

27. Schenker S, Henderson GI, Hoyumpa AM Jr, McCandless DW: Hepatic and Wernicke's encephalopathies: current concepts of pathogenesis. *Am J Clin Nutr* 22:229, 1980.

28. Henderson GI, Schenker S: Reversible impairment of cerebral DNA synthesis in thiamine deficiency. *J Lab Clin Med* 86:77, 1975.

29. Heroux M, Butterworth RF: Reversible alterations of gamma-amino-butyric acid in pyrithiamine-treated rats: implications for the pathogenesis of Wernicke's encephalopathy. *J Neurochem* 51:1221, 1988.

30. Itokawa Y, Schulz RA, Cooper JR: Thiamine in nerve membranes. *Biochim Biophys Acta* 266:293, 1972.

31. Schroth G, Wichmann W, Valavanis A: Blood-brain barrier disruption in acute Wernicke's encephalopathy: MR findings. *J Computer Assist Tomogr* 15:1059, 1991.

32. Kwee IL, Nakada T: Wernicke's encephalopathy induced by tolazamide. *N Eng J Med* 297:1367, 1977.

33. Mukherjee AB, Ghazanfari A, Svoronos S, et al: Transketolase abnormality in tolazamide-induced Wernicke's encephalopathy. *Neurology* 36:1508, 1986.

34. Butterworth RF: Effects of thiamine deficiency in brain metabolism: implications for the pathogenesis

of the Wernicke-Korsakoff syndrome. *Alcohol Alcoholism* 24:274, 1989.

35. Butterworth RF: Pathophysiology of cerebellar dysfunction in the Wernicke-Korsakoff syndrome. *Can J Neurol Sci* 20(suppl 3): S123, 1993.

36. Torvik A: Two types of brain lesions in Wernicke's encephalopathy. *Neuro Exp Neurobiol* 11:179, 1985.

37. Harper CG, Giles M, Finlay-Jones R: Clinical signs in the Wernicke-Korsakoff complex: a retrospective survey of 131 cases diagnosed at autopsy. *J Neurol Neurosurg Psychiatry* 49:341, 1986.

38. Donnan GA, Seeman A: Coma and hypothermia in Wernicke's encephalopathy. *Aust NZ J Med* 10:438, 1980.

39. De La Paz MA, Chung SM, McCrary JA III: Bilateral internuclear ophthalmoplegia in a patient with Wernicke's encephalopathy. *J Clin Neuro-ophthalmol* 12:116, 1992.

40. Chez C: Vestibular paresis: a clinical feature of Wernicke's disease. *J Neurol Neurosurg Psychiatry* 32:134, 1969.

41. Philip G, Smith JF: Hypothermia and Wernicke's encephalopathy. *Lancet* 2:122, 1973.

42. Ackerman WJ, Stupor, bradycardia and hypothermia—a presentation of Wernicke's encephalopathy with rapid response to thiamine. *West Med* 121:428, 1974.

43. Heier MS, Fossa SD: Wernicke-Korsakoff-like syndrome in patients with colorectal carcinoma treated with high dose oxifludrine (5'-dFUrd). *Acta Neurol Scand* 73:449, 1986.

44. Vanneste J, Hage J: Acute severe hypophosphatemia mimicking Wernicke's encephalopathy. *Lancet* 1:44, 1986.

45. Szcsepanska-Sjerej A: Paogenetyczne i kliniczne aspekty zespolu Fishera. *Neurol Neurosurg Pol* 27:239, 1993.

46. D'Aprile P, Gentile MA, Carella A: Enhanced MR in the acute phase of Wernicke's encephalopathy. *AJNR* 15:591, 1994.

47. Doraiswamy PM, Massey EW, Enright K, et al: Wernicke-Korsakoff syndrome caused by psychogenic food refusal: MRI findings. *AJNR* 15:594, 1994.

48. Chan Y-W, McLeod JG, Tuck RR, Feary PA: Brain stem auditory evoked responses in chronic alcoholics. *Neurol Neurosurg Psychiatr* 48:1107, 1985.

49. Charness ME, Simon RP, Greenberg DA: Ethanol and the nervous system. *N Eng J Med* 321:442, 1989.

50. Marchiafava E, Bignami A: Spora un' arterazione del corpo calloso osservata in soggetti alcoolisti. *Riv Patol Nerv Ment* 8:544, 1903.

51. Victor M: Neurologic disorders due to alcoholism and malnutrition, in Joynt RF (ed): *Clinical Neurology*, vol 61. Philadelphia, Lippincott-Raven, 1986, pp 1–94.

52. Baron R, Heuser K, Marioth G: Hallazgos de la tomografia computadorizada en la forma aguda de la enfermedad de Marchiafava-Bignami. *Neurologia* 5:62, 1990.

53. Tomasini P, Guillot D, Sabbah P, et al: Marchiafava-Bignami disease with a favorable course. A popos of a case. *Ann Radiol* 36:319, 1993.

54. Nicoli F, Vion-Dury J, Chave B, et al: Maladie de Marchiafava-Bignami: disconnexion interhemispherique, syndrome de Balint, evolution spontaniment favorable. *Rev Neurol* 150:157, 1994.

55. Pappata S, Chabriat H, Levasseur M, Lagault-Demare F, Baron JC: Marchiafava-Bignami disease with dementia: severe cerebral metabolic depression revealed by PET. *J Neural Trans Park Dis Dement Sect* 8:131, 1994.

56. Tchelingerian JL, Quinonero J, Booss J, Jacque C: Localization of TNF alpha and IL-1 alpha in striatal neurons after surgical injury to the hippocampus. *Neuron* 10:213, 1993.

57. Kido G, Wright JL, Merchant RE: Acute effects of human recombinant tumor necrosis factor-alpha on the cerebral vasculature of the rat in both normal brain and in an experimental glioma model. *NeuroOncol* 10:95, 1991.

58. Brion S, Jedynak CP: Troubles du transfert interhémispherique (callosal disconnection). A propos de trois observations de tumeurs du corpus calleux. Le seigne de la main étrangère. *Rev Neurol* 126:257, 1972.

59. Kalckreuth W, Zimmerman P, Preilowski B, Wallesch CW: Incomplete split-brain syndrome in a patient with chronic Marchiafava-Bignami disease. *Behav Brain Res* 64:219, 1994.

60. Berek K, Wagner M, Chemelli AP, Aichner F, Benke T: Hemispheric disconnection in Marchiafava-Bignami disease: clinical, neuropsychological and MRI findings. *Neurol Sci* 123:2, 1994.

61. Kamaki M, Kawamura M, Moriya H, Hirayama K: "Crossed homonymous hemianopia" and "crossed hemispatial neglect: in a case of Marchiafava-Bignami disease." *J Neurol Neurosurg Psychiatry* 56:1027, 1993.

62. Caparros-Lefebvre D, Pruvo JP, Josien E, et al: Marchiafava-Bignami disease: use of contrast media in CT and MRI. *Neuroradiology* 36:509, 1994.

63. Marjama J, Yoshino MT, Reese C: Marchiafava-Bignami disease. Premortem diagnosis of an acute case utilizing magnetic resonance imaging. *J Neuroimaging* 4:106, 1994.

64. Kawamura M, Shiota J, Yagishita T, Hirayama K: Marchiafava-Bignami disease: computed tomographic scan and magnetic resonance imaging. *Ann Neurol* 18:103, 1985.

65. Chang KH, Han MH, Park SH, et al: Marchiafava-Bignami disease: serial changes in corpus callosum on MRI. *Neuroradiology* 34:480, 1992.

66. Serdau M, Hausser-Hau C, Laplane D, et al: The clinical spectrum of alcoholic pellagra encephalopathy. *Brain* 111:829, 1988.

67. Teleerman-Toppet N, Noël S: Alcoholic pellagra. *Neurology* 41:609, 1991.

68. Still CN: Nicotinic acid and nicotinamide deficiency: pellagra and related disorders of the nervous system, in Vinken PJ, Bruyn GW (eds): *Handbook of Clinical Neurology*, vol 28. Amsterdam, North Holland Publishing, 1976, pp 59–104.

69. Freundlich E, Slatter M, Yatziv S: Familial pellagra-like skin rash with neurologic manifestations. *Arch Dis Child* 56:146, 1981.

70. Clayton PT, Bridges NA, Atherton DJ, et al: Pellagra with colitis due to a defect in tryptophan metabolism. *Eur T Pediatr* 150:498, 1991.

71. Kieburtz K, Feigin A: Neurologic complications of vitamin and mineral disorders, in Joynt R, Griggs RC (eds): *Clinical Neurology*, vol 60. Philadelphia, Lippincott-Raven, 1993, p 5

72. Hauw J-J, De Baecque C, Hauser-Hauw C, Serdaru M: Chromatolysis in alcoholic encephalopathies. *Brain* 111:843, 1988.

73. Victor M, Adams RD: The neuropathology of experimental B_6 deficiency in monkeys. *Am J Clin Nutr* 4:346, 1956.

74. Joliffe N, Bowman KM, Rosenblum LA, Fein HD: Nicotinic acid deficiency encephalopathy. *JAMA* 114:307, 1940.

75. Healton EB, Savage DG, Brust JCM, et al: Neurologic aspects of cobolamin deficiency. *Medicine* 70:229, 1991.

76. Shorvon SD, Carney MWP, Chanarin I, Reynolds EH: The neuropsychiatry of megaloblastic anemia. *Br Med J* 281:1036, 1980.

77. Higginbottom MC, Sweetman L, Nyhan WL: A syndrome of methylmalonic aciduria, homocysteinuria, megaloblastic anemia and neurologic abnormalities in a vitamin B_{12}-deficient breast-fed infant of a strict vegetarian. *N Eng J Med* 299:317, 1978.

78. Kosik KS, Mullins TF, Bradley WG, et al: Coma and axonal degeneration in vitamin B_{12} deficiency. *Arch Neurol* 37:590, 1980.

79. Pearson HA, Vinson R, Smith RT: Pernicious anemia with neurologic involvement in childhood. *J Pediatr* 65:334, 1964.

80. Wighton MC, Manson JI, Speed I, Robertson E, Chapman E: Brain damage in infancy and dietary vitamin B_{12} deficiency. *Med J Aust* 2:1, 1979.

81. Mayfrank L, Thoden U: Downbeat nystagmus indicates cerebellar or brainstem lesions in vitamin B_{12} deficiency. *J Neurol* 233:145, 1970.

82. Sandyk R: Paralysis of upward gaze as a presenting symptom of vitamin B_{12} deficiency. *Eur Neurol* 23:198, 1984.

83. Kandler RH Davies-Jones GAB: Internuclear ophthalmoplegia in pernicious anemia. *BMJ* 297:1583, 1988.

84. Pruthi RK, Tefferi A: Pernicious anemia revisited. *Mayo Clin Proc* 69:144, 1994.

85. Battersby AR: How nature builds the pigments of life: the conquest of vitamin B_{12}. *Science* 264:1551, 1994.

86. Pruthi RK, Tefferi A: Pernicious anemia revisited. *Mayo Clin Proc* 69:144, 1994.

87. Tefferi A, Pruthi RK: The biochemical basis of cobolamin deficiency. *Mayo Clin Proc* 69:181, 1994.

88. Ferraro A, Arieti S, English WH: Cerebral changes in the course of pernicious anemia and their relationship to psychic symptoms. *J Neuropath Exp Neurol* 4:217, 1945.

89. Green R, Kinsella IJ: Cobolamin deficiency. *Neurology* 47:310, 1997.

90. Norman EJ, Cronin C: Cobolamin deficiency. *Neurology* 47:310, 1997.

91. Fine EJ, Soria ED: Myths about vitamin B_{12} deficiency. *South Med J* 84:175, 1991.

92. Mayer RF: Peripheral nerve function in vitamin B_{12} deficiency. *Arch Neurol* 13:355, 1965.

93. Kayser-Gatchalian MC, Neundorfer B: Peripheral neuropathy with vitamin B_{12} deficiency. *J Neurol* 214:183, 1977.

94. Jones SJ, Yu YL, Rudge P, et al: Central and peripheral SEP defects in neurologically symptomatic and asymptomatic subjects with low vitamin B_{12} levels. *J Neurol Sci* 82:55, 1987.

95. Babior BM, Bunn HF: Megaloblastic anemias, in Braunwald E, Isselbacher KJ, Petersdorf RG, Wilson JD, Martin JB, Fauci AS (eds): *Harrison's Principles of Internal Medicine*, 11th ed. New York, McGraw-Hill, 1987, pp 1498–1506.

Chapter 15

ANOXIC AND ISCHEMIC BRAIN INJURY

G. Bryan Young

Compared with other organs, the human brain, especially the cerebral cortex, has enormous requirements for energy, blood flow, and oxygen. With an average weight of 1.3 kg (less than 2 percent of the mass of a 70-kg person), the brain receives 20 percent of the cardiac output and consumes 60 percent of the body's glucose and 20 percent of the metabolized oxygen.[1] The cells of the cerebral cortex, which take up 20 percent of the brain mass, account for 75 percent of the brain's metabolic requirements.[1]

Hypoxia is a decrease in oxygen delivery to tissues, whatever the cause. Ischemia is a decrease in the blood flow to an organ. Hypoxemia is a decrease in the oxygen-carrying capacity of the blood. Hypoxic and/or ischemic states of the brain have been traditionally classified as follows[2]:

1. Focal ischemia (ischemic stroke).
2. Generalized ischemia or hypoxia.
   a. Ischemic hypoxia: complete disruption of blood flow, usually from cardiac arrest.
   b. Oligemic hypoxia (partial ischemia): incomplete reduction of blood flow that may be generalized or focal.
   c. Anoxic hypoxia: arterial oxygen concentration is zero.

d. Hypoxic hypoxia: arterial oxygen tension is reduced below the threshold level of 40 mmHg.
e. Anemic hypoxia: oxygen delivery to tissues is reduced because of reduced ability of the blood to carry the oxygen. The example discussed is carbon monoxide poisoning.
f. Histiotoxic hypoxia: poisoning of the mitochondial system involved in oxidative metabolism. The example discussed is cyanide poisoning. Inherited mitochondrial encephalopathies (e.g., MELAS, Chap. 13) would also produce this type of energy failure.

Oxygen extraction reserve, or the ability of the tissues to extract more oxygen from the circulating blood, is conveniently estimated by measuring the oxygen content of venous blood draining the organ. The brain and heart each use about 60 to 65 percent of their available oxygen under normal circumstances, compared with an extraction of 20 percent by most organs. Thus, the oxygen extraction *reserve* of the brain and heart is more limited than other organs. There are a number of mechanisms that are compensatory for a drop in oxygen concentration or blood pressure. With hypoxemia, brain blood flow increases through vasodilatation and an augmentation of the stroke volume of the heart. (Brain blood flow is normally tightly auto-regulated, but this is overcome by marked hypox-emia or hypercarbia; see Fig. 3-18). The extraction of oxygen from blood is maximized. Blood flow is redistributed, away from the extremities and non-vital organs, to maintain flow to the brain. There are limits to which the brain can compensate for hypoxemia. Below a Pa_{O_2} of 40 mmHg, especially if acutely lowered from a higher value, there is mea-surable cerebral dysfunction.[1] Nonlethal degrees of hypoxemia (Pa_{O_2} values of 20 to 40 mmHg) are associated with altered neuronal activity, increases in extracellular potassium and glutamine, and a decrease in extracellular sodium concentration.[3-5] Lactate and free fatty acids increase, while phos-phatidylinositol, involved in some secondary mes-senger systems that do not involve cyclic adenine monophosphate, is decreased.[6] There is not, how-ever, a decrease in stores of high-energy phosphate; significant brain swelling does not occur.[7,8]

Hypoxia as an isolated phenomenon is an uncommon cause of encephalopathy. Most often, there is a combination of hypoxia and ischemia. Decompensation occurs in severe hypoxemia, in that the heart will fail, causing a drop in cardiac output and blood pressure. This leads to a drop in cerebral perfusion. Below a mean arterial pressure of 60 mmHg, the brain cannot autoregulate its blood pressure; cerebral perfusion falls passively with further decreases in cerebral blood flow (Fig. 3-18).

Figure 15-1 illustrates the current understand-ing of the sequence of events in neuronal death from ischemia. The same processes occur in focal ische-mia or stroke, in global ischemia with cardiac arrest and, probably, with lethal hypoxia. The prevailing hypothesis is that increased extracellular concentra-tions of excitatory amino acids, particularly gluta-mate, lead to toxicity mediated by ion-channel linked receptors, that, in turn, allow large amounts of calcium ions to enter the neuron. Ionized calcium may activate a number of intracellular enzymes, including neuronal nitric oxide synthetase that gen-erates nitric oxide. The toxic effects of nitric oxide are due to its interaction with the superoxide anion to form peroxynitrite, a cytotoxic compound.[9,10]

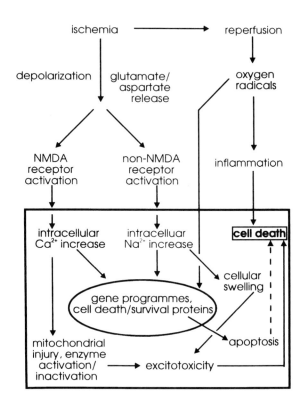

Figure 15-1

The sequence of events in acute brain ischemia lead-ing ultimately to cell death. NMDA = N-methyl-D-aspar-tate. (Redrawn from Korsohetz WJ, Moskowitz MA, Emerging treatment for stroke in humans. TIPS 17:227, 1996, with permission.)

This may be the most important "final common pathway" leading to cell death.[11]

ISCHEMIC STROKE (FOCAL ISCHEMIA)

Definition and Significance

In ischemic stroke, there is complete loss of circula-tion affecting a circumscribed region in which all tissue elements, neurons, glia, and vessels are infarcted. Some infarcts are surrounded by an ischemic "penumbra" with a relative, but incom-plete, reduction in blood flow with preserved struc-tural integrity.[12] There is, thus, a graded reduction in blood flow that is complete in the center of the ischemic region (infarcted region) and milder in the periphery (penumbra). Focal ischemic strokes are usually classified into embolic or thrombotic categories.

In the United States, 550,000 strokes occur annually.[13] The incidence has declined in recent years, probably due to reduction of risk factors: better control of hypertension and hyperlipidemia, and reduced smoking. Further, proper management of patients with transient ischemic attacks, or threatened strokes, may have reduced the occurrence of frank strokes. The morbidity and mortality have enormous societal cost, besides the loss of dignity, productivity, and enjoyment of life.

Although animal experiments indicate that only minutes to a few hours of such ischemia are sufficient to produce neuronal and glial death, in humans the process is more variable. The process may not be complete for several hours or even days.[14,15] The central core of the lesion is densely ischemic and probably dies in the shortest time. Surrounding the ischemic core, the "penumbra" may be vulnerable to the effects of excitatory neurotransmitters or free radicals that increase the metabolic demand beyond the threshold for infarction, or cause direct toxic damage in themselves. Castillo and colleagues have recently shown that patients with progressive strokes show higher cerebrospinal fluid (CSF) and plasma glutamate and glycine than patients with nonprogressive strokes.[16] Hyperthermia and hyperglycemia may also add metabolic stress to the penumbra. If the penumbra infarcts, the stroke is said to have "progressed" or "extended."[17] Recent evidence suggests that if the penumbra region does not undergo infarction, it often remains permanently hypometabolic, because of either partial ischemic neuronal loss or disconnection.[18]

STROKE AND IMPAIRED CONSCIOUSNESS

Frank coma is uncommon after single artery territory ischemic stroke, except in basilar territory ischemia with rostral brainstem or thalamic infarction, or in single internal carotid or middle cerebral artery occlusion with massive hemispheric ischemia that causes brain edema with secondary mass effect. Bilateral internal carotid ischemia may lead to abrupt coma without signs of brainstem or cranial nerve dysfunction. While coma is expected with severe global ischemia, impairment of consciousness with focal strokes depends on the dysfunction of specific regions involved in consciousness (see below and Chap. 2). These can be directly affected by the ischemia or hemorrhage, or indirectly affected by compression, disruption of blood-brain barrier function or by diaschisis (remote metabolic suppression—see Chap. 1). Complications, such as seizures, superimposed infections or sepsis, or coincidental metabolic derangements, should also be considered.

In the following discussion, the common causes of embolism from atherosclerotic large arterial or cardiac disease are emphasized. Less common causes of ischemic stroke, e.g., migraine and hypercoagulable states, are considered briefly later. The sites of infarction that cause coma or coma-like states, along with the corresponding clinical pictures, are given below:

1. *Anterior cerebral territory infarction*: Bilateral lesions in the distribution of the anterior cerebral arteries (Fig. 15-2) are often the consequence of vasospasm from the rupture of an anterior communicating artery aneurysm. Akinetic mutism is the main manifestation of ischemia in the total territories of both anterior cerebral arteries (see Chap. 2).[19] Such patients open the eyes and visually track, but do not initiate speech of other voluntary movements. Patients may show catalepsy, or the tendency to maintain postures for extended periods of time, resembling a catatonic state. Bilateral lesions of the anterior cingulate gyri or the anterior limbs of the internal capsule constitute the more restricted lesions that may produce this syndrome or various degrees of abulia (loss of motivation and spontaneous activity), even if the latter is transient.[20] Most lesions are considerably larger. Infarction of the supplementary motor area (the medial aspect of areas 6: see Fig. 1-3), even unilaterally, may produce abulia, failure to move the contralateral limbs, a prominent forced grasp

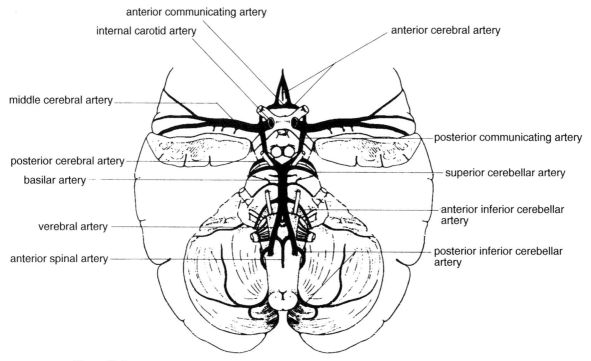

Figure 15-2
The arteries of the brain.

response of the contralateral hand, and motionless facies; these symptoms are usually transient, clearing in about 2 weeks.[21,22] An anterior disconnection syndrome may occur with infarction of the anterior corpus callosum.[23]

2. *Basilar system ischemia:* The basilar system is illustrated in Fig. 15-3.

Impairment of consciousness or akinetic mutism occurs in about 6 percent of thalamic infarcts, in contrast to 13 percent of thalamic hemorrhages and 62 percent of thalamic hemorrhages that extend into the ventricular system.[24] Impairment of alertness is more likely if the paramedian areas of the thalamus are affected bilaterally; unilateral or bilateral anterior and posterior thalamic strokes are not commonly associated with stupor or coma unless there is bilateral extension of the stroke.[24]

Ocular movement abnormalities are also more likely with paramedian thalamic lesions than with involvement of other sites.[24] These include horizontal gaze palsy to the contralateral side, "wrong-way eyes" (gaze palsy to the opposite side), skew deviation, and vertical gaze palsy.[24] Nystagmus does not occur.

If the thalamic infarcts are restricted to the paramedian or dorsal regions, there is usually no motor deficit.[24] The latter is common, however, if infarcts are more extensive anterior and posterior lesions.[24]

The 90-day survival for ischemic thalamic strokes is 87 percent compared with 48 percent for thalamic hemorrhages.[24] On recovery, there is commonly neglect contralateral to the thalamic lesion.[24] Watson and colleagues argue that hemineglect reflects involvement of the paramedian thalamus.[25] Transcortical sensory, Wernicke's, and Broca's aphasias are uncommon, but have been described.[24] Hemianopsia is not uncommon with posterior thalamic lesions. Contralateral sen-

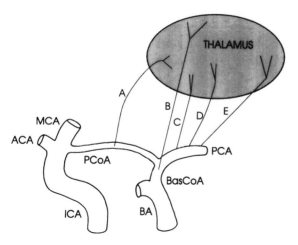

Figure 15-3

Arterial supply to deep cerebral structures arising from the posterior communicating artery (PCoA), basilar communicating artery (BasCoA) and the posterior cerebral artery (PCA). The anterior (ACA), middle (MCA) and internal carotid (ICA) arteries are also shown. A, polar artery; B, paramedian artery; C, thalamogeniculate pedicle; D, posteromedial choroidal artery; E, posterolateral choroidal artery. (From Castaigne et al,[27] with permission.)

sory deficits and the thalamic pain syndrome sometimes follow thalamic strokes.

Impaired consciousness results primarily from lesions of the ascending reticular activating system, either bilateral paramedian thalamic structures or the rostral brainstem tegmentum (see Chap. 1).[26] The most detailed studies of posterior circulation disorders affecting paramedian structures in the diencephalon and rostral midbrain were by Castaigne and colleagues and Tatu et al.[27,28] Unilateral paramedian infarctions involving medial thalamic structures resulted in confusion, disorientation, and behavioral changes. Acute, bilateral paramedian thalamic infarcts (Fig. 15-3) consistently caused initial marked impairment in consciousness, either coma or akinetic mutism, behavior, memory loss, or a combination of these. Some patients with initial coma evolved into an amnestic state. Some showed marked mental slowing with decreased attention, slow ideation, and apathy. These lesions related to

ischemia in the territory of the paramedian arteries that arise from the initial portion of the posterior cerebral arteries, before being joined by the posterior communicating arteries. The midline and intralaminar thalamic nuclei were affected. Memory problems were related to bilateral lesions of the mammillothalamic tract or the medial dorsal thalamic nuclei.

Paramedian thalamopeduncular infarcts, related to the paramedian thalamo-subthalamic artery, affect the rostral midbrain and medial thalamus.[27] (In contrast, lesions in the distribution of the thalamogeniculate artery do not.[35]) Most patients, especially those with bilateral lesions, are obtunded. Hypersomnolence seems related to lesions of the ascending noradrenergic pathway through the brainstem.[27] Third nerve nuclear lesions, with ocular paralyses, convergence or vertical gaze paralysis, ptosis, and Parinaud syndrome, are common and related to rostral mesencephalic tegmental lesions. Pupillary abnormalities are expected with rostral midbrain–diencephalic lesions. Involvement of the Edinger-Westphal nucleus of the oculomotor nuclear complex results in dilated, fixed pupils. If the descending sympathetic pathways are also involved, the pupils become "cadaveric," midposition, and nonreactive. Occasionally, oval pupils may be found transiently in evolving third nerve palsies and in rostral herniation.[29] Thalamic lesions are commonly associated with small, poorly reactive pupils.

Bilateral lesions of the rostral tegmentum are always associated with impaired consciousness.[26] Such lesions are commonly accompanied by signs of damage to surrounding structures, including pupillary abnormalities, abnormal extraocular movements, other cranial nerve abnormalities, (often bilateral) corticospinal motor deficits, and ataxia. The "top of the basilar" syndrome is characterized by initial symptoms and signs of brainstem ischemia (e.g., diplopia followed by hemiparesis or tetraparesis, then coma).[30] Most such strokes are embolic; about one-quarter are atherothrombotic.

Eye movements: A variety of ocular movement disorders have been described in basilar occlusion. These are discussed in Chap. 3 in the section on neurologic evaluation. They include internuclear ophthalmoplegia, conjugate gaze palsy, and ocular bobbing. Ptosis may also occur, especially with rostral, "top of the basilar" strokes that involve the Edinger-Westphal nucleus in the midbrain.

Peduncular hallucinations: Vivid visual hallucinations have been described in association with lesions of the rostral brainstem–hypothalamic region. All such patients have suffered sleep disturbances; it is of interest that patients who are deprived of rapid-eye-movement (REM) sleep may experience similar visual hallucinations. Perhaps both reflect a disturbance in the centers that govern aspects of REM sleep.[31]

Exceptionally, coma without focal findings occurs in strokes involving the thalamus and midbrain.[32] This closely simulates the picture in metabolic encephalopathy. However, there are abnormalities involving vertical eye movements with basilar ischemia.[32]

Thalamic strokes are usually ischemic, but hemorrhage accounts for 8 to 35 percent, depending on the series studied.[33–35] Those with hemorrhages tend to do worse than do those with infarcts.[35] Patients with thalamic strokes tend to be younger than those with other strokes.[35] Most ischemic thalamic strokes are associated with strokes in other vascular territories. Atherosclerosis-promoting factors are important, as in other strokes.

3. The occurrence of acute unilateral cerebral hemispheric dysfunction with loss of consciousness or alertness, coincident with the *onset* of ischemia, is debated in the literature.[36,37] Large, acute, dominant cerebral hemisphere strokes have been reported to impair alertness and responsiveness transiently.[38] Albert and colleagues found coma or "semicoma" in 10 percent of patients (2 of 23) with acute left, but in none of the 24 patients with acute right, hemispheric lesions.[38] This could not be explained on the basis of lesion size, based on clinical signs. Careful studies of unilateral intracarotid amytal injections have noted unconsciousness in a minority of patients. Whether such patients are truly unconscious is not clear. Lesser and colleagues reported that patients could later recognize objects presented during the confusional, mute phase.[39] It is likely that some patients have diminished alertness with amnesia and lack of responsiveness. The explanation may be an alteration of interhemispheric communication with resultant bihemispheric dysfunction or "diaschisis." Alternatively, there may be some bilaterality of ischemia of both hemispheres; e.g., both frontal lobes may be affected if the anterior cerebral arteries are supplied from the left carotid system.

4. Bilateral middle cerebral artery territory strokes may occur nearly simultaneously, e.g., with cardiogenic embolism, or sequentially. In such situations, there is sparing of thalamic and brainstem function. The patient is usually deeply comatose with normal pupils and continuously roving horizontal eye movements. With large bilateral infarcts, the possibility of recovery beyond a persistent vegetative state (PVS) is poor.

Diagnostic Workup

The initial step is the localization of the deficit. The absence of any intrinsic brainstem signs (i.e., normally sized and reacting pupils, normal eye movements with caloric testing, and intact corneal reflexes in the unconscious patient) implies that the stroke is probably not in the brainstem.

The etiology often is assisted by the history and other physical findings. Historically, if there have been prior symptoms of transient neurologic deficits of a similar nature, the focal ischemia is likely to be ischemic rather than hemorrhagic.

Within focal ischemic stroke, it is important therapeutically to determine whether the stroke was embolic, especially cardioembolic. Some clinical clues for a cardioembolic mechanism include: occurrence in young adults; sudden, maximal-at-onset symptoms; evidence of previous strokes in different vascular territories; evidence of systemic embolism; abnormal cardiac examination; and no large artery source for emboli found.[40]

The general exam can give clues as to risk factors: i.e., hypertension, cardiac status, and other features. The presence of a fever, a cardiac murmur, and focal or multifocal neurologic deficits raises the possibility of bacterial endocarditis. Other conditions, including sepsis, meningitis, herpes simplex encephalitis, or drug abuse, need to be excluded.

Immediately after stabilization and clinical assessment, a computed tomography (CT) scan of the head is necessary to exclude intracranial hemorrhage (intraparenchymal, subdural or subarachnoid), venous thrombosis, and nonvascular lesions (such as brain tumors) that may mimic ischemic stroke.[41] Such findings have important therapeutic implications. If doubt remains, a contrast-enhanced or magnetic resonance imaging (MRI) scan should be performed.

The following should be performed in all patients with ischemic stroke: complete blood count, including platelets, and differential white blood cell count; prothrombin time (INR: international normalized ratio), partial thromboplastin time; serum creatinine, electrolytes and glucose; electrocardiogram (ECG); CT scan of the brain; and chest film.[42] Liver function tests are also useful in excluding hepatic disease and as a prelude to starting anticoagulants. Forty-eight-hour Holter monitoring and echocardiography (transesophageal in cases where there is a high suspicion of a cardiac source and the transthoracic echocardiogram is negative) are often necessary to exclude a cardiac source.

Occasionally, stroke may be mimicked by severe hypoglycemia, hyponatremia, or hepatic failure. Postictal paralysis, migraine and hypertensive encephalopathy should be excluded clinically and with appropriate laboratory tests. With fever, blood cultures and CSF analyses may be necessary to exclude endocarditis or a primary central nervous system (NS) infection.

The EEG can occasionally be useful in differential diagnosis, e.g., nonconvulsive seizures or a metabolic encephalopathy versus stroke. Also, the EEG can be used as a rough but readily accessible and dynamically responsive test of regional or diffuse thalamocortical function. The test is useful only if specific questions (seizures, trending of conscious level, differential diagnosis, and monitoring during carotid surgery) are asked of the electroencephalographer; it should not delay investigation or treatment in clinically or radiologically obvious cases.[43]

In the workup of established ischemic stroke or transient ischemia, cardiac, arterial, and hematologic workup are necessary. Focal ischemic stroke in young individuals is often cardiogenic or related to arterial embolism, e.g., arterial dissection or fibromuscular hyperplasia, or oral contraceptive use in women.[44] In older individuals, atherosclerotic arterial or cardiac disease is much more likely than other causes.

To determine the vascular pathogenesis, Doppler ultrasound of the carotids, with or without transcranial Dopplers, and sonification of the vertebral arteries are useful screening procedures. "Pseudo-occlusion" from tight stenosis is a problem with Doppler studies that usually requires angiography to resolve. Computed tomographic (spiral CT with digital reconstruction) and MRI angiography are emerging as potentially useful noninvasive techniques. Diffusion-weighted MRI or CT may ultimately prove to be useful in differentiating infarcted from noninfarcted tissue.[45] These may be difficult to perform in the restless, acutely ill patient, however. Cerebral angiography is still the gold standard and is used when the patient is a surgical candidate or if an unusual arterial cause is suspected, e.g., vasculitis.

Management

Management of Focal Ischemia The management of stroke can be divided into the following categories: (1) primary stoke prevention; (2) secondary prevention; (3) acute stroke therapy, including the amelioration of secondary mass effect from edema; and (4) rehabilitation.

It is well known that primary prevention is the most ideal measure and involves risk factor identification and modification. Risk factors include hypertension, cigarette smoking, diabetes mellitus, hyperlipidemia, and excessive alcohol consumption.[46] These factors alone and in isolation may interact with age and heart disease, especially atrial fibrillation, to increase the risk of stroke.[47]

Patients who have had transient ischemic attacks (TIAs), threatened strokes with symptoms lasting less than 24 h, have a significant risk of stroke and require investigation to determine the source. For TIAs associated with greater than 70 percent stenosis of the appropriate proximal internal carotid artery, endarterectomy at a good center significantly reduces stroke risk.[48] Vertebrobasilar TIAs and patients who are not candidates for endarterectomy may reduce stroke risk with acetylsalicylic acid or ticlopidine.[49] Patients at significant risk from a cardiac source, e.g., chronic atrial fibrillation and rheumatic valvular disease, are best treated prophylactically with oral anticoagulants, unless there are contraindications.[50]

Emergency Management

Ideally, patients with acute strokes should be seen promptly in an emergency room at a referral center with (1) expertise in the diagnosis of ischemic stroke (misdiagnosis occurs 13 to 19 percent of the time), (2) prompt neuroimaging availability, (3) provision for interventional therapy for selected patients, and (4) neurosurgical intervention if hemorrhagic complications arise.[51]

Recent strategies include thrombolysis, rheological strategies, and metabolic salvage with the use of neuroprotective agents. Of these, the recent National Institute of Neurological Disorders and Stroke multicenter study supports intravenous thrombolytic therapy with recombinant tissue plasminogen activator (rt-PA) in patients with acute ischemic stroke.[52] A subsequent subgroup analysis of the European Cooperative Acute Stroke Study (ECASS) showed benefit for those treated within 6 h, providing that normal CT scans did not show early changes of edema.[53]

Despite a 12 percent increased chance of improvement in neurologic outcome at 3 months, there is a 3 to 6 percent chance of early death from rt-PA-induced hemorrhage (beyond the control group for both benefit and hemorrhage).[54] The identification of subgroups that benefit most, and the exclusionary criteria for those in whom the risk is too great, requires further refinement.[55] At present, recommended contraindications for

thrombolysis include: (1) duration of ischemic symptoms of more than 3 h (this time window may increase with certain provisos); (2) large (greater than one-third of middle cerebral artery territory) ischemic lesions clinically or with early signs of edema or loss of gray-white matter distinction on CT scan; (3) arterial hypertension with systolic presures >180 mmHg; and (4) coexistent coagulopathy or anticoagulated state.

Intra-arterial thrombolysis, with rt-PA or urokinase appears to be better than systemic therapy in achieving recanalization of acute middle cerebral artery occlusions.[56] Streptokinase should not be used because of prohibitively high risks of intracerebral hemorrhage.[57,58]

Neuroprotective strategies that hold promise include: the use of blockers of N-methyl-D-aspartate NMDA receptors, non-NMDA-glutamate receptor antagonists, drugs to reduce release of glutamate and aspartate (e.g., lamotrigine, fosphenytoin), therapeutic hypothermia, calcium channel antagonists (either to prevent calcium influx or to improve perfusion through a vasodilatatory effect), and antioxygen free radical therapy.[59–68] In addition, anti-inflammatory drugs (agents that produce transient leukopenia or antibodies against leukocyte adhesion molecules or P-selectin) offer promise.[69–71] Combinations of these may also be worthwhile, but definitive results from randomized clinical trials on single and combinations of agents are awaited.[72]

Potential new agents/techniques that may be a generation away from the above include: agents that increase nitric oxide in the vasculature (but not within neurons or glia),[73] neurotropic factors (e.g., fibroblast growth factor),[74] and stimulation of genes that suppress apoptosis.[75]

Stroke Management Patients are best managed in a co-ordinated fashion in which physicians, nurses, and allied health professionals work together to prevent complications (cardiac problems, infections, deep vein thromboses, etc.) and to enroll the patient promptly in the rehabilitative process.[76–80]

The neurologic status should be trended and charted. Sedation and analgesia should be administered only when necessary to allow for adequate clinical monitoring.

Adequate oxygenation and hemoglobin concentration should be assured. In the obtunded patient, maintaining the airway is vital, but assisted ventilation is rarely necessary. Prevention of aspiration may require endotracheal intubation in patients with severe obtundation or marked dysphagia. Also, pulmonary embolism is a frequent complication of acute stroke; appropriate preventive and screening measures are needed.

Monitoring the ECG, blood pressure, and breathing should be routine. Arrhythmias are not uncommon and should be treated appropriately. To perfuse the penumbra region adequately, the blood pressure may need to be greater than normal; it is best not to lower the blood pressure unless it becomes markedly elevated, e.g., values greater than 220/120. Patients should be screened clinically, with chest films taken for aspiration, atelectasis, and deep venous thrombosis. Chest physiotherapy and passive limb movements should be routine.

Up to one-third of stroke patients are volume-depleted. Correction of hypovolemia and optimization of cardiac output are important measures in aiding cerebral perfusion.[81]

Hyperthermia should be prevented, as there is evidence that elevated temperature increases tissue damage in ischemia and hypoxemia.[82] It is very important that hyperthermic patients be carefully screened for underlying cause, and the latter should be promptly and specifically treated. About one-third of stroke patients have a preceding infectious illness.[83] Hyperglycemia should be prevented, as stroke volume is correlated with the severity of hyperglycemia.[84,85] The relative importance of hyperglycemia in worsening the stroke has recently been called into question.[86]

Clinically apparent seizures occur in about 10 percent of patients with acute stroke and are more common when the Rolandic region is involved. These are usually partial seizures with variable spread or secondary generalization. Nonconvulsive seizures are almost certainly underrecognized in this population. There is evidence that nonconvulsive seizures contribute to brain damage

(see Chap. 17). Furthermore, they can prolong the duration of unresponsiveness and prolong stay in special care areas. In patients with fluctuating responsiveness EEGs should be ordered liberally; continuous EEG, if available, may be worthwhile in some patients.

Intracranial pressure (ICP) monitoring is not of proven value, but is advisable in patients with extensive cerebral hemispheric infarction or large cerebellar (without significant brainstem) infarcts. This may allow for control of cerebral perfusion pressure or the relief of raised pressure if CSF can be withdrawn from an intraventricular catheter. Daily head CT scans may be necessary in patients with large cerebellar infarcts to look for progressive hydrocephalus related to mass effect.

Anticoagulation is used primarily in cardiogenic embolism to prevent intracardiac thrombus formation and further embolism, and to prevent deep venous thrombosis. Heparin is used acutely; later, this is switched to coumadin. Recommended INR should be 1.5 to 2 for nonvalvular disease and 2.5 to 3.0 for natural or artificial valvular sources. Relative contraindications to acute anticoagulation include a large ischemic infarct with edema on CT, advanced patient age, the presence of blood on CT or MRI, and very early infarction (less than 3 h). For deep venous thrombosis, the use of antiembolism stockings and subcutaneous heparinization is recommended.

Cerebral Edema Cerebral edema can be life-threatening, especially in younger individuals with large hemispheric lesions. Elevation of the head of the bed to 30° improves venous drainage and may prevent worsening of brain edema. Hyperventilation to P_{CO_2} values between 25 and 30 mmHg (lower values may be associated with a detrimental decrease in cerebral perfusion) and osmotic agents are the first-line measures. Hypothermia has not been adequately assessed thus far, but this is difficult to achieve in clinical situations. Animal and tissue culture studies show that glucocorticoids enhance neuronal and glial loss in the presence of anoxia or hypoglycemia.[87,88] Since there is evidence that exogenous corticosteroids do not improve outcome in patients with ischemic stroke or hypoxia, it seems best to avoid their administration.[89]

Decompressive craniectomy should be considered in large cerebral or cerebellar hemispheric lesions with mass effect that is not responding to the above measures (see Figs. 15-4 and 15-5).[90,91] "Malignant middle cerebral artery (MCA) infarctions," in which massive edema develops, carry a mortality rate of 80 percent; survivors often have significant morbidity.[92] Parenchymal hypodensity that occupies more than 50 percent of the MCA territory on the initial CT scan has a 85 percent likelihood of evolving into malignant MCA infarction.[93] The above-mentioned standard measures, including osmotic diuretics and hyperventilation, are usually ineffective. Uncontrolled clinical trials and anecdotal case reports suggest that decompressive craniotomy can be life-saving, at least with some younger patients surviving with minor deficits.[94–99] Such decompressive surgery has usually been reserved for younger patients with nondominant hemispheric infarcts, but this could be extended to older individuals and those with dominant hemispheric lesions. Recent controlled studies, using an ischemic model in rats, have confirmed the value of craniotomy in reducing mortality and the volume of infarcted tissue.[100,101] The earlier the craniotomy, the better the outcome, but the optimum timing cannot be directly extrapolated from rats to humans. Some centers perform craniectomies as soon as it is obvious that compliance on ICP monitoring begins to decline, or with a decline in the Glasgow Coma Scale or with ipsilateral pupillary dilatation indicating herniation.[94]

It is unclear whether the removal of apparently nonviable brain tissue requires resection with cerebral infarcts; decompression alone may suffice. Removal of necrotic cerebellar tissue and intraventricular drainage are additional options in patients with large cerebellar infarcts.

Prognosis

Prognosis for survival is mainly dependent on the level of consciousness and the density of the paresis.[102] Coma as a direct consequence of the stroke itself shows a strong relationship to mortality in the acute phase.[103] The odds ratio is 30.7 for death, comparing those patients with stroke in coma with noncomatose patients.[103] Depressed level of consciousness also correlates independently with infarct size.[104] Age is not an independent risk factor for survival of an acute stroke.

With thalamic stroke, either ischemic or hemorrhagic, mortality is significantly increased in the presence of coma, a Glasgow Coma Scale value of < 9, a weakness score of >15/30, abnormal ocular movements, and loss of pupillary reactivity.[105] For prediction of survival and high morbidity for longer periods (e.g., 6 months to 3 years), the level of consciousness and other factors, such as age, residence at the time of stroke (institution versus home), marital status, and previous history of stroke, are important.[106,107] Combinations of factors have increased predictive value. Only 5 percent of chronically institutionalized patients who lost consciousness with strokes were alive 3 years later.[106]

Patients who require mechanical ventilation after stroke, either ischemic or hemorrhagic, have a mortality rate of about 90 percent.[108] It has been argued that such intervention is not worthwhile. However, endotracheal intubation and ventilation seem appropriate for those patients with potentially reversible complications, e.g., status epilepticus (convulsive or nonconvulsive), problems protecting the airway with vertebrobasilar strokes, and those with complications such as pneumonia or metabolic disturbances. Thus, it seems inappropriate to make general policy decisions on this matter; each case should be considered individually.

POST ANOXIC-ISCHEMIC ENCEPHALOPATHY

Significance

The overall 1-year survival rate of initially unconscious survivors resuscitated from cardiac arrest has been variably quoted to be between 10 and 25 percent.[109,110] Anoxic-ischemic encephalopathy is the principal cause of mortality in at least 30 to 40

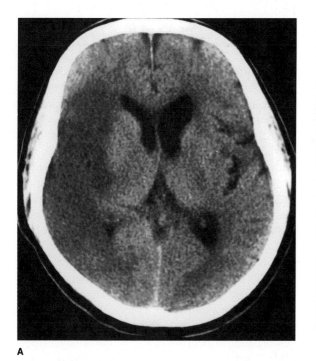

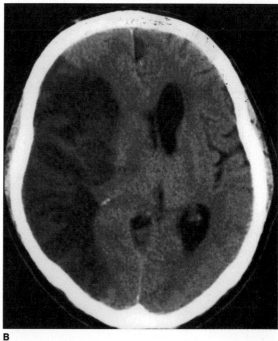

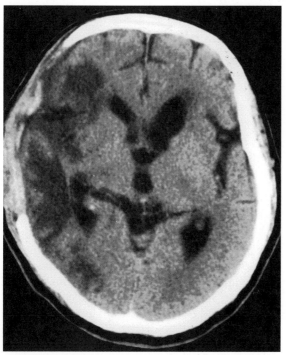

Figure 15-4
A. *Mass effect from edema 3 days after the onset of an ischemic infarct in right middle cerebral artery territory.* B. *Two days later the mass effect has markedly increased, associated with obtundation.* C. *A craniectomy and duraplasty were performed and by the next day the mass effect was much less. The patient had a good outcome.*

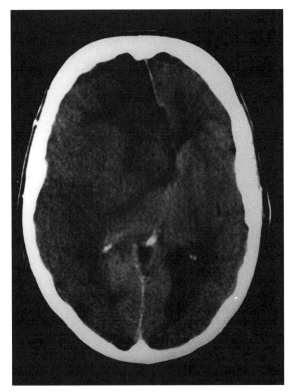

Figure 15-5
Malignant cerebral edema with a stoke affecting both the anterior and the middle cerebral artery territories.

percent of those who die; only 3 to 10 percent of survivors return to their previous life-styles including employment.[111] Well under 1 percent survive in a PVS.[112]

Pathology and Pathogenesis

Certain neurons show a "selective vulnerability" to anoxic/ischemic insults. The large cell layers (3, 5, and 6) of the neocortex, the CA1, and the end folium (CA4–6) of the hippocampus are especially vulnerable.[113–117] Other relatively vulnerable regions include the Purkinje cells of the cerebellum, and the putamen, caudate, and thalamus.[118] If the patient survives for a sufficient time, the neurons are replaced by a gliotic reaction. Transsynaptic degeneration may affect thalamic nuclei and brainstem nuclei such as the inferior olivary complex.[119]

If the insult is sufficiently severe, all neurons may die, producing brain death.[120]

It is, thus, not surprising that patients who are comatose after cardiac arrest often show intact central respiratory drive and brainstem functions (some of the latter may be enhanced as "release phenomena"), even though the vulnerable regions (frequently all cell layers of the neocortex) may have no viable neurons.[121,122]

With widespread neocortical damage, patients may develop a PVS, in which wake and sleep cycles return, but there is no response, awareness, or meaningful interaction with the environment. On clinical grounds alone, it is difficult to estimate the prognosis in the early stages of such "recovery" of function, as discussed below.

The pathogenesis of anoxic-ischemic encephalopathy is incompletely understood. Hypotheses include: excitotoxic damage from excitatory amino acids (notably glutamate and aspartate), disturbance in neuronal calcium homeostasis (possibly related to excitotoxic amino acids), the relative balance of various excitatory and inhibitory neurotransmitters, impaired synthesis of proteins, damage from oxygen-derived free radicals, the no-reflow phenomenon, and neuronal sodium-potassium pump and energy failure.[123–127] Many of these insults relate to damage following reperfusion.[128] There are some problems with each of these in serving as a complete explanation for neuronal death; it is likely that a number of mechanisms operate together.

The main unifying hypothesis involves initial insult from excitotoxic amino acids. Activation of NMDA receptors opens a voltage-dependent ion channel, allowing sodium and calcium to enter the neuronal cytoplasm from the extracellular fluid. This causes acute osmotic swelling of the neuron, which may be lethal. Delayed neuronal death may result from subsequent actions resulting from the increase in intracellular calcium ions. This results in activation of the following: (1) various enzymes that cause proteolysis of the cytoskeleton; (2) protein kinase C, leading to further calcium entry into the cell; (3) phospholipase C, responsible for the generation of inositol triphosphate, in turn, causing release of ionized calcium from internal stores;

(4) diacylglycerol, which activates protein kinase C; (5) phospholipase A_2, which contributes to free radical production; (6) calcium/calmodulin-dependent protein kinase II, causing more glutamate release; and (7) the inducible form of nitric acid synthetase, leading to the formation of nitric oxide which interacts with superoxide to produce a highly toxic free-radical species.[129] (It should be noted that, in the early phase of ischemia, neuronally produced nitric oxide increases regional blood flow through effects on the microcirculation and on larger vessels.[130]) In cells with alpha-amino-3-hydroxy-5-methyl-4-isoxazole propionic acid (AMPA) receptors, e.g., cerebellar Purkinje cells, the initiation of at least some of these destructive processes also occurs.[129]

Management

Management of Generalized Anoxic-Ischemic Encephalopathy Patients resuscitated from cardiac arrest require immediate, high-quality intensive care.[131] Along with optimal general care, it is important to minimize ongoing or subsequent brain damage by (1) preventing hyperglycemia and hyperthermia; (b) maintaining adequate blood pressure (because of loss of autoregulation, adequate systemic blood pressure is essential; on the other hand, hypertension may lead to cerebral edema); and (3) achieving normal arterial concentrations of oxygen and carbon dioxide (excessive oxygen may contribute to increased free radical damage; hypocapnia reduces cerebral perfusion and hypercapnia raises ICP).[132–136]

Assessment of Prognosis

1. Clinical Predictors A number of clinical studies have shown that it is possible to predict a poor outcome in a subset of patients. "Poor outcome" includes not only the PVS but also conditions with various degrees of awareness and disability, including dementia and motor deficits. This is less definitive than a prediction of an outcome no better than PVS, a condition from which withdrawal of care would not be controversial.

Coma lasting more than 3 days carries a greater than 90 percent risk of poor outcome.[137] Levy and colleagues, in their series of 210 patients with anoxic-ischemic encephalopathy, found that independent existence did not occur with absence of pupillary light reflexes at the time of initial evaluation.[138] Only 1 of their 93 patients with no response or decorticate or decerebrate posturing to stimulation at 24 h recovered. A number of algorithms were constructed for prediction at postarrest days 3, 7, and 14. Longstreth's group found the following four variables upon admission gave a positive predictive value for awakening of 0.84: motor response, pupillary light response, spontaneous eye movements, and serum glucose.[139] False prediction of nonawakening occurred in 16 patients, but 12 of these were unable to live independently. Edgren and colleagues found predictive accuracy, at resuscitation, for those with poor outcome ranged from 52 to 84 percent.[140] At 3 days, using the Glasgow and Glasgow-Pittsburgh Coma Scales, clinical predictors for poor outcome were reliable (severe cerebral disability, PVS, or death), with absence of motor response being the best predictor (see Fig. 15-6). Unless there is considerable compromise of brainstem function, one cannot make a certain, early prediction of an outcome of PVS or death in coma using clinical predictors alone. Severe cerebral disability may not be definitive enough; prediction of PVS, persistent coma, or death would be more useful. An accompanying editorial comment recommended a further prospective study and that 4 to 6 weeks should elapse before a decision is made to withdraw care.[141] This seems excessively long, when there are better predictors of an outcome no better than PVS (see below).[142]

2. Electrophysiologic Predictors A markedly suppressed or "flat" EEG correlates with severe damage to the neocortex associated with death in coma or PVS.[143] The significance of lesser degrees of suppression, burst-suppression, alpha coma, and generalized periodic complexes (see Chap. 3) were each initially thought to have an invariably poor prognosis, but exceptions have been found.[144,145] An invariant pattern on

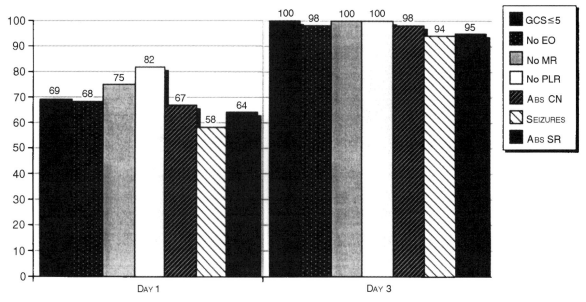

Figure 15-6

Predictive value (percentage) for poor outcome examining several variables. Poor outcome is described as either severe cerebral disability, PVS, clinical death, or brain death. Abbreviations: GCS= Glasgow Coma Score; No EO= no eye opening to painful stimuli; No MR= no motor response to pain; No PLR= absent pupillary light reflex; Abs CN= absence of selected cranial nerve reflexes; Seizures= epileptic seizures or myoclonus; Abs SR= absence of spontaneous respirations. (Figure constructed from paper by Edgren et al.[140])

the continuously monitored EEG may turn out to be a reliable indicator of PVS or worse outcome, but more work is needed.[146]

Evoked responses, especially early somatosensory evoked responses, have high predictive value but rather low sensitivity for determining a prognosis no better than PVS. The bilateral absence of the N20 response with median nerve stimulation is highly predictive of PVS or death in coma, but, not uncommonly, patients with preserved N20s also die in coma.[147–149] More recently, the N70, a longer latency evoked response, was shown to be predictive.[150] It is hoped that the latter may have higher sensitivity than the N20 somatosensory evoked potential (SEP) response, but further confirmatory work is needed. The use of evoked responses is of greatest usefulness and prognostic accuracy when carried out in the first 10 days following the event.[151] A relatively

favorable outcome is suggested by normal somatosensory, visual, and auditory evoked responses within this time.[151] The prognostic role of transcranial motor stimulation remains to be adequately assessed.

Jorgensen and Malchow-Moller showed the value of *combining* clinical and electroencephalographic (EEG) predictors.[152] This appears to be the most promising strategy. The author of this chapter and colleagues are in the process of developing algorithms that may be linked to the APACHE II or III score for improving prognostic accuracy.

3. Other Tests Nuclear magnetic resonance (NMR) spectroscopy allows a noninvasive, in vivo examination of high-energy phosphate in both neurons and glia. Following severe anoxic insult, there is a decrease of 40 to 60 percent of this phosphate. It is difficult-to-impossible, in an individual case, to know the proportion of loss that is due to neuronal death. N-acetylaspartate (NAA) and N-acetylaspartylglumatate are compounds found only in neurons.[153] These can be detected by NMR spectroscopy. Although absence of these N-acetylaspartyl compounds is conceivably reversible, preliminary evidence indicates that NAA reduction by 7 days after insult shows a strong correlation with neuronal loss.[154] This technology holds considerable promise for prognosis following cardiac arrest, but conclusive studies are needed.

POST ANOXIC-ISCHEMIC STATUS MYOCLONICUS

Significance

Of comatose survivors of cardiac arrest with generalized myoclonus, only 3 percent recover conscious awareness (see Table 15-1).[155–158] The mortality of 97 percent associated with seizures from anoxic-ischemic encephalopathy contrasts sharply with the rate of 6 to 35 percent associated with generalized convulsive status epilepticus due to other causes.[159]

Pathology and Pathogenesis

It thus appears that there is a fatal post anoxic-ischemic status myoclonicus (FSM) that differs from conventional status epilepticus (with any

Table 15-1

Outcome of myoclonic status epilepticus after cardiac arrest

Authors	Number of cases	survivors (%)
Snyder et al[158]	4	1 (25%)
Celesia et al[155]	13	1 (8%)
Krumholz et al[157]	19	0 (0%)
Jumao-as and Brenner[156]	15	0 (0%)
Wijdicks et al[354]	40	0 (0%)
Personal cases	18	1 (6%)
Total	**109**	**3 (3%)**

etiology) in which individuals recover consciousness (SE). This is supported by neuropathologic data. The extent of cortical damage is greater in patients dying from anoxic-ischemic insult than from epileptic seizures.[160] Meldrum and Brierley found that when baboons with SE were ventilated, with control of blood pressure, arterial oxygen, and temperature, the cerebellum was not affected.[161] Since patients with FSM are similarly managed, and since they uniformly have severe damage to the Purkinje cells of the cerebellum, the damage is likely due to the initial anoxic-ischemic insult, rather than to the seizures.[160] Although the gray matter of the spinal cord is commonly affected by cardiac arrest, there are no reports of SE causing such damage.[162] Spinal gray matter damage occurred in 9 of 10 patients with fatal post-anoxic myoclonic status epilepticus.[160] This, again suggests that the neuronal damage in FSM is due to the anoxic-ischemic insult rather than to SE.[160]

The differences between FSM and SE may have a physiologic basis. Many cases of FSM do not have associated EEG spikes, while SE cases usually do. There may be a subcortical origin for those cases that do not have spikes. The brainstem reticular formation, with a possible role of cerebellar dysfunction, may be the site of origin for these cases of FSM. This has been confirmed in those cases that show an "upwards" pattern of activation of brainstem motor nuclei—e.g., the muscles innervated by the facial nerve fire before those supplied by the trigeminal motor nucleus.[163] It is likely that there are fundamental differences between SE and FSM in the mechanisms for production and synchronization of epileptiform discharges. Synaptic mechanisms are responsible for the synchronization of discharges in SE.[164] Seizures after anoxic encephalopathy may occur through synaptic mechanisms because of increased release of excitatory amino acids which act on NMDA receptors.[165,166] This could make the seizures difficult to treat and could contribute to neuronal damage.

Ephaptic transmission may be operative in FSM. Populations of neurons depolarize in synchrony without synaptic communication, depending on field effects.[167] Partially depolarized neurons damaged by hypoxia may be susceptible.[168] Neuronal death may evolve over several days, allowing membrane function to continue temporarily. Neurons, even if fated to suffer delayed death,[169] may continue to undergo membrane oscillations for a time.[170] The increase in extracellular potassium markedly enhances synchronous epileptiform discharges in populations of neurons.[170] It is possible that ephaptic transmission is the sole mechanism for synchronized bursts in some cases of FSM, e.g., those without cortical spikes or cases refractory to antiepileptic drugs, but, in other cases, it could operate in concert with synaptic mechanisms.

Electrotonic coupling is another method of cell-to-cell spread of depolarization. Although such communication does occur in the hippocampus[171] and neocortex,[172] it is of uncertain importance in the postanoxic state. The profound swelling of apical dendrites found in the CA1 region of the hippocampus, which occurs beyond 12 h after reperfusion may provide an opportunity for electrotonic coupling.[173] This requires further study.

The author and colleagues have found that FSM patients have absent thalamocortical SEPs, suggesting that synaptic mechanisms are dysfunctional. This gives support to a nonsynaptic mechanism such as the ephaptic or electrotonic transmission for synchronous depolarizations. The mechanisms are not mutually exclusive.

The management implications are clear: SE deserves vigorous treatment,[174] but, in the FSM group, such vigorous measures would not be warranted. The aim is to reliably identify FSM. Clinical, electrophysiologic, and other tests are discussed below.

Clinical Aspects

Some clinical factors favor FSM over SE, but they are not sufficiently reliable. After prolonged seizures of either type, the generalized myoclonic movements may become more subtle or may disappear.[175] In SE, there is often a generalized tonic component before the clonic movements, while the seizures of FSM are typically myoclonic from the onset.[156] The clonic movements of FSM tend to involve the face and axial structures: platysma,

eyes, diaphragm, and trunk more than the limbs.[176,177] This pattern may reflect primary involvement of the brainstem reticular formation.[163]

Investigations (Present and Future)

Electrophysiologic Studies The EEG features of SE have been divided into five sequential stages by Treiman and colleagues[175]: (1) Discrete seizures: epileptiform activity occurs in discrete epochs separated by postictal slow-frequency waves. (2) Merging seizures: epileptiform activity persists throughout, but the discharges wax and wane in frequency and amplitude. (3) Continuous seizures: spikes and spike-waves are rhythmic and relatively constant throughout the seizure. (4) Continuous with flat periods: ongoing epileptiform activity is interrupted by generalized attenuation of voltage from 0.5 to 8 s. (5) Periodic epileptiform discharges on a flat background: high-voltage, repetitive epileptiform discharges occur regularly against a flat or suppressed background.

In FSM, EEGs often show patterns similar to the above categories 3, 4 and 5 of Treiman.[175] While the EEG in SE rarely evolves to electrocerebral silence, this is not uncommon in FSM. In some cases, the EEG fails to show epileptiform activity during the myoclonus, likely reflecting a subcortical mechanism or ephaptic transmission (see below).[178]

With anoxic-ischemic encephalopathy, the bilateral absence of the N20 SEP component to median nerve stimulation at the wrist is associated with a strong likelihood of an outcome no better than PVS.[179] Dr. Kenneth Jordan (personal communication) and the current author and colleagues have independently observed intact N20 responses during conventional SE, indicating that synaptic activation of primary sensory cortex still occurs during active seizure activity. Thus, SEPs may be a reliable method of establishing a hopeless prognosis in patients with FSM.

Metabolic and Blood Flow Studies In both FSM and SE, lactate production in the brain is increased.[180] Neuronal death in both conditions may be related to calcium influx due to activation of NMDA receptors.[181] Cerebral blood flow likely shows an increase, with poor autoregulation in both conditions.[182] In SE, there is increased activity of the sodium-potassium pump and increased synthesis of neurotransmitters and other compounds. The cerebral metabolism of oxygen is increased by 200 to 400 percent in various animal models; marked increases in glucose metabolism have been demonstrated.[66,183] Adenosine triphosphate (ATP), the principal high-energy compound, and the energy charge potential, an aggregate value of high-energy phosphates, are well maintained.[180]

In severe hypoxic-ischemic encephalopathy, ATP stores are reduced, as revealed by in vivo magnetic resonance spectroscopy.[184] After the condition stabilizes, cerebral blood flow is consistently reduced; cerebral oxygen and glucose metabolism are also diminished to about 40 to 60 percent of normal.[185]

Management

At present, there are no established guidelines for the precise determination of FSM, but these need to be formally developed. The following suggest a diagnosis of FSM over SE: (1) partial or complete cranial nerve areflexia between seizures; (2) a flat or totally suppressed EEG during or between seizures (unless large doses of anesthetic barbiturates have been used); (3) absent N20 response with SEP testing; and (4) < 50 percent of normal ATP stores or low levels of N-methyl-aspartic acid (NMAA), a compound found only in neurons, on NMR spectroscopy. Hopefully further work on commonly available blood flow studies [e.g., technetium^{99m} hexamethyl propyleneamineoxime–single photon emission computed tomography (HMPAON–SPECT)] or invariant patterns on continuous EEG monitoring may be useful.

Treatment of the myoclonic seizures in the unconscious patient after cardiac arrest should be conducted with the prognosis in mind. Valproic acid syrup, given down the nasogastric tube or by retention enema at 500 mg every 8 h, is often effective. Clonazepam, 0.5 mg tid, administered per nasogastric tube as crushed tablets dissolved or suspended in tepid water, is less effective but is often better than other benzodiazepines, phenytoin, or phenobarbital. If the seizures stop, the prognosis is dependent on the underlying anoxic-ischemic damage. Vigorous treatment with anesthetic barbiturates is not warranted if the prognosis can be established as hopeless for meaningful recovery. Skeletal muscle relaxants are sometimes necessary to stop the myoclonus to allow for adequate ventilation. Stopping the myoclonus without attempting to stop cerebral seizures is only justifiable in patients with a hopeless prognosis, however. Stopping the myoclonus in such cases may lessen the stress on families and nurses.

In patients for whom the prognosis is uncertain or favorable, full treatment for SE, including midazolam and anesthetic agents if necessary, appears advisable.[186,187]

Some patients become brain dead; brain death and its criteria are discussed in Chap. 2.

ANOXIC-ISCHEMIC COMPLICATIONS OF OPEN HEART SURGERY

Incidence and Significance

More than 300,000 cardiac procedures are performed annually in the United States.[188] Thus, even with a low percentage of cerebral complications, the burden in numbers is significant. Although death from generalized hypoxic-ischemic damage is rare and usually results from recognizable disasters, encephalopathy or strokes commonly occur without recognized intra- or postoperative misadventures.[189]

A multicenter prospective American study found adverse neurologic outcomes in 6.1 percent of cases.[190] These were equally divided into deaths from brain injury and nonfatal strokes and deficits, including decreased intellectual function, disorientation, memory deficit, or seizure. Risk factors for strokes included an atherosclerotic ascending aorta, a history of pre-existing neurologic problems, and older age. Cognitive worsening was more likely with older age, systolic hypertension on admission, pulmonary disease, and excessive alcohol consumption. Prolonged depression of conscious level was found in 10 of 312 (3 percent) of patients in a prospective British study, delirium occurred in 3 patients (1 percent).[189] Fifteen (5 percent) of patients suffered clinically significant strokes. Neuropsychologic abnormalities are common in cardiac postoperative patients: 60 to 80 percent of patients if tested within a week of surgery.[191] However, these subside to 20 to 40 percent by 8 weeks postsurgery and almost certainly improve further with time.[188]

Type I outcomes (focal injury) are more commonly related to single or multiple embolic strokes, while type II outcomes (general deterioration) were more likely to be due to relative hypoperfusion. Most focal or multifocal vascular complications appear to be related to the cardiopulmonary bypass procedure. Potential mechanisms include: macroembolism of atherosclerotic material in the ascending aorta, air, or particulate matter; and microembolism of air, fat, platelet or white cell aggregates, and particles from the tubing, and inadequate cerebral perfusion pressure.[188,192] Emboli are more common with valvular replacement compared with coronary bypass grafts, and are proportional to the number of embolic particles detected by transcranial Doppler testing.[188]

Clinical Approach

Neurologists are often asked to evaluate patients after open heart surgery when they fail to recover consciousness in the expected time. Details of the surgery can be of help: e.g., periods of severe hypotension, or observations of the surgeon re the severity of disease in the ascending aorta. The general health of the patient before the operation (e.g., previous strokes, alcohol abuse, drug history) may be helpful. On examination, the detailed neurologic assessment, including funduscopic examination for atherosclerotic emboli (Hollenhurst plaques), may offer clues of multiple atherosclerotic emboli to the brain. Any localizing neurologic findings indicate the site of problems. The lack of brainstem findings implies bicerebral dysfunction that may be from emboli, or watershed infarcts

from ischemia, anoxia or metabolic problems. Seizures are occasionally found and nonconvulsive seizures may be suspected clinically (see Chap. 17).

Investigation

Neuroimaging with CT scanning may be helpful, especially with focal findings. Even without focal features, the CT may show embolic or watershed lesions that can be helpful. The EEG may offer clues as to the mechanism for impaired consciousness—seizures or metabolic encephalopathy—and can give early prognostic information if the etiology is known.

Management

Symptomatic treatment is necessary for seizures or to limit the damage from strokes (see above and Chap. 17).

Protective strategies require further research: changes in the operative procedure (avoidance of—or greater care in clamping—the ascending aorta, graft replacement of the ascending aorta in high-risk patients), use of pharmacologic agents (thiopental, insulin, perfluocarbon, superoxide dismutase, nimodepine, GM_1 ganglioside, prostacyclin), hypothermia, and special filters.[191] None has yet been proven to be effective.

CEREBRAL ARTERIAL GAS EMBOLISM

Cerebral arterial gas embolism (CAGE) will be discussed under its two main categories; decompression sickness and intraoperative and traumatic air embolism.

Decompression Sickness

Cerebral arterial gas embolism is an uncommon but serious condition when it occurs as a major event. Minor degrees of CAGE may not be clinically apparent or may cause minor or transitory brain dysfunction. Cerebral complications are present in about one-third of cases of decompression sickness.[193]

The embolism of gas to brain arteries and capillaries may occur in several contexts. In patients with neurologic complications, it is more common for the spinal cord to be clinically affected than the brain.[194] However, single photon emission computed tomography (SPECT) indicates that the brain is affected whenever a myelopathy is present.[194] Thus, decompression sickness with neurologic complications should be thought of as a diffuse or multifocal CNS disease with variable severity. Decompression sickness is most common in divers who surface too quickly from the depths.[195] Other causes include sudden altitude rise in unpressurized aircraft and in divers working at fish farms.[196,197]

Clinical Features

Neurologic features include confusional state with impaired concentration, neglect syndromes, aphasia, focal motor signs (such as hemiparesis), or focal special sensory and somatosensory symptoms and signs. Myelopathy is common. More severe cases may show focal or multifocal seizures and coma. The syndrome typically onsets within 15 min of surfacing from a dive, but can be delayed by several to 48 h, especially in the presence of a patent foramen ovale.[198]

Nonneurologic features include joint pains, rashes, cardiorespiratory problems with dyspnea and chest pains. Some develop shock and die.

Pathogenesis

Decompression sickness relates to the formation of bubbles of gas (nitrogen, if the diver is breathing air) as a result of reduction in ambient pressure.[199] Intravascular bubbles, the most common cause of brain dysfunction, may form de novo in the cerebral circulation. Alternatively, they may enter the vascular system because of pulmonary barotrauma. In this instance, gas expanding in pulmonary alveoli may enter torn pulmonary veins and gain access to the general circulation. Because of their buoyancy, gas bubbles tend to go into the cerebral circulation.[200,201] Autochthonous or in situ extravascular bubbles may also form, especially in the spinal cord.[202,203]

In retrospective studies, the presence of, or the potential for, interarterial shunts, e.g., a patent foramen ovale, appears to be a risk factor for cerebral or spinal decompression sickness, although this is a statistical association only and not a proven mechanism.[204,205]

Risk factors for decompression sickness from diving include: uncontrolled rapid ascents, dives to more than 50 m, duration of time at such depths and multiple dives in a single day (especially "yo-yo diving," in which gas bubbles may not redissolve and thus accumulate), or failure to take "decompression stops" during ascent.[194,206,207] Additionally, advanced age, obesity, and hypothermia may further increase individual susceptibility.

The exact mechanism by which intravascular bubbles cause neurologic dysfunction is uncertain.[208] Nitrogen bubbles likely cause a mechanical tissue disruption, triggering a cascade of complement, histamine, and prostaglandins, as well as activation of platelets and leukocytes. Air gas embolism, as a consequence of pulmonary barotrauma, may lead to frank occlusion of small cerebral arteries, with subsequent ischemia. Gas-induced disruption of the blood-brain barrier probably occurs in some patients and may play a contributory role.

Investigation

Cerebral arterial gas embolism can be confirmed with SPECT, which shows multifocal perfusion defects.[209] Other causes of cerebral embolism should be excluded. Although CT may reveal gas in the arterial system with major embolism, it is relatively insensitive.[210]

Management

Recommendations for scuba divers to have an ECG, to determine if they have an interatrial defect that puts them at risk for CAGE, are still debated.[194,211] Precautions, at least, can be taken, e.g., avoiding deep dives and taking precautions in ascending from dives.

The immediate management of decompression sickness includes hyperbaric therapy with oxygen. Since hyperbaric oxygen itself can be injurious if high pressures (>2.5 atm) are allowed for too long, treatment is limited to a maximum of 2 to 3 atm for no more than 3 h.[212]

Traumatic and Intraoperative Air Embolism

Air embolism may also occur with pulmonary barotrauma and as a complication of neurosurgical procedures when cranial venous sinuses are inadvertently entered.

Intraoperative air embolism is widely recognized as a major, life-threatening intraoperative complication of neurosurgical operations.[213] The risk is greatest for operations in which the patient is sitting, because of the maximal negative pressure differential between the right atrium and the venous channels. Posterior fossa operations and transsphenoidal hypophysectomies are the most common procedures associated with venous or paradoxical air embolism.[214,215] If the cut venous channel (especially dural venous sinuses, emissary veins, or intraosseous venous lakes or veins) does not collapse, air can enter the vasculature.[216] Air then can enter the heart in large amounts, which may cause cardiac arrest, or air can enter the pulmonary capillaries and thence the left side of the heart. Paradoxical air embolism is significantly more likely in the presence of a patent foramen ovale.[217] This could then enter the cerebral arteries and capillaries, causing ischemic damage if the blockade of circulation is of sufficient magnitude and duration. One would expect this to be a multifocal phenomenon.

Clinically, one can auscultate a "washing machine murmur" over the heart in massive air embolism. The brain may be directly affected by gas embolism or rendered globally ischemic by loss of effective cardiac output.

It may be wise to screen with ECG those candidates for a "sitting" neurosurgical procedure, and to avoid the sitting posture if possible or to take precautions.[213,217] Transesophageal or transcranial Doppler screening may help in the detection of air embolism.[217]

The principles of therapy for venous air embolism include: (1) closure of the point of air access to the venous system, (2) removal of air from the vascular system, and (3) cardiorespiratory stability.[213] Suction via a Swan-Ganz catheter is helpful in removing the air.[213] Air within the heart chambers can be removed by such catheters or by direct cardiac puncture in an extreme situation.[218]

CARBON MONOXIDE INTOXICATION

Carbon monoxide (CO) intoxication is the most common form of serious anemic hypoxia, causing death in at least 3500 Americans yearly.[219] Most CO exposure occurs by accidental poisoning at home, either from building fires or from incomplete combustion by furnaces, or from gas leaks. Other cases include attempted suicide by exposure to automobile exhaust or domestic cooking fumes. Approximately 35 percent of fire victims have concomitant exposure to CO and cyanide (CN) gas.[220]

Clinical Features and Outcome

The acuity of onset and progression of symptoms depend on the concentration of CO in the inspired air. High concentrations of CO may produce abrupt coma, without warning, while lower concentrations cause a more protracted prodrome to coma. A concentration of CO of 0.05% in the inspired air for more than 1 h will produce a concentration of carboxyhemoglobin of 30 to 50%. Mild, chronic exposure may result in headache, shortness of breath with exertion or at rest, or vague, "flu-like symptoms." Bleeding diatheses, fever and hepatomegaly are described. Early acute symptoms include generalized, throbbing headaches, confusion, irritability, dizziness, visual disturbances, nausea, and vomiting. Exertion may produce loss of consciousness. An exposure for 1 h at concentrations of $\geq 0.1\%$ of CO in inspired air will result in serum carboxyhemoglobin concentrations of 50 to 80%, resulting in coma, brainstem compromise with ventilatory failure, convulsions and, usually, death.

The most characteristic sign is a cherry-red discoloration of the lips and mucous membranes. This is not always present, however. Comatose patients may show focal neurologic signs; some may progress to impairment of brainstem function and cranial nerves, including pupillary reflexes.

Delayed neurologic deterioration, following apparent improvement or recovery, occurs in about 12 percent of such patients who present in coma.[221,222] This deterioration begins 2 days to 3 weeks after initial resuscitation.[223] The onset is typically an acute confusional state accompanied by behavioral change or apathy, often mistaken for a psychiatric illness.[224] This may be associated with cognitive changes, including agnosia and apraxia.[225] These may be followed by severe deterioration in responsiveness with, extrapyramidal features resembling Parkinson disease with marked rigidity. Patients may develop akinetic mutism. Coma may develop and can be followed by a PVS.

The prognosis is worse for patients who present in coma. Patients who regain responsiveness are often (i.e., at least 50 percent) left with severe motor and cognitive deficits.[226,227] Motor disability involves akinetic mutism, extrapyramidal complications with parkinsonian rigidity, akinesia, spasticity, and lateralized weakness.[228] Cognitive problems include apathy, defective memory, apraxia, visual agnosia, executive frontal lobe dysfunction, and impairments in concentration, attention, perception, and calculation.[229]

Pathophysiology and Pathology

The toxic effects of CO are due to tissue hypoxia caused by inactivation of the oxygen-carrying capacity of hemoglobin. Carbon monoxide combines (with an affinity of 200 times greater than oxygen) with hemoglobin to form carboxyhemoglobin. Carboxyhemoglobin also prevents the release of oxygen from oxyhemoglobin. These effects cause tissue hypoxia. The concentration of carboxyhemoglobin in the blood is a function of CO in the inhaled gas and the duration of exposure.

The lack of oxygen may set up the cycle of neuronal death, as shown in Fig. 14-1. Ginsberg has suggested that anemic hypoxia from CO usually is accompanied by cerebral ischemia and lactic acidosis.[230] Free radical production and lipid peroxidation have been proposed clinically and demonstrated experimentally in rats.[231,232] It is possible that CO may also be a mitochondrial poison; in any case, CO may act synergistically with cyanide when there is coexposure, e.g., with wood fires.[233]

Patients with delayed deterioration usually have symmetric damage to deep cerebral white matter.[234] This may be truly demyelinative, with sparing of the axons. Gray matter damage, the most common being necrosis of the globus pallidus, is usually accompanied by white matter disease (Fig. 15-7).[234] Neuronal loss in the vulnerable

Figure 15-7

Initial T2-weighted image at 2.0 Tesla from a 35-year-old woman with carbon monoxide intoxication. She was in a confusional state with Parkinsonian features and urinary and fecal incontinence. The white matter shows altered signal. (From Chang KH, Han MH, Kim HS et al: Delayed encephalopathy after acute carbon monoxide intoxication: MR imaging features and distribution of cerebral white matter lesions. Radiology *184:117, 1992.)*

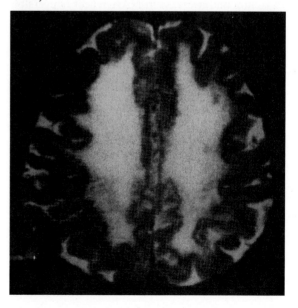

sections of the hippocampus and layers of the neocortex is found in about 50 percent of autopsied cases.[234]

Functional neuroimaging was performed, using technetium[99m] HMPAO–SPECT scanning, on a patient in the early phase of delayed deterioration following CO poisoning.[235] This revealed a diffuse but frontally predominant hypoperfusion involving both gray matter and white matter. There was transient improvement in blood flow to these regions with hyperbaric oxygen therapy, but the patient showed no significant clinical recovery, remaining in a PVS.

Investigations

A blood carboxyhemoglobin concentration should be performed; more than 20% is significant. Arterial or capillary blood gases can help in the assessment of the insult and resultant metabolic acidosis.

Computed tomographic and MRI scanning, especially with fluid attenuated inversion recovery (FLAIR) pulse imaging, have a role in determining prognosis.[236,237] Early changes in the basal ganglia and white matter may be found. Nuclear magnetic resonance spectroscopy may have greater prognostic value: increased choline in the white matter correlates with early demyelination and an increase in lactate and decrease in NAA reflect irreversible neuronal injury.[238] Although these hold promise, their use has to be tempered with practical aspects of patient management.

Treatment

The half-life of carboxyhemoglobin is inversely proportional to the pressure and concentration of oxygen in the inspired air.[239] It is about 5 h with ordinary room air, 90 min with 100% oxygen at 1 atm pressure, and 20 min for 100% O_2 at 2 atm. It follows that 100% O_2 should be delivered promptly. The airway should be secured; endotracheal intubation should be performed if the patient is unconscious. Assisted ventilation may also be necessary.

Hyperbaric oxygen is not necessary for patients without impaired consciousness. A randomized controlled trial in which patients were randomized to 100% O_2 at normal pressure or at 2 atm pressure for 2 h, followed by normal pressure for 4 h, showed no difference in outcome between the two groups.[240] Several large trials claiming benefit for hyperbaric oxygen therapy were uncontrolled, retrospective, or based on historical controls.[241–244] There are no controlled studies comparing normal-pressure oxygen with hyperbaric oxygen in humans. A comparison of one versus two sessions of hyperbaric oxygen in patients with impaired consciousness did not show a difference in outcome between the two groups.[240] The use of hyperbaric oxygen seems advisable for comatose CO-poisoned patients. Its use seems safe even in infants and in pregnancy, in the face of CO-intoxication.[245,246]

Patients should be monitored carefully in an intensive care unit. Cerebral edema is a risk and any deterioration should prompt a CT scan. Baseline CT scanning is probably worthwhile in comatose patients, once stabilized.

CYANIDE POISONING

Background and Pathophysiology

Cyanide is a metabolic poison (see Chap. 16).[247] It causes cellular histiotoxic hypoxia by paralyzing the electron transfer in mitochondria by binding with the trivalent form of iron. There are also actions on various enzyme systems.[248]

Cyanide poisoning can occur through inhalation or by oral ingestion. Sources include: inhalation of hydrocyanic acid, or swallowing soluble inorganic cyanide salts or cyanide-releasing substances, including cyanamide, cyanogen chloride and nitroprusside, certain plants (stone fruits of chokecherry, pincherry peach, apricot and bitter almond; cassava roots, jet berry bush berries, leaves and shoots of elderberry, and all parts of hydrangia), and the drug Laetrile. Cyanide is contained within the smoke of wood fires, but its concentration is much less than the carbon monoxide that is also present. The mortality and morbidity from such inhalations are almost always related more to CO than CN.[249]

Clinical Significance

There is a characteristic "bitter almond" smell to the breath. The patient may be unconscious with the picture of a metabolic encephalopathy. Cyanosis is not seen until ventilatory failure occurs. There may be a history of inhalation or ingestion of one of the above agents.

Treatment

Methemoglobin (Fe^{3+}) competes with cytochrome for cyanide. This constitutes the rationale for the conversion of hemoglobin to methemoglobin by nitrites as the specific therapy. Death occurs quickly unless the antidote is rapidly administered. Amyl nitrite perles are administered by inhalation. These should be given at a rate of one every 2 min, followed by an intravenous injection of 10 mL sodium nitrite in a 3% solution, then sodium thiosulfate (50 mL of 25% solution) is administered over 10 min. Further doses of nitrites may be necessary, but methemoglobin concentration should not exceed 40% or the delivery of oxygen to tissues is compromised.

Supportive measures include endotracheal intubation, administration of 100% O_2, and blood pressure support with norepinephrine if necessary.

Prognosis

The recovery is often all-or-none. If the victim survives for 4 h, a complete recovery is expected, but occasionally some residual cerebral damage may be present.

OTHER CAUSES OF BRAIN ISCHEMIA AND IMPAIRED CONSCIOUSNESS

MIGRAINE

Definition

Migraine headaches affect 250 of every 100,000 persons yearly.[250] Neurologic symptoms, including impairment of alertness or cognitive function, occur in the subcategory known as migraine with aura, formerly called "classical migraine."[251] Diagnostic criteria are:

A. At least two attacks fulfilling B.

B. At least three of the following characteristics:
1. One or more fully reversible aura symptoms indicating focal cerebral and/or brainstem dysfunction.
2. At least one aura symptom develops over 4 min, or two or more symptoms occur in succession.
3. No aura symptom lasts more than 60 mins. If more than one aura symptom is present, accepted duration is proportionately increased.
4. Headache follows aura with a free interval of less than 60 min. (It may also begin before or simultaneously with the aura).

C. At least one of the following:
1. History, physician and neurologic examinations do not suggest one of the following disorders: acute or chronic posttraumatic headache, intracranial hemorrhage, unruptured vascular malformations, ischemic cerebrovascular disease, arteritis, carotid or vertebral artery pain, venous thrombosis, severe hypertension, high CSF pressure, low CSF pressure, intracranial infection or noninfectious inflammation, substance use or withdrawal (e.g., monosodium glutamate, ergotamine withdrawal), systemic inflammation, matabolic disorders (e.g., hypoxia, hypercapnia, hypoglycemia), and disorders of the cranium, neck, eyes, nose, sinuses, teeth, or mouth.
2. History and/or physical and/or neurologic examinations suggest such a disorder, but this is ruled out by appropriate investigations.
3. Such disorder is present, but migraine attacks do not occur for the first time in close temporal relation to the disorder.

Migraine headaches are usually unilateral and pulsating and have moderate to severe intensity. They are often aggravated by physical activity and are frequently accompanied by sensitivity to light or sound, nausea, or vomiting.

Pathogenesis of Clinical Features

Migraine with aura is associated with vasospasm and reduced regional blood flow, usually in the vertebrobasilar circulation.[252] This is typified by the "Bickerstaff syndrome" in which young persons, usually adolescent girls, develop symptoms of ischemia of the brainstem and occipital regions: visual field disturbances, vertigo, diplopia, ataxia, dysarthria, tinnitus or hearing loss, bilateral sensory or motor disturbances, and loss of consciousness, confusion, or stupor.[253] Migrainous marches of symptoms are usually, but not always, slower than embolic phenomena, often taking tens of minutes to evolve. The vasospasm of migraine can sometimes lead to infarction of tissue, if the ischemia is sufficiently prolonged. Rarely, the internal carotid territory may be affected; this is always a diagnosis of exclusion, especially of cardiogenic emboli, dissection, or vasospasm following subarachnoid hemorrhage. Infarction of one cerebral hemisphere in a young individual may produce life-threatening cerebral swelling.[254]

Migraine is occasionally associated with recurrent delirium, sometimes provoked by mild head injury.[255] The EEG is diffusely slow, reminiscent of a metabolic encephalopathy. Patients make a spontaneous, complete recovery.

A "malignant variant" of familial migraine, with coma, has been described.[256] The syndrome is characterized by episodes of impaired consciousness progressing to coma, meningeal signs, fever, and focal neurologic signs. Coma may last up to several days. Attacks are precipitated by minor head trauma, vigorous work, and angiography. Some patients have been left with persistent cerebellar ataxia.

Occasionally, patients with migraine have prolapsing mitral valves, a potential (although controversial) source of embolism.[257]

Occasionally, patients may have both migraine and epilepsy.[258] This can take several forms:[258]

1. Attacks of migraine with aura are complicated by seizure activity, either simple partial, complex partial, or secondary generalized. This may happen in both adolescents and adults.

2. Confusion due to seizures may occur during migraine with transient global amnesia.

3. Seizures, especially temporal lobe seizures, may occur after years of migraine with aura.

4. Occipital lobe epilepsy may develop in patients with a past history or strong family history of migraine.

5. Complicated migraine may produce cerebral infarction that, in turn, leads to seizures.

The EEG is often helpful in showing abundant interictal epileptiform activity in the posterior head.[259]

Management

Prevention is the best strategy. Migraine is aggravated by, and migrainous infarction is more likely in the presence of, the birth control pill, smoking, and, possibly, hypertension.[260,261] These factors should be eliminated in young persons at risk. Reduction in identified provoking factors may also help. These vary among individuals but include: stress, irregular sleep habits, and certain foods, beverages, and medicines. Most treatments of acute migrainous attacks do not address the vasospastic component. In severe cases, prophylactic medications are used: beta blockers; calcium channel blockers; antidepressants including tricyclics, fluoxetine, and monoamine oxidase inhibitors; nonsteroidal anti-inflammatory drugs, and some anticonvulsants including valproate. Cases in which migraine and seizures coexist may be treated with valproate or carbamazepine, which may help both conditions, or each can be treated separately.

DISSEMINATED INTRAVASCULAR COAGULATION

Disseminated intravascular coagulation (DIC) is a complex disorder of the hemostatic system, in which a central feature is the excess of intravascular thrombin.[262] This is followed by further activation of the coagulation system, with deposition of fibrin within the microcirculation. This can affect organ function. The brain may be directly involved or a metabolic encephalopathy may follow the failure of other organs such as the kidney, liver, or lungs. Large-vessel occlusions may occur. The plasmin system is also activated, leading to disruption/lysis of fibrin thrombi. The net effect is consumption of the coagulation system that leads to a bleeding diathesis.

Pathogenesis

Disseminated intravascular coagulation is often secondary to underlying diseases, such as trauma (including head trauma), sepsis, burns, obstetric catastrophes, postoperative states, malignancy, and other systemic disorders.[262–265]

THROMBOTIC THROMBOCYTOPENIC PURPURA

Definition

Thrombotic thrombocytopenic purpura (TTP) is a hematologic disorder, mainly occurring in adults, consisting of a microangiopathic hemolytic anemia with formation of thrombi in small vessels and resultant organ dysfunction, including the brain and kidneys.

Hemolytic uremic syndrome (HUS) is a closely related syndrome that occurs primarily in children, and in which there is no neurologic involvement, but the kidneys are consistently and often severely affected. The prevailing view is that HUS and TTP are different endpoints of the same disease process, as supported by their similar precipitants, hematologic features, and microscopic pathology.[266,267]

Incidence and Significance

This is a rare disease. The incidence in Olmsted and Filmore counties in Minnesota was calculated to be one per million over a 30-year period.[268] The peak incidence is in the fourth decade; 60 percent of cases occur in women.[269] One or more relapses occur in 36 percent of TTP survivors over 10 years.[270]

Clinical Features

Thrombotic thrombocytopenic purpura is usually an acute, fulminant illness that evolves over days to weeks, but, occasionally, it can be more protracted. Fever is present in most patients and petechiae in the skin are often present, but are not essential.

The classic pentad is moderate-to-severe thrombocytopenia, microangiopathic hemolytic anemia, varying neurologic symtoms and signs, renal impairment, and fever.[269] Less than 50 percent of patients have all five features, but more than 90 percent have the combination of decreased platelets, neurologic complications, and anemia.

Neurologic complications consist of focal or multifocal brain dysfunction. Alterations of consciousness consist of confusion, stupor, or coma. Focal deficits, including hemiparesis, aphasia, and visual field defects, are common during the illness. There may be considerable fluctuation from hour-to-hour or day-to-day. Focal seizures with varied secondary generalization are common. Nonconvulsive status epilepticus may also account for impaired cognitive function, fluctuating signs, and declining alertness in TTP, despite otherwise successful treatment of the disease.[271] Many signs clear but permanent neurologic deficits or a persistent seizure disorder may result from strokes.[272]

Renal involvement includes any of the following: proteinuria, a fall in urine output, mild-to-moderate renal insufficiency, and, occasionally, acute renal failure.

The hematologic manifestations include anemia (hemoglobin less than 5.5 g/L in 30 percent of patients), hemorrhages in the skin (petechiae and purpura) and retina, and epistaxis related to thrombocytopenia.[273] Hemolysis may produce jaundice.

Etiology, Pathogenesis, and Pathology

The etiology is unknown. The vessels are filled with hyaline material, presumably fibrin and platelets mixed with red blood cells. These may transiently block various end arterioles causing transient deficits and a dynamically shifting clinical picture.

Sometimes, TTP is associated with various immunologic disorders, pregnancy, toxins, and drugs. Tissue necrosis (as in an injury, infection, or surgical procedure) often precedes TTP.[274] Although there are many hypotheses based on hematologic observations of nonspecific tissue factors, loss of fibrinolytic activity, endothelial damage, prostacyclin deficiency, lack of inhibitors of platelet aggregation, and the presence of unusually large multimers of factor VIII–von Willebrand factor (factor VIII:vWF), the initiating cause and the specific sequence of events are still debated.[275]

Successful management with plasma exchange underlines the key role of a "toxic substance" that causes platelets to aggregate. Plasma from patients with TTP will aggregate platelets in the blood from normal individuals. A predisposing cause appears to be the presence of large multimeric forms of factor VIII:vWF complexes in the plasma.[276] These substances promote the aggregation of platelets. It has been proposed that stresses, e.g., tissue necrosis, release cationic polyamines that neutralize the negative charges on platelet membranes.[275] The large factor VIII:vWF multimers then attach to the platelets and vigorous platelet aggregation occurs.

Conversely, the benefit of plasma infusion suggests that there is a "missing substance" that is replaced by the transfused material.[277] The Fc fragment of infused immunoglobulin binds to platelet membrane and helps to prevent aggregation.[278] It has been proposed that this or a similar immunogobulin component, normally interferes with platelet aggregation.[279] A deficiency of factor VIII:vWF depolymerase, which normally degrades the large multimers, may be a predisposing factor in some patients.[275]

The failure of reduction of factor VIII:vWF multimers to produce remission in the chronic relapsing form of TTP suggests that these multimers may not be the cause of at least this form of TTP.[280]

Recently, the role of calpain, a cysteine proteinase, in TTP has been emphasized.[281] The platelet aggregating ability of plasma from TTP patients is closely matched by calpain. Depletion of calpain from TTP blood destroyed its platelet-aggregating activity, while depletion of other proteinases did not.

Laboratory Features

The blood smear is usually diagnostic and reveals a microangiopathic anemia, with fragmented red blood cells (schistocytes, helmet cells), this being evidence of intravascular trauma to the blood elements (Fig. 15-8). Review of the blood smear is probably the most important laboratory test.[282] The increased output of reticulocytes and nucleated red blood cells into the systemic circulation is also a feature. With the destruction of red blood cells, serum concentrations of lactic acid dehydrogenase (LDH) and indirect (unconjugated) bilirubin are elevated. Hemolysis leads to increased hemoglobin in the serum or plasma and decreased or absent measured haptoglobin. Thrombocytopenia, with platelet counts usually less than $20,000 \times 10^9$/L, is due to increased consumption of platelets in the intravascular thrombotic process. Megakaryocytes in the bone marrow are normal or increased.

There is usually preservation of normal coagulation tests; i.e., the features of DIC, e.g., fibrin degradation products or D-dimer, are absent.

With renal impairment, there is mild-to-moderate elevation of serum creatinine and urea.

Biopsies of the gingiva, skin, or kidneys confirm the above-mentioned pathologic features, but are usually not necessary, nor are they specific for TTP or HUS.

Computed tomographic scans of the brain are of prognostic usefulness.[283] Positive scans

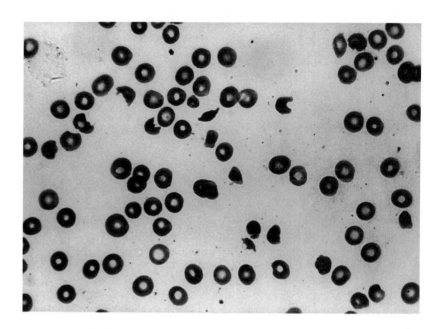

Figure 15-8

A blood smear showing features typical of TTP or microangiopathic anemia. Note the fragmented red blood cells.

showed varied features in different patients including: intraparenchymal hemorrhages of various sizes and numbers; diffuse areas of white matter attenuation; and ischemic infarcts, often multiple, in various locations. Coma was more common in patients with such findings than in patients with normal CT scans. Over 80 percent of patients with such lesions either died or had significant neurologic deficits. In contrast, most of the patients with normal scans made complete recoveries, without apparent deficits. The study was, however, retrospective; it is unclear how carefully the patients were examined and followed.

The MRI is a more sensitive test than CT and may replace it as the imaging test of choice.[272] Hyperintensities on spin-echo T2-weighted MRI images (not seen on T1-weighted pictures) may completely resolve along with clinical recovery.[284] Thus, these lesions likely do not reflect infarcted tissue, but reversible tissue edema.

Differential Diagnosis

The nosologic relationship to HUS was discussed above. Other conditions that may mimic TTP include: Evans syndrome [immune-mediated

destruction of red blood cells (schistocytes may be present) and platelets, with positive direct Coomb's test and a large amount of antibody production), systemic lupus erythematosus (underlies some cases of TTP), DIC (abnormal coagulation tests including decreased fibrinogen, D-dimer, or FDP, which are not features of TTP), meningococcemia, bacterial or non-bacterial endocarditis, disseminated carcinomatosus, malignant hypertension, and eclampsia and the HELLP (hemolysis, with elevated liver enzymes and low platelets) pre-eclamptic syndrome. The lack of fibrinolytic activity in the thrombosed vascular lesions helps to differentiate TTP from most of the disseminated intravascular coagulopathies.[285]

Treatment

The timely recognition of the disorder in its early stages, and prompt, appropriate treatment, has dramatically reduced the mortality and morbidity of TTP. Multiple therapies are almost always utilized simultaneously, making it difficult to weigh the relative effectiveness of each. It is also possible that TTP is a syndrome with different emphases on the various pathogenetic mechanisms discussed above. The following seem to have made a difference:

1. *Plasma exchange*[286]: This was significantly more effective than plasma infusion in a randomized controlled study.[287]

2. *Fresh-frozen plasma or immunoglobulin infusion*: rationale discussed above.

3. *Antiplatelet drugs* (acetylsalicylic acid and/or dipyridamole): these prolong the half-life of platelets in TTP; whether they influence outcome is uncertain.

Other measures have included: platelet transfusions, splenectomy, glucocorticoids, Vinca alkaloids, dextran infusion, prostacyclin infusion, and antithrombin III infusion.[275,284]

As mentioned, TTP may relapse. In the prevention of relapse, splenectomy or immunosuppressive therapy (including cyclophosphamide, prednisolone, azathioprine, and vincristine) have been reported to be effective.[288–293] In some of these cases an immune-mediated mechanism may be operative.

Symptomatic treatment of seizures, supportive care for reduced level of consciousness, and management of acute renal failure and other complications are carried out as needed, often in special care units. In contrast to HUS, dialysis for renal failure is rarely necessary in TTP.

OTHER COAGULOPATHIES

Antiphospholipid antibody syndrome is discussed in Chap. 12.

Myeloproliferative disorders may be associated with brain ischemia. Essential thrombocythemia and polycythemia rubra vera are sometimes associated with hyperaggregability and focal or multifocal strokes.[294] In contrast, reactive thrombocytosis is usually well tolerated.

Hypereosinophilic syndrome is a heterogeneous group of disorders in which increased numbers of eosinophils are present in the blood or tissues. The release of toxic compounds (eosinophil cationic protein and eosinophil major basic protein) may damage tissues, e.g., endothelium or

endocardium, and lead to ischemic (especially cardioembolic) brain ischemia.

Antithrombin III, an intrinsic anticoagulant that binds to thrombin and activated factor X, has rarely been associated with ischemic stroke.[295]

Deficiency of proteins C or S, also intrinsic anticoagulants, is occasionally implicated in some cases of intracranial venous thrombosis (see Chap. 5), but they are rarely, if ever, causes of ischemic stroke.

Bacterial endocarditis is discussed in Chap. 12.

FIBROMUSCULAR HYPERPLASIA

Fibromuscular dysplasia is a nonatherosclerotic angiopathy of small-to-large arteries. The arterial wall shows proliferation of fibrous connective tissue, destruction of the internal elastic lamina, and either hyperplasia or thinning of smooth muscle. The prevalence is unknown, but probably under 1 percent of the population is affected; the occurrence is greatest in white women between the ages of 30 and 50 years.

Clinical Features

Neurologic problems relate to ischemic stroke, emboli or dissection, or intracranial hemorrhage. The latter is most often due to the increased association with intracranial "berry" aneurysms or, less commonly, to dissection or disruption of the arterial wall caused by the disease, or to associated severe hypertension. The carotid territories are usually involved but the vertebrobasilar system can also cause symptomatic disease, from either intra- or extracranial involvement.[296]

Patients may have focal symptoms from ischemia or hemorrhage or may suffer syncope or anoxic seizures. The latter sometimes correlate with severe stenosis of both internal carotid arteries and may be associated with head turning.[297] Head turning may occlude a vertebral artery and compromise the already threatened intracranial perfusion. Carotid sinus sensitivity might account for some cases.

Investigations

Cerebral angiography shows involvement of the one or both internal carotid arteries in their mid-portion, in the majority of cases, although any of the four major arteries to the brain can be affected, in either their extra- or intracranial aspects. The following have been described: a "string-of-beads" appearance with alternating areas of constriction and normality or dilatation, long (tubular) stenosis, diverticula from the wall, dissection with a "string sign," severe stenosis, or, rarely, complete occlusion.

Management

Most patients are managed conservatively. Oral contraceptives should be stopped. Transient ischemic attacks are treated with antiplatelet therapy; dissection is usually managed with anticoagulation. Occasionally, severe stenosis has been managed surgically, but angioplasty with stenting may prove to be useful. Four-vessel angiography should be carried out on all patients to look for intracranial berry aneurysms. Those over 7 to 10 mm should be clipped prophylactically.[298]

CEREBRAL VEIN THROMBOSIS

Classification

Intracranial venous thrombosis can be divided into nonseptic and septic forms. Large venous channels and/or their draining (especially cerebral cortical) veins from the brain parenchyma may be affected.

Significance and Incidence

Cerebral or cortical vein thrombosis is an uncommon but underrecognized cause of acute neurologic dysfunction.[299] A fatal outcome occurs in 10 percent of noninfectious forms.[300] However, a complete recovery is expected in over 70 percent of cases.[301]

Pathophysiology

Thrombosis in intracranial veins or venous sinuses occurs in a variety of conditions in which there is a hypercoagulable state, venous stasis, or damage to the vessel wall (Table 15-2). Such coagulation tends to involve the superior sagittal and lateral sinuses with or without extension into the cortical veins; involvement of deep cerebral or posterior fossa veins is much less common.[300] Recent studies indicate that the most common predisposing factor for cerebral venous sinus thrombosis is a point mutation in the coagulation factor V gene, called the Leiden mutation.[302,303] This mutation renders activated protein C, a natural anticoagulant, ineffective. The factor V Leiden mutation, either heterozygous or homozygous, poses a risk for venous thrombosis that is further increased by other risk factors, such as factor C or S deficiency, heterozygous homocysteinuria or antiphospholipid antibodies.[304]

A congenital deficiency of protein C or protein S, which acts as a cofactor for the natural anticoagulant action of activated protein C, predisposes to venous thromboses in the above factor V Leiden mutation and other procoagulant conditions: pregnancy, the birth control pill, trauma (including neurosurgical operations near the venous sinuses or other surgery), electrical injury, Behçet disease, inflammatory bowel disease (ulcerative colitis and Crohn disease), underlying cancer, polycythemia, sickle cell anemia or trait, acquired plasminogen deficiency, or paroxysmal nocturnal hemoglobinuria.[305–313] Each of the latter conditions may be the only identifiable predisposing cause in individual cases. The antiphospholipid antibody syndrome, with or without systemic lupus erythematosis, may also be responsible.[314] There is one report of cerebral venous thrombosis with the use of androgenic steroids in a previously healthy male.[315] Minor head injury may precipitate venous sinus thrombosis in predisposed patients, e.g., those with protein S deficiency.[316] Dural arteriovenous fistulae may occasionally be accompanied by venous sinus thrombosis, presumably because of endothelial damage.[317]

Septic thrombophlebitis affects mainly the cavernous sinus. With cavernous sinus infections, risk factors include infections of the middle third (muzzle area) of the face, upper teeth, paranasal

Table 15-2
Causes of cerebral vein thrombosis

Hematologic disorders
Polycythemia
Hemolytic anemia
Thrombocytosis
Protein C deficiency
Protein S deficiency
Antithrombin III deficiency
Cryofibrinogenemia
Antiphospholipid antibodies
Paroxysmal nocturnal hemoglobinuria
Sickle cell disease
Cancer

Inflammatory conditions
Infection of the venous sinus
Sarcoidosis
Otitis media
Meningitis
Wegener's granulomatosis
Fungal infections: aspergillosis
Disseminated intravascular coagulation
Behçet disease

Other hypercoagulable states
Pregnancy or puerperium
Oral contraceptives
Inflammatory bowel disease
Nephrotic syndrome
Excess androgen use

Stasis
Dehydration
Cachexia and marasmus
Cardiac failure

Vessel wall damage
Trauma
Mechanical: complications of neurosurgery of mastoid surgery
Arteriovenous malformations
Systemic lupus erythematosis
Indwelling venous catheters
Infection or inflammation

Other
Carcinomatous or lymphomatous infiltration
Electrical injury
Carbon monoxide poisoning
Adriamycin chemotherapy

(especially sphenoid) sinusitis, ocular infections, or diabetes (risk of aspergillosis or mucormycosis). In the preantibiotic era, facial infection was the most common source, with spread to the cavernous sinus via the superior and inferior ophthalmic veins. In recent years, advanced infection of the paranasal sinuses is the main cause; intracranial spread occurs through small emissary veins.[318] The most common organism is *Staphylococcus aureus*, followed by other gram-positive bacteria including *Steptococcus* spp. and anaerobic bacteria. Occasionally, gram-negative, polymicrobial or fungal infections are found. Septic thrombosis of the superior sagittal sinus may occasionally complicate bacterial meningitis or paranasal sinusitis. The responsible organisms are usually *Strep. pneumoniae*, *Staph. aureus*, and anaerobes. Lateral sinus thrombosis may occur as a result of adjacent mastoiditis or purulent otitis media, with *Proteus*

spp., *Escherichia coli*, *Staph. aureus* and anaerobes.[318]

The effect of the occlusion of an intracranial vein depends on the site, propagation and acuity of the thrombosis, with the resultant effect on transcapillary pressure and tissue perfusion. If there are alternate routes of drainage, there may be no effect or minimal effect. The integrity of the vessel wall may be disrupted, causing a hemorrhage into tissue and the CSF spaces. In cerebral sinus thrombosis, large areas of brain may be functionally disturbed metabolically, but are not necessarily irreversibly damaged.[319] Lack of perfusion may lead to cytotoxic edema.[320]

Experimental studies suggest that involvement of the *cortical veins* is necessary before the microcirculation of the cortex is affected.[321] Sinus thrombosis alone does not lead to tissue hemorrhage or necrosis; it is only when the final pathway, via bridging and cortical veins, is occluded that this evolves. There is a resultant reduction in arterial perfusion of the regional tissue; local areas of ischemia develop along with petechial bleedings and disruptions in the blood-brain barrier, and vasogenic as well as cytotoxic edema.[321,322]

Clinical Features

The signs and symptoms of intracranial venous or sinus occlusion have remarkable variability and the consequences reveal a spectrum of severity.[323]

With multifocal involvement, defects in attention, concentration, or consciousness may occur. With cortical venous occlusion, partial epileptic seizures are commonly the first indication.[296] These may be followed by focal deficits, such as hemiparesis or aphasia. Loss of consciousness is uncommon, brief, and usually relates to epileptic seizures. Septic thrombophlebitis may be associated with impaired consciousness as part of a general response to sepsis (see Chap. 12). Occasionally, episodes of loss of consciousness may be unexplained and are probably not always due to an epileptic mechanism. Recurrent episodes over months or years have been described.[324]

Headaches are sometimes present, but do not necessarily relate to raised ICP. They are not associated with nausea, vomiting, or papilledema.[299] Nuchal rigidity may be found with bleeding into the subarachnoid space, or with tonsillar herniation.

Superior sagittal sinus thrombosis may lead to hemorrhages and infarction of cerebral tissue in both cerebral hemispheres, or may be restricted to one side. Occlusion of the superior sagittal sinus may be asymptomatic if just the anterior portion is occluded and there is no thrombosis of draining cortical veins. Alternatively, the patient may manifest features of raised ICP, including headache, visual obscurations, and papilledema. Superior sagittal sinus thrombosis is usually bland or nonseptic. Septic thrombosis of the superior sagittal sinus is usually a complication of meningitis, mainly with *Strep. pneumoniae* infection.[318]

Thrombosis of deep cerebral veins is rare.[325] Recurrent headaches and visual obscurations, even for several months, may be the only warning. Patients may present with confusion or various degrees of impaired consciousness. The most devastating complications are coma, decerebration, and death related to massive, bilateral thalamic and basal ganglionic hemorrhagic infarction.[326-328] This may be asymmetric.[329] This is a preventable complication if a stuttering progression is caught early in the course and if anticoagulation with heparin is instituted promptly.

Other types of intracranial venous thrombosis (cavernous sinus, petrosal sinus, and internal jugular vein and lateral sinus occlusion) are uncommonly associated with impairment of consciousness unless complications occur. Some cases of septic cavernous sinus thrombosis may be complicated by internal carotid artery occlusion and ipsilateral hemispheric infarction. Septic cases may be complicated by meningitis, subdural empyema, septic arterial emboli, systemic sepsis with encephalopathy, pituitary insufficiency (pituitary infarction), and the syndrome of inappropriate antidiuretic hormone secretion.[330-333] Septic emboli and cerebellar abscess are uncommon in the antibiotic era.

Cavernous sinus thrombosis causes a characteristic picture of palsy of cranial nerves III, IV, and VI and the ophthalmic division of V that traverse the structure, along with chemosis and signs of raised venous ocular pressure (see Fig. 15-9). It is common for thrombosis to start unilaterally and become bilateral within a few days due to spread of the thrombosis through the intercavernous sinuses. Septic thrombosis of the cavernous sinus is a true emergency. Such presentations are usually acute, but may be chronic with less aggressive organisms. In contrast to bland thrombosis, septic thrombosis is accompanied by toxic or septic encephalopathy. Symptoms include severe regional headache, orbital or periorbital pain, facial pain, fever, and diplopia. On examination, fever, periorbital edema, chemosis, proptosis, ocular movement (initially abducens) palsies, ptosis, parasympathetic pupillary paralysis, and facial sensory loss in V1 with or without V2 distribution are found. There may be venous engorgement and hemorrhages on funduscopy;

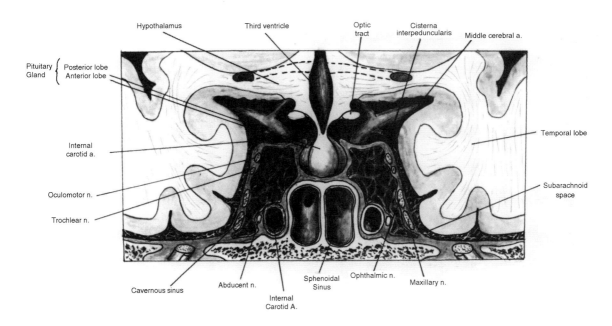

Figure 15-9

A coronal section through the cavernous sinuses, showing cranial nerves III, IV, and VI and the ophthalmic and maxillary divisions of V, as well as their relationship to the internal carotid artery and the pituitary gland.

patients may have reduced visual acuity. Septic cases may show purulent nasal discharge or infection of the upper half of the face. Meningismus or distended veins in the frontal region of the forehead have been described.[318]

Differential diagnosis of septic cavernous sinus thrombosis includes bland (noninfectious) cavernous sinus thrombosis, orbital cellulitis, the Tolossa-Hunt syndrome, superior orbital fissure syndrome, orbital apex syndrome, carotid-cavernous fistula, giant intracavernous carotid artery aneurysm, and intracavernous or intraorbital tumor (e.g, meningioma or nasopharyngeal carcinoma with intracranial spread). Cogan syndrome consists of polyarteritis with intracranial venous thrombosis.

Investigation

Magnetic resonance imaging has emerged as the principal noninvasive diagnostic procedure of choice (Fig. 15-10).[334] With MRI there is absence

Figure 15-10

MRI showing a high signal on the T2-weighted image, with the lesion in the right parietal region showing some cortical hypodense regions (arrows) *due to petechial bleeding in a patient with cortical vein thrombosis. (From Jacobs et al,[299] with permission.)*

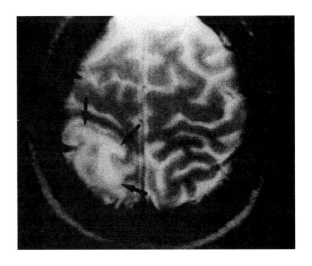

of flow void in the thrombosed vessels, which appear hypodense on T2-weighted images. In several days, this is followed by increased signal in the thrombosed vessels on T1 and T2-weighted images due to the production of intravenous methemoglobin.[335] With time, the veins may recanalize and flow void reappears. There can be false positives and false negatives with MRI, however.[336] The occluded vein may show a decreased signal on T2-weighted images that can be confused with patency. There may be an absence of signal if there is some flowing blood. The MRI scans help in most cases of cortical venous thrombosis by at least showing the location of infarcts.[299]

Scanning by CT may detect the thrombosed veins and venous infarcts before fatal infarction occurs.[328] An unenhanced CT may rarely reveal the thrombosed vein (cord sign) as a transient linear hyperdensity, related to recent intravenous thrombus.[337,338] The thrombus then becomes hypodense and contrast enhancement produces the "empty delta sign," as contrast outlines the thrombus in the superior sagittal or other major sinuses.[339] Dilated cortical veins may also be a helpful finding.[338] With progression of thrombosis, cortical hemorrhages may appear, often in the parasagittal regions.

One should be suspicious of cortical vein thrombosis if the lesion does not fall into a single arterial territory and/or if there is a hemorrhagic component to the lesion on CT or MRI (Fig. 15-10).[299]

Cerebral angiography still has a role in cases of limited cortical or deep venous thrombosis, especially when MRI or CT is not definitive.[340,341] There is lack of filling of the venous system on the late phase of the angiogram (Fig. 15-11).[342]

Figure 15-11

A. *Cerebral angiogram during the venous phase: the short arrow indicates an interrupted vein while the long arrows indicate marked slowing or nonfilling of nearby cortical veins.*
B. *Repeat angiography 3 days later shows that the same veins* (at arrows) *are now patent. (From Jacobs et al,[299] with permission.)*

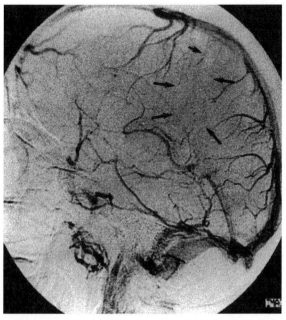

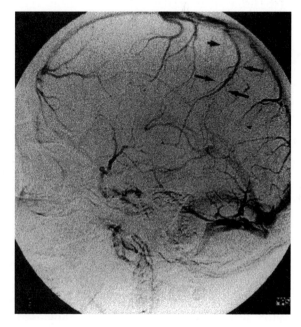

A   B

Cavernous sinus thrombosis is often associated with narrowing of the carotid artery on the arterial phase. Veinography has been used in the past, but it is difficult to perform and probably impractical.

Other investigative results that are less useful include: raised CSF pressure with increased red blood cells, anemia, increased erythrocyte sedimentation rate, and EEG—showing focal slowing with cortical vein thrombosis and more widespread rhythmic delta with symptomatic occlusion of the larger sinuses.[343] With septic cavernous sinus thrombosis, the CSF picture of a parameningeal infection (increased white blood cells with a mixture of lymphocytes and polymorphonuclear leukocytes; increased protein and normal glucose) is typically present.

Tomography is useful in demonstrating sphenoid sinusitis in cases of septic cavernous sinus thrombosis.[318] Plain skull films commonly show an ipsilateral mastoiditis in cases of lateral venous sinus thrombosis.[318]

Causes or associated risk factors are listed in Table 15-2. In about a third of cases, no cause is found.[344] Patients with protein C or S deficiency, as if such are present, are at risk for recurrence of thromboses. It seems reasonable to screen patients who develop intracranial venous thromboses to test their coagulation status. Girls with protein S or C deficiency should avoid the birth-control pill.

Therapy

Anticoagulation has reduced morbidity and mortality over earlier, less aggressive approaches. Earlier studies however, may have been biased towards inclusion of the sickest patients.[344,345] Even with hemorrhage, anticoagulation with heparin and then coumadin can produce satisfactory outcomes, presumably because the prevention of thrombotic progression and subsequent opening of venous channels lessens the venous and capillary back pressure.[346]

Local or systemic infusion of thrombolytic agents, such as streptokinase or plasminogen activator, have been attempted more recently, with some favorable results.[347–349] Direct surgical removal of the thrombus has also been used in refractory cases.[350] Because of the rarity of the condition, clinical trials to assess effective therapy adequately are unlikely. There is a need, however, for animal models.

The use of mannitol or other hyperosmolar agents may be dangerous, as fluid is withdrawn from the brain into the capillary and thence the venous vascular compartments. This may aggravate the already elevated venous back pressure and transcapillary pressure gradient and aggravate or precipitate cerebral edema or hemorrhage. There is one report of the successful use of barbiturate therapy to lower ICP in a desperate situation with sinus thrombosis.[351]

A suspicion of septic thrombophlebitis should lead to culture and prompt, vigorous antibiotic therapy. The choice of antimicrobial therapy depends on the material available for Gram stain and culture, the primary site of infection, and the presence or absence of associated meningitis. In general, a penicillinase-resistant penicillin, such as methicillin, is indicated. If there is a possibility of methicillin-resistant *Staph. aureus*, vancomycin should be used. Vancomycin is also useful in the context of penicillin allergy. (Most cases of septic cavernous sinus thrombosis are due to *Staph. aureus*, while septic lateral sinus thrombosis is more commonly associated with *Proteus* spp., anaerobes *E. coli*, and *Staph. aureus*.[318]) In the case of an unknown pathogen, metronidazole or chloramphenicol can be added to increase the spectrum of coverage. Impenem and cilastatin may also be useful. Prompt surgical drainage of infected paranasal sinuses or mastoids should be undertaken.

Heparin is commonly avoided in septic thrombophlebitis because of concern for hemorrhagic complications. Such therapy, however, may prevent spread of the thrombosis to other sites, such as the petrosal sinuses and cerebral veins. If heparin is started early, before hemorrhagic complications occur, the outcome is improved.[352] It is best not to anticoagulate excessively (partial thromboplastin time [PTT] less than twice normal) and to be ready to reverse the anticoagulation promptly if bleeding complications arise. Some argue strongly that anticoagulation should be avoided in more advanced septic cases when cortical hemorrhages are present, and in septic lateral sinus thrombosis.[318] This, however, remains controversial.

The use of corticosteroids is controversial, but coverage is wise if there is concern re pituitary insufficiency. Serial lumbar punctures may be helpful in reducing ICP in cases where visual acuity is threatened, e.g., certain cases of lateral sinus thrombosis.[318]

Prognosis

The prognosis is better in younger patients and those with isolated intracranial hypertension than in those with cortical lesions or brain swelling.[353] Probably, the promptness of anticoagulation will be found to be important as well. The prognosis of septic thrombophlebitis of the cavernous sinus is worse, especially with advanced infections and complications. The overall mortality is about 30 percent.[333] About one-third of patients suffer from permanent complications, including ocular palsies, diminished visual acuity, chronic pituitary insufficiency, or hemiparesis.[318]

REFERENCES

1. Griggs RC, Arieff AI: Hypoxia and the central nervous system, in Arieff AI, Griggs RC (eds): *Metabolic Brain Dysfunction in Systemic Disorders.* Boston, Little, Brown, 1992, pp 39–51.
2. Brierley JB: Experimental hypoxic brain damage. *J Clin Invest* 30:181, 1977.
3. Paulson OB, Newmau EA: Does the release of potassium from the astrocyte endfeet regulate cerebral blood flow? *Science* 237:896, 1987.
4. Hossman KA, Sakaki S, Zimmerman V: Cation activities in reversible ischemia of the cat brain. *Stroke* 8:77, 1977.
5. Kirshner HS, Blank WF Jr, Myers RE: Brain extracellular potassium activity during hypoxia in the cat. *Neurology* 25:1001, 1975.
6. Ikeda M, Busto R, Yoshida S, et al: Cerebral phosphoinositide, triacylglycerol and energy metabolism during severe hypoxia and recovery. *Brain Res* 459:344, 1988.
7. Norris JW, Pappius HM: Cerebral water and electrolytes: effect of asphyxia, hypoxia and hypercapnia. *Arch Neurol* 23:248, 1970.
8. Behar KL, Den Hollander JAD, Stromski ME, et al: High resolution 1H-nuclear magnetic resonance study of cerebral hypoxia in vivo. *Proc Natl Acad Sci USA*, 80:4945, 1983.
9. Dawson VL, Dawson TM, Bartley DA, Uhl GR, Snyder SH: Mechanisms of nitric oxide-mediated neurotoxicity in primary brain cultures. *J Neurosci* 13:2651, 1993.
10. Xia Y, Dawson VL, Dawson TM, Snyder SH, Zweier JL: Nitric oxide synthetase generates superoxide and nitric oxide in arginine-depleted cells leading to peroxynitrite-mediated cellular injury. *Proc Natl Acad Sci USA* 93:6770, 1996.
11. Dawson VL, Dawson TM, London ED, Bredt DS, Snyder SH: Nitric oxide mediates glutamate neurotoxicity in primary cortical cultures. *Proc Natl Acad Sci USA* 88:6368, 1988.
12. Pulsinelli W, Levy D, Duffy T: Regional cerebral blood flow and glucose metabolism following transient forebrain ischemia. *Ann Neurol* 11:499, 1982.
13. Moskowitz MA, Kaplan LR: *Cerebrovascular Disease. Nineteenth Princeton Conference.* Butterworth-Heinemann, 1995.
14. Bodsch W, Barbier A, Oehmichen M, Grosse Ophoff B, Hossmann KA: Recovery of monkey brain after prolonged ischemia. II. Protein synthesis and morphological alterations. *J Cereb Blood Flow* 6:22, 1986.
15. Petito CK, Feldman E, Pulsinelli WA, Plum F: Delayed hippocampal damage in humans following cardiorespiratory arrest. *Neurology* 37:1281, 1987.
16. Castillo J, Dávalos A, Noya M: Progression of ischaemic stroke and excitoxic aminoacids. *Lancet* 349:79, 1997.
17. Fisher M, Garcia JH: Evolving stroke and the ischemic penumbra. *Neurology* 47:884, 1996.
18. Baron JC, Furlan M, Marchal G: The metabolic status of the ultimately noninfarcted penumbra: a positron emission tomography study in humans. Presented at 121st Meeting of the American Neurological Association, Miami, October 14, 1996.
19. Freeman FR: Akinetic mutism and bilateral anterior cerebral artery occlusion. *J Neurol Neurosurg Psychiatry* 34:693, 1971.
20. Nielsen JM, Jacobs LL: Bilateral lesions of the anterior cingulate myri. *Bull Los Angeles Neurol Soc* 16:231, 1951.

21. Penfield W, Welch K: The supplementary motor area of the cerebral cortex. A clinical and experimental study. *Arch Neurol Psychiatry* 66:289, 1931.

22. Laplane D, Talairach J, Meininger V, et al: Clinical consequences of corticectomies involving the supplementary motor area in man. *J Neurol Sci* 34:301, 1977.

23. Geschwind N, Kaplan E: A human cerebral disconnection syndrome. A preliminary report. *Neurology* 12:675, 1962.

24. Steinke W, Sacco RL, Mohr JP, et al: Thalamic stroke. Presentation and prognosis of infarcts and hemorrhages. *Arch Neurol* 49:703, 1992.

25. Watson RT, Valenstein E, Heilman KM: Thalamic neglect. *Arch Neurol* 38:301, 1981.

26. Chase T, Moretti L, Presnky A: Clinical and electroencephalographic manifestations of vascular lesions of the pons. *Neurology* 18:357, 1968.

27. Castaigne P, Lhermitte F, Buge A, et al: Paramedian thalamic and midbrain infarcts: clinical and neuropathological study. *Ann Neurol* 10:127, 1981.

28. Tatu L, Moulin T, Bogousslavsky J, Duvernoy H: Arterial territories of the human brain: brainstem and cerebellum. *Neurology* 47:11, 1996.

29. Fisher CM: Oval pupils. *Arch Neurol* 37:502, 1980.

30. Caplan LR: "Top of the basilar" syndrome: selected clinical aspects. *Neurology* 30:72, 1980.

31. Caplan LR: "Top of the basilar" syndrome: selected clinical aspects. *Neurology* 30:72, 1980.

32. Shuaib A, Farah S: Stroke involving the midbrain and thalamus and causing "nonfocal" coma. *South Med J* 85:49, 1992.

33. Del Brutto OH, Mosquera A, Sanchez X, et al: Stroke subtypes among Hispanics living in Guayaquil, Equador: results from the Luis Vernaza Hospital stroke registry. *Stroke* 24:1833, 1993.

34. Sacco RL: Current epidemiology of stroke, in Fisher M, Bogousslavsky J (eds): *Current Review of Cerebrovascular Diseases*. Philadelphia, Current Medicine, 1993, pp 3–14.

35. del Mar Sáez de Ocariz M, Nader JA, Santos JA, Baustista M: Thalamic vascular lesions: risk factors and clinical course for infarcts and hemorrhages. *Stroke* 27:1530, 1996.

36. Ahern GL, Herring AM, Tackenberg J: The association of multiple personality and temporolimbic epilepsy. *Arch Neurol* 50:1020, 1993.

37. Serafetinides EA: Cerebral laterality and consciousness. *Arch Neurol* 52:337, 1993.

38. Albert ML, Silverberg R, Reches A, Berman M: Cerebral dominance for consciousness. *Arch Neurol* 33:453, 1976.

39. Lesser RP, Dinner DS, Lüders H, Morris HH: Memory loss for objects presented soon after intracarotid ampobarbital sodium injections in patients with medically intractable partial seizures. *Neurology* 36:895, 1986.

40. Love B, Biller J: Stroke in the young. *Stroke Clin Updates* 4:13, 1990.

41. Mazza C, Pasqualin A, Cavazzani P, Dalla Bemardina B, Da Pian R: Childhood cerebrovascular diseases not associated with arteriovenous malformations. *Child's Nerv Syst* 1:268, 1985.

42. Hanson SK Grotta JC: Acute stroke, in Grotta JC (ed): *Managment of the Acutely Ill Neurological Patient*. London, Churchill Livingstone, 1993, pp 17–37.

43. Faught E: Current role of electroencephalography in cerebral ischemia. *Stroke* 24:609, 1993.

44. Hund E, Grau A, Hacke W: Neurological care for acute ischemic stroke, in Jordan K (ed): Neurological Critical Care. *Neurol Clin* 13:511, 1995.

45. Schabitz WR, Fisher M: Diffusion weighted imaging for acute cerebral infarction. *Neurol Res* 17:270, 1995.

46. Sandercock P, Willems H: Medical treatment of acute ischemic stroke. *Lancet* 339:337, 1992.

47. Wolf PA, D'Agostino DB, Belanger AJ, Kannel WB: Probability of stroke: a risk profile from the Framingham study. *Stroke* 22:312, 1991.

48. North American Symptomatic Carotid Endarterectomy Trial (NASCET) Collaborators: Beneficial effect of carotid endarterectomy in symptomatic patients with high grade carotid stenosis. *N Eng J Med* 325:445, 1991.

49. Barnett HJM: 35 years of stroke prevention: challenges, disappoinments and successes. *Cerebrovasc Dis* 1:61, 1991.

50. Hart RG: Cardiogenic embolism to the brain. *Lancet* 339:589, 1992.

51. Hachinski V: Thrombolysis in stroke. Between the promise and the peril. *JAMA* 276:993, 1996.

52. The National Institute of Neurological Disorders and Stroke rt-TPA Stroke Study Group: Tissue plasminogen activator for acute ischemic stroke. *N Eng J Med* 333:1381, 1993.

53. Hacke W, Kaste M, Fieschi C, et al: Intravenous thrombolysis with recombinant tissue plasminogen activator for acute hemispheric stroke. *JAMA* 274:1058, 1995.

54. Riggs JE: Tissue plasminogen activator should not be used in acute ischemic stroke. *Arch Neurol* 53:1306, 1996.

55. Tarr R, Taylor CL, Selman WR, et al: Good clinical outcome in a patient with a large CT scan hypodensity treated with intra-arterial urokinase after an embolic stroke. *Neurology* 47:1076, 1996.

56. Kummer VR, Holle R, Rosin L, Forsting M, Hacke W: Does arterial recanalization improve outcome in carotid territory stroke? *Stroke* 26:581, 1995.

57. Donnan GA, Davis SM, Chambers BR, et al: Trial of streptokinase in severe acute hemispheric stroke. *Lancet* 345:578, 1995.

58. The Multicenter Acute Stroke Trial—Europe Study Group: Thrombolytic therapy with streptokinase in acute ischemic stroke. *N Eng J Med* 335:145, 1996.

59. Ginsberg MD, Pulsinelli WA: The ischemic penumbra, injury thresholds, and the therapeutic window for acute stroke. *Ann Neurol* 36:553, 1994.

60. Scatton B, Carter C, Benavides J, Giroux C: N-methyl-D-aspartate antagonists: a novel therapeutic perspective for the treatment of ischemic brain injury. *Cerebrovasc Dis* 1:121, 1991.

61. Sheardown MJ, Nielsen E, Hansen AJ, Jacobsen P, Honore T: 2,3-Dihydroxy-6-nitro-7-sulfamoyl-benzo (F)quinoxaline: a neuroprotectant for cerebral ischemia. *Science* 247:571, 1990.

62. Valentino K, Newcomb R, Gadbois T, Singh T, et al: A selective N-type channel antagonist protects against neuronal loss after global cerebral ischemia. *Proc Natl Acad Sci USA* 90:7894, 1993.

63. Busto R, Dietrich WD, Globus MY-T, et al: Small differences in intraischemic brain temperature critically determine the extent of ischemic neuronal injury. *J Cereb Blood Flow Metab* 7:729, 1987.

64. Steen PA, Newberg LA, Milde JH, Michenfelder JD: Nimodepine improves cerebral blood flow and neurologic recovery after complete cerebral ischemia in the dog. *J Cereb Blood Flow Metab* 3:38, 1983.

65. Hossmann K-A: Calcium antagonists for the treatment of brain ischemia: a critical appraisal, in Krieglstein J (ed): *Pharmacology of Cerebral Ischemia 1988—Proceedings of the Second International Symposium on Pharmacology of Cerebral Ischemia.* Stuttgart, Wissenschatl Verlagsgesellschaft, 1989, pp 53–63.

66. Hall ED: Lazaroids: efficacy and anti mechanism in experimental cerebral ischemia, in Krieglstein J (ed): *Pharmacology of Cerebral Ischemia 1988—Proceedings of the Second international Symposium on Pharmacology of Cerebral Ischemia.* Stuttgart, Wissenschatl Verlagsgesellschaft 1989.

67. Xue D, Slivka A, Buchan AM: Tirilizad reduces cortical infarction after transient but not permanent focal ischemia in rats. *Stroke* 23:894, 1992.

68. Ginsberg MD, Globus MY, Dietrich WD, Busto R: Temperature modulation of ischemic brain injury—a synthesis of recent advances. *Prog Brain Res* 96:13, 1993.

69. Dutka AJ, Kochanek PM, Hallenbeck JM: Influence of granulocytopenia on canine cerebral ischemia produced by air embolism. *Stroke* 20:390, 1989.

70. Zhang RL, Chopp M, Li Y, et al: Anti-ICAM-1 antibody reduces ischemic cell damage after transient middle cerebral artery occlusion in the rat. *Neurology* 44:1747, 1994.

71. Weyrich AS, Ma X, Lefer DJ, Albertine KH, Lefer AM: In vivo neutralization of P-selectin protects feline heat and endothelium in myocardial ischemia and reperfusion injury. *J Clin Invest* 91:2620, 1993.

72. Ginsberg MD, Globus MY-T, Busto R, Dietrich WD: The potential of combination pharmacotherapy in cerebral ischemia, in Krieglstein J, Oberpichler H (eds): *Pharmacology of Cerebral Ischemia 1990.* Stuttgart, Wissenschaftl Verlagsgesellschaft, 1990, pp 343–350.

73. Huang Z, Huang PL, Panahian M, et al: Effects of cerebral ischemia in mice deficient in neuronal nitric oxide synthetase. *Science* 26:1883, 1994.

74. Koketsu N, Berlove DJ, Moskowitz MA, et al: Pretreatment with intraventricular basic fibroblast growth factor decreases infarct size following focal cerebral ischemia in rats. *Ann Neurol* 33:451, 1994.

75. Linnik MD, Zobrist RH, Hatfield MD: Evidence supporting a role for programmed cell death in focal cerebral ischemia in rats. *Stroke* 24:2002, 1993.

76. Hachinski V, Norris JW: *The Acute Stroke.* Philadelphia, FA Davis, 1985.

77. Langhorne P, Williams BO, Gilchrist W, Howe K: Do stroke units save lives? *Lancet* 342:395, 1993.

78. Strand T, Asplund K, Eriksson S, et al: A non-invasive stroke unit reduces functional disability and the need for long-term hospitalization. *Stroke* 16:29, 1985.

79. Jørgensen HS, Nakayama H, Raaschou HO, et al: The effect of a stroke unit: reductions in mortality, discharge rates to nursing home, length of hospital stay, and cost. *Stroke* 26:1178, 1995.

80. Wood-Dauphinee S, Shapiro S, Bass ER, et al: A randomized trial of team care following stroke. *Stroke* 15:864, 1984.

81. Grotta JC, Pettigrew LC, Allen S, et al: Baseline hemodynamic state and response to hemodilution in patients with acute cerebral ischmia. *Stroke* 16:790, 1985.

82. Adams HP, Brott T, Crowell R, et al: Guidelines for the management of patients with acute ischemic stroke. *Circulation* 3:1588, 194.

83. Ameriso SF, Wong VLY, Quismorio FP Jr, Fisher M: Immunohematological causes of infection-associated cerebral infarction. *Stroke* 22:1004, 1991.

84. Pulsinelli WA, Levy DE, Sigsbee B, Scherer P, Plum F: Increased damage after ischemic stroke in patients with hyperglycemia with or without established diabetes mellitus. *Am J Med* 74:540, 1983.

85. de Falco FA, Sepe Visconti O, Fucci G, Caruso G: Correlation between hyperglycemia and cerebral infarct size in patients with stroke. A clinical and x-ray computed tomography study in 104 patients. *Schweiz Arch Neurol Psychiatr* 144:233, 1993.

86. Matchar DB, Divine GW, Heyman A, Feussner JR: The influence of hyperglycemia on outcome of cerebral infarction. *Ann Intern Med* 117:449, 1992.

87. Sapolsky RM, Pulsinelli WA: Glucocorticoids potentiate ischemic injury to neurons: therapeutic implications. *Science* 229:1397, 1985.

88. Tombaugh GC, Yang SH, Swanson RM, Sapolsky RM: Glucocoticoids exacerbate hypoxic and hypoglycemic hippocampal injury in vitro: biochemical correlates and a role for astrocytes. *J Neurochem* 59:137, 1992.

89. WHO Task Force on Stroke and other Cerebrovascular Disorders: Recommendations on stroke prevention, diagnosis and therapy. *Stroke* 20:1407, 1989.

90. Ropper AH, Shafran B: Brain edema after stroke. Clinical syndrome and intracranial pressure. *Arch Neurol* 41:26, 1984.

91. Rieke K, Krieger D, Adams HP, et al: Therapeutic strategies in space-occupying infarctions based on clinical, radiological and neurophysiological data. *Cerebrovasc Dis* 3:45, 1993.

92. Hacke W, Schwab S, De Georgia M: Intensive care of acute ischemic stroke. *Cerebrovasc Dis* 4:385, 1994.

93. von Kummer R, Meyding-Lamadé U, Forsting M, et al: Sensitivity and prognostic value of early CT in occlusion of the middle cerebral artery trunk. *AJMR* 15:9, 1994.

94. Rieke K, Schwab S, Krieger D, et al: Decompressive surgery in space-occupying hemispheric infarction: results of an open prospective trial. *Crit Care Med* 23:1576, 1995.

95. Renachary SS, Batinzky S, Morantz RA, et al: Hemicraniectomy for acute massive cerebral infarction. *Neurosurgery* 8:321, 1981.

96. Young PH, Simith KR Jr, Dunn RC: Surgical decompression after cerebral hemispheric stroke: indication and patient selection. *South Med J* 75:473, 1982.

97. Kondziolka D, Fazl M: Functional recovery after decompressive craniectomy for cerebral infarction. *Neurosurgery* 23:143, 1988.

98. Kalia KK, Yonas H: aggressive approach to massive middle cerebral artery infarction. *Arch Neurol* 50:1293, 1993.

99. Delashaw JB, Broaddus WC, Kassell NF, et al: Treatment of right cerebral hemispheric infarction by hemicraniectomy. *Stroke* 21:874, 1990.

100. Forsting M, Reith W, Schäbitz WR, et al: Decompressive craniectomy for cerebral infarction. An experimental study in rats. *Stroke* 26:259, 1995.

101. Doerfler A, Forstine M, Reith W, et al: Decompressive craniotomy in a rat model of "malignant" cerebral hemispheric stroke: experimental support for an aggressive therapeutic approach. *J Neurosurg* 85:833, 1996.

102. Anderson CS, Jamrozik KD, Stewart-Wynne EG: Predicting survival after stroke: experience from the Perth Community Stroke Study. *Clin Exp Neurol* 29:117, 1992.

103. Ahmed OI, Orchard TJ, Sharma R, Mitchell H, Talbot E: Declining mortality from stroke in Allegheny County, Pennsylvania. Trends in case fatality and severity of disease, 1971–1980. *Stroke* 19:181, 1988.

104. de Falco FA, Mastoroberto G, Mazzei G, et al: Atrial fibrillation and infarct area in ischemic stroke. A clinical and radiological study in 104 patients. *Acta Neurol* 13:249, 1991.

105. Steinke W, Sacco RL, Mohr JP, et al: Thalamic stroke. Presentation and prognosis of infarcts and hemorrhages. *Arch Neurol* 49:703, 1992.

106. Bonita R, Ford MA, Stewart AW: Predicting survival after stroke: a three year follow-up. *Stroke* 19:669, 1988.

107. Dignan MB, Howard G, Toole JF, Becker C, McLeroy KR: Evaluation of the North Carolina Stroke Care Program. *Stroke* 17:382, 1986.

108. Baruch E-A, Bornstein NM, Fuchs P, Korczyn AD: Mechanical ventilation in stroke patients—is it worthwhile? *Neurology* 47:657, 1996.

109. Thomassen A, Wernberg M: Prevalenee and prognostic significance of coma after cardiac arrest outside intensive care and coronary care units. *Acta Anaesth Scand* 23:143, 1979.

110. Longstreth W, Diehr P, Inui TS: Prediction of awakening after out-of-hospital cardiac arrest. *N Eng J Med* 308:1378, 1983.

111. Edgren E, Kelsey S, Sutton K, et al: The presenting ECG pattern in survivors of cardiac arrest and its relation to long-term survival. *Acta Anaesth Scand* 33:1, 1989.

112. Stephenson HE, Reid CL, Hinton W: Some common denominators in 1200 cases of cardiac arrest. *Ann Surg* 137:731, 1952.

113. Brierley JB, Graham DI, Adams JH, Simpson JA: Neocortical death after cardiac arrest: a clinical, neurophysiological, and neuropathological report of two cases. *Lancet* 2:560, 1971.

114. Dougherty JH Jr, Rawlinson DG, Levy DE, Plum F: Hypoxic-ischemic brain injury and the vegetative state: clinical and neuropathological correlations. *Neurology* 3:31, 1981.

115. Ingvar DH, Brun A, Johansson L, Samuelsson SM: Survival after severe cerebral anoxia with destruction of the cerebral cortex: the apallic syndrome. *Ann NY Acad Sci* 315:184, 1978.

116. French JD: Brain lesion associated with prolonged unconsciousness. *Ach Neurol Psychiatry* 68:727, 1952.

117. Brierley JB, Miller AA: Fatal brain damage after dental anaesthesia: its nature, etiology, and prevention. *Lancet* 2:869, 1966.

118. Kinney HC, Korein J, Panigraphy A, Dikkes P, Goode R: Neuropathological findings in the brain of Karen Ann Quinlan. *N Eng J Med* 330:1469, 1994.

119. Cole G, Cowie VA: Long survival after cardiac arrest: case report and neuropathological findings. *Clin Neuropathol* 6:104, 1987.

120. Korein J, Maccario M: On the diagnosis of cerebral death: a prospective study on 55 patients to define irreversible coma. *Clin Electroencephalogr* 2:178, 1971.

121. Dougherty JH, Rawlinson DG, Levy DE, Plum F: Hypoxic-ischemic brain injury and the vegetative state: clinical and neuropathological correlation. *Neurology* 31:991, 1981.

122. Bonvallet M, Hugelin A: Influence de la formation réticulare et du cortex cérébral sur l'éxitabilité motrice au cours de l'hypoxie. *Electroenceph Clin Neurophysiol* 13:270, 1961.

123. Wieloch T: Neurochemical correlates to selective neuronal vulnerability. *Prog Brain Res* 63:69, 1985.

124. Nowycky MC, Fox AP, Tsien RW: Three types of neuronal calcium channels with different calcium agonist sensitivity. *Nature* 316:440, 1985.

125. McCord JM: Oxygen-derived free oxygen radicals in postischemic tissue injury. *N Eng J Med* 312:159–163, 1985.

126. Michenfelder JD, Theye RA: The effects of anesthesia and hypothermia on canine cerebral ATP and lactate during anoxia produced by decapitation. *Anesthesiology* 33:430, 1970.

127. Ames A III Wright RL, Kowada M, et al: Cerebral ischemia. II. The no-reflow phenomenon. *Am J Pathol* 52:437, 1968.

128. White BC, Grossman LI, Krause GS: Brain injury by global ischemia and reperfusion. *Neurology* 43:1656, 1993.

129. Meldrum B, Garthwaite J: Excitatory amino acid toxicity and neurodegenerative disease. *TIPS* 11:379, 1990.

130. Faraci FM, Brian JE Jr: Nitric oxide and the cerebral circulation. *Stroke* 23:692, 1994.

131. Lee WL: Managment of hypoxic-ischemic encephalopathy. *Ann Acad Med Sinapore* 24:242, 1995.

132. Kuriowa T, Bonnekoh P, Hossmann K-A: Prevention of postischemic hyperthermia prevents ischemic injury of CA_1 neurons in gerbils. *J Cereb Blood Flow Metab* 10:550, 1990.

133. Pulsinelli WA, Lev DE, Sigsbee B, et al: Increased damage after ischemic stroke in patients with hyperglycemia with or without established diabetes mellitus. *Ann J Med* 74:540, 1983.

134. Nemoto EM, Snyder JV, Carrol RG, Morita H: Global ischemia in dogs: cerebrovascular CO_2 reactivity and autoregulation. *Stroke* 6:425, 1975.

135. Hossman K-A, Lechtape-Gruter H, Hossman V: The role of cerebral blood flow for the recovery of the brain after prolonged ischemia. *Z Neurol* 204:281, 1973.

136. Yoshida S, Inoh S, Asanoet T, et al: Effect of transient ischemia on free fatty acids and phospholipids in the gerbil brain. Lipid peroxidation as a possible cause of postischemic injury. *J Neurosurg* 53:323, 1980.

137. Bell JA, Hodgson HJF: Coma after cardiac arrest. *Brain* 97:361, 1974.

138. Levy DE, Caronna JJ, Singer BH, et al: Predicting outcome from hypoxic-ischemic coma. *JAMA* 253:1420, 1985.

139. Longstreth WT, Diehr P, Inui TS: Prediction of awakening after out-of-hospital cardiac arrest. *N Eng J Med* 308:1378, 1983.

140. Edgren E, Hedstand U, Kelsey S, Sutton-Tyrell K, Safar P: Assessment of neurological prognosis in comatose survivors of cardiac arrest. *Lancet* 343:1055, 1994.

141. Saltuan L, Marori M: Coma after cardiac arrest: will he recover all right? *Lancet* 343:1052, 1994.

142. Wijdicks EF, Young GB: Myoclonus status in comatose patients after cardiac arrest. *Lancet* 343:1642, 1994.

143. Pollack MA, Kellaway P: Cortical death with preservation of brainstem function: Correlations of clinical, electrophysiologic and CT scan findings in 3 infants and 2 adults with prolonged survival. *Trans Am Neurol Assoc* 103:36, 1978.

144. Hockaday JM, Potts F, Epstein EM, Bonazzi A, Schwab RS: Electroencephalographic changes in acute cerebral anoxia from cardiac or respiratory arrest. *Electroenceph Clin Neurophysiol* 18:575, 1965.

145. Brenner RP, Schwartzman RJ, Richey ET: Prognostic significance of episodic low amplitude or relatively isoelectric EEG patterns. *Dis Nerv Syst* 36:582, 1975.

146. Tsubokawa T, Yamamoto T, Katayama Y: Prediction of outcome of coma caused by brain damage. *Brain Injury* 4:329, 1990.

147. Brunko E, Zegers de Beyl D: Prognostic value of early cortical somatosensory evoked potentials after resuscitation from cardiac arrest. *Electroenceph Clin Neurophysiol* 66:15, 1987.

148. Rothstein TL, Thomas EM, Sumi SM: Predicting outcome in hypoxic-ischemic coma. A prospective clinical and electrophysiologic study. *Electroenceph Clin Neurophysiol* 79:101, 1991.

149. Eisenhuber E, Madl C, Kramer L, et al: Prediction of individual outcome in patients with nontraumatic coma by somatosensory evoked potentials. *Crit Care Med* 24(suppl 1):A38, 1996.

150. Madl C, Grimm G, Kramer L, et al: Early prediction of individual outcome after cardiopulmonary resuscitation. *Lancet* 341:855, 1993.

151. Guerit JM, de Tourtchaniniff M, Soveges L, Mahieu P: The prognostic value of three-modality evoked potentials in anoxic and traumatic comas. *Neurophysiol Clin* 23:209, 1993.

152. Jorgensen EO, Malchow-Moller A: Natural history of global and critical brain ischemia. *Resuscitation* 9:133, 1981.

153. Younkin DP: Magnetic resonance spectroscopy in hypoxic-ischemic encephalopathy. *Clin Invest Med* 16:116, 1993.

154. Nakano M, Ueda H, Li J-Y, et al: Regional N-acetyl aspartate level as an index for neuronal viability in experimental ischemic/postischemic injury. Presented as a poster at the American Neurological Association Meeting, Miami, October 15, 1996.

155. Celesia GG, Grigg MM, Ross E: Generalized status myoclonicus in acute anoxic and toxic-metabolic encephalopathies. *Arch Neurol* 45:781, 1988.

156. Jumao-as A, Brenner RP: Myoclonic status epilepticus: a clinical and electrographic study. *Neurology* 40:1199, 1990.

157. Krumholz A, Stern BJ, Weiss HD: Outcome from coma after cardiopulmonary resuscitation (CPR): relation to seizures and myoclonus. *Neurology* 38:401, 1988.

158. Snyder BD, Hauser WA, Loewenstein RB, et al: Neurologic prognosis after cardiac arrest: III. Seizure activity. *Neurology* 30:1292, 1980.

159. Hauser WA: Status epilepticus. Etiology and neurological sequelae. *Adv Neurol* 34:3, 1983.

160. Young GB, Gilbert JJ, Zochodne DW: The significance of myoclonic status epilepticus in postanoxic coma. *Neurology* 40:1843, 1990.

161. Meldrum BS, Brierley JB: Prolonged epileptic seizures in primates: ischemic cell change and its relation to ictal physiological events. *Arch Neurol* 28:10, 1973.

162. Azzerrelli B, Roessmann U: Diffuse anoxic myelopathy. *Neurology* 27:1049, 1977.

163. Hallett M, Chadwick, Adam J, Marsden CD: Reticular reflex myoclonus: a physiological type of human post-anoxic myoclonus. *J Neurol Neurosurg Psychiatry* 40:253, 1977.

164. Schwartzkroin PA, Prince DA: Cellular and field potential properties of epileptogenic hippocampal slices. *Brain Res* 147:117, 1978.

165. Nakanishi H, Kamata O, Katsuda N: 2-amino-5-phosphovaleric acid blocks induction of an epileptiform discharge following a brief hypoxic episode in the hippocampal slices prepared from dietary Mg-deficient mouse. *Japan J Pharmacol* 50:31, 1989.

166. Young RSK, During MJ, Aquial WJ, Tendler D, Ley E: Hypoxia increases extracellular concentrations of excitatory and inhibitory neurotransmitters

in subsequently induced seizure: in vivo microdialysis study in the rabbit. *Exp Neurol* 117:204, 1992.

167. Taylor CP, Dudek FE: Synchronous neural after discharges in rat hippocampal slices without active chemical synapses. *Science* 218:810, 1982.

168. Schwartzkroin PA: Mechanisms of cell synchronization in epileptiform activity. *TINS* 6:157, 1983.

169. Kirino T: Delayed neuronal death in the gerbil hippocampus. *Brain Res* 239:57, 1982.

170. Yaari Y, Konnerth A, Heinemann U: Nonsynaptic epileptogenesis in the mammalian hippocampus in vitro. II. Role of extracellular potassium. *J Neurophysiol* 56:424, 1986.

171. McVicar BA, Dudek FE: Dye-coupling between CA3 pyramidal cells in slices of rat hippocampus. *Brain Res* 196:494, 1980.

172. Gutnick MJ, Prince DA: Dye-coupling and possible electrotonic coupling in the guinea pig neocortical slice. *Science* 211:67, 1981.

173. Yamamoto K, Hayakawa T, Mogami H, Akai F, Yanagihara T: Ultrastructural investigation of the CA1 region of the hippocampus after transient cerebral ischemia in gerbils. *Acta Neuropathol* 80:487, 1990.

174. Lowenstein DH, Aminoff MJ, Simon RP: Barbiturate anesthesia in the treatment of status epilepticus: clinical experience with 14 patients. *Neurology* 38:395, 1988.

175. Treiman DM, Walton NY, Kendrick C: A progressive sequence of electroencephalographic changes during generalized convulsive status epilepticus. *Epilepsy Res* 5:49, 1990.

176. Nathanson N, Krumholz A, Biddle B: Seizures of axial structures. Presumptive evidence for brainstem origin. *Arch Neurol* 35:445, 1978.

177. Simon RP, Aminoff MJ: Electrographic status epilepticus in fatal anoric coma. *Ann Neurol* 20:351, 1986.

178. Westmoreland BF, Klass DW, Sharbrough FW, Reagan TJ: Alpha-coma. Electroencephalographic, clinical, pathologic and etiologic correlations. *Arch Neurol* 32:713, 1975.

179. Goldie WD, Chiappa KH, Young RR, Brooks EB: Brainstem auditory and short-latency somatosensory evoked responses in brain death. *Neurology* 31:248, 1981.

180. Howse DC: Cerebral energy metabolism during experimental status epilepticus. *Adv Neurol: Status Epilepticus* 34:209, 1983.

181. Choi DW: Glutamate neurotoxicity and diseases of the nervous system. *Neuron* 1:623, 1988.

182. Deutsch G, Eisenberg HM: Frontal blood flow changes in recovery from coma. *J Cereb Blood Flow Metab* 7:29, 1987.

183. Plum F, Posner JB, Troy B: Cerebral metabolic and circulatory responses to induced convulsions in animals. *Arch Neurol* 18:1, 1968.

184. Younkin DP: Magnetic resonance spectroscopy in hypoxic-ischemic encephalopathy. *Clin Invest Med.* 16:115, 1993.

185. Shalit MN, Beller AJ, Feinsod M: Clinical equivalents of cerebral oxygen consumption in coma. *Neurology* 22:673, 1972.

186. Lowenstein DH, Aminoff MJ, Simon RP: Barbiturate anesthesia in the treatment of status epilepticus: clinical experience with 14 patients. *Neurology* 38:395, 1988.

187. Parent JM, Lowenstein DH: Treatment of refractory status epilepticus with continuous infusion of midazolam. *Neurology* 44:1837, 1994.

188. Mills SA: Cerebral injury and cardiac complications. *Ann Thorac Surg* 56:S86, 1993.

189. Shaw PJ, Bates D, Cartlidge NE, et al: Early neurological complications of coronary artery bypass surgery. *BMJ* 291:1384, 1985.

190. Roach GW, Kanchuger M, Mangano CM, et al: Adverse cerebral outcomes after coronary bypass surgery. *N Eng J Med* 335:1857, 1996.

191. Mills SA: Cerebral injury and cardiac complications. *Ann Thorac Surg* 56:S86, 1993.

192. Blauth CI, Cosgrove DM, Webb BW, et al: Atheroembolism from the ascending aorta. An emerging problem in cardiac surgery. *J Thorac Cardiovasc Surg* 103:1104, 1992.

193. Francis TJR, Pearson RR, Robertson AG, et al: Central nervous system decompression sickness: latency of 1070 human cases. *Undersea Biomed Res* 15:102, 1988.

194. Adkisson GH, Macleod MA, Hodgson M, et al: Cerebral perfusion deficits in dysbaric illness. *Lancet* 2:119, 1989.

195. Wilmhurst P: Medical aspects of scuba diving. Decompression sickness may be due to paradoxical embolism. *BMJ* 309:340, 1994.

196. Rudge FW: Decompression sickness in a private pilot. *South Med J* 88:227, 1995.

197. Douglas JD, Milne AH: Decompression sickness in fish farm workers: a new occupational hazard. *BMJ* 302:1244, 1991.

198. Wilmshurst PT, Byrne JC, Webb-Peploe MM: Neurological decompression sickness. *Lancet* 1:731, 1989.

199. Spencer MP: Decompression limits for compressed air determined by ultrasonically detected blood bubbles. *J Appl Physiol* 40:229, 1976.

200. Pearson RR: *The Aetiology, Pathophysiology, Presentation and Therapy of Pulmonary Barotrauma and Arterial Gas Embolism Resulting from Submarine Escape Training and Diving.* Newcastle upon Tyne, The University of Tyne Press, 1981.

201. Fries CC, Levowitz B, Alder S, et al: Experimental gas embolism. *Ann Surg* 243:461, 1957.

202. Douglas JDM: Medical problems of sport diving. *BMJ* 291:1224, 1983.

203. Francis TJR, Pezeshpour GH, Dutka AJ, et al: Is there a role for the autochthonous bubble in the pathogenesis of spinal cord decompression sickness? *J Neuropathol Exp Neurol* 47:371, 1988.

204. Wilmhurst PT, Byrne JC, Webb-Peploe MM: Relation between interatrial shunts and decompression sickness in divers. *Lancet* 2:1302, 1989.

205. Smith DJ: Interatrial shunts and decompression sickness. *Lancet* 336:879, 1990.

206. Smith DJ, Francis TJR, Hodson M, Murrison JJW, Sykes JJW: Interatrial shunts and decompression sickness in divers. *Lancet* 335:914, 1990.

207. Bartlop AH: Decompression sickness. *BMJ* 303:250, 1991.

208. Ah-See AK: Permeability of the blood-brain-barrier to FITC labelled dextran in massive cerebral air embolism, in Hallenbeck JM, Greenbaum LJ (eds): *Air Embolism and Acute Stroke.* Bethesda, US Medical Service, 1977, pp 43–48.

209. Adkinsson GH, Macleod MA, Hodson M, et al: Cerebral perfusion deficits in dysbaric illness. *Lancet* 2:119, 1989.

210. Hodson M, Beran RG, Shirtley G: The role of computed tomography in the assessment of neurologic sequelae of decompression sickness. *Arch Neurol* 45:1033, 1988.

211. Cross SJ, Thomson LF, Jennings KP, Shields TG: Right-to-left shunt and neurological decompression sickness in divers. *Lancet* 1:568, 1990.

212. Strauss RH: Diving medicine. *Am Rev Respir Dis* 119:1001, 1979.

213. Sato S, Toya S, Ohira T, Mine T, Greig NH: Echocardiographic detection and treatment of intraoperative air embolism. *J Neurosurg* 64:440, 1986.

214. Marshall BM: Air embolus in neurosurgical anaesthesia, its diagnosis and management. *Can Anaesth Soc J* 12:255, 1965.

215. Newfield P, Albin MS, Chestnut JS, et al: Air embolism dring trans-sphenoidal pituitary operations. *Neurosurgery* 2:39, 1978.

216. Frost EAM: Some inquiries in neuroanesthesia and neurological supportive care. *J Neurosurg* 60:673, 1984.

217. Papadopoulous G, Kuhly P, Brock M, et al: Venous and paradoxical air embolism in the sitting position. A prospective study with transoesophageal echocardiography. *Acta Neurochir* 126:140, 1994.

218. Stallworth JM, Martin JB, Postlethwait RW: Aspiration of the heart in air embolisin. *JAMA* 143:624, 1930.

219. Gajdos PH, Korach JM, Conso F, et al: Epidemiological investigation of acute carbon monozide poisoning (A-CMP) in the Hauts-De-Seine departement. Results of a 3 year survey. *Intens Care Med* 14:324, 1988.

220. Moore SJ, Norris JC, Walsh DA, Hume AS: Antidotial use of methylhemoglobin forming cyanide antagonists in concurrent carbon monoxide/cyanide intoxication. *J Pharmacol Exp Ther* 242:70, 1987.

221. Ginsberg MD: Delayed neurological deterioration following hypoxia. *Adv Neurol* 26:21, 1979.

222. Choi IS: Delayed neurological sequelae in carbon monoxide intoxication. *Arch Neurol* 40:433, 1983.

223. Zagami AS, Lethlean AK, Mellick R: Delayed neurological deterioration following carbon monoxide poisoning: MRI findings. *J Neurol* 240:113, 1993.

224. Min SK: A brain syndrome associated with delayed neuropsychiatric sequelae following acute carbon monoxide intoxication. *Acta Psychiatr Scand* 73:80, 1986.

225. Garland H, Pearce J: Neurological complications of carbon monoxide poisoning. *QJM* 36:445, 1967.

226. Vieregee P, Klostermann W, Blümm RG, Borgis KJ: Carbon monoxide poisoning: clinical, neurophysiological, and brain imaging observations in acute disease and follow-up. *J Neurol* 236:478, 1988.

227. Deckel AW: Carbon monoxide poisoning and frontal lobe pathology: two case reports and a discussion of the literature. *Brain Inj* 8:345, 1994.

228. Min K: A brain syndrome associated with delayed neuropsychiatric sequelae following acute carbon monoxide intoxication. *Acta Psychiatr Scand* 73:77, 1986.

229. Garland H, Pearce J: Neurological complications of carbon monoxide poisoning. *QJM* 36:445, 1967.

230. Ginsberg MD: Carbon monoxide intoxication: clinical features, neuropathology and mechanisms of injury. *Clin Toxicol* 23:281, 1985.

231. James PB: Hyperbaric oxygen in the treatment of carbon monoxide and smoke inhalation: a review. *Intens Care World* 6:399, 1989.

232. Thom SR: Carbon monoxide-mediated brain lipid peroxidation in the rat. *J Appl Physiol* 68:997, 1990.

233. Penney DG: Acute carbon monoxide poisoning: animal models—a review. *Toxicology* 62:123, 1990.

234. Lapresle J, Fardeau M: The central nervous system and carbon monoxide poisoning. II. Anatomical study of brain lesions following intoxication with carbon monoxide (22 cases). *Prog Brain Res* 24:31, 1967.

235. Maeda Y, Kawasaki Y, Jibiki I, et al: Effect of oxygen under high pressure in regional cerebral blood flow in the interval form of carbon monoxide poisoning: observation from subtraction of HMPAO-SPECT technetium^{99m} brain imaging. *Eur Neurol* 31:380, 1991.

236. Silver DA, Cross M, Fox B, Parton RM: Computed tomography of the brain in acute carbon monoxide poisoning. *Clin Radiol* 51:480, 1996.

237. Murata T, Itoh S, Loshino Y, et al: Serial cerebral MRI with FLAIR sequences in acute carbon monoxide poisoning. *J Comput Assist Tomogr* 19:631, 1995.

238. Murata T, Itoh S, Koshino Y, et al: Serial proton magnetic resonance spectroscopy in a patient with the interval form of carbon monoxide poisoning. *J Neurol Neurosurg Psychiatry* 58:100, 1995.

239. Gabb G, Robin ED: Hyperbaric oxygen. A therapy in search of diseases. *Chest* 92:1074, 1987.

240. Raphael J-C, Elkharrat D, Jars-Guinestre M-C, Chastand C, et al: Trial of normobaric and hyperbaric oxygen for acute carbon monoxide intoxication. *Lancet* 2:414, 1989.

241. Barois A, Crosbuis S, Goulon M: Les intoxications aigües par l'oxyde de carbone et les gaz de chauffage. *Rev Prat* 29:1211, 1979.

242. Norkool DM, Kirkpatick JN: Treatment of acute carbon monoxide poisoning with hyperbaric ozygen: a review of 115 cases. *Ann Emerg Med* 14:1168, 1985.

243. Larcan A, Lambert H: Aspects épidémiologique, clinico-biologique et thérapeurtique actuels de l'intoxication oxycarbonée aiguë. *Bull Acad Nat Med* 165:471, 1981.

244. Mathieu D, Nolf M, Durocher A, et al: Acute carbon monoxide poisoning, risk of late sequelae and treatment by hyperbaric oxygen. *Clin Toxicol* 23:315, 1985.

245. Rudge FW: Carbon monoxide poisoning in infants: treatment with hyperbaric oxygen. *South Med J* 86:334, 1993.

246. Van Hoesen KB, Camporesi EM, Moon RE, Hage ML, Piantadosi CA: Should hyperbaric oxygen be used to treat the pregnant patient for acute carbon monoxide poisoning? A case report and review of the literature. *JAMA* 261:1039, 1989.

247. Salkowski AA, Penney DG: Cyanide poisoning in animals and humans: a review. *Vet Hum Toxicol* 36:455, 1994.

248. Isom GE, Borowitz JL: Modification of cyanide toxicodynamics: mechanistic-based antidote development. *Toxicol Lett* 82–83:795, 1995.

249. Barillo DJ Goode R, Esch V: Cyanide poisoning in victims of fire: analysis of 364 cases and review of the literature. *J Burn Care Rehabil* 15:46, 1994.

250. Garrison LP, Bowman MA, Perrin MB: Estimating physician requirements for neurology: a needs based approach. *Neurology* 34:1218, 1984.

251. Headache Classification Committee of the International Headache Society. Classification and diagnostic criteria for headache disorders, cranial neuralgias, and facial pains. *Cephalgia* 8(suppl 7):1, 1988.

252. Olesen J: The classification and diagnosis of headache disorders, in Mathew NT (ed): *Neurologic Clinics*. Philadelphia, Saunders, 1990, pp 793–799.

253. Bickerstaff ER: The basilar artery and the migraine-epilepsy syndrome. *Roy Soc Med Proc* 55:167, 1962.

254. Buckle RM, DuBoulay G, Smith B: Death due to vasospasm. *J Neurol Neurosurg Psychiatry* 27:440, 1964.

255. Haan J, Ferraii MD, Brouwer OF: Acute confusion migraine. Case report and review of the literature. *Clin Neurol Neurosurg* 90:275, 1988.

256. Munte TF, Muller-Vahl H: Familial migraine coma: a case study. *J Neurol* 237:59, 1990.

257. Centonze V, Amat G, Loisy C, Vena G, Pelage S: Considerations sur les accidents vasculaires cerebraux chez les migraineux. *Sem Hop Paris* 56:1908, 1980.

258. Andermann F: Clinical features of migraine-epilepsy syndromes, in Andermann F, Lugaresi E (eds): *Migraine and Epilepsy*. Boston, Butterworth, 1987, pp 3–30.

259. Camfield PR, Metrakos K, Andermann F: Basilar migraine, seizures and severe epileptiform EEG abnormalities: a relatively benign syndrome in adolescents. *Neurology* 28:584, 1978.

260. Collaborative Group for the Study of Stroke in Young Women: Oral contraception and increased risk of cerebral ischemia or thrombosis. *N Eng J Med* 288:871, 1973.

261. Collaborative Group for the Study of Stroke in Young Women: Oral contraception and increased risk of stroke in young women. Assocated risk factors. *JAMA* 231:718, 1975.

262. Bick RL: Disseminated intravascular coagulation and related syndromes. *Am J Hematol* 5:265, 1978.

263. Kaufman HH, et al: Delayed and recurrent intracranial hematomas related to disseminated intravascular clotting and fibrinolysis in head injury. *Neurosurgery* 7:445, 1980.

264. Barnett AH, Harrison JH: Disseminated intravascular coagulation in diabetic ketoacidosis. *Lancet* II:103, 1979.

265. Esmon CT, Owen WG: Identification of an endothelial cell cofactor for thrombin catalyzed activation of protein C. *Proc Natl Acad Sci USA* 78:2249, 1981.

266. Remuzzi G: HUS and TTP: variable expression of a single entity. *Kidney Int* 32:292, 1987.

267. Kovacs MJ, Roddy J, Grégoire S, et al: Thrombotic thrombocytopenic purpura following hemorrhagic colitis due to *Escherischia coli* 0157:H7. *Am J Med* 88:177, 1990.

268. Petitt RM: Thrombotic thrombocytopenic purpura: a thirty year review. *Semin Thromb Hemost* 6:350, 1980.

269. Ridolfi RL, Bell WL: Thrombotic thrombocytopenic purpura: report of 25 cases and review of literature. *Medicine* 60:413, 1981.

270. Shumak KH, Rock GA, Nair RC: Late relapses in patients successfully treated for thrombotic thrombocytopenic purpura: Canadian Apheresis Group. *Ann Intern Med* 122:569, 1995.

271. Blum AS, Drislane FW: Nonconvulsive status epilepticus in thrombotic thrombocytopenic purpura. *Neurology* 47:1079, 1996.

272. Rinkel JGE, Widjicks EFM, Hené RJ: Stroke in relapsing thrombotic thrombocytopenic purpura. *Stroke* 22:1087, 1991.

273. Amorosi EL, Ultmann JE: Thrombotic thrombocytopenic purpura: report of 16 cases and review of the literature. *Medicine* 45:139, 1966.

274. Moake JL, Rudy CK, Troll JH, et al: Unusually large plasma factor VIII: von Willebrand factor multimers in chronic relapsing thrombotic thrombocytopenic purpura. *N Eng J Med* 307:1432, 1982.

275. Schmidt JL: Thrombotic thrombocytopenic purpura: successful treatment unlocks etiologic secrets. *Mayo Clin Proc* 64:965, 1989.

276. Chintagumpala MM, Hurwitz RL, Moake JL, Mahoney DH, Steuber CP: Chronic relapsing thrombotic thrombocytopenic purpura in infants with large von Willebrand factor multimers during remission. *J Pediatr* 120:49, 1992.

277. Ruggenenti P, Galbusera M, Plata Cornejo R, Bellavita P, Remuzzi G: Thrombotic thrombocytopenic purpura: evidence that infusion rather than removal of plasma induces remission of the disease. *Am J Kidney Dis* 21:314, 1993.

278. Lian EC-Y, Mui PTK, Siddiqui FA, Chiu AYY, Chiu LLS: Inhibition of platelet-aggregating activity in thrombotic thrombocytopenic purpura by normal adult immunologlobulin G. *J Clin Invest* 73:548, 1984.

279. Siddiqui FA, Lian EC-Y: Novel platelet agglutinating protein from a thrombotic thrombocytopenic purpura plasma. *J Clin Invest* 76:1330, 1985.

280. Galbusera M, Ruggenenti P, Noris M, et al: Alpha 1 antitrypsin therapy in a case of thrombotic thrombocytopenic purpura. *Lancet* 345:224, 1995.

281. Kelton JG, Moore JC, Warkentin TE, Hayward CPM: Isolation and characterization of cysteine proteinase in thrombotic thrombocytopenic purpura. *Br J Haematol* 93:421, 1996.

282. Olenich M, Schattner E: Postpartum thrombotic thrombocytopenic purpura (TTP) complicating pregnancy-induced immune thrombocytopenic purpura (ITP). *Ann Intern Med* 120:843, 1994.

283. Kay AC, Solberg LA, Nichols DA, Petitt RM: Prognostic significance of computed tomography in the brain in thrombotic thrombocytopenic purpura. *Mayo Clin Proc* 66:602, 1991.

284. D'Aprile P, Farchi G, Pagliarulo R, Carella A: Thrombotic thrombocytopenic purpura: MR demonstration of reversible brain abnormalities. *AJNR* 15:19, 1994.

285. Kwaan HC: The role of thrombolysis in thrombotic thrombocytopenic purpura. *Semin Hematol* 24:101, 1987.

286. Lichtin AE, Schreiber AD, Hurwitz S, Willoughby TL, Silberstein LE: Efficacy of intensive plasmapheresis in thrombotic thrombocytopenic purpura. *Arch Intern Med* 147:2122, 1987.

287. Rock GA, Shumak KH, Buskard NA, et al: Comparison of plasma exchange with plasma infusion in the treatment of thrombotic thrombocytopenic purpura. *N Eng J Med* 325:393, 1991.

288. Byrnes JJ, Moake JL: Thrombotic thrombocytopenic purpura and the hemolytic-uremic syndrome: evolving concepts of pathogenesis and therapy. *Clin Haematol* 15:413, 1985.

289. Moake JL, Rudy CK, Troll JH, et al: Therapy of chronic relapsing thrombotic thrombocytopenic purpura with prednisone and azathioprine. *Am J Hematol* 20:73, 1985.

290. Gutterman LA, Stevenson TD: Treatment of thrombotic thrombocytopenic purpura with vincristine. *JAMA* 247:1433, 1982.

291. Wallach HW, Oren ME, Herkowitz A: Treatment of thrombotic thrombocytopenic purpura with plasma infusion and cyclophosphamide. *South Med J* 72:1346, 1979.

292. Bird JM, Cummins D, Machin SJ: Cyclophosphamide for chronic relapsing thrombotic thrombocytopenic purpura. *Lancet* 336:565, 1990.

293. Udvardy M, Rak K: Cyclophosphamide for chronic relapsing thrombotic thrombocytopenic purpura. *Lancet* 336:1508, 1990.

294. Wu K: Platelet hyperaggregability and thrombosis in patients with thrombocythemia. *Ann Intern Med* 88:7, 1978.

295. Thalen EM, Lechner K: Antithrombin III deficiency and thromboembolism. *Clin Haematol* 10:369, 1981.

296. Frens DB, Petajan JH, Anderson R, DeBlanc HJ Jr: Fibromuscular dysplasia of the posterior cerebral artery: report of a case and review of the literature. *Stroke* 5:161, 1975.

297. Collins GJ, Rich NM, Clagett GP, et al: Fibromuscular dysplasia of the internal carotid arteries. *Ann Surg* 194:89, 1981.

298. Ojemann RG, Crowell RM: Intracranial aneurysms and subarachnoid hemorrhage: Incidence, pathology, clinical features and medical management, in Ojemann RG, Crowell RM (eds): *Surgical Management of Cerebrovascular Disease*. Baltimore Williams and Wilkins, 1983, p 128.

299. Jacobs K, Moulin T, Bougousslavsky J, et al: The stroke syndrome of acute cortical vein thrombosis. *Neurology* 47:376, 1996.

300. Ameri A, Bousser MG: Cerebral venous thrombosis. *Ann Radiol* 37:101, 1994.

301. Ameri A, Bousser MG: Cerebral venous thrombosis. *Neurol Clin* 10:87, 1992.

302. Zuber M, Toulon P, Marnet L, Mas JK-L: Factor V Leiden mutation in cerebral venous thrombosis. *Stroke* 27:1721, 1996.

303. Deschiens M-A, Conrad J, Horellou MH, et al: Coagulation studies, factor V Leiden, and cardiolipin antibodies in 40 cases of cerebral venous thrombosis. *Stroke* 27:1724, 1996.

304. Brey RL, Coull BM: Cerebral venous thrombosis. Role of activated protein C resistance and factor V gene mutation. *Stroke* 27:1719, 1996.

305. Koelman JHTM, Bakker CM Plandsoen WCG Peeters FLM, Barth PG: Hereditary protein S deficiency presenting with cerebral sinus thrombosis in an adolescent girl. *J Neurol* 239:105, 1992.

306. Kajs-Wyllie M: Venous stroke in the pregnant and postpartum patient. *J Neurosci Nursing* 26:204, 1994.

307. Donaldson JO, Lee NS: Arterial and venous stroke associated with pregnancy. *Neurol Clin* 12:383, 1994.

308. Talbot RW Heppell J, Dozois RR, Beart RW Jr: Vascular complications of inflammatory bowel disease. *Mayo Clin Proc* 61:140, 1986.

309. Musio F, Older SA, Jenkins T, Gregorie EM: Case report: cerebral venous thrombosis as a manifestation of acute ulcerative colitis. *Am J Med Sci* 305:28, 1993.

310. al-Hakim, Katirji B, Osorio I, Weisman R: Cerebral venous thrombosis in paroxysmal nocturnal hemoglobinuria: report of two cases. *Neurology* 43:742, 1993.

311. Wechsler B, Vidailhet M, Piette JC, et al: Cerebral venous thrombosis in Behcet's disease: clinical study and long-term follow-up of 25 cases. *Neurology* 42:614, 1992.

312. Schutta HS, Williams EC, Baranski BG, Sutula TP: Cerebral venous thrombosis with plasminogen deficiency. *Stroke* 22:401, 1991.

313. Schneiderman JH, Sharpe JA, Sutton DMC: cerebral and retinal vascular complications of inflammatory bowel disease. *Ann Neurol* 5:331, 1979.

314. Brey RI., Gharavi AE, Lockshin MD: Neurologic complications of antiphospholipid antibodies. *Rheum Dis Clin North Am* 19:833, 1993.

315. Jaillard AS, Hommel M, Mallaret M: Venous sinus thrombosis associated with androgens in a healthy young man. *Stroke* 25:212, 1994.

316. Rich C, Gill JC. Wernick S, Konkol RJ: An unusual cause of cerebral venous thrombosis in a four-year-old child. *Stroke* 24:603, 1993.

317. Convers P, Michel D, Brunon J, Sindou M: Dural arteriovenous fistulas of the posterior cerebral fossa and thrombosis of the lateral sinus. Discussion of their relations and treatment a propos of 2 cases. *Neurochirurgie* 32:495, 1986.

318. Southwick FS, Richardson EP Jr, Swartz MN: Septic thrombosis of the dural venous sinuses. *Medicine* 65:82, 1986.

319. Villringer A, Mehraein S, Einhaupl KM: Pathophysiological aspects of cerebral sinus venous thrombosis. *J Neuroradiol* 21:72, 1994.

320. Frerichs KU, Deckert M, Kempski O, et al: Cerebral sinus and venous thrombosis in rats induces long-term deficits in brain function and morphology—evidence for a cytotoxic process. *J Cereb Blood Flow Metab* 14:289, 1994.

321. Ungersbock K, Heimann A, Kempski O: Cerebral blood flow alterations in a rat model of cerebral sinus thrombosis. *Stroke* 24:563, 1993.

322. Frerichs KU, Deekert M, Kempski O, et al: Cerebral and venous thrombosis in rats induces long-tenn deficits in brain function and morphology—evidence for a cytotoxic genesis. *J Cereb Blood Flow Metab* 14:289, 1994.

323. Cantú C, Barinagarrementeria F: Cerebral venous thrombosis associated with pregnancy and puerperium. *Stroke* 24:1880, 1993.

324. Ichyama T, Houdou S, Tomita Y, Yoshiokaa K, Ohno K: Cerebral venous thrombosis associated with recurrent eplilepsy-like attacks. *Brain Dev* 11:326, 1989.

325. Rahman NU, al-Tahan AR: Computed tomographic evidence of an extensive thrombosis and infarction of the deep venous system. *Stroke* 24:744, 1993.

326. Brown JI, Coyne TJ, Hurlbert RJ, Fehlings MG, Ter Brugee KG: Deep cerebral venous system thrombosis: case report. *Neurosurgery* 33:911, 1993.

327. Brown JI, Coyne TJ, Hurlbert RJ, Fehlings MG, Ter Brugge KG: Deep cerebral venous system thrombosis: case report. *Neurosurgery* 33:911, 1993.

328. Rahman NU, Al-Tahan AR: Computed tomographic evidence of an extensive thrombosis and infarction of the deep venous system. *Stroke* 24:74, 1993.

329. Milandre L, Pellissier JF, Vincentelli F, Khalil R: Deep cerebral venous system thrombosis in adults. *Eur Neurol* 30:93, 1990.

330. Gupta A, Jalali S, Bansal RK, Grewal SP: Anterior ischemic optic neuropathy and branch retinal artery occlusion in cavernous sinus thrombosis. *J Clin Neuroophthalmol* 10:193, 1990.

331. Silver HS, Morris LR: Hypopituitarism secondary to cavernous sinus thrombosis. *South Med J* 76:642, 1983.

332. Domenici R, Stefani G, Fiorini V et al: Thrombophlebitis of the cavernous sinus and inappropriate ADH seeretion syndrome. *Pediatr Med Chir* 7:841, 1985.

333. DiNubile MJ: Septic thrombosis of the cavernous sinus. *Arch Neurol* 43:367, 1988.

334. Perkin GD: Cerebral venous thrombosis: developments in imaging and treatment. *J Neurol Neurosurg Psychiatry* 59:1, 1995.

335. Ameri A, Bpousser LIG: Cerebral venous thrombosis. *Neurol Clin* 26:87, 1992.

336. McMurdo S, Brant-Zawadzki H, Bradley M: Dural sinus thrombosis study using intermediate field strength MRI. *Radiology* 161:83, 1986.

337. Rao KCVG, Knipp HC, Wagner EJ: Computed tomographic findings in cerebral sinus and venous thrombosis. *Radiology* 140:391, 1981.

338. Anxionnat R, Blanchet B, Dormont D, et al: Preseut status of computed tomography and angiography in the diagnosis of cerebral thrombophlebitis, cavernous sinus thrombosis excluded. *J Neuroradiol* 21:59, 1994.

339. Shimazaki H, Ogawa M, Takiyama Y, Nishizawa M, Yoshida M: Cerebral sinuis thrombosis in a young man with hereditary protein C deficiency. *Rinsho Shikeigaku* 33:1083, 1993.

340. Anxionnat R, Blanchet B, Dormont D, et al: Present status of computerized tomography and angiography in the diagnosis of cerebral thrombophlebitis cavernous sinus thrombosis excluded. *J Neuroradiol* 21:59, 1994.

341. Buonanno FS, Moody DM, Ball MR, et al: Computed cranial tomographic findings in cerebral sinovenous occlusion. *J Comput Assist Tomogr* 2:271, 1978.

342. McLean BN: Dural sinus thrombosis. *Br J Hosp Med* 45:226, 1991.

343. Bousser MG, Barnett HJM: Cerebral venous thrombosis, in Barnett HJM, Morh JP, Stein BM, Yatsu (eds): *Stroke: Pathophysiology, Diagnosis and Management*. New York, Churchill Livingstone, 1992.

344. Barnett HJM, Hyland HH: Non-infective intracranial venous thrombosis. *Brain* 76:36, 1953.

345. Buchanan DS, Brazinska JH: Dural sinus and cerebral venous thrombosis. Incidence in young women receiving oral contraceptives. *Arch Neurol* 22:440, 1970.

346. Einhaupl KM, Villringer A, Meister W, et al: Heparin treatment in sinus venous thrombosis. *Lancet* 338:597, 1991.

347. Tsai FY, Higashida RT, Matovitch V, Alferi K: Acute thrombosis of the intracranial dural sinus: direct thrombolytic treatment. *AJNR* 13:1137, 1992.

348. Alexander LF, Yamamoto Y, Ayoubi S, al-Mefty O, Smith RR: Efficacy of tissue plasminogen activator in the lysis of thrombosis of the cerebral venous sinuses. *Neurosurgery* 26:559, 1990.

349. Khoo KB, Long FL, Tuck RR, Allen RJ, Tymms KE: Cerebral venous sinus thrombosis assocated with the primary antiphospholipid syndrome. Resolution with local thrombolytic therapy. *Med J Aust* 162:30, 1995.

350. Persson L, Lilja A: Extensive dural sinus thrombosis treated by surgical removal and local streptokinase infusion. *Neurosurgery* 143:441, 1990.

351. Maruishi M, Kato H, Nawashiro H, et al: Successful treatment of increased intracranial pressure by barbiturate therapy in a patient with severe sinus thrombosis after failure of osmotic therapy. A case report. *Acta Neurochir* 120:88, 1993.

352. Southwick FS, Richardson EP Jr, Swartz MN: Septic thrombosis of the dural venous sinuses. *Medicine* 65:82, 1986.

353. Rondepierre P, Hamon M, Leys D, et al: Cerebral venous thrombosis: study of the course. *Rev Neurol* 151:100, 1995.

354. Wijdicks EFM, Parisi JE, Sharbrough FW: Prognostic value of myoclonic status epilepticus in comatose survivors of cardiac arrest. *Ann Neurol* 35:239, 1994.

Chapter 16

DRUGS
PART A: POISONING

Rocco V. Gerace

> *...every substance is a poison.*
> Paracelsus

In this chapter, designated as *toxins* are various poisons (or substances) that impair consciousness and perception. In a review of 500 causes of coma, initially of unknown etiology, almost two-thirds (326) were subsequently classified as diffuse-metabolic encephalopathies.[1] Of these, the largest single group (149 cases) were drug intoxications. Thus, it is important to consider toxins in cases of coma of unknown cause. However, even if the clinical picture suggests a toxic cause, it may initially be difficult to identify the agent. Hence, it is imperative to establish a systematic investigative approach. Often, we rely inappropriately heavily on the laboratory to make our diagnosis. One study revealed that a careful history and physical examination with routine laboratory analysis was sufficient to identify the principal drug cause in 86 percent of cases.[2]

It is not possible to describe the clinical features and management of all toxins capable of altering consciousness, so the reader is referred to suitable references.[3,4] Here, the clinical features and routine laboratory analysis of selected toxins will be described. The purpose is to emphasize the clinical approach.

Historical features are often thought to be unreliable. However, this may reflect the unwillingness of the physician or nurse to pursue details of the history with the patient, the family, friends, and others. For example, illness of the patient, family, or friends may implicate medications that are available to the patient. Similarly, hospital records may reveal the patient's maintenance medications. Information from ambulance drivers, police, or hospital personnel may implicate other substances, chemicals, or over-the-counter preparations. Possible industrial exposures necessitate an occupational history from either the patient or coworkers and supervisors.

The physical examination can be very useful. For example, altered body temperature narrows the differential diagnosis. Individual toxins resulting in autonomic nervous system dysfunction produce characteristic constellations of clinical features or "toxidrome." They may be classified as sympathomimetic, sympatholytic, parasympathomimetic, and parasympatholytic. Within each of these, two major major classes—altered temperature and autonomic dysfunction—are subgroups of agents with characteristic clinical features.

Judicious use of the laboratory extends and refines the clinical assessment. As mentioned, over-reliance on the laboratory may be misleading. Most "toxic screens" assess only a few toxins, and a "negative screen" may be mistakenly interpreted as excluding toxic exposure. On the other hand, routine biochemical tests may provide clues for a wide range of categories of toxins. Some life-threatening toxins, however, produce nonspecific clinical and biochemical alterations, yet they are treatable. Noteworthy in this regard is acetaminophen. Because of this, it is wise to measure acetaminophen concentrations in any patient with undifferentiated toxic exposure and to consider early administration of N-acetylcysteine.

The subsequent sections discuss poisonings under the following headings: "Autonomic Disturbances," "Toxic Seizures," "Toxic Temperature Alterations," "Arterial Blood Gas Disorders," and "Anion and Osmolar Gap Derangements."

AUTONOMIC DISTURBANCES

Physical assessment of the poisoned patient may reveal features, other than a depressed level of consciousness, that serve to assist in the identification of the toxin responsible. There are numerous drugs that either primarily or in conjunction with other sites of toxicity directly affect the autonomic nervous system (ANS). Many of these agents will also act centrally and lead to an alteration of consciousness in addition to other central nervous system (CNS) symptomatology, e.g., behavioral changes, seizures, and ischemic or hemorrhagic stroke. These autonomic toxins produce *toxidromes* related to their specific autonomic action and assist in the clinical diagnosis of the involved toxin.

The ANS is illustrated in Fig. 16A-1. In order to understand the clinical syndromes, it is necessary to recall the physiology of the peripheral ANS.[5] The two components of the ANS, the sympathetic and parasympathetic systems, are normally in balance. The effects of stimulation of one are generally the opposite in the other. Conversely, blockade of one system allows unopposed activity of the other. Neurotransmitters involved in stimulation may be classified as preganglionic (between the pre- and postganglionic fibers) or postganglionic (at the site of the ultimate receptor). The neurotransmitters acetylcholine and norepinephrine are shown in Fig. 16A-1. Cholinergic (associated with acetylcholine) receptors are either muscarinic or nicotinic (see Fig. 16A-1). Muscarinic receptors are postganglionic parasympathetic receptors, as well as some selected sympathetic receptors, e.g., on sweat glands. Nicotinic receptors include all preganglionic receptors and the neuromuscular junction. The sympathetic postganglionic neurotransmitter is norepinephrine.

Sympathomimetic Syndrome

The following is an illustrative case:

Case 1

A 20-year-old man was brought to the emergency department by ambulance, having suffered a seizure. According to his girlfriend, 10 min prior to their arrival, the patient's eyes rolled back and he had violent movements of all his extremities and started to "foam at the mouth."

On arrival, the patient was agitated and disoriented, appearing to be "postictal." His pupils were dilated (8 mm) but reactive to light. Extraocular movements and funduscopic examination were normal. Deep tendon reflexes were hyperactive. Vital signs were: blood pressure 220/130, pulse 120 beats per minute, respiration 28 per minute, and temperature 38.9°C. His skin was diaphoretic and flushed. The head and neck revealed no evidence of trauma. The lateral aspect of the tongue was bruised, suggestive of a recent convulsive seizure. His chest was clear and heart sounds were normal, with occasional extrasystoles. Examination of the abdomen revealed high-pitched, hyperactive bowel sounds, mild tenderness throughout without rebound, and no organomegaly. The patient subsequently vomited bilious material. A complete blood count (CBC), serum electrolytes, urea, creatinine, are blood sugar were all normal.

The above case illustrates typical features of the sympathomimetic syndrome. Mental status changes include agitation and paranoia. Hallucinations and convulsive or nonconvulsive seizures sometimes occur. Strokes, either hemorrhagic or ischemic, may result from acute or chronic abuse. The heart rate and blood pressure are typically markedly elevated. Pupils are widely dilated but reactive. There is often sweating, but not to excess. Gastrointestinal smooth muscle hyperactivity leads

Autonomic Nervous System   **Central Nervous System**

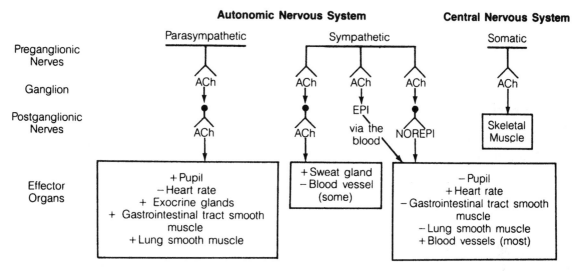

Figure 16A-1

Anatomic arrangement, receptors, and neurotransmitters in the peripheral autonomic nervous system. (From Taferi J, Roberts J: Organophosphate poisoning. Ann Emerg Med *16:196, 1987.)*

to nausea, vomiting, diarrhea, and abdominal cramping. There are numerous agents of abuse in this class, including cocaine, amphetamines, and over-the-counter sympathomimetics (ephedrine and phenylpropanolamine), that will be reviewed here briefly:

Cocaine Cocaine is readily available and can be ingested orally, inhaled nasally (snorted), or injected. The alkaloid form, "crack," is more heat stable with a lower vaporization point and can be smoked. Neurologic and cardiovascular features predominate among a wide range of pharmacologic effects. In addition to agitated, paranoid behavior, tactile hallucinations ("cocaine bugs") and visual hallucinations (halo lights around objects) are described. Cumulative use is associated with seizures as repeated dosing of the drug effects a progressive increase in central neuronal activity until the seizure threshold is reached and the patient suffers a tonic-clonic seizure. Cocaine use can be associated with status epilepticus, especially in the absence of treatment. In the "agitated delirium syndrome," patients exhibit bizarre paranoid behavior with unusual physical strength (it may require many persons to subdue the individual) and an elevated temperature.[6] The victim may then suffer a cardiopulmonary arrest from which resuscitation is impossible. Postmortem blood levels are subtoxic. It has been postulated that this syndrome is a variant of neuroleptic malignant syndrome.[7] Hypertension and vasoactive response can cause either ischemic or hemorrhagic stroke. Because of its membrane-stabilizing effects, cocaine can cause arrhythmias. Other cardiovascular effects include coronary spasm, myocardial infarction, and sudden cardiac death.[8,9]

Amphetamines Amphetamines are another class of sympathomimetics with central and peripheral effects that are typical of the sympathomimetic toxidrome. Many "designer" variants [e.g., methylenedioxyamphetamine (MDA) and methylenedioxymetamphetamine (MDMA)] have been synthesized in an attempt to maximize hallucinogenic properties. However, in overdose, these agents tend to lose specificity. Like cocaine, use is associated with confusion, agitation, and seizures. Death is secondary to cardiac events or intracerebral hemorrhage. Over-the-counter sympathomimetics, such as pseudoephedrine and phenylpro-panolamine, are associated with similar features.[10]

Lysergic Acid Diethylamide and Other Hallucinogens Lysergic acid diethylamide (LSD) has sympathomimetic activity. While intoxicated patients show widely dilated pupils, there is only a mild elevation of heart rate and blood pressure. Unlike the paranoid type of behaviour associated with classic sympathomimetics, LSD users tend to experience sensory misperceptions and/or synesthesias (hearing lights or seeing sounds).

A similar array of clinical features are produced by several plants, including psilocybin (magic mushrooms), peyote, and morning glory seeds. Depressed level of consciousness is limited to large ingestions of such substrates. Treatment is generally not necessary in recreational doses.

Sympatholytic Syndrome

The following is an illustrative case:

> **Case 2**
> The parents brought a 23-month-old child in a stuporous state to the emergency room. Shortly after arrival, the patient was pale and responsive to painful stimuli only. Pupils were pinpoint; vital signs were: heart rate 88 beats per minute, blood pressure 50/0, and respiratory rate 12 per minute. Shortly after arrival, the patient suffered a brief apneic episode. Initial treatment with inotropes was effective, but the patient continued to suffer apneic spells and bradycardia. It was subsequently learned that the patient had consumed his grandmother's "heart pill."

The above case of clonidine intoxication is typical of the sympatholytic syndrome.[11] The physical features, generally the reverse of the sympathetic syndrome, are due to inhibition of the central sympathetic outflow tract. These include the α_2-sympathetic agonists (clonidine and the imidazoline derivatives), the opiates, and, occasionally, high doses of other agents such as the sedative

hypnotics and ethanol. The mechanism of these toxic effects is outlined in the subsequent section on opiates (see "Opioids" in the second part of this chapter). The typical clinical features, exemplified in this case, are a depressed level of consciousness, pupillary constriction (miosis), bradycardia, hypotension, and respiratory depression.

Sedative Hypnotic Agents

Benzodiazepines Benzodiazepines are the most common sedative hypnotics encountered in drug overdose. Their pharmacology is discussed in detail with other anesthetic agents in the second part of this chapter. While their effects are reversible with flumazenil, antidotal treatment can be associated with seizures and arrhythmias.

Chloral Hydrate Chloral hydrate is rapidly metabolized to trichloroethanol, the agent responsible for coma. The metabolic interaction with ethanol (a "Mickey Finn") leads to more rapid and sustained blood levels and resultant coma. This intoxication can be associated with malignant ventricular arrhythmias. Both the parent drug and its metabolite are amenable to removal by extracorporeal techniques.

Glutethimide Glutethimide intoxication is manifested by prolonged coma with dilated fixed or reactive pupils due to its anticholinergic effects.

Meprobamate Meprobamate can produce profound and persistent hypotension due to direct myocardial depression. Large doses have been associated with gastric concretions necessitating aggressive gastrointestinal decontamination. Like chloral hydrate, it is amenable to extracorporeal removal by hemodialysis.

Anticholinergic Syndrome

The following is an illustrative case:

> **Case 3**
> A 14-year-old stuporous girl was brought to the emergency room by friends who related that she had been depressed and had

consumed a bottle of an over-the-counter sleep preparation. When roused, the patient was confused, disoriented, and mumbled incoherently. Pupils were 8 mm and reactive. Vital signs were: heart rate 130 beats per minute, blood pressure 140/90, respiratory rate 20 per minute, and temperature 38.5°C. Her skin was flushed and dry. Mucous membranes likewise were dry. Bowel sounds were absent and the bladder was palpable midway between the pubic symphysis and the umbilicus. Shortly after arrival, the patient suffered a generalized tonic-clonic seizure.

This case typifies the anticholinergic syndrome. With blockade of the parasympathetic receptors, there is unopposed sympathetic activity. However, unlike the sympathetic syndrome, there is usually only mild tachycardia and hypertension. Exocrine secretions are blocked and the lack of sweating contributes to the increased temperature (as does the central effect) and flushed dry skin. There can be an associated ileus and/or urinary retention. The mental status of awake patients is one of delirium with confusion and disorientation. The pupils are dilated and, at high doses, their reaction to light may be lost. Life-threatening complications include seizures, arrhythmias, and severe hallucinosis.

Numerous agents are capable of producing anticholinergic toxicity. Examples include over-the-counter antihistamines (e.g., diphenhydramine, which is also common in over-the-counter sleep preparations as exemplified in this case) and anti-nauseants such as dimenhydrinate and scopola-mine patches. Other agents include atropine, the antiparkinsonian agents (such as benztropine), skeletal muscle relaxants (orphenadrine), neuro-leptic agents (chlorpromazine), and cyclic anti-depressants (see below). Plants such as *Datura stramonium* (jimson weed) and *Atropa belladonna* (deadly nightshade) contain agents with anticho-linergic toxicity and may be abused. Treatment is generally supportive with airway control and ventilation as needed. Standard treatment for coma, seizures, and hyperthermia are impli-mented as necessary (see Chap. 20). While

physostigmine may reverse anticholinergic toxicity, it can produce severe complications, e.g., seizures and cardiac arrhythmias, in its own right. Its use should be reserved for life-threatening complica-tions (including delirium, hyperthermia, or tachy-cardia) that are unresponsive to conventional therapy.

Cyclic (Tricyclic and Tetracyclic) Antide-pressants Cyclic antidepressants are the most common class of drugs leading to intensive care unit (ICU) admission for intoxication. Because of their potential for lethality, they deserve special attention. While early intoxication with cyclic antidepressants often produces anticholinergic toxicity, of greater concern is their potential for cardiotoxicity. They block sodium channels in myocardial tissue, leading to slowing of electrical conduction [widening of the QRS complex on the echocardiograph (ECG)] and decreased con-tractility. Life-threatening complications include ventricular arrhythmias, heart block, and hypo-tension. The CNS manifestations include coma, seizures, and myoclonus. While physostigmine may be useful in reversing anticholinergic toxi-city, its use in conjunction with cyclic antidepres-sant toxicity, on the other hand, is sometimes associated with fatal outcomes and should be avoided.[12]

Cholinergic Syndrome

The following is a typical case of cholinergic toxi-city:

Case 4
A 33-year-old male was brought to the emergency department following an apparent suicide attempt. The patient had consumed an unknown amount of insecticide, later found to be an organophosphate. He had been previously healthy.

On arrival, he was unconscious, salivating excessively, and markedly diaphoretic. Vital signs were: heart rate 48 per minute and regular, blood pressure 90/60, respirations 30 per minute, and temperature 37.5°C. Pupils were 1 mm and nonreactive. His neck was supple. On chest examination, air entry was decreased and there were diffuse crackles and wheezes. There were also noted to be fine fasciculations in the intercostal muscles. Bowel sounds were hyperactive. Skin was diffusely moist.

Organophosphates Organophosphates and carbamate insecticides exert their toxicity by inhibiting acetylcholinesterase. This results in accumulation of acetylcholine at receptor sites, producing cholinergic toxicity. Unlike organophosphates, carbamates are quaternary compounds and do not cross the blood-brain barrier; their toxic symptoms are limited to peripheral effects. As nonspecific enhancers of cholinergic activity, these agents can have both muscarinic and nicotinic effects. Muscarinic stimulation results in miosis, diffuse exocrine secretion with sweating, salivation, lacrimation, urination, defecation, and bronchorrhea, bradycardia, and hypotension. Nicotinic stimulation can result in both sympathetic and parasympathetic stimulation, as well as muscle fasciculations as demonstrated by the patient in Case 4. The resultant clinical response can be somewhat confusing, with a mixed nicotinic/muscarinic toxicity. Organophosphate intoxication can result in tachycardia and hypertension when nicotinic features predominate. Central effects include confusion, delirium, seizures, and coma. Death is commonly secondary to respiratory failure. Long-term sequelae of organophosphate intoxication include peripheral neuropathy and behavioral and memory impairment.[13] Other agents capable of causing parasympathetic stimulation include bethanechol and pilocarpine.

Treatment includes the maintenance of vital signs and the administration of atropine to block the cholinergic excess. Large doses of atropine may be necessary to reverse the cholinergic crisis. In organophosphate intoxication, cholinesterase activity can be reactivated by the use of pralidoxime, which serves to unbind the toxin from the acetylcholinesterase. Over a period of several hours, the organophosphate becomes irreversibly bound and pralidoxime treatment becomes ineffective.

TOXIC SEIZURES

Numerous agents can cause seizures, including pharmaceuticals, plants, industrial agents, heavy metals, substances of abuse, and certain household agents. Generally, the seizure alone is not useful in the diagnosis of the offending agent. However, associated physical features may give a clue. Several cardiovascular toxins will cause seizures in addition to their cardiovascular effect. These include cyclic antidepressants, certain beta blockers (lipid soluble with membrane-stabilizing effects, e.g., propranolol), lidocaine, and calcium antagonists (rarely). Many of the autonomic agents can cause seizures, including sympathomimetics (cocaine, amphetamines), anticholinergics (diphenhydramine), and cholinergics (organophosphate insecticides). Each of these agents will produce an associated "toxidrome" with features that assist in the clinical diagnosis.

Some toxin-induced seizures may not respond to conventional treatment. For example, theophylline-induced seizures respond poorly to phenytoin and are better treated with a benzodiazepine followed by phenobarbital. Isoniazid-induced seizures are refractory to conventional treatment unless large doses of pyridoxine are administered. Seizure activity may aggravate the problem, e.g., in cyclic-antidepressant intoxication, the resultant metabolic acidosis exacerbates the cardiovascular effects of the drug.

Heavy metal toxicity may occasionally be associated with seizures. Severe lead toxicity in children may present as seizures with associated symptoms of lead toxicity, such as anemia and abdominal pain (lead colic). Heavy metal toxicity is often insidious and requires a careful history of occupational and environmental exposures.

TOXIC TEMPERATURE ALTERATIONS

Agents that will increase heat production include uncouplers of oxidative phosphorylation. The most common agent in this category is the family of salicylates but also included are the dinitrophenols, pentachlorophenols, and the chlorphenoxy herbicides (weak uncouplers). Other agents that increase temperature are those causing seizures or increased motor activity. Agents implicated in the latter category include the sympathomimetics, phencyclidine, and the monoamine oxidase inhibitors. Drugs, e.g., anticholinergics and neuroleptics, may also impair temperature exchange by impairing subsequent heat loss through perspiration. The serotonin syndrome or neuroleptic syndrome, described below, can also cause elevated temperature through additional or combined mechanisms.

Agents causing a decrease in temperature are generally CNS depressants. As part of their depressant effects, they allow passive heat loss and suppress heat production. Examples of agents causing hypothermia include barbiturates (and other sedatives/hypnotics), carbon monoxide, phenothiazines, and opiates.

Salicylates

Salicylate intoxication, chronic and/or acute, continues to be a serious clinical problem. Chronic toxicity often goes unrecognized.[14] Salicylates produce both metabolic (fever and an anion gap acidosis) and respiratory (primary respiratory alkalosis and noncardiac pulmonary edema) abnormalities. These commonly produce marked dehydration. Other metabolic effects include altered glucose metabolism with early hyperglycemia and late hypoglycemia. Animal models have demonstrated decreased cerebral glucose in the presence of normoglycemia.[15] The CNS manifestations of salicylate intoxication include early lethargy or delirium but, with increasing severity, can progress to seizures and coma with cardiovascular collapse. Treatment of salicylate intoxication involves stabilization of vital signs, aggressive gastrointestinal decontamination, and rehydration with correction of metabolic abnormalities and efforts to remove the toxin from the circulation. Salicylate elimination may be enhanced by urinary alkalinization but, in

more serious toxicity, hemodialysis may be indicated.[16]

Neuroleptic Malignant Syndrome

This idiosyncratic syndrome, associated with the therapeutic use of neuroleptic agents, is clinically manifest by fever, rigidity, and autonomic dysfunction. The muscle rigidity, associated with fever, contributes to the diffuse rhabdomyolysis with elevated creatinine phosphokinase and potential for renal failure. Other features of the syndrome include acute confusion or delirium, dystonic reactions, various degrees of muscular rigidity, dysphagia, and dysarthria. Risk factors in the triggering of the disease include existing cognitive dysfunction, the use of high-potency neuroleptics, especially with depot administration, dehydration, agitation, and concurrent infections. Clinicians must maintain a high index of suspicion in making the diagnosis as the onset of the rigidity and fever can be subtle. The differential diagnosis of systemic and CNS infection should be considered. Mortality is high in the untreated patient. In addition to aggressive supportive care (i.e., reversal of hyperthermia and correction of dehydration), treatment may include dantrolene and bromocriptine.[17,18] A similar syndrome may be seen in parkinsonian patients who suddenly withdraw from taking dopaminergic agents.

Serotonin Syndrome

The serotonin (5-hydroxytryptamine) syndrome is the result of increased serotonin availability at the receptor site. Agents may increase availability by increasing production of serotonin (tryptophan), blocking of serotonin reuptake at the synapse (e.g., selective serotonin reuptake inhibitors, cyclic antidepressants, and selected opioids), and reducing serotonin metabolism (monoamine oxidase inhibitors). The syndrome is commonly seen in patients who receive a combination of agents which increase serotonin availability by separate mechanisms. In addition to fever, this syndrome may be associated with confusion, ataxia, movement disorders, incoordination, diaphoresis, shivering, and diarrhea. It can, rarely, produce severe hyperthermia, seizures, ventricular arrhythmias, respiratory arrest, and death. With mild symptoms, treatment is directed to removal of the offending agent. In more severe cases, aggressive systemic support may be coupled with the administration of nonspecific serotonin blocking agents (methysergide or cyproheptadine) or propranolol.[19]

ARTERIAL BLOOD GAS DISORDERS

In addition to providing simple information related to acid-base status, blood gases can give other key information related to toxic exposures. General aspects of the various hypoxias are discussed in Chap. 10 and alterations in arterial concentrations of carbon dioxide (Pa_{CO_2}) are discussed in Chap. 11. The salient features due to toxins are described here.

Hypoxia

A low Pa_{O_2}, coupled with a rising Pa_{CO_2}, represents hypoventilation and is commonly seen with exposure to toxins causing CNS depression. These include the sedative hypnotics, narcotics, and numerous other centrally acting agents. Conversely, hypoxia in the presence of a widened alveolar-arterial oxygen gradient (A-a DO_2) is suggestive of shunting and can be seen with a variety of toxins which, in addition to causing an alteration in consciousness, can lead to noncardiac pulmonary edema [adult respiratory distress syndrome (ARDS)]. These include, but are not limited to, narcotics, salicylates, products of combustion, and cocaine.

Hypocapnia

Some toxins produce a metabolic acidosis and compensatory hyperventilation, characterized by a low Pa_{CO_2}. In addition, a number of toxins, along with their other effects, can cause direct stimulation of the respiratory center and a primary respiratory alkalosis. These include salicylates, dinitrophenol, and, to a lesser extent, stimulants, such as theophylline.

Alterations in Oxygen Saturation

When assessing oxygen-hemoglobin saturation, it is helpful to determine the difference between measured (laboratory co-oximeter) and calculated values. A significant difference between measured and calculated O_2 saturation (O_2 saturation gap) suggests a toxin which may be bound to hemoglobin, causing an alteration of the oxygen-carrying capacity of hemoglobin. Possibilities include carbon monoxide or the presence of methemoglobinemia. Bedside pulse oximetry is not reliable in determining these differences. Carbon monoxide intoxication can give a spuriously high bedside O_2 saturation levels while methemoglobinemia can cause spuriously low Pa_{O_2}, readings.

Methemoglobinemia Methemoglobinemia produces the appearance of "cyanosis" in a patient who appears to be otherwise systemically healthy. Numerous drugs and chemicals are capable of inducing methemoglobinemia.[20] Methemoglobin results from oxidation of the iron in hemoglobin (Hb) from the Fe^{2+} to the Fe^{3+} form. The primary toxicity of this condition is the direct interference of hemoglobin oxygen-carrying capacity, as well as a shift to the left in the O_2-hemoglobin (O_2-Hb) dissociation curve, further compromising O_2-carrying capacity. The brownish color of methemoglobin gives a cyanotic appearance to the patients and, at low levels, can be quite pronounced in the absence of other symptoms. Blood with methemoglobin can be distinguished from normal blood by its chocolate brown appearance when samples are put next to one another on filter paper and compared. High levels can result in marked cerebral hypoxia, with alteration in consciousness. Treatment includes removal of the offending agent and, in the presence of severe symptoms or high levels, the administration of methylene blue. This antidote enhances an alternate metabolic pathway that facilitates the reduction of methemoglobin to hemoglobin.

Carbon Monoxide Carbon monoxide (CO) toxicity is discussed in Chap. 10.

ANION AND OSMOLAR GAP DISORDERS

The following is an illustrative case:

Case 5

A 60-year-old man was brought to the emergency department by the police, having been arrested in the restaurant at the train station. Apparently, the man had walked into the restaurant and was putting chocolate bars into his pocket so the cashier phoned the police. The police found the man to be somewhat confused and disoriented and unable or unwilling to relate any information. He did not resist arrest and followed them willingly to a nearby hospital where the police requested a psychiatric assessment in the emergency room.

Any attempt to secure further history from the patient was fruitless. His personal effects were not contributory to his past history. There was no suggestion of toxic exposure. On examination, the patient was diaphoretic, short of breath, and somewhat restless, continuously adjusting his hospital gown and giving darting glances in all directions. He was disoriented to person, place, or time, disorganized, and unable to concentrate. His pulse was 92 beats per minute and blood pressure 110/72. Temperature was elevated at 38.5°C and respirations were regular at 30 per minute. He was somewhat thin. Head and neck examination was normal, with the neck being supple and nontender. Examination of the chest demonstrated good air entry, with occasional diffuse crackles in all fields. The cardiovascular system was normal. With the exception of mental status, the neurologic examination was normal as well.

The patient soon became progressively more agitated and restless. Increased respiratory compromise due to ARDS necessitated endotracheal intubation and assisted ventilation.

The initial blood work revealed: CBC normal, urea nitrogen 6 mmol/L (17 mg/dL), glucose 7 mmol/L (126 mg/dL), sodium 143 mmol/L (meq/L), potassium 3.1 mmol/L (meq/L), bicarbonate 12.7 mmol/L (meq/L), and chloride 108 mmol/L (meq/L). Arterial blood gases: pH 7.48, P_{CO_2} 13.8 mmHg, P_{O_2} 118 mmHg (F_{iO_2} 0.40). Urinalysis: pH 6.0; sugar, blood, and protein-negative; ketones 4+. Other: calcium 2.14 mmol/L (8.85 mg/dL), magnesium 0.68 mmol/L (1.65 mg/dL), serum osmolality 295 mmol/kg (mosmol/kg), lactate 2.1 mmol/L (meq/L).

The initial investigations in revealing the anion gap metabolic acidosis and superimposed respiratory alkalosis and fever prompted the laboratory testing for salicylates, which confirmed the diagnosis of salicylate intoxication. The patient did not respond to early aggressive medical management and was subsequently dialyzed. He recovered without further problems.

An anion gap metabolic acidosis, as revealed by electrolyte assessment, can be associated with various intoxications. This toxin-induced acidosis may be either a primary result of the toxin or secondary to lactic acidosis (Table 16A-1). There are numerous toxic conditions that are able to induce lactic acidosis by interfering with normal circulation, resulting in tissue hypoxia. On the other hand, toxins such as cyanide and hydrogen

Table 16A-1

Calculation and causes of an anion gap metabolic acidosis

Calculation of anion gap:

$$\text{Anion gap} = Na^+ - (Cl^- + HCO_3^-)$$
$$[\text{Normal} = 12\text{–}15]$$

Causes of positive anion gap metabolic acidosis:

Endogenous	Exogenous
Uremia	Salicylates
Ketoacidosis	Methanol
Lactic acidosis[a]	Ethylene glycol
Cyanide	Iron
Carbon monoxide	Paraldehyde
Isoniazid	Others

[a] Cyanide, carbon monoxide, and isoniazid produce a lactic acidosis.

sulfide interfere with aerobic metabolism at the cellular level. With the resultant anaerobic metabolism, large amounts of lactate are generated.

Group I: Toxin-Induced Acidosis

Cyanide Cyanide (CN) is a metabolic poison that causes cellular histiotoxic hypoxia by paralyzing the electron transfer in mitochondrial cytochrome oxidase through binding of the trivalent form of iron (Fe^{3+}).[21] This causes a shift from aerobic to anaerobic metabolism, leading to lactic acidosis.[22] There are also actions on various enzyme systems.[23]

Cyanide (CN) poisoning can occur through inhalation or by oral ingestion. It is found as a by-product of multiple industrial processes, in certain drugs, and has been used as a homicidal agent. Sources include the following: inhalation of hydrocyanic acid, and swallowing soluble inorganic cyanide salt or cyanide-releasing substances including cyanamide, cyanogen chloride and nitroprusside, certain plants (stone fruits of chokecherry, pincherry peach, apricot and bitter almond, cassava roots, jet berry bush berries, leaves and shoots of elderberry, and all parts of hydrangia), Laetrile (the controversial "anticancer drug"), and nitrile compounds (acetonitrile is a component of some cosmetic nail preparations). Cyanide is contained within the smoke of wood fires, but its concentration is much less than the carbon monoxide that is also present. The mortality and morbidity from such inhalations are almost always related more to CO than CN.[24] However, cyanide toxicity is synergistic with carbon monoxide.

There may be a history of inhalation or ingestion of one of the above agents. There is a characteristic "bitter almond" smell to the breath (many individuals are genetically incapable of smelling this). The patient may be unconscious, with the picture of a metabolic encephalopathy. In severe intoxication, cyanide can lead to a rapid loss of consciousness and seizures. Cyanosis is not seen until ventilatory failure occurs. Similar to other toxins, cyanide is able to cause a variety of cardiovascular effects, as well as noncardiac pulmonary

edema. Because of the inability of cells to utilize oxygen, hemoglobin is unable to release oxygen at the capillary, which causes the venous P_{O_2} to approach arterial P_{O_2} levels. Clinically, equivalent venous and arterial P_{O_2} can be appreciated by funduscopic examination: the visualized arterioles and venules have the same color. Similarly, measuring arterial and venous blood gases taken concurrently (almost equivalent oxygen partial pressures) assists in the diagnosis of cyanide poisoning.

The management of cyanide intoxication involves the administration of 100% oxygen, blood pressure support with norepinephrine if necessary, and the use of the Lily Cyanide Antidote Kit. The active components of the kit are amyl nitrite, sodium nitrite, and sodium thiosulphate. The first two facilitate the conversion of hemoglobin to methemoglobin which competes for the cyanide radical. Under enzymatic influence of rhodenese, sodium thiosulphate combines with cyanide to form thiocyanate which is readily excreted. While sodium thiosulphate has a low order of toxicity, amyl nitrite and sodium nitrite can be associated with toxicity and have been fatal in their own right.[25] If nitrites are used, methemoglobin concentration should not exceed 40% or the delivery of oxygen to tissues is compromised.

Recovery is often all-or-none. If treatment is prompt and the victim survives for 4 h, a complete recovery is expected; occasionally, some residual cerebral damage may be present.[26]

Toluene and Other Volatile Hydrocarbons

Toluene, another substance capable of producing an anion gap, typifies the volatile substances of abuse. Toluene is composed of a benzene ring with a single methyl group. It is readily available in multiple commercial products, including paints and glues. It is one of many substances commonly abused by inhalation ("huffing, bagging," or putting into a rag or plastic bag and inhaling). Like inhalational anesthetics, toluene-containing substances are rapidly absorbed and cause a wide variety of clinical presentations in association with a depressed level of consciousness. When metabolized to benzoate, toluene may be associated with an anion gap metabolic acidosis. Alternately, it can cause a non anion gap metabolic acidosis (renal tubular acidosis). Clinical syndromes include neuropsychiatric manifestations, ataxia, confusion, muscle weakness with profound hypokalemia, and abdominal discomfort.[27] Some halogenerated hydrocarbons (e.g., 1,1,1-trichloroethane, a widely used solvent) cause similar neurologic impairment and are associated with ventricular arrhythmias and sudden cardiac death.[28] Six-carbon-chain hydrocarbons (e.g., *n*-hexane, methylbutylketone) produce similar depressant effects acutely, while chronic abuse or industrial exposure can cause a severe peripheral neuropathy.[29]

Group II: Osmotically Active Agents

Calculated serum osmolarity is compared with measured serum osmolarity to determine the osmolar gap due to unmeasured osmols, including low-molecular-weight toxins (Table 16A-2).[30] For this calculation to be reliable, one must ensure that the laboratory uses the freezing-point depression technique for osmolarity determination rather than vaporization point. While the presence of an osmolar gap is helpful in determining etiology, its absence does not rule out the presence of toxic alcohols.

Table 16A-2
Calculation and causes of osmolar gap

Calculated serum osmolarity (Os) =

$2 \times Na^+ + BUN(mmol/L) + glucose(mmol/L)$
or $2 \times Na + BUN/2.8\,(mg\%) + glucose/18\,(mg\%)$

Calculation of osmolar gap:

Osmolar gap = measured Os − calculated Os
[Normal <10]

Causes of increased osmolar gap:

Ethanol	Ethylene glycol
Methanol	Isopropyl alcohol
Acetone	Mannitol

Ethanol *Ethanol is the most commonly encountered intoxicant associated with a positive osmolar gap.* Wines, beers, and spirits may have characteristic odors, but alcohol itself, e.g. vodka, is odorless. In the ethanol-intoxicated patient, it is essential to consider other causes of depressed level of consciousness, e.g., trauma and infection. Ethanol use may also be associated with varied metabolic abnormalities, e.g., alcoholic ketoacidosis with an anion gap, Wernicke's encephalopathy, and withdrawal symptoms, e.g., seizures or delirium tremens. One must be aware of the toxicity of the other alcohols described below.

Isopropyl Alcohol and Acetone. Isopropyl alcohol intoxication is similar to that of ethanol in its presentation, but, unlike most ethanol intoxications, it may be associated with deep coma following exposure.[31] This substance is readily available over-the-counter in many rubbing alcohol preparations. It can also lead to shock and hemorrhagic gastritis. It is readily detectable by the laboratory, along with its major metabolite, acetone. Acetone is also metabolically active and will contribute to the osmolar gap. Because the half-life of acetone is longer than that of isopropyl alcohol (IPA), the osmolar gap may stay elevated in the face of falling IPA levels. Isopropyl alcohol is readily dialysable, but, generally, intoxications can be managed with aggressive support of vital signs.

Methanol and Ethylene Glycol Methanol and ethylene glycol, in addition to producing an osmolar gap, are also associated with a profound anion gap-type metabolic acidosis. This acidosis is the result of metabolism of the parent compound: from methanol to formate; and, in the case of ethylene glycol, to glycolate.[32,33] Glycolate is further metabolized to oxalic acid which crystallizes in the urine and contributes to renal toxicity. Laboratory identification of oxalate crystalluria is helpful in distinguishing these toxins. The parent compound is relatively nontoxic. Like ethanol, both substances are initially metabolized by alcohol dehydrogenase. Given that this metabolic pathway is effectively blocked by concurrent ethanol exposure, coingestion of ethanol with methanol or ethylene glycol may delay the appearance of toxic signs. Methanol is associated with a classic clinical triad of optic neuropathy, abdominal pain, and metabolic acidosis. It is directly toxic to the optic nerve, leading to blurred vision, "snowfield vision" optic disc, and retinal edema and demyelination of the optic nerve.[34] Often objective funduscopic findings lag behind progressive visual impairment. Direct toxicity to the putamen has resulted in a parkinsonian syndrome.

Ethylene glycol is described in three stages.[35] Stage I can resemble ethanol intoxication and can last up to 12 h. Central nervous system toxicity with coma and seizures may occur. Stage II, the cardiopulmonary stage, lasts from 12 to 36 h and is associated with progressive tachypnea, cyanosis, pulmonary edema, and cardiomegaly. Stage II, the renal stage, develops by 72 h and can progress to acute renal failure and death. A fourth stage consisting of cranial nerve abnormalities has been suggested.

Management of both methanol and ethylene glycol intoxication involves the therapeutic use of ethanol to block the metabolism, hemodialysis to remove the parent compound, and metabolites and sodium bicarbonate to buffer the severe acidosis. Cofactors—folic acid for methanol and thiamine, and pyridoxine for ethylene glycol—are also administered. By increasing the metabolism and eliminating toxic metabolites, the aforementioned substances may serve to attenuate toxicity.

SUMMARY

Poisoning is a common cause of depressed level of consciousness. The source may be intentional, recreational, occupational, or inadvertent. The diagnosis can often be a made on the basis of a careful history and a physical examination with judicious use of standard biochemical testing. Treatment of the intoxicated patient may be specific for the offending agent. The clinician must maintain a high index of suspicion when considering toxic causes of coma.

REFERENCES

1. Plum F, Posner JB: *The Diagnosis of Stupor and Coma.* Philadelphia, F. A. Davis, 1980, pp. 1–86.
2. Rygnestad T: Evaluation of benefits of drug analysis in the routine clinical management of acute self poisoning. *Clin Toxicol* 22:51, 1984.
3. Goldfrank LR, Flomenbaum NE, Lewin NA: *Goldfrank's Toxicologic Emergencies.* Norwalk, Conn. Appleton and Lange, 1994.
4. Haddad LM, Winchester JF: *Clinical Management of Poisoning and Drug Overdose.* Philadelphia, WB Saunders, 1990.
5. Lefkowitz RJ, Hoffman BB, Taylor P: Neurohumoral transmission: the autonomic and somatic motor nervous systems, in Gilman AG, Rall TW, Nies AS, Taylor P (eds): *Goodman and Gilman's: The Pharmacological Basis of Therapeutics.* New York, Pergamon Press, 1990, pp 84–121.
6. Wetli CV, Fishbain DA: Cocaine-induced psychosis and sudden death in recreational cocaine users. *J Forensic Sci* 30:873–800, 1985.
7. Kosten TR, Kleber HD: Rapid death during cocaine abuse: a variant of the neuroleptic malignant syndrome. *Am J Drug Alcohol Abuse* 14:335, 1988.
8. Lange RA, Cigarroa RG, Yancy CW, Willard JE, Popma JJE: Cocaine-induced coronary-artery vasoconstriction. *N Engl J Med* 321:1557, 1989.
9. Isner JM, Estes NA, Thompson PD, Costanzo-Nordin MR, Subramanian RE: Acute events temporally related to cocaine abuse. *N Engl J Med* 315:1438, 1986.
10. Aaron C: Sympathomimetics. *Emerg Med Clin N Am* 8:513, 1990.
11. Artman M, Boerth RC: Clonidine poisoning: a complex problem. *Am J Dis Child* 137:171, 1983.
12. Smilkstein MJ: Reviewing cyclic antidepressant cardiotoxicity: wheat and chaff. *J Emerg Med* 8:645, 1990.
13. Namba T, Nolte CT, Jackrel J, Grob D: Poisoning due to organophosphate insecticides: acute and chronic manifestations. *Am J Med* 50:475–492, 1971.
14. Anderson RJ, Potts DE, Gabow PA, Rumack BH, Schrier RW: Unrecognized adult salicylate intoxication. *Ann Intern Med* 85:745, 1976.
15. Thurston JH, Pollock PG, Warren SK, Jones EM: Reduced brain glucose with normal plasma glucose in salicylate poisoning. *J Clin Invest* 49:2139, 1970.
16. Temple AR: Acute and chronic effects of aspirin toxicity and their treatment. *Arch Intern Med* 141:364, 1981.

17. Harpe C, Stoudemire A: Aetiology and treatment of neuroleptic malignant syndrome. *Medic Toxicol* 2:166, 1987.

18. Guze BH, Baxter LR: neuroleptic malignant syndrome. *N Engl J Med* 313:163, 1985.

19. Sporer KA: The serotonin syndrome: implicated drugs, pathophysiology and management. *Drug Safety* 13:94, 1995.

20. Curry S: Methemoglobinemia. *Ann Emerg Med* 11214, 1982.

21. Salkowski AA, Penney DG: Cyanide poisoning in animals and humans: a review. *Vet Hum Toxicol* 36:455, 1994.

22. Hall AH, Rumack BH: Clinical toxicology of cyanide. *Ann Emerg Med* 15:067, 1986.

23. Isom GE, Borowitz JL: Modification of cyanide toxicodynamics: mechanistic-based antidote development. *Toxicol Lett* 82–83:795, 1995.

24. Barillo DJ, Goode R, Esch V: Cyanide poisoning in victims of fire: analysis of 364 cases and review of the literature. *J Burn Care Rehabil* 15:46, 1994.

25. Berlin CM: The treatment of cyanide poisoning in children. *Pediatrics* 46:793, 1970.

26. Chen KK, Rose CL: Nitrite and thiosulfate therapy in cyanide poisoning. *JAMA* 149:113, 1952.

27. Streicher HZ, Gabow PA, Moss AH: Syndromes of toluene sniffing in adults. *Ann Intern Med* 94:758, 1981.

28. Flanagan RJ, Ruprah M, Meredith TJ, Ramsey JD: An introduction to the clinical toxicology of volatile substances. *Drug Safety* 5:359, 1990.

29. Garrettson LK: n-Hexane and 2-Hexanone, in Sullivan JB, Krieger GR (eds): *Hazardous Materials Toxicology*. Baltimore, Wilkins and Wilkins 1992, pp 1124–1126.

30. Glaser DS: Utility of the serum osmolar gap gap in the diagnosis of methanol or ethylene glycol ingestion. *Ann Emerg Med* 27:343, 1996.

31. Lacouture PG, Wason S, Abrams A, Lovejoy FH: Acute isopropyl alcohol intoxication: diagnosis and management. *Am J Med* 75:680, 1983.

32. Mcmartin KE, Ambre JJ, Tephley TR: Methanol poisoning in human subjects: role for formic acid accumulation in the metabolic acidosis. *Am J Med* 68:414, 1980.

33. Gabow PA, Clay K, Sullivan JB, Lepoff R: Organic acids in ethylene glycol intoxication. *Ann Intern Med* 105:16, 1986.

34. Jacobsen D, McMartin KE: Methanol and ethylene glycol: mechanism of toxicity, clinical course, diagnosis and treatment. *Medic Toxicol* 1:309, 1986.

35. Burkhart KK, Kulig KW: The other alcohols: methanol, ethylene glycol, and isopropanol. *Emerg Med Clin N Am* 8913, 1990.

DRUGS

PART B: PHARMACOLOGIC CONSIDERATIONS IN IMPAIRED CONSCIOUSNESS

Christopher G. Wherrett

Consider the following clinical cases:

Case 1

A 57-year-old male is transferred from a referring hospital. One week previously, he had sustained an anterior wall myocardial infarction. He had been recovering uneventfully until the morning of transfer, when he suddenly developed pulmonary edema and hypotension. His resuscitation was difficult and he required endotracheal intubation and hemodynamic support with dopamine. He was sedated with diazepam during intubation and later during transport. The amount of diazepam given was not specified in the transfer notes. On arrival in the intensive care unit (ICU) he remained intubated and ventilated with 100% O_2. His pulse was 85 beats per minute and his blood pressure was 100/60. Oxygen saturation was 95% by pulse oximetry. His eyes were closed. There was no posturing. Pupils were 2 mm and reacted sluggishly to light. Corneal reflexes were absent. There was no response to pain. The house officer made a diagnosis of hypoxic

encephalopathy and suggested further diagnostic testing.

What was the significance of the sedative medications that were administered?

Case 2

A 67-year-old female developed gram-negative septicemia from a perforated appendix 2 weeks previously. She developed multiple organ dysfunction syndrome, which included respiratory failure, hemodynamic instability, hepatic dysfunction, and renal failure. She still required ventilatory support and hemodialysis. Morphine, midazolam, and vecuronium infusions were discontinued 24 h previously. She was receiving parenteral nutrition, subcutaneous heparin, and sucralfate. She was found to be hemodynamically stable. On examination, where was no spontaneous movement but she withdrew sluggishly to deep pain. Her pupils were equal and reactive. Corneal reflexes were present. Deep tendon reflexes were absent. A neurologic opinion was requested regarding her depressed level of consciousness.

Table 16B-1

Anesthetic drugs commonly used in critically ill patients

Class	Drugs	Mechanism of action	Antagonists
Benzodiazepines	Diazepam Midazolam	Facilitates action of GABA at GABA receptors	Flumazenil
Induction agents			
Barbiturates	Thiopental	Decreases rate of dissociation from GABA receptor	
Phencyclidine	Ketamine	Produces dissociative anesthesia	
Other intravenous anesthetics	Propofol	Enhances GABA action	
Opioids	Morphine Meperidine Fentanyl	Opioid receptor agonist	Naloxone
Muscle relaxants			
Depolarizing	Succinylcholine	Sustained depolarization of nicotinic postjunctional membrane	
Nondepolarizing	Pancuronium Vecuronium Atracurium	Blocks nicotinic cholinergic receptors	Neostigmine Edrophonium Pyridostigmine
Inhaled anesthetics	Nitrous oxide Halothane Enflurane Isoflurane Desflurane Sevoflurane	Incompletely understood	

Impaired consciousness is a common problem in critically ill patients. Often there are multiple possible causes, including effects of sedative drugs. Critically ill patients frequently receive multiple sedative and analgesic agents. Many ICU patients have undergone surgical procedures; the effects of anesthetic agents may persist into the postoperative period. The effects of these agents on critically ill patients can be profound and unpredictable.

In this chapter, the term anesthetic agent will apply to drugs having sedative, hypnotic, or potent analgesic effects. Examples include commonly used drugs such as thiopental, propofol, midazolam, diazepam, fentanyl, and morphine (Table 16B-1). Muscle relaxants, such as vecuronium, will also be discussed. The first half of this chapter will discuss the pharmacology of anesthetic agents as applied to the critically ill or postoperative patient. This discussion is subdivided into two parts: (1) agents given intravenously, and (2) inhaled anesthetic agents. The second half of the chapter will discuss the diagnosis and management of patients with impaired consciousness who have received sedative drugs.

PHARMACOLOGIC PRINCIPLES

Intravenous Agents

A brief review of the basic pharmacokinetic principles of anesthetic drugs is necessary in order to understand their clinical characteristics. Pharmacokinetics is the study of the absorption, distribution, metabolism, and excretion of drugs. The intravenous route provides nearly immediate and complete absorption of drugs. Oral, intramuscular, and transdermal routes may have unreliable absorption, especially in critically ill patients.

The onset of an intravenous drug is determined largely by its initial rapid distribution characteristics and its membrane solubility. Organs such as the brain, heart, kidney, liver, and lung comprise only 10 percent of body mass yet they receive 75 percent of the cardiac output. These tissues are termed the "vessel-rich group"; distribution of injected drugs to the vessel-rich group is rapid. With most drugs, the plasma concentration generally correlates with pharmacologic effect. This is because lipid-soluble drugs readily cross capillary membranes, including the blood-brain barrier, thus allowing rapid brain uptake and a rapid onset of action.

The duration of a drug's effect on the central nervous system (CNS) (in addition to potential unwanted effects on the cardiovascular and respiratory systems) depends largely on distribution away from these organs. A two- or three-compartment model can be used to describe this concept (Fig. 16B-1).[1] The central compartment is essentially the intravascular space and the vessel-rich group of organs. The peripheral compartments include the lean tissue group (made up of muscle and skin), the fat tissue group, and the vessel-poor group (bone and cartilage). These peripheral compartments can be thought of as large, inactive storage depots. In a two-compartment model, the peripheral compartments are all combined as one compartment; in a three- or four-compartment model, they are subdivided into the previously described peripheral compartments.

Intravenous drug boluses rapidly reach a peak concentration in the central compartment (Fig. 16B-2). This creates a concentration gradient that causes the drug to move from the central to the peripheral compartments. The rate of this distribution, or intercompartmental transfer, determines the rate of fall in concentration at the receptor site, and therefore is a major determinant in the duration of action.

Drug excretion via hepatic metabolism or renal elimination occurs from the central compartment. Clearance is the theoretic volume of plasma that is completely cleared of a drug by hepatic, renal, or other mechanisms during a specific time period. The units for clearance are mL/min. Excretion has a minor effect on plasma concentration during the distribution phase. Once equilibration between the compartments occurs, the concentration gradient reverses and the drug transfers back into the central compartment from where it

Figure 16B-1

A two-compartment pharmacokinetic model. The drug is injected intravenously into the smaller volume central compartment. Intercompartmental transfer is governed by the rate constants K_{12} and K_{21}. The elimination rate constant K_e describes elimination of drug from the central compartment. (From Stanski and Watkins,[1] with permission.)

Figure 16B-2

A plasma concentration versus time curve for a drug given by rapid intravenous injection. The steep slope of the distribution phase is primarily due to the transfer of drug from the central compartment to the peripheral compartment. The slope of the elimination phase reflects the rate of elimination from the central compartment. (From Stanski and Watkins,[1] with permission.)

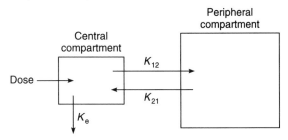

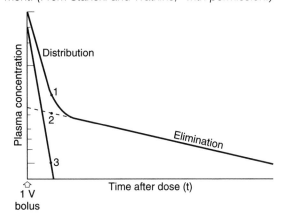

is eliminated. At this point, the plasma concentration has decreased significantly; the decline in plasma concentration is much slower in the elimination phase than during the distribution phase. The elimination half-life quantifies this phase and is inversely proportional to the clearance.[1]

Some of these pharmacokinetic principles are illustrated in the following examples. Thiopental is an ultra-short-acting, highly lipid-soluble barbiturate. Its onset, with resultant loss of consciousness, occurs within 30 s of intravenous administration (i.e., arm-to-brain circulation time). Benzodiazepines, such as diazepam and midazolam, do not act as quickly, but large doses (i.e., induction doses) can produce unconsciousness in 1 to 2 min. In contrast, morphine, which is much less lipid-soluble, requires 20 min to reach its peak effect. This is primarily due to its slower passage across the blood-brain barrier. Recovery from a single "sleep dose" of thiopental is very rapid, occurring within approximately 5 to 15 min. This is due to its rapid distribution half-time of 8.5 min.[2] However, the elimination half-time of thiopental is 11.6 h. Therefore, a long time is required to clear the drug completely from the body. This likely explains why the residual effects of thiopental may persist long after return to consciousness. These effects can interfere with postoperative recovery and mobilization. Impairment of psychomotor function has been demonstrated 8 h after the administration of thiopental.[3]

Inhaled Agents

Inhaled anesthetic agents include nitrous oxide and the volatile agents halothane, enflurane, isoflurane, desflurane, and sevoflurane. These agents are frequently used during the maintenance phase of general anesthetics. The term "balanced anesthetic" describes a general anesthetic technique where opioids; intravenous hypnotics, and inhaled agents are combined. The pharmacokinetics of inhaled agents differ from those of intravenous agents because the primary route of absorption and excretion is the lung.

Although the mechanism of action of inhaled anesthetics remains poorly understood, it is accepted that the magnitude of the effect depends on the partial pressure of the gas in the brain. Concentration in the brain is not easily measured; however, the concentration of exhaled gas can be monitored routinely in the operating room. The exhaled concentration reflects alveolar concentration. Over time, there is equilibration between alveolar partial pressure and the blood and brain partial pressures. Therefore, once a steady-state depth of anesthesia is obtained, the concentration in the alveoli reflects brain concentration. The factors that modify this relationship affect the induction and recovery from inhaled anesthetics.

The concentration of an anesthetic gas in the alveoli depends on both the inspired concentration and the alveolar ventilation. Gases diffuse easily across the alveolar-capillary membrane. The main determinant of gas transfer across the membrane is the solubility of the gas in the blood. Solubility is quantified by the blood/gas partition coefficient. Highly soluble drugs have high partition coefficients and a large amount of gas must transfer into the blood to saturate the blood compartment. Therefore, a longer time is required to reach equilibrium. Similarly, there is a blood/tissue partition coefficient which characterizes transfer of anesthetic gas from the blood into tissues such as the brain. Agents with low blood and tissue solubility are taken up in smaller amounts but reach equilibrium faster. Therefore, the induction and emergence from anesthesia are more rapid for less soluble gases. Nitrous oxide is the least soluble gas; it equilibrates within minutes. Isoflurane, a commonly used volatile agent, is more soluble than nitrous oxide and therefore equilibrates more slowly. Desflurane and sevoflurane are two newer agents that have lower solubilities and faster equilibration properties.

Rates of change in brain partial pressure are also influenced by global cardiac output, cerebral blood flow, the inspired concentration itself, and the addition of another anesthetic gas.

The metabolism of volatile agents is quite variable. Older agents, such as halothane, undergo up to 11 to 25 percent metabolism. This does make a small contribution to the speed of recovery. However, less than 1 percent of isoflurane is metabolized; the rest is excreted unchanged.[4]

The primary route of elimination is via the lungs; elimination is affected by the same factors that influence uptake. During drug elimination, the gradient from brain to alveoli is reversed. The higher the brain concentration (i.e., a greater depth of anesthesia), the longer the time required for recovery. Another major determinant of recovery is the duration of administration. Longer anesthetic exposure results in greater uptake into the peripheral compartments. Thus, recovery is slower after a longer anesthetic.

One measure of the speed of emergence from inhalational anesthesia is the time from the discontinuation of an inhalational agent to the patient's response to command. After 2 h of steady-state anesthesia, the time to recovery from isoflurane administration was 15.6 and 30.0 min after moderate and deep levels of anesthesia, respectively.[5] When desflurane, a less soluble agent, was used, these times were reduced to 8.8 and 16.1 min, respectively. In clinical practice, the depth of anesthesia is often decreased and the agent is discontinued prior to the end of a routine operation. Thus, most patients emerge from anesthesia less than 15 min after the end of surgery. However, a critically ill patient often requires postoperative mechanical ventilation. Usually, intravenous agents are given to maintain adequate sedation and analgesia during transport to the ICU.

Effects of Age and Coexisting Disease

Elderly patients are more sensitive to the effects of anesthetic drugs. Also, duration of action is prolonged in the elderly. This is due to both the effects of age on organ systems and a greater prevalence of coexistent illness in the elderly. Changes in receptor responsiveness occur with age for some, but not all, drugs. For example, there was no change found in plasma concentrations of thiopental required to suppress the electroencephalogram (EEG) in the elderly to that of other patients to a similar degree.[6] However, an increase in sensitivity of the CNS to midazolam with age has been shown.[7] Suppression of the EEG occurs at lower plasma levels of opioids in the elderly.[8] Elderly patients also require lower concentrations of volatile agents.[9]

Several changes in pharmacokinetic factors occur with age. The distribution of lipid-soluble drugs from the central to the peripheral compartments is slower, allowing more drug to reach the brain. An increase in the body fat compartment allows greater accumulation of lipid-soluble drugs, such as diazepam and thiopental.[10] When combined with decreased protein binding, this factor results in an increase in the volume of distribution of many drugs. An age-related decrease in cardiac output has an associated decrease in hepatic blood flow, which slows hepatic elimination. Hepatic microsomal activity also decreases with age. All these factors result in a decrease in plasma clearance rates. For example, large doses of fentanyl have a prolonged elimination half-life in the elderly due to decreased clearance (hepatic blood flow and hepatic microsomal activity).[11] This results in a longer duration of action after administration of larger doses. Finally, the decrease in renal function with age is associated with a slower elimination of drugs and their metabolites. The clinical implications of all these factors are that the elderly generally require lower doses of premedication, sedatives, and anesthetic agents to achieve the same effect. Also, side effects, especially cardiac and respiratory ones, are proportionally greater in the elderly.

Liver disease can affect drug metabolism because of hepatocellular dysfunction and/or altered blood flow. Cirrhosis is associated with decreased hepatic blood flow as well as shunting of blood around the liver. This affects the actions of intravenous drugs and orally administered drugs that have a high first-pass hepatic metabolism. These drugs will achieve a greater peak plasma concentration. Decreased plasma proteins results in an increased free fraction of drugs; therefore, when giving drugs by intravenous bolus, smaller doses are required to achieve the same clinical effect. In general, liver dysfunction prolongs the elimination half-life because of decreased clearance and increased volume of distribution.[12] This has little effect on small doses of drugs that depend on redistribution for the termination of their effect. However, larger doses or prolonged infusions of drugs depend on elimination for termination of their effect. The result can be a greatly prolonged clinical duration.

Renal disease may also affect drug distribution and excretion. Decreased albumin associated with renal disease may increase the free fraction of drugs such as morphine[13] and diazepam.[14] This factor can actually increase the clearance, which shortens elimination time. Renal drug excretion depends on glomerular filtration, tubular secretion, and tubular reabsorption.[15,16] Renal drug clearance is proportional to creatinine clearance. Therefore, as creatinine clearance decreases, renal drug clearance decreases proportionately. Many drugs have active metabolites that are excreted renally; some examples are pancuronium,[17] vecuronium,[18] and meperidine.[19]

Cardiac dysfunction, including congestive heart failure, shock, and low output states, results in impaired drug metabolism and excretion because both renal and hepatic blood flow are decreased.[20] Severe hepatic ischemia impairs intrinsic hepatic clearance.[21]

Several drugs increase the metabolism of other drugs by inducing hepatic enzymes. Examples include the barbiturates, phenytoin, macrolides, and corticosteroids. Cigarette smoking and chronic ethanol ingestion also induce enzymes, resulting in tolerance to anesthetic drugs. Acute alcohol ingestion can inhibit drug metabolism.

Several genetic factors have implications for the use of certain anesthetic drugs. Patients with atypical plasma cholinesterase have a very slow metabolism of succinylcholine. Malignant hyperthermia-susceptible patients can have a fatal reaction to triggering agents. These agents include all the volatile anesthetics and succinylcholine. Barbiturates, such as thiopental, can precipitate a crisis in patients with an acute porphyria.[22]

PHARMACOLOGY OF ANESTHETIC DRUGS

Mehanisms of Action

Pharmacodynamics is the study of the interaction of a drug with its receptors, as well as its mechanism of action. Unfortunately, we have a limited understanding of the mechanisms of action of the sedative/hypnotic drugs used in general anesthesia. Recently, there have been several developments in receptor pharmacology that will be discussed here. The clinical pharmacology of these agents is dealt with in the following section.

In general, one would expect that all anesthetic agents might inhibit synaptic transmission in a number of pathways, but particularly in the reticular activating system. Different mechanisms have been proposed for different classes of agents. Early work was directed at the interactions of volatile agents with the neuronal lipid membrane. It was shown that there is a strong correlation between the potency of volatile anesthetics and their solubility in oil. This suggests that volatile anesthetics act at a hydrophobic site, such as the cellular lipid membrane itself. The anesthetic could alter membrane structure, which would then impair ion channel function and thereby reduce synaptic transmission.[23]

More recently, the gamma-aminobutyric acid (GABA) receptor has been proposed as a site of action for several intravenous agents; GABA is a major inhibitory neurotransmitter in the CNS. The $GABA_A$ receptors are located primarily in the neocortex, hippocampus, hypothalamus, cerebellum, midbrain, medulla, and spinal cord. The GABA subtype A ($GABA_A$) receptor is a ligand-gated ion channel receptor. This receptor-chloride ionophore complex consists of five subunits clustered around a hydrophobic core. Binding of GABA to the beta subunit enhances the opening of the chloride ion channel. This increases channel chloride conductance, which causes the neuronal membrane to become hyperpolarized and therefore resistant to excitation.[24] Numerous intravenous agents, including the benzodiazepines, propofol, barbiturates, etomidate, and steroid anesthetics, interact with $GABA_A$ receptors.[25]

Glutamate is a major excitatory neurotransmitter. It activates the *N*-methyl D-aspartate (NMDA) receptor, which can also be found widely throughout the CNS. This receptor is also a ligand-gated ion channel; it conducts predominantly sodium and calcium ions. Ketamine and phencyclidine are examples of drugs that interact with the NMDA receptor.

Benzodiazepines bind to a specific benzodiazepine receptor on the $GABA_A$ receptor complex. This results in an increase in chloride ion flux. The presence of GABA is required for the benzodiazepine to exert its effects. Recently, a group of endogenous peptides that positively modulate GABA have been described.[26] These ligands have been called endozepines. Endozepines may have a causal role in the central neurologic symptoms of hepatic encephalopathy. In this condition, there is an increase in brain content of endozepines.[27] Also, flumazenil, a benzodiazepine antagonist, has been shown to reverse central neurologic symptoms in hepatic encephalopathy.[28]

Propofol is another intravenous anesthetic that enhances the effects of GABA at the $GABA_A$ receptor. Two or more molecules of propofol are required to bind to the $GABA_A$ receptor–chloride ionophore complex. This increases chloride conductance, which results in suppression of neuronal activity.[25,29] Propofol's effects, however, are not reversed by flumazenil. This suggests that propofol has a different binding site on the receptor complex. Also, diazepam augments the effect of propofol.[25] This synergistic effect is used in clinical practice; e.g., the two drugs can be combined during induction of anesthesia, allowing a lower dose of both drugs to be administered.[30]

Barbiturates also bind to the $GABA_A$ receptor. Once again, this different class of sedative/hypnotic drug is thought to have a distinct recognition site on the receptor complex.[31] Unlike benzodiazepines, the barbiturates do not require the presence of GABA to open the chloride channel.

Ketamine has been shown to be a noncompetitive antagonist at the NMDA receptor.[32] Its sedative effect may result from inhibition of excitatory amino acid.[33–35] Ketamine also binds to opioid receptors, which may provide a mechanism for its analgesic effect.[37] These effects are attenuated by naloxone, an opioid receptor antagonist.[36,37] Ketamine also interacts with the sigma receptor; this action may be responsible for the dysphoria sometimes induced by ketamine.[37]

The GABA receptor is not the only possible site of action of anesthetics. Other neurotransmitters and receptors have proposed roles. For example, brain concentrations, as well as the presynaptic release of dopamine, are affected by thiopentone, ketamine, and the volatile anesthetics.[38] An alternative mechanism of action has been suggested for propofol. It has been shown to alter cellular communication mediated by gap junctions between astrocytes. Propofol produces an increase in intracellular calcium concentration, which then causes closure of the gap junction.[39,40] Ketamine also affects intracellular calcium by inhibiting calcium influx through voltage-gated calcium channels;[41] this may have a role in the hypnotic action of ketamine. Finally, the hypnotic (as opposed to the anticonvulsant) effects of benzodiazepines may result from calcium ion flux.[40]

The nicotinic acetylcholine receptor is another receptor modulated by general anesthetics.[42,43] Numerous agents bind to channel proteins and block the flow of ions through the channel. Different agents produce different patterns of blockade; this may explain some of the different pharmacodynamic characteristics of these agents.

In summary, interactions with the $GABA_A$ complex serve as a model for the site of action of general anesthetics. However, it is not known if this is the primary site of action. The clinical significance of many of these proposed mechanisms remains to be defined. Much debate still exists about whether a single mechanism exists for all general anesthetics. Nonetheless, several of these models are consistent with a theory of a unitary mechanism of action for general anesthetic.[43]

Benzodiazepines

The clinical effects of benzodiazepines on the CNS include sedation, anxiolysis, anterograde to amnesia, mild muscle relaxation, and an anticonvulsant effect. The EEG shows a decrease in alpha (8 to 13 Hz) activity and an increase in beta (>13 Hz) activity. It is estimated that the anxiolytic effect occurs with receptor occupancy of less than 20 percent, sedation occurs with occupancy of 30 to 50 percent, and unconsciousness occurs when greater

Table 16B-2

Benzodiazepines commonly used in critically ill patients

Drug	Distribution half-life (min)	Elimination half-life (h)	Elimination route	Uses in ICU patients
Midazolam	15	1.7–4.0	Liver	Sedation Amnesia Anxiolysis Induction of anesthesia Anticonvulsant
Lapazepam	—	12-15	Conjugation with glucuronide	Same
Diazepam	30–60	24–57	Liver	Same

Table compiled from data from Refs. 14 and 108.

than 60 percent of receptors are occupied.[44] Amnesia may occur despite minimal sedative effects.[45]

Benzodiazepines have widespread clinical use in anesthesia and intensive care (Table 16B-2). They can be given orally, intramuscularly, or intravenously for premedication, and induction of, and maintenance of, general anesthesia. They are frequently used alone or in combination with opioids for sedation in the ICU. Benzodiazepines have a rapid anticonvulsant action. They are used to manage alcohol withdrawal syndrome. Their muscle relaxant properties are of little use in anesthesia or the ICU.

Sedative doses of benzodiazepines usually cause minimal cardiac or respiratory depression. However, large doses can cause apnea and/or hypotension.[46] Patients with underlying chronic disease, especially critically ill patients with cardiac or respiratory instability, are more susceptible to these side effects. Also, when benzodiazepines are combined with opioids, they can produce hypotension that would not occur if either drug were used alone.[47] The means to support the ventilatory and circulatory systems should always be available when these drugs are given intravenously.

Midazolam, diazepam, and lorazepam are the most commonly used benzodiazepines in anesthesia and intensive care (Table 16B-3).

Table 16B-3

Opiods commonly used in critically ill patients

Drug	Distribution half-life (min)	Elimination half-life (h)	Elimination route	Uses in ICU patients	Potency ratio (relative to morphine)
Morphine	9–13.3	1.7–2.2	Liver	Sedation Analgesia	1.0
Fentanyl	13–28	3.1–7.9	Liver	Sedation Analgesia	100
Sulfentanil	17.1	2.7	Liver	—	500–1000
Alfentanil	8.2–16.8	1.2–1.9	Liver	—	10–20
Meperidine	—	3.2–7.9	Liver	Infrequent	0.1

Table compiled from data from Ref. 109.

Midazolam has a short elimination half life (1.7 to 4 h), whereas for diazepam it is 24 to 57 h.[48] Both drugs have active metabolites. Desmethyldiazepam has a half-life of 48 to 96 h and accumulates in the tissues after prolonged use. Note that the clinical effect of diazepam is much shorter than its half-life because of rapid tissue redistribution. Lorazepam has an intermediate half-life of 12 to 15 h and does not have active metabolites. Because it is conjugated with glucuronic acid, its metabolism is less dependent on the function of hepatic microsomal enzymes.[49] Dosage of benzodiazepines depends on a number of factors. For example, sedative doses of midazolam are usually 1 to 2.5 mg, while general anesthesia can be induced with 5 to 10 times this amount. In the ICU, these drugs can be given by intermittent intravenous bolus or infusion. Prolonged recovery times have been reported in ICU patients. Malacrida et al found that the half-life of midazolam was over twice that of healthy volunteers, probably because of a greater volume of distribution in ICU patient.[50] Also, tolerance can develop; dosages should always be individualized.

Opioids

The term opioid refers to all exogenous substances that bind to opioid receptors and produce morphine-like effects. The more specific term *narcotic* (from the Greek for stupor) also refers to morphine-like properties but has the connotation of being a substance that produces dependence.

In 1976, Martin et al described three types of opioid receptors[51]; mu, kappa, and sigma. This was based on the discovery of three separate agonist drugs that had three characteristic pharmacologic profiles. Since then, a delta and an epsilon receptor have been added and the mu receptor has been subdivided into mu-1 and mu-2.[52] The presence of opioid receptors prompted the search for, and discovery of, endogenous ligands for them. These include the beta-endorphins and enkephalins, which are thought to play a role in the modulation of pain and also to have effects on mood and the cardiovascular and respiratory systems.

Mu receptors are found in forebrain, midbrain, and hindbrain structures, including the periaqueductal grey matter, nucleus raphe magnus, and locus ceruleus. Their actions include supraspinal analgesia, respiratory depression, bradycardia, euphoria, physical dependence, and ileus.

Kappa receptors are concentrated in the caudate putamen, nucleus accumbens, amygdala, hypothalamus, neural lobe of the pituitary gland, median eminence, and nucleus tractus solitarius. Their actions include analgesia, sedation, respiratory depression, and meiosis. Meiosis is caused by an excitatory action on the Edinger-Westphal nucleus.

Sigma receptors are responsible for the dysphoric effect of opioids, as well as other excitatory effects including tachycardia, tachypnea, and mydriasis. Delta receptors are thought to be important in spinal analgesia. Spinal opioid receptors are concentrated in the substantia gelatinosa of the spinal cord.

Opioids, in doses used for analgesic effects, usually produce mild sedation. Higher doses of morphine (1 mg/kg) were previously used in cardiac anesthesia in an attempt to produce an adequate depth of anesthesia. However, this dose (and even doses several-fold higher) did not produce unconsciousness in all patients. Therefore, an opioid cannot be used as the sole agent to produce general anesthesia. In situations where the patient becomes hypercarbic secondary to the respiratory depressant effects of opioids, the hypercarbia will have an additional sedative effect.

Opioids are commonly used both during and after surgery (Table 16B-3). In the ICU, morphine is the most commonly used agent for relief of discomfort due to trauma, endotracheal tubes, suctioning, etc.[53] It is usually given by intermittent intravenous bolus or by infusion. Dosing depends on the intensity of the painful stimulus and factors such as the patient's age, general condition, and tolerance of opioids. Wide variations in requirements exist, ranging from 1 to 2 mg/h to more than 20 mg/h. The numerous side effects of opioids are described elsewhere.[54] Side effects of special concern in ICU patients are respiratory depression and hypotension. Respiratory depression is not a problem in the mechanically ventilated patient. In fact, it may decrease subjective feelings of respiratory distress and prevent the patient from fighting the ventilator. All opioids can cause hypotension by blunting compensatory cardiovascular reflexes, which are especially important in hypovolemic patients. Large doses of morphine cause histamine release. Nausea and vomiting are common side effects of opioids. Important CNS effects include decreased cerebral blood flow (provided hypercarbia is prevented[55,56]), sedation, and miosis. Large doses of synthetic opioids can cause skeletal muscle rigidity. The effects on the EEG include replacement of alpha (8 to 13 Hz) waves with delta (≤ 4 Hz) waves. Tolerance and physical dependence can develop and will require weaning opioids over several days or longer.

Fentanyl, a synthetic opioid, is approximately 100 times more potent than morphine. Its main advantages are a more rapid onset and a shorter duration of action due to rapid distribution. Therefore, it is useful for short procedures such as endotracheal intubation and bronchoscopy. Fentanyl is frequently used as the opioid component of balanced general anesthesia. Unlike morphine, large doses of fentanyl do not cause histamine release or vasodilatation. When infused over longer periods of time, its duration of action is prolonged and so it offers little advantage over morphine.[57]

Meperidine has several disadvantages that preclude its routine use in ICU patients. Hypotension is more frequent than with other opioids; myocardial contractility can be decreased by large doses. Meperidine is structurally similar to atropine; because of this, meperidine toxicity can present with anticholinergic features such as mydriasis and tachycardia. The metabolite normeperidine can produce delirium and seizures due to its stimulating effects on the CNS.[58] The half life of normeperidine is much longer than that of the parent compound; therefore, its excitatory effects may occur after the depressant effects of meperidine have subsided. This is especially important after prolonged administration or in the presence of renal dysfunction.

Epidural administration of opioids is an alternative means of managing postoperative or traumatic pain. Advantages include superior analgesia, lower dosage requirements, and fewer systemic effects.[59] Sometimes, a dilute concentration of local anesthetic is added to the opioid which results in a synergistic analgesic effect. However, systemic absorption still occurs, especially with lipid-soluble opioids. A single dose of epidural morphine provides analgesia for up to 24 h; however, delayed respiratory depression can occur, typically 6 to 12 after administration.[60] Therefore, appropriate monitoring of respiratory function is necessary when using epidural opioids.

Induction Agents

Thiopental, propofol, and ketamine are three agents used for induction of anesthesia (Table 16B-4). Other drugs, such as etomidate, thiamylal, midazolam, and even diazepam, are also used but will not be discussed here. An ideal induction agent would rapidly produce unconsciousness without side effects such as cardiovascular depression. It would be short-acting, leaving few residual neurologic effects.

Thiopental (or sodium pentothal) has been in use since 1934 and meets some of the previously mentioned criteria. It is an ultra-short-acting barbiturate; the pharmacokinetics of thiopental have already been discussed.

The most significant side effect of thiopental is hypotension, caused by myocardial depression and pooling of venous blood. The venodilatation is thought to be caused by depression of transmission in sympathetic ganglia. Thiopental also causes transient apnea. Laryngospasm and bronchoconstriction can occur if the airway is stimulated under light anesthesia. Thiopental can also precipitate a crisis in patients with porphyria.

The primary indication for thiopental is induction of general anesthesia. Because of its rapid redistribution, frequent supplemental doses or an infusion would be required to maintain anesthesia for more than a few minutes. This would lead to cumulation of the drug and a greatly prolonged effect. Thiopental is an effective anticonvulsant; however, because of its sedative and hypotensive effect, other barbiturates or

Table 16B-4
Anesthetic induction agents

Drug	Distribution half-life (min)	Elimination half-life (h)	Elimination route	Uses in ICU patients	Major adverse effects
Thiopental	8.5 + 6.1	11.6 + 6.0	Liver	Seizures, Intracranial hypertension	Depression of consciousness Hypotension Immune suppression
Propofol	2–4	1–3	Liver ? Other	Sedation Anesthesia for brief procedures	Depression of consciousness Hypotension
Ketamine	4.7	2.2	Liver	Analgesia Anesthesia in hemodynamically unstable patients	Respiratory depression Sympathetic stimulation Emergence phenomena

Table compiled from data from Refs. 2 and 61.

benzodiazepines are usually preferred. Because anesthetists are very familiar with thiopental, it is occasionally used for treatment of perioperative seizures or status epilepticus. Thiopental reduces intracranial pressure by causing cerebral vasoconstriction and decreasing cerebral oxygen consumption. Therefore, thiopental is currently the drug of choice for induction of anesthesia prior to endotracheal intubation in patients at risk of intracranial hypertension.

Propofol, an intravenous anesthetic/hypnotic, was approved for use in the United States in 1989. It is an alkylphenol compound and therefore is in a different class than the barbiturates and benzodiazepines. Propofol is highly lipid-soluble and therefore is formulated in an emulsion of intralipid (also used in parenteral nutrition solutions). The intralipid gives it a distinctive white colour.

Recovery from propofol anesthesia is very rapid, due to both rapid redistribution and elimination. This results in a more rapid awakening with fewer residual CNS effects. Thus, it is commonly used for short operative procedures and in day-surgery patients. Propofol can be used for induction of anesthesia and also for maintenance of anesthesia during long procedures. Unlike thiopental and pentobarbital, it has a short elimination

half-life and therefore large doses do not accumulate in peripheral compartments. Thus, its duration remains short, even after prolonged infusions. This characteristic makes it a unique sedative in the operating room and the ICU.

As with many anesthetics, propofol causes myocardial depression and vasodilatation. During induction of anesthesia, a decrease in blood pressure of 24 to 45 percent often occurs.[61] Propofol should only be used when the expertise to manage the respiratory and cardiovascular side effects is available. Propofol probably has both anticonvulsant and proconvulsant actions.[62] Animal studies have shown its anticonvulsant effects; propofol has been used successfully to treat status epilepticus. However, a wide variety of motor phenomena have been reported in human patients: i.e., grand-mal convulsions, opisthotonus, tonic-clonic movements, muscle rigidity, and athetoid movements. These have occurred during induction of anesthesia and even several hours after recovery. This excessive motor activity may be related to abnormal subcortical electrical activity.[63]

Ketamine is a dissociative anesthetic chemically related to phencyclidine (PCP). It creates a functional and electrophysiologic dissociation between the thalamoneocortical and limbic systems.[64] Ketamine produces what is described as a "cataleptic state," Nystagmus is often present. Hypertonus, purposeful movement, and vocalizations can occur. Corneal and light reflexes are maintained. Ketamine causes central sympathetic stimulation, which can increase heart rate and blood pressure and also intracranial pressure. A major disadvantage of ketamine is the frequent occurrence of emergence phenomena, such as floating sensations, vivid dreams, dysphoria, delirium, and hallucinations. The incidence of these reactions is decreased by coadministration of a benzodiazepine such as midazolam.[64,65] Because of this potential for emergence reactions, ketamine is only used in special circumstances. For example, the cardiovascular stimulant effects are beneficial in hypovolemic critically ill patients. Ketamine also causes bronchodilatation and therefore is useful in acute severe asthma cases for sedation prior to endotracheal intubation. It is also used in pediatric cardiac surgery. Ketamine is also the only induction agent with analgesic properties.

CENTRAL NERVOUS SYSTEM DEPRESSANTS: AN APPROACH TO DIAGNOSIS AND MANAGEMENT

Causes of Postoperative Alterations of Consciousness

The majority of postoperative abnormalities of consciousness are apparent soon after arrival in the postanesthesia care unit (PACU) or ICU. Reactions to recovery from anesthesia range from prolonged somnolence to extreme combativeness. When a patient is allowed to recover from the anesthetic slowly (e.g., after cardiac or prolonged surgery), problems may not be apparent until long after the surgery. The causes of prolonged emergence can be classifed as systemic, drug-related, or CNS-related (see Table 16B-5).

Systemic problems affect the metabolic milieu of the nervous system. Hypoxemia and hypercarbia should always be considered first. Hypercarbia secondary to CNS depression is generally not associated with respiratory distress or agitation. In the presence of normal respiratory drive, hypercarbia or hypoxia can produce severe agitation.

Examples include airway obstruction, pulmonary edema, pneumothorax, and bronchospasm. Retained secretions or inappropriate ventilator settings in mechanically ventilated patients can cause distress. Cardiac dysfunction with cerebral hypoperfusion can impair consciousness. Metabolic problems can present postoperatively, especially hyponatremia, metabolic acidosis, and hyper- or hypoglycemia. Underlying medical problems can become unmasked during periods of perioperative stress. Examples include thyroid dysfunction, adrenal insufficiency, and renal and hepatic insufficiency. A high index of suspicion is required to detect these problems. Hypothermia and hyperthermia can also impair consciousness and decrease drug elimination rates.

Drug effects are probably the most common causes of abnormalities of consciousness in the general postoperative population. Postoperative somnolence is commonly caused by residual effects of anesthetic agents.[66] It is more common after long-duration anesthetics, in elderly patients, after high concentrations of inhaled agents have been used, or after long-acting intravenous agents have been used. Patients who are fatigued or sleep-deprived can also have a slower recovery.

Recovery can be affected by preoperative medications, especially psychotropic medications in long-term use. Benzodiazepines can cause paradoxical excitement reactions. Scopolamine is an anticholinergic drug sometimes used for its anti-sialogogue and sedative properties. It can produce disorientation, paranoia, and combativeness, as well as other manifestations of the central anticholinergic syndrome.[67] Central anticholinergic syndromes can potentially be caused by any medication with anticholinergic actions (e.g., atropine,[68] or tricyclic antidepressants). The toxic CNS effects of anticholinergic medications include delirium, restlessness, irritability, confusion, obtundation, hallucinations, and seizures. Other drugs have been reported to cause this syndrome, including meperidine[58] and benzodiazepines. An example of this syndrome occurred in a young male who underwent upper limb surgery under regional anesthesia. He was sedated with midazolam, 2 mg, and fentanyl, 75 μg. Postoperatively, he

Table 16B-5
Causes of postoperative agitation and alterations of consciousness

I. Systemic
  A. Respiratory
    1. Hypoxemia
    2. Hypercarbia
  B. Cardiovascular
    1. Circulatory failure (i.e., hypotension, shock)
  C. Metabolic
    1. Hypoglycemia/hyperglycemia (including diabetic ketoacidosis, hyperosmolar states)
    2. Hyponatremia/hypernatremia
    3. Hypocalcemia
    4. Hypermagnesemia
    5. Renal failure
    6. Hepatic failure
    7. Endocrine (e.g., myxedema, adrenal insufficiency)
    8. Hypothermia/hyperthermia (including maligaant hyperthermia crisis)
II. Drug-related
  A. Opioids
  B. Benzodiazepines
  C. Neuromuscular blocking agents (persistent neuromuscular blockade)
  D. Inhaled anesthetic agents
  E. Miscellaneous psychotropic agents (e.g., phenothiazines, anticholinergic agents, ketamine)
  F. Intoxicants (e.g., alcohol, street drugs)
III. CNS-related
  A. Pre-existing organic brain disorders
  B. Noxious stimuli
    1. Surgical pain
    2. Other (e.g., endotracheal tubes, nasogastric catheters, other invasive devices)
  C. Acute CNS insults
    1. Ischemia and/or anoxia
    2. Mass lesions
    3. Vascular events, embolism
    4. Seizures
  D. Psychiatric (e.g., extreme anxiety, pre-existing psychiatric dysfunction)

was initially agitated but by the fourth postoperative day he had developed coma. Rapid and complete resolution of all symptoms occurred after physostigmine, 2 mg, was given.[69] Chronic benzodiazepine use was thought to be a causative factor in the development of this patient's anticholinergic syndrome.

Prolonged effects of neuromuscular blocking agents can result in a patient who is conscious, yet profoundly weak or unable to move at all. There are rare reports of patients being aware during a surgical procedure and yet unable to move because of neuromuscular blockade. It is obvious why this situation would be extremely unpleasant. Patients with incomplete reversal of neuromuscular blockade usually have unco-ordinated, flailing movements, sometimes described as "flopping like a fish out of water." The patient is at risk of airway obstruction, aspiration, hypoventilation, and hypoxemia. Persistent neuromuscular blockade can be caused by excessive doses of nondepolarizing (or competitive) neuromuscular blockers or inadequate reversal with acetylcholinesterase (AChE) inhibitors. Patients with neuromuscular disease may decompensate in the presence of residual neuromuscular blocking drugs and/or sedative drugs. Patients in the ICU are at risk of accumulation of neuromuscular blocking agents and their active metabolites. There are also reports of patients receiving large doses of corticosteroids and neuromuscular blockers who developed a myopathy.[53] Succinylcholine, a depolarizing neuromuscular blocker, has a prolonged duration of action (8 to 16 h) in patients with atypical plasma cholinesterase.[70]

Recovery from anesthesia can be associated with profound emotional swings and agitation. There are many non-drug factors associated with untoward reactions. These types of emergence reactions are more common in children and young adults. Patients with pre-existing psychiatric disorders, mental retardation, or organic brain dysfunction can decompensate during recovery. Patients who are hostile preoperatively often maintain their aggressive tendencies postoperatively. Language barriers impair communication with a disoriented or confused patient. Emotionally charged procedures, such as breast biopsy, are also associated with emergence reactions. Also, the elderly have a slower recovery of cognitive function after general anesthesia.[71] Of the individual anesthetic agents, ketamine has the greatest incidence of emergence phenomena (as previously described).

Pain is a common cause of agitation. There are numerous sources of pain in critically ill patients. Pain and discomfort can arise from a surgical site, endotracheal and nasogastric tubes, or even a distended urinary bladder. However, if communication with the patient is impaired, the assessment of pain can be difficult. The psychologic stress of illness and the multiple noxious stimuli in the ICU can cause agitation and delirium. Loss of the day-night cycle and the absence of natural light can contribute to delirium.[72]

Primary neurologic causes occasionally present postoperatively. Anesthetic complications causing CNS injury are, fortunately, very rare. With the current standard of intraoperative monitoring and vigilance, many episodes of hypoxia and ischemia are brief and do not result in cardiac or neurologic sequelae. Intracranial mass lesions are unlikely to develop intraoperatively, but acute deterioration may occur due to hemorrhage or edema. Status epilepticus is another diagnosis to be considered, especially in patients at risk of alcohol withdrawal or who have underlying seizure disorders.

Perioperative stroke is a serious complication since it carries a mortality of approximately 26 percent[73,74] The reported incidence ranges from 0.07 percent in the general surgical population to 3.2 percent in a population of surgical patients over 90 years of age 75.[75] Stroke is more likely after high-risk procedures, such as carotid endarterectomy—where the incidence of permanent CNS complications ranges from 1.0 to 5.2 percent.[76] The incidence of stroke associated with cardiopulmonary bypass is about 5 percent for coronary artery surgery and slightly higher for cardiac valve surgery.[77] For cardiopulmonary bypass surgery, stroke occurs more commonly in patients with clinical or laboratory evidence of carotid disease.

In noncardiac, noncarotid surgery, the risk factors for stroke include a history of hypertension, smoking, previous neurologic symptoms, and an abnormal rhythm on the echocardiogram (ECC).[73] The majority of strokes occur postoperatively, after a lucid interval.[78,79] The mechanism can be difficult to ascertain, but a significant number of strokes are thought to be cardioembolic in origin, especially if atrial fibrillation is present. In most cases, the onset of a neurologic deficit occurs several days postoperatively. A causative role for intraoperative hypotension has not been clearly demonstrated.[78,79,74] Many of these patients have other significant factors, such as atrial fibrillation, or they have a hemorrhagic stroke. The postoperative hypercoagulable state may be a factor in thrombotic or embolic stroke. Unusual causes of perioperative stroke include events such as paradoxical cerebral emboli in patients with a patent foramen ovale.[80]

Clinical and Laboratory Assessment

The patient with impaired consciousness in the PACU could simply be "slow to wake up" or could have a life-threatening problem. Therefore, assessment should begin with simultaneous assessment and management of the airway, breathing, and circulation (the ABCs). Vital signs, including continuous ECG, blood pressure, temperature, and pulse oximetry, should be assessed. The previously discussed systemic problems should be ruled out.

Following cardiopulmonary stabilization, the CNS can be assessed. The patient's level of consciousness may change rapidly; if the patient is simply recovering from anesthesia, there should be noticeable improvement within 30 to 60 min. A patient who has received a significant amount of opioid may appear to be asleep but respond appropriately when stimulated. An agitated patient is often calmed by initial attempts at reassurance and "reorientation" to the PACU. The Glasgow Coma Scale was designed to assess level of consciousness in patients with head injury. It is less reliable in patients with nontraumatic causes of impaired consciousness. It also has limitations in patients who are intubated or cannot open their eyes. The Reaction Level Scale is an alternative clinical measurement tool for assessing level of consciousness in patients with acute brain disorders, including self poisoning.[81] There are also scales specifically designed to assess levels of sedation in ICU patients.[82]

Motor examination may note a generalized increase in tone and/or tremor that may have a clonic pattern or resemble normal shivering.[83] This commonly occurs after the use of volatile anesthetics. In a co-operative patient, motor power should be assessed (e.g., hand grip strength). The most sensitive sign of residual neuromuscular blockade is an inability to sustain a head lift off the pillow for 5 s.[84] Testing of vital capacity is not practical in an unstable patient. If the patient cannot co-operate, a peripheral nerve stimulator should be used to test for residual neuromuscular blockade.

Postoperatively, the pupils are usually small when opioids have been used. Atropine is often given intravenously with an anticholinesterase drug to reverse nondepolarizing muscle relaxants. This combination of drugs does not have a significant effect on pupillary size.[85] Corneal reflexes are abolished by deep levels of anesthesia. Cough and gag reflexes are important, not just as clinical signs, but also as mechanisms of protecting the airway from aspiration of gastric contents. Airway protection can be assessed by the patient's response to oral suctioning or to the presence of an endotracheal tube or oral airway.

In general, physical findings in patients with a depressant-induced coma are similar to those of coma from other metabolic causes. Deep tendon reflexes, corneal reflexes, and caloric responses are all depressed or absent with deep levels of drug intoxication. Also, motor tone becomes flaccid, and there may be decorticate posturing. Spontaneous eye movement is decreased. There are a few key signs, however. Opioids cause hypoventilation, miosis, and bradycardia. The pupils are pinpoint with severe opioid intoxication; reaction to light may require a magnifying glass to observe. Pupil size was used to assess depth of anesthesia when ether was used. With current anesthetic agents, there is not a dose-response relationship. Instead, pupil size depends on the presence of opioids and the amount of sympathetic activity present.

The patient's past medical and surgical history should be reviewed, including medications and drug intolerances. Intoxication with street drugs or alcohol should be considered. The anesthetic record should be checked for specific details. For example, the induction drugs and doses may provide information about the patient's sensitivity to hypnotics. The amounts of opioids and volatile agents given during the maintenance phase are important, as is the duration of the anesthetic and the surgery. Additional drugs may have been given (e.g., mannnitol for raised intracranial pressure). The use of muscle relaxants and their reversal is important. Finally, intraoperative complications and any general comments should be noted.

Laboratory assessment is initially aimed at systemic derangements, and therefore a systems approach can guide testing. Arterial blood gases and a chest film (using a portable x-ray machine) can be quickly obtained. An ECG may show signs of myocardial ischemia. Of note, ECG abnormalities have been well-characterized in patients with head injury, tumors, meningitis, cerebral infarction, and especially subarachnoid hemorrhage. These include large upright T waves, T wave inversion, QT prolongation, and ST segment depression or elevation. These abnormalities have an association with potentially fatal ventricular dysrhythmias.[86] Blood tests that may be obtained include hemoglobin and coagulation parameters, electrolytes, urea, creatinine, serum osmolality (especially if osmotic or loop diuretics are used), and glucose. There is little role for testing levels of specific sedative drugs. In this author's hospital, only qualitative tests are routinely available to screen for the presence of benzodiazepines, barbiturates, and opioids. Clinical experience with quantitative assays is limited.

Specific CNS testing depends on the clinical situation and is discussed in Chap. 3. There may be special situations, such as after neurosurgical procedures, where CT scanning or angiography are required. Electroencephalographic assessment may be useful in the patient with a known seizure disorder or an unusual emergence reaction.

General and Specific Management

As mentioned in the previous section, the initial management should always follow the "airway, breathing, and circulation" (ABC) approach. This focuses attention on the most life-threatening problems first. The reader is referred to standard texts of critical care for information on cardiopulmonary management.

The patient with significant muscle weakness should be oxygenated and ventilated by mask, with consideration given to urgent intubation. Management should follow the "ventilate, sedate, and wait" principle. This situation has many features in common with a myasthenic crisis or severe Guillain-Barré syndrome. If the patient is obtunded, there is usually no need for further anesthetic drugs during the initial management.

The agitated patient can be difficult to manage. Underlying systemic or drug-related problems are frequently present. Hypoxemia, hypercarbia, and hypovolemia should be identified and managed promptly. Administration of anesthetic drugs may be necessary to control an aggressive patient, yet the drugs can cause further disorientation and agitation. Once the situation is under control, a more thorough assessment can be carried out.

There are three specific reversal agents commonly available: physostigmine, naloxone, and flumazenil. Physostigmine is a reversible inhibitor of AChE. It has a tertiary amine structure and therefore crosses the blood-brain barrier. Thus, it is used to antagonize central anticholinergic syndromes by increasing the amount of acetylcholine (ACh) available at receptors in the CNS. The primary indication for physostigmine is treatment of a central anticholinergic syndrome associated with drugs such as atropine and scopolamine. It has also been used to antagonize the effects of other drugs that have anticholinergic side effects (e.g., phenothiazines and tricylic antidepressants).

Physostigmine has also been reported to antagonize the sedative effects of the benzodiazepines.[87,88] There are reports that it also has a reversal effect on ventilatory depression from opioids.[89,90] Also, there is evidence that physostigmine decreases postoperative somnolence after volatile anesthetics have been used.[91]. This evidence suggests that ACh receptor blockade need not be present for an effect from physostigmine to be seen. Perhaps, baseline cholinergic activity can still be potentiated by physostigmine, resulting in a stimulating effect on consciousness. Other drugs possibly antagonized by physostigmine include diphenhydramine, benztropine, haloperidol, and meperidine.[92]

Physostigmine can be given in 1 mg doses to a maximum of 3 mg. The duration of action is short due to its rapid metabolism by ester hydrolysis. All cholinesterase inhibitors allow accumulation of ACh in the heart, which can cause bradycardia. Physostigmine is contraindicated in the presence of cyclic antidepressant toxicity because of its propensity to cause asystole. Therefore, it should be used with caution, particularly when the patient's drug history is not completely known. In clinical practice, central anticholinergic syndromes are not common and the specific instances when this drug is useful are limited.

Naloxone, a derivative of oxymorphone, is a pure competitive antagonist at all opioid receptors. There are other antagonists and agonist-antagonists, which will not be discussed here. When given intravenously, the peak effect of naloxone occurs in 1 to 2 min. Naloxone has a half-life of 60 to 90 min and is metabolized in the liver. It is not given orally because of a first-pass effect. The duration of action is dose dependent but averages at 30 to 45 min; this is, in part, due to rapid removal of the drug from brain.[93]

Naloxone is used to treat a known or suspected opioid overdose. This can occur after self-intoxication, after general anesthesia, or after opioid administration for pain. Naloxone is used in the depressed neonate who has received opioids across the placenta. It can also be used to diagnose opioid tolerance. Adverse effects include severe pain and agitation, especially in the postoperative or intubated patient. Severe hypertension,[94,95] pulmonary edema,[96–98] cardiac dysrhythmias, and cardiac arrest[99,100] have occurred with naloxone use, even in young, healthy patients. These effects are thought to be caused by the reversal of the beneficial effects of opioids, particularly sedation and analgesia. This can lead to sympathetic hyperactivity and cardiovascular complications. An acute withdrawal syndrome can be precipitated in addicts. Therefore, caution is advised in the patient who might be tolerant of opioids. This can even occur in the neonate of an opioid-addicted mother. Nausea and vomiting can occur with rapid intravenous administration. Finally, return of respiratory depression and sedation (i.e., "renarcotization") are a possibility because the duration of action of most opioids is longer than that of naloxone. Thus, the patient should be observed carefully until the opioid has cleared from the plasma. Naloxone can be infused to maintain adequate plasma levels. This can avoid the need for ventilatory support. In patients with iatrogenic intoxication, standard doses can provoke the adverse reactions previously mentioned. Therefore, titrating smaller doses is best (e.g., 40 to 80 µg/L

increments in the postoperative patient) until the desired effect is seen. In the postoperative patient, an attempt is made to reverse the respiratory depression while maintaining analgesia.

Naloxone is used in the emergency department as both a diagnostic and a therapeutic agent in patients with impaired consciousness. However, benefit is only likely if at least one of the following criteria is also present: (1) respiratory rate ≤ 12, (2) pinpoint pupils, or (3) circumstantial evidence of opioid use (e.g., needle tracks, bystander corroboration).[101] Withholding naloxone in the agitated patient who does not have any of these clinical criteria is appropriate. Naloxone has a safe record in the emergency department; however, there are a few precautions. The opioid-dependent patient is at risk of developing the withdrawal syndrome. If this occurs, the patient might then reinject opioid after leaving the hospital, resulting in an overdose. Also, the patient should not be discharged shortly after receiving naloxone. The duration of action of most street opioids is longer than that of naloxone; therefore, the patient is at risk of renarcotization.[102] The dose in the opioid-dependent patient is an initial 0.1 mg to a maximum of 0.8 mg intravenously. In the patient with impaired consciousness but no respiratory depression, the dose range is also 0.1 to 0.8 mg. If respiratory depression is present, the dose range is 2.0 to 10 mg. Higher doses are generally required in patients who have taken synthetic opioids (e.g., propoxyphene, fentanyl or pentazocine). This author recommends that the dose of naloxone be titrated, guided by the particular drug and dose, to a desired effect. The aim is for reversal of respiratory depression without precipitation of withdrawal, loss of analgesia, or even complete return of consciousness (which might result in an uncooperative patient). Once an appropriate dose has been found, an infusion can be initiated to maintain the desired effect.

Flumazenil, an imidobenzodiazepine, is a specific, competitive benzodiazepine receptor antagonist. It does not reverse sedation caused by other sedatives such as ethanol, opioids, or barbiturates. Onset of action occurs within minutes and the half-life is 42 to 72 min. Therefore, resedation can occur when long-acting benzodiazepine, or when large doses of a short-acting drug such as midazolam, have been given. The average dose to reverse sedative effects is 0.3 to 0.6 mg, titrated in 0.1 to 0.2 mg increments. The maximum recommended dose is 2.0 mg.

Adverse effect, such as nausea, vomiting, and headache, have been reported with flumazenil. Seizures and cardiac arrhythmias can occur in patients who have also ingested epileptogenic drugs, such as theophylline, or cyclic antidepressants.[103] It is thought that the anticonvulsant action of the benzodiazepine protects against seizures that would otherwise be caused by the other proconvulsant drugs. Antagonism of the benzodiazepine action then unmasks the seizure potential of the other drugs. A withdrawal syndrome can occur in patients physically dependent on benzodiazepines. Also, flumazenil reverses other beneficial effects of the benzodiazepine, such as anxiolysis or the favourable effect on cerebral metabolic rate and cerebral blood flow. Interestingly, flumazenil may not completely reverse the respiratory depression caused by benzodiazepines: its effect has been inconsistent and sometimes short-lived. The improvement in ventilation may be a result of improved level of consciousness.[104] Therefore, the drug is not recommended for reversal of respiratory depression.

Flumazenil is effective for reversal of sedation from benzodiazepines used with regional anesthesia and other invasive procedures. It may also hasten recovery from sedation in ICU patients, but it is somewhat less effective in this situation.[105] It may also be helpful in differentiating sedative effects of benzodiazepines from other causes of impaired consciousness.[102] This may avoid the need for interventions such as computed tomography (CT) scanning and intubation.[106] It may even permit history-taking from a previously unconscious patient.[107] However, rapid changes in the level of consciousness are not without risk. One patient awakened after administration of flumazenil but became resedated 10 min later, vomited, and developed aspiration pneumonia.[107]

In the emergency department, flumazenil has not shared the same success as naloxone. Benzodiazepines do not produce the same degree of respiratory depression that opioids do. They can also have some beneficial effects. Controversy exists as to the appropriate use of flumazenil in the emergency department. There are several considerations when contemplating the use of flumazenil in this situation. Basic supportive measures and toxicology management should always be carried out first. The clinical features should be consistent with a significant benzodiazepine component to the toxicity. Tachycardia, hypotension, increased muscle tone, hyperreflexia, and ECG abnormalities are not caused by benzodiazepines. The reversal of the benzodiazepine effect is not always desirable. For example, the patient could require sedation for mechanical ventilation.[102] Flumazenil is contraindicated if coingestion of cyclic antidepressants or other epileptogenic substances is suspected. It should be used with caution, if at all, in patients with any potential for seizures or a withdrawal syndrome. Therefore, this author recommends that flumazenil not be routinely used in patients with impaired consciousness in the emergency department. However, its use should be based on a careful clinical and laboratory evaluation of the patient. Considering how the drug will specifically improve the management of the patient is important.

DISCUSSION OF CASES

Please refer to Cases 1 and 2 presented at the beginning of this chapter. The first patient experienced a cardiorespiratory emergency. The degree and duration of hypoxia and hypotension were not documented; however, he did not have a cardiac arrest. Therefore, hypoxic-ischemic encephalopathy could not be diagnosed with any degree of certainty. Also, documentation of the sedatives and doses administered was not provided. Sometimes, in an emergency, patients are heavily sedated to facilitate mask ventilation and intubation. The clinical duration of the sedative action depends on the pharmacokinetics the drugs and the individual patient's response. Even when a drug with a short duration of action is used (e.g., midazolam), large doses may have a prolonged duration of action. This patient was in cardiogenic shock, which slows the redistribution of drugs. Also, since hepatic and renal blood flow are decreased in this condition, drug clearance is impaired. Thus, in critically ill patients, prolonged effects should be anticipated, though they cannot be accurately predicted. Knowledge of the exact doses given to the patient may not change the management. The options here are the following: (1) to wait until the drugs are metabolized while supporting ventilation, or (2) to administer a specific antagonist in addition to respiratory support. Since this patient had been given diazepam, administration of flumazenil was chosen. Within minutes the patient opened his eyes spontaneously and responded to questions. It was then possible to rule out a major hypoxic-ischemic event or structural lesion. A transesophageal ECG revealed a ruptured papillary muscle with mitral valve incompetence. The patient underwent successful mitral valve replacement.

The second case illustrates many problems typical of an ICU patient. Important historical facts to obtain include the duration and doses of anesthetic drugs. The degree of renal and hepatic dysfunction is important. Residual neuromuscular blockade should be ruled out with a peripheral nerve stimulator. This patient's age, female sex, and renal dysfunction placed her at risk of prolonged muscle weakness. These factors can also prolong the duration of morphine and midazolam for hours or days.

Further investigation was carried out to rule out treatable causes of this patient's depressed consciousness. A CT scan of the brain was normal. The CSF examination was also normal. An EEG showed diffuse slow-wave abnormalities. A peripheral nerve stimulator demonstrated persistent blockade of the neuromuscular junction. Because of this, flumazenil and naloxone were not given; these drugs could leave the patient conscious but unable to move. Over the following days, there was a progressive improvement in consciousness. Eventually, the patient made a full recovery. Retrospectively, it was felt that her impaired consciousness was multifactorial. The most significant factors were probably prolonged effects of sedative drugs and septic encephalopathy.

REFERENCES

1. Stanski DR, Watkins WD: *Drug Disposition in Anesthesia.* New York, Grune and Stratton 1982.
2. Hudson RJ, Stanski DR, Burch PG: Pharmacokinetics of methohexital and thiopental in surgical patients. *Anesthesiology* 59:215, 1983.
3. Kortilla K, Linnoila M, Ertama P: Recovery and simulated driving after intravenous anesthesia with thiopental, methohexital, propanidid, or alphadione. *Anesthesiology* 43:291, 1975.
4. Carpenter RL, Eger EL, Johnson BH, et al: The extent of metabolism of inhaled anesthetics in humans. *Anesthesiology* 65:201, 1986.
5. Smiley RM: An overview of induction and emergence characteristics of desflurane in pediatriac, adult, and geriatric patients. *Anesth Anal* 75:s38, 1992.
6. Homer TD, Stanski DR: The effect of increasing age on thiopental disposition and anesthetic requirement. *Anesthesiology* 62:714, 1985.
7. Greenblatt DJ, Sellers EM, Shader RI: Drug disposition in old age. *N Engl J Med* 306:1081, 1982.
8. Kaiko RF, Wallenstein SL, Rogers AG, et al: Narcotics in the elderly. *Med Clin North Am* 66:1079, 1982.
9. Munson ES, Hoffman JC, Eger EI: Use of cyclopropane to test generality of anesthetic requirement in the elderly. *Anesth Anal* 63:998, 1984.
10. Jung D, Mayersohn M, Perrie D, Calkins J, Saunders R: Thiopental disposition as a function of age in female patients undergoing surgery. *Anesthesiology* 56:163, 1982.
11. Bentley JB, Borel JD, Nad RE, Gillespie TJ: Age and fentanyl pharmacokinetics. *Anesth Analg* 61:968, 1982.
12. Barash PG, Cullen BF, Stoelting RK: *Clinical Anesthesia*, 2nd ed. Philadelphia, JB Lippincott, 1992, p 309.
13. Olsen GD, Bennet WM, Porter GA: Morphine and phenytoin binding to plasma proteins in renal and hepatic failure. *Clin Pharmacol Ther* 17:677, 1975.
14. Grossman SH, Davis D, Kitchell BB, et al: Diazepam and lidocaine plasma protein in renal disease. *Clin Pharmacol Ther* 31:350, 1982.

15. Duchin KL, Schrier RW: Interrelationship between renal hemodynamics, drug kinetics, and drug action. *Clin Pharmacokinet* 3:58, 1978.

16. Garrett ER: Pharmacokinetics and clearances related to renal processes. *Int J Clin Pharmacol* 16:155, 1978.

17. Miller RD, Agoston S, Booij LHDJ, et al: The comparative potency and pharmacokinetics of pancuronium and its metabolites in anesthetized man. *J Pharmacol Exp Ther* 207:539, 1978.

18. Segredo V, Caldwell JE, Matthay MA, Sharma ML, Gruenke L: Persistent paralysis in critically ill patients after long-term administration of vecuronium. *N Engl J Med* 327:524, 1992.

19. Szeto HH, Inturnsi CE, Houde R, et al: Accumulation of normeperidine, an active metabolite of meperidine, in patients with renal failure or cancer. *Ann Intern Med* 86:738, 1977.

20. Stenson RE, Constantino RT, Harrison DC: Interrelationships of hepatic blood flow, cardiac output, and blood levels of lidocaine in man. *Circulation* 43:205, 1971.

21. Benowitz NL, Meister W: Pharmacokinetics in patients with cardiac failure. *Clin Pharmacokinet* 1:389, 1976.

22. Jensen NF, Fiddler DS, Stroepe V: Anesthetic considerations in prophyrias. *Anesth Analg* 80:591–599, 1995.

23. Koblin DD: Mechanisms of action. In Miller RD (ed): *Anesthesia*, 4th ed. New York, Churchill Livingstone, 1994.

24. Stoelting RK: *Pharmacology and Physiology in Anesthetic Practice*. Philadelphia, JB Lippincott, 1991, p 118.

25. Hara M, Kai Y, Ikemoto Y: Propofol activates GABAA receptor-chloride ioophore complex in dissociated hippocampal neurons in the rat. *Anesthesiology* 79:781–788, 1993.

26. Rothstein JD, Garland W, Puia G, et al: Purification and characterization of naturally occurring benzodiazepine receptor ligands in rat and human brain. *J Neurochem* 58:2102–2115, 1992.

27. Olasmaa M, Rothstein JD, Guidotta, et al: Endogenous benzodiazepine receptor ligands in human and animal hepatic encephalopathy. *J Neurochem* 55:2015–2023, 1990.

28. Jones EA, Basile AS, Yurdaydin C, Skolnich P: Do benzodiazepine ligands contribute to hepatic encephalopathy? *Adv Exp Med Biol* 341:57–69, 1993.

29. Hales TG, Lambert JJ: The actions of propofol on inhibitory amino acid receptors of bovine adrenomedullary chromaffin cells and rodent central neurons. *Br J Pharmacol* 104:619–628, 1991.

30. Amrein R, Hetzel W, Allen SR: Co-induction of anaesthesia: the rationale. *Eur J Anaesthesiology* 12:5–11S, 1995.

31. Prince RJ, Simmonds MA: Temperature and anion dependence of allosteric interaction of the gamma-aminobutyric acid-benzodiazepine receptors. *Biochem Pharmacol* 44:1297–1302, 1992.

32. Carla V, Moroni F: General anesthetics inhibit the responses induced by glutamate receptor agonists in the mouse cortex. *Neurosci Lett* 146:21–24, 1992.

33. Anis NA, Berry SC, Burton NR, Lodge D: The dissociative anesthetics, ketamine and phencyclidine, selectively reduce excitation of central mammalian neurones by N-methyl-aspartate. *Br J Pharmacol* 79:565, 1983.

34. Thomson AM, West DC, Lodge D: An N-methyl-aspartate receptor-mediated synapse in rat cerebral cortex: a site of ketamine? *Nature* 313:479, 1985.

35. Lodge D, Anis NA: Effects of ketamine and three other anaesthetics on spinal reflexes and inhibitions in the cat. *Br J Anaesth* 56:1143–1151, 1984.

36. Finck AD, Ngai SH: Opiate receptor mediation of ketamine analgesia. *Anesthesiology* 56:291–729, 1982.

37. Smith DJ, Bouchal RL, deSanctis CA, et al: Properties of the interaction between ketamine and opiate binding siters in vivo and in vitro. *Neuropharmacology* 26:1253–1260, 1987.

38. Mantz J, Varlet C, Lecharney JB, et al: The effects of volatile anesthetics, thiopental, and ketamine on spontaneous and depolarization-evoked dopamine release from striatal synaptosomes in the rat. *Anesthesiology* 80:352–363, 1994.

39. Mantz J, Delumeau JC, Cordier J, Petitet F: Differential effects of propofol and ketamine on cytosolic calcium concentrations of astrocytes in primary culture. *Br J Anaesth* 72:351–355, 1994.

40. Mendelson WB: Neuropharmacology of sleep induction by benzodiazepines. *Crit Rev Neurobiol* 6:221–232, 1992.

41. Wong BS, Martin CD: Ketamine inhibition of cytoplasmic calcium signalling in rat pheochromocytoma (PC-12) cells. *Life Sci* 53:PL359–364, 1993.

42. Tonner PH, Miller KW: Molecular sites of general anesthetic action on acetylcholine receptor. *Eur J Anaesthesiol* 12:21, 1995.

43. Dilger JP, Vidal AM, Mody HI, Liu Y: Evidence for direct actions of general anesthetics on an ion channel protein. *Anesthesiology* 81:431–442, 1994.

44. Amrein R, Hetzel W, Harmann D, Lorscheid T: Clinical pharmacology of flumazenil. *Eur J Anesthesiol* 2:65, 1988.

45. George KA, Dundee JW: Relative amnestic actions of diazepam, flunitrazepam and lorazepam in man. *Br J Pharmacol* 4:45, 1977.

46. Lebowitz PW, Cote ME, Daniels AL, et al: Comparative cardiovascular effects of midazolam and thiopental in healthy patients. *Anesth Analg* 61:661, 1982.

47. Tomichek RL, Roscow CE, Philbin DM, et al: Diazepam-fentanyl interaction: hemodynamic and hormonal effects in coronary arteries. *Anesth Analg* 62:881, 1983.

48. Reves JG, Fragen RJ, Vinik HR, Greenblatt DJ: Midazolam: pharmacology and uses. *Anesthesiology* 62:310, 985.

49. Stoelting RK: *Pharmacology and Physiology in Anesthetic Practice.* Philadelphia, JB Lippincot, 1991, pp 129, 118.

50. Malacrida R, Fritz ME, Suter PM, Crevoisier C: Pharmacokinetics of midazolam administered by continuous infusion to intensive care patients. *Crit Care Med* 20:1122, 1991.

51. Martin WR, Eades CG, Thompson JA, et al: The effects of morphine- and nalophine-like drugs in the nondependent and morphine-dependent spinal dog. *J Pharmacol Exp Ther* 197:517, 1976.

52. Pasternak GW: Multiple morphine and enkephalin receptors in the relief of pain. *JAMA* 266:1362, 1988.

53. Hansen-Flaschen JH, Brazxinsky S, Basile C, et al: Use of sedating and neuromuscular blocking agents in patients requiring mechanical ventilation for respiratory failure; a national survey. *JAMA* 266:2870, 1991.

54. Goodman LS, Gilman A, Gilman AG: *Pharmacological Basis of Therapeutics.* New York, Pergamon Press, 1990, p 490.

55. Ropper AH: *Neurological and Neurosurgical Intensive Care,* 3rd ed. New York, Raven Press, 1993, p 38.

56. Cottrell JE, Smith DS: *Anesthesia and Neurosurgery,* 3rd ed. St. Louis, Mosby-Year Book, 1994, p 159.

57. Murphy MR, Olson WA, Hug CC: Pharmaco-kinetics of 3H-fentanyl in the dog anesthetized with enflurane. *Anesthesiology* 50:13, 1979.

58. Eisendrath SJ, Goldman B, Douglas J, et al: Meperidine induced delirium. *Am J Psychiatry* 144:1062, 1987.

59. Etches RC: Postoperative epidural analgesia: is it worth the effort? *Can J Anesth* 42:R20, 1995.

60. Chaney MA: Side effects of intrathecal and epidural opioids. *Can J Anaesth* 42:891, 1995.

61. Sebel PS, Lowdon JD: Propofol: a new intravenous anesthetic. *Anesthesiology* 71:260, 1989.

62. Bevan JC: Propofol-related convulsions. *Can J Anaesth* 40:805, 1993.

63. Reynolds LM, Koh JL: Prolonged spontaneous movement following emergence from propfol/nitrous oxide anesthesia. *Anesth Analg* 76:192, 1993.

64. Reich DL, Silvay G: Ketamine: an update on the first twenty-five years of clinical experience. *Can J Anaesth* 36:186, 1989.

65. Cartwright PD, Pingel SM: Midazolam and diazepam in ketamine anaesthesia. *Anaesthesia* 59:439, 1984.

66. Denlinger JK: Prolonged emergence and failure to regain consciousness, in Orkin FK, Cooperman LH (eds): *Complications in Anesthesiology.* Philadelphia, Lippincott, 1983, p 368.

67. Barash PG, Cullen BF, Stoelting RK: *Clinical Anesthesia,* 2nd ed. Philadelphia, JB Lippincott, 1992, p 1541.

68. Hammon K, Demartino BK: Postoperative delirium secondary to atropine premedication. *Anesth Progress* 32:107, 1985.

69. Carras PM, Mion G, Pats B: A postoperative syndrome of confusion and stupor or a central anticholinergic syndrome. *Cahiers D'Anesthesiologie* 40:112, 1992.

70. Whittaker M: Plasma cholinesterase variants and the anesthetist. *Anaesthesia* 35:174, 1980.

71. Chung F, Seyone C, Dyck B, et al: Age related cognitive recovery after general anesthesia. *Anesth Analg* 71:217, 1990.

72. Wilson LM: Intensive care delirium. The effect of outside deprivation in a windowless unit. *Arch Intern Med* 130:225, 1972.

73. Parikh S, Cohen JR: Perioperative stroke after general surgical procedures. *NY State J Med* 93:162, 1993.

74. Harris EJ, Moneta GL, Yeager RA, et al: Neurologic deficits following noncarotid vascular surgery. *Am J Surgery* 163:537, 1992.

75. Hoskin MP, Lobdell CM, Warner MA, Offord KP, Melton W: Anesthesia for patients over 90 years of age: outcome after regional and general anesthetic techniques for two common surgical procedures. *Anaesthesia* 44:142, 1989.

76. Wong DHW: Perioperative stroke. Part I: General surgery, carotid artery disease, and carotid endarterectomy. *Can J Anaesth* 38:347, 1991.

77. Wong DHW: Perioperative stroke. Part II: Cardiac surgery and cardiogenic embolic stroke. *Can J Anaesth* 38:471, 1991.

78. Hart R, Hindman B: Mechanisms of perioperative cerebral infarction. *Stroke* 137:66, 1982.

79. Landercasper J, Metz BJ, Cogbill TH, et al: Perioperative stroke risk in 173 consecutive patients with a past history of stroke. *Arch Surg* 125:986, 1990.

80. Liu S, Holley S, Stulberg SD, Cohen B: Failure to awaken after general anesthesia secondary to paradoxical venous embolus. *Can J Anaesth* 38:335, 1991.

81. Starmark J-E, Stalhammar D, Holmgren E: The Reaction Level Scale (RLS 85), manual and guidelines. *Acta Neurochirurgica* 91:12, 1988.

82. Ramsay MAE, Savage TM, Simpson BRJ, Goodwin R: Controlled sedation with alphaloxone-alphadolone. *Br M J* 2:56, 1974.

83. Sessler DI, Rubinstein EH: Hypothermia triggers spontaneous post-anesthetic tremor. *Anesthesiology* 73:A173, 1990.

84. Pavlin EG, Holle RH, Schoene RB: Recovery of airway protection compared with ventilation in humans after paralysis with curare. *Anesthesiology* 70:381, 1989.

85. Balamoutsos NG, Drossou FR, Alevizou FR, et al: Pupil size during reversal of muscle relaxants. *Anesth Analg* 59:615, 1980.

86. Marion DW, Segal R, Thompson ME: Subarachnoid hemorrhage and the heart *Neurosurgery* 18:101, 1986.

87. Caldwell CB, Gross JB: Physostigmine reversal of midazolam-induced sedation. *Anesthesiology* 57:125, 1982.

88. Bidwai AV, Stanley TH, Rogers C, Riet EK: Reversal of diazepam-induced postanesthetic somnolence with physostigmine. *Anesthesiology* 51:256, 1979.

89. Bourke DL, Rosenberg M, Allen PD: Physostigmine: effectiveness as an antagonist of respiratory depression and pyschomotor effects caused by

90. Snir-Mor I, Weinstock M, Davidson JT, Bahar M: Physostigmine antagonizes morphine-induced respiratory depression in human subjects. *Anesthesiology* 59:6, 1983.

91. Hill GE, Stanley TH, Sentker CR: Physostigmine reversal of postoperative somnolence. *Can Anaesth Soc J* 24:707, 1977.

92. Barash PG, Cullen BF, Stoelting RK: *Clinical Anesthesia*, 2nd ed. Philadelphia, JB Lippincott, 1992, p 348.

93. Stoeltin RK: *Pharmacology and Physiology in Anesthetic Practice*. Philadelphia, JB Lippincott, 1992, pp 96, 118.

94. Azar I, Turndorf H: Severe hypertension and multiple atrial premature contractions following naloxone. *Anesth Analg* 58:524, 1979.

95. Tanaka GY, Hypertensive reaction to naloxone. *JAMA* 228:25, 1974.

96. Flacke JW, Flaccke WE, William GD: Acute pulmonary edema following naloxone reversal of high dose morphine anesthesia. *Anesthesiology* 47:376, 1977.

97. Schwartz JA, Koenigsberg MD: Naloxone-induced pulmonary edema. *Ann Emerg Med* 161:294, 1987.

98. Taff RH: Pulmonary edema following naloxone administration in a patient without heart disease. *Anesthesiology* 59:76, 1983.

99. Andree RA: Sudden death following naloxone administration. *Anesth Analg* 59:782, 1980.

100. Cuss FM, Colaco CB, Baron JH: Cardiac arrest after reversal of effects of opiates with naloxone. *BMJ* 299:63, 1984.

101. Hoffman JR, Schriger DL, Luc JS: The empiric use of naloxone in patients with altered mental status: a reappraisal. *Ann Emerg Med* 20:246, 1991.

102. Doyon S, Roberts JR. Reappraisal of the "coma cocktail". Dextrose, flumazenil, naloxone, and thiamine. *Emerg Med Clinics N Am* 12:301, 1994.

103. Spivey WH: Flumazenil and seizures: analysis of 43 cases. *Clin Therapeutics* 14:12, 1992.

104. Shalansky SJ, Naumann TL, Englander FA: Effect of flumazenil on benzodiazepine-induced respiratory depression. *Clin Pharmacy* 12:483, 1993.

105. Amaha K, Tsunoda Y, Hashimoto Y, et al: A study on the utility of flumazenil for patients in the ICU (in Japanese). *Masui—Japanese J of Anesth* 39:1101, 1990.

106. Chern TL, Hu C, Lee CH, Deng JF: The role of flumazenil in the management of patients with acute alteration of mental status in the emergency department. *Hum Exper Toxicol* 13:45, 1994.

107. Chern TL, Hu SC, Lee CH, Deng JF: Diagnostic and therapeutic utility of flumazenil in comatose patients with drug overdose. *Am J Emerg Med* 11:122, 1993.

108. Ativan product monograph. Montreal, Wyeth-Ayerst Co, 1995.

109. Barash PG, Cullen BF, Stoelting RK: *Clinical Anesthesia*, 2nd ed. Philadelphia, Lippincott, 1992, p 421.

Part 5

EPISODIC IMPAIRMENT OF CONSCIOUSNESS

Chapter 17

SEIZURES AND STATUS EPILEPTICUS

G. Bryan Young
Eelco F.M. Wijdicks

Casca: *He fell down in the market-place and foamed at the mouth, and was speechless.*
Brutus: *'Tis very like: he hath the falling sickness.*

William Shakespeare, *Julius Caesar*

SEIZURES

Definition of Seizures

A seizure is a paroxysmal disorder of the central nervous system (CNS) characterized by an abnormal, excessive neuronal discharge that results in dysfunction of the brain, including impairment of content of consciousness and alertness.[1] A seizure may be a single, isolated phenomenon, often symptomatic of an acute illnesses, such as head injury, metabolic abnormality, intoxication or systemic or central nervous system inflammation. Unless seizures recur after the acute event or provoking cause has passed, they are not considered to be epilepsy. Therefore, febrile seizures in children or alcohol withdrawal seizures in adults are not considered to be epilepsy. Thus, epilepsy consists of spontaneous, recurring seizures in which the attacks are not acutely symptomatic of a proximate brain insult or of physical or chemical stress. The most extreme ictal motor manifestation is the "convulsion," or generalized convulsive seizure, consisting of loss of consciousness, arrest of ventilation, and tonic contraction of the body's musculature, then generalized rhythmic clonic jerks and autonomic changes.

Epidemiology

The annual incidence rate for seizures is between 73 and 86 per 100,000 people, based on careful case ascertainment in Rochester, Minnesota.[2] Of these cases, about 62 percent represent epilepsy.[2] The peak times for both the occurrence of seizures and for the onset of epilepsy is in childhood and at over 50 years of age.[2]

Classification and Clinical-Electroencephalographic Manifestations

The nature and severity of dysfunction of the brain form the basis for the International Classification of Epileptic Seizures (Table 17-1).[3] Partial seizures are those that begin within one cerebral hemisphere. Generalized seizures appear to begin in both hemispheres simultaneously and reflect a diffuse excitability.

Partial Seizures

Simple Partial Seizures Although consciousness (alertness) is, by definition, preserved in simple partial seizures in those with psychic symptoms, the cognitive function, sensory

Table 17-1
International Classification of Epileptic Seizures

I. Partial (focal, local) seizures
  A. Simple partial seizures (consciousness preserved)
  B. Complex partial seizures (consciousness and memory impaired, but no convulsion)[a]
  C. Secondary generalized (evolve from simple or complex partial seizure into generalized tonic-clonic seizure)[b]

II. Generalized seizures
  A. Absence (formerly petit mal) seizures: typical or atypical[a]
  B. Tonic-clonic seizures[b]
  C. Myoclonic seizures[b]
  D. Clonic seizures[b]
  E. Tonic seizures[b]
  F. Atonic seizures[a]

III. Unclassified seizures (incomplete data)

[a] Nonconvulsive seizures with impaired consciousness.
[b] Convulsive (generalized clonic or tonic movements) seizures with impaired consciousness.
Source: Modified from Ref. 3.

processing, or memory are often dysfunctional. Such a patient may be caught up in hallucinations, illusions, or emotional change with transiently impaired mental function. Furthermore, strictly focal seizures may occur during obtundation from bilateral cerebral lesions or may be superimposed upon a metabolic encephalopathy; such seizures are difficult to classify using the International Classification of Epileptic Seizures (Fig. 17-1).

The associated psychic, motor, sensory, or autonomic symptoms reflect the region of the brain from which the seizure arises; sometimes, there is an evolution of symptoms as the seizure spreads via cortical-cortical circuits or through white matter connections within or between cerebral hemispheres.

Partial seizures have the characteristic that they are often associated with focal interictal spikes between seizures. Recorded seizures may have a variety of manifestations, including spikes that augment in amplitude and frequency, attenuation of voltage, or rhythmic waves that continually

change in amplitude and frequency.[4] There is often an identifiable structural cause, especially in adult-onset cases; some childhood varieties may not have an obvious substrate, e. g., benign Rolandic epilepsy of childhood.[5]

Complex Partial Seizures Complex partial seizures are, by definition, associated with impaired consciousness, but generally not with coma. This is surmised because of the lack of either responsiveness to commands or meaningful interaction with others during the event, and the absence of any memory for the event. However, patients may still interact with the environment to some extent, e.g., resisting physical restraint, so that the "unconsciousness" is not always complete (see Case 2, Chap. 1, p. 29). The main features include profound impairment of cognitive and memory functions during the attack. The patient often demonstrates automatisms, or co-ordinated, involuntary, (usually) repetitive motor activity. With seizures of mesial temporal origin, automatisms often consist of repetitive chewing, lip smacking, or swallowing movements. More complex, interactive, or perseverative (in which the patient repeats a motor act that happened just before the seizures) activities exemplify more elaborate automatisms, implying responsiveness to the environment or activation of stored programs, respectively.

Most complex seizures begin in the mesial-inferior temporal region, but some arise from the poles of the temporal lobe, the opercular-insular region, or the frontobasal-cingulate region.[6] Others have an extratemporal origin, e.g., other parts of the frontal or occipital lobes.[7,8] The impairment of consciousness and memory and the occurrence of automatisms usually reflects spread of the seizure discharge throughout the limbic system bilaterally.[9–11] However, documented impairment in responsiveness and recall occasionally occurs with strictly unilateral seizures.[12] The temporal lobe is nearly always involved. Presumably, the ictal discharge either suspends interpretive and memory functions or distracts the patient sufficiently, while preventing recollection, to preclude responsiveness.

Complex partial seizures recorded from scalp electrodes are quite variable. Patterns include bitemporal or lateralized temporal spikes or rhythmic wave of 8 to 20 Hz, low-voltage high-frequency discharges alternating with diffuse slow frequencies, anterior temporal spikes on a normal background, or, occasionally, little on the electroencephalogram (EEG) change.[13]

Secondary Generalized Seizures Simple or complex partial seizures may evolve into generalized tonic-clonic convulsions (secondary generalization, Table 17-1). Seizure discharges spread from the focus to other regions by existing anatomic pathways.[14] Certain pathways appear to be "preferred" in individual patients, judging by clinical manifestations. These favored paths depend on the seizure intensity, anatomic connections, different susceptibilities of regions to after-discharges, sensitization from previous seizures, and facilitation.[15] Spread or extension of seizures to other sites can be intracortical through synaptic connections or association fibers, intercortical via commissures, or to deeper structures via projections to the thalamus, limbic structures, and the reticular formation.[14] Patients become unconscious as a result of bilateral or diffuse ictal involvement of the cerebral hemispheres or deeper structures (see later). The motor manifestations relate to spread to deeper structures, which are then "driven" by the more rostrally firing neurons. Tonic extension is mediated by the mesencephalic or pontine reticular formation and its descending projections; synchronous clonic contraction of axial and proximal limb muscles in a convulsive seizure are probably also mediated by the brainstem reticular formation and reticulospinal pathways.[2,16]

The EEGs may show focal spikes or slow frequencies interictally. The seizure begins like simple partial seizures, but shows greater spread and synchrony of rapid discharges or generalized attenuation followed by generalized spike-wave as with primary generalized tonic-clonic seizures.

Generalized Seizures

Absence Seizures Absence (formerly "petit mal") seizures usually begin in childhood, but may appear in late life as absence status epilepticus (see later). They occur abruptly, without warning, and similarly terminate in an instant, without confusion postictally. They usually last several seconds only and occur many times a day. Consciousness, as measured by responsiveness, is impaired maximally in the first few seconds and then returns, along with memory and interaction, to various degrees.[17] Absence seizures may be unaccompanied by motor phenomena or there may be only myoclonus of the face (especially of the eyelids) or the limbs, brief atonic phenomena (rarely sufficient to produce falls), brief extensor tonic movements, automatisms similar to those described above for complex partial seizures.[18] The EEG shows a generalized, usually 3 per second, spike-and-wave pattern that begins and ends abruptly. Consciousness, including alertness and cognitive function, returns instantly to normal with cessation of the spike-wave discharges. If the attack persists for several minutes, the repetition rate of the spike-wave slows to 2.5 or even 2 Hz (see Fig. 17-2).

In patients with absence seizures, attention is dysfunctional: continuous performance tasks and auditory (not visual) performance in event-related potentials that depend on detection of unusual stimuli (P300; see Chap. 1) are abnormal.[19] These abnormalities are found even when spike-and-wave discharges are not active. These findings give some evidence to brainstem reticular formation involvement, although bilateral cerebral cortical involvement could also be relevant when there is widespread cortical involvement in the spike-and-wave activity.[20] In general, the degree of impairment of responsiveness is directly related to the extent of generalization of the spike-wave discharges on the EEG.[17,21]

Generalized Tonic-Clonic Seizures Generalized tonic-clonic (formerly "grand mal" seizures may begin with a nonspecific subjective premonitory feeling (aura) or, more typically, without

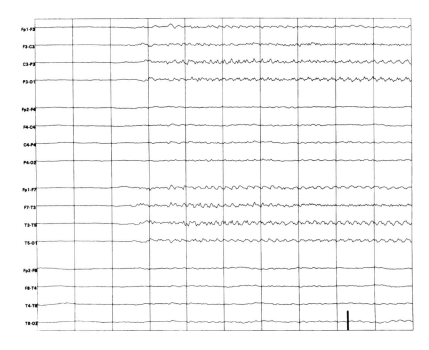

A

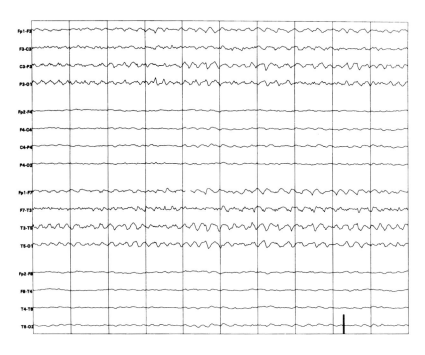

B

Figure 17-1
A. *Evolutionary changes of a partial seizure beginning in the left cerebral hemisphere (odd numbers after the letters) as rapid rhythmic waves.*
B. *and* C. *These change to progressively slower frequencies and show some spread to the right hemisphere (even numbers after the letters) in part* C. *The patient was unconscious with recurrent nonconvulsive seizures due to bilateral subdural hematomas.*

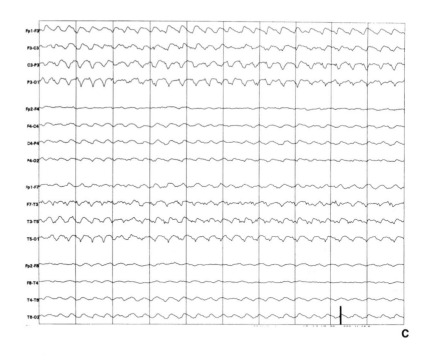

Figure 17-1 (*Continued*)

C

Figure 17-2

An EEG showing generalized spike-and-wave associated with an absence seizure. Note the abrupt onset and recovery, and the slowing of frequency of the spike-and-wave complexes toward the latter part of the epoch.

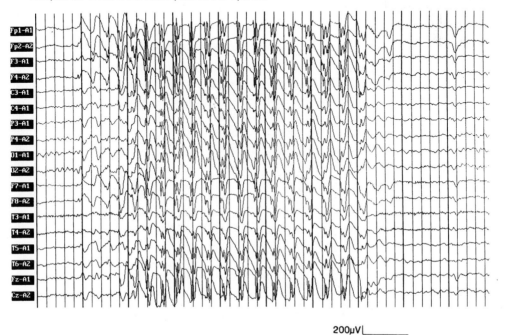

200µV

1 second

warning. Often, one or more brief jerks of one or all of the limbs and the face are followed by generalized tonic contraction of all muscles (air forced through a closed glottis may cause a cry at the onset). There follows a widespread extensor, tonic, vibratory movement and then a generalized clonic phase with symmetric jerking movements of the limbs and jaw, commonly with tongue biting. Loss of consciousness is usually complete, although occasionally patients may recall some features, including their own movements, environmental sounds, auditory hallucinations, or vertigo.[22] The convulsions gradually lessen and are followed by hyperventilation that is related to combined respiratory and metabolic acidoses. The patient remains deeply unconscious for minutes to tens of minutes (usually less than 1 h), then is confused or sleeps for the subsequent minutes to hours. The EEG shows generalized spike-wave followed by generalized rhythmic waves (epileptic recruiting rhythm) at about 10 Hz during the tonic phase; this is interrupted by generalized spikes (related to excitation of a large population of neurons) and slow waves (related to inhibition in the deeper cortical layers.) After the convulsion, the EEG shows generalized suppression of background activity, followed by the return of rhythmic waves that gradually increase in frequency until the patient's usual interictal pattern is achieved.

Other Generalized Seizure Types *Generalized myoclonic seizures* are brief, sudden symmetric jerks of the limbs or face that are single or repetitive. Individual jerks, associated with generalized spikes or polyspikes and waves on EEG, are too brief to allow for testing of responsiveness. However, they sometimes evolve into longer duration seizures or repetitive jerks that usually cause a brief period of impaired consciousness.

Generalized tonic seizures are defined by the sudden but sustained contractions of both sides of the body. There is sometimes a predominance of contraction on one side, causing the head or body to turn. During the tonic seizure, the EEG resembles that of the tonic phase of generalized tonic-clonic seizures (Fig. 17-3).

In *atonic seizure,* a sudden decrease in muscle tone occurs, causing the head or the body to drop forwards. There may be an initial, very brief jerk before the "drop seizure" occurs. At the onset of the atonic seizure, the EEG can show either generalized polyspike-and-wave or suppression of voltage (electrodecremental response).

Pathophysiology of Seizures

The fundamental mechanism of seizures is still uncertain. There is no satisfactory unifying hypothesis and several mechanisms may apply. The suitability of animal models for human seizures is also debated, but there are many useful similarities in EEG and clinical features. The initiation of seizures and their spread appear to relate to burst generation in neuronal populations, a loss of inhibitory influences, increased synchronization of firing, and the propagation of electrical activity along anatomic pathways. Field or electronic effects may play a role, as do neurotransmitters, modulator, and the extracellular concentrations of ions, especially potassium. These and other putative mechanisms are addressed in a number of excellent reviews.[23–26]

Evaluation and Differential Diagnosis

Other conditions that can cause transient impairment of consciousness may mimic seizures. These are discussed in Chap. 18. Among the most common are syncope, transient vascular events including migraine, concussion, transient metabolic disorders including hypoglycemia, intoxications, trauma, transiently raised intracranial pressure, and certain psychiatric disorders. Rarely, mechanisms are combined, e.g., the ictal bradycardia syndrome, in which epileptic seizures trigger cardiogenic syncope or apnea and bradycardia.[27–29]

Usually, the patient is evaluated by a physician *after* a seizure, so that first-hand medical observations or intraictal investigations are not possible. In patients suffering repeated attacks, videotaping, even with a home camera, can be valuable. It is most useful to obtain as much

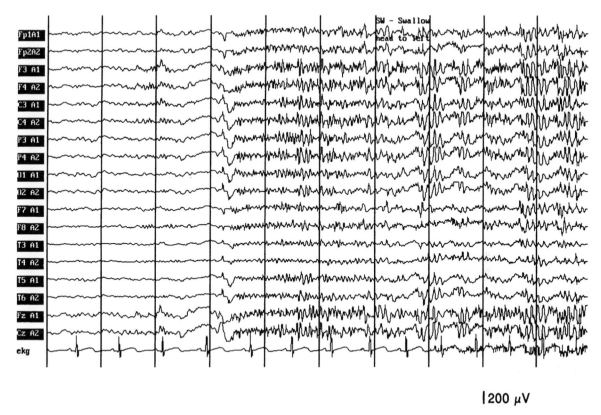

Figure 17-3

A recorded generalized seizure during sleep in a 30-year-old woman with primary generalized epilepsy. The discharge begins in the fourth second as a sharp wave followed by a high-frequency discharge that tends to slow in frequency and augment in amplitude with time. The patient swallowed and showed tonic deviation of the head to the left during the seizure.

information as possible from the patient and from eyewitnesses. The patient should be questioned about the presence or absence of a warning before the loss of consciousness and the nature of any such aura. It is helpful to know if there have been other events of impaired consciousness and how they resembled the current episode. Great variability in manifestations of the episodes raises the possibility of pseudoseizures or more than one condition. Activity preceding the events may help to identify precipitants.

A recent febrile illness, a history of alcohol or illicit drug use, past and current medical illnesses (especially hospitalizations and head injuries), and medications (e.g., theophylline) may reveal causes or precipitants.

During the postictal recuperative phase, the examination can be revealing. Postictal hemiplegia implies a focal origin for the convulsive seizure. If the patient is alert, aphasia denotes an origin in the dominant hemisphere. Pathologic limb withdrawal or extensor motor responses suggest diffuse brain injury or a large intracranial mass that has caused substantial brainstem dysfunction (usually in association with unreactive pupils).

Failure of full awakening or arousability within an hour should lead to a suspicion of underlying factors other than the convulsive seizure

Table 17-2

Some causes of prolonged coma after a single seizure or series of seizures

1. Nonconvulsive status epilepticus
2. Encephalitis
3. Fulminant meningitis
4. Ethanol withdrawal
5. Hypernatremia
6. Hyponatremia
7. Hypoglycemia
8. Nonketotic and hyperosmolar ketotic hyperglycemia
9. Hypocalcemia
10. Hypomagnesemia
11. Uremia
12. Substantial hypoxic or hypoxic-ischemic insult
13. Continued dysfunction from the condition that caused the seizures, e.g., enlarging hemispheric lesion with brainstem compression, hypertensive encephalopathy, trauma, intracranial hemorrhage, CNS infection or other inflammation, stroke, cortical vein thrombosis, or the advanced phase of a neurodegenerative process
14. Substantial hypoxic or hypoxic-ischemic insult
15. Drug withdrawal
16. Intoxication with AEDs, especially repeated doses of barbiturates or benzodiazepines
17. Substance abuse
18. Complications: sepsis

itself, especially the evolution of nonconvulsive status epilepticus (Table 17-2). The differential diagnosis should be possible based on clinical features and selected confirmatory diagnostic laboratory tests.

Investigations

The EEG is a key investigative test, but it has limitations that are reviewed in Chap. 3. The main role of interictal EEG is to aid in the classification of the type of seizure disorder, especially in patients who do not have aurae. Focal EEG abnormalities, notably consistently localized interictal spikes, favor a partial seizure disorder. Generalized epileptiform discharges support a diagnosis of a generalized seizure disorder (see Table 17-1.) Thus the EEG can be indispensable in the differentiation of absence from complex partial seizures and in differentiating primary generalized convulsions from secondary generalized seizures that occur without warning. The EEG features of each major seizure type have been reviewed earlier. A recorded seizure is of enormous diagnostic assistance, but this is uncommon, given the usual 20 to 30-min period of routine recordings. The yield is increased by prolonging the duration of the recording, e.g., using ambulatory recording or prolonged inpatient monitoring, and by activating procedures such as hyperventilation, photic stimulation, sleep recordings, and reduction of antiepileptic drugs (AEDs).

The cause of a seizure in any individual is related to the clinical context, e.g., head injury, stroke, complications of pregnancy, immunosuppression, or age. These give direction to subsequent specific investigations. Magnetic resonance imaging (MRI) or computed tomographic (CT) scanning is advisable in all adult-onset, focally originating seizures; the MRI is superior to CT for most conditions.[30,31] About 60 percent of scans are abnormal, but many show only atrophic changes. Tumors are found in about 10 percent of patients, but the yield is higher in partial seizures of adult onset that do not have a clinically identifiable cause. Other structural causes, including vascular or traumatic lesions, may also be detected. The probability of finding a single structural lesion exceeds 50 percent if there are focal neurologic findings and if the EEG shows a localized abnormality.

Laboratory screening for metabolic abnormalities is helpful in determining the cause for some acute convulsive seizures (e.g., theophylline toxicity, hyponatremia, hypoglycemia, uremia) and in the differential diagnosis of some toxic and metabolic conditions (e.g., impaired functioning from drug intoxication or hypoglycemia) from seizures (see Chaps. 13 and 16). Drug and metabolic analyses can be broad or focused, depending on the possibilities. It has been stated that an elevated serum prolactin concentration gives support to the event being a seizure rather than a syncopal attack or pseudoseizure.[32] However, the specificity of such chemical elevation has been questioned. The level of creatine kinase (CK) in the hours after the episode of loss of consciousness can, however, be quite helpful in establishing that a convulsion has occurred. Inflammation of the CNS should be considered when seizures accompany an acute febrile illness with altered cognitive functioning, focal signs, or meningeal irritation (see Chap. 11). Neuroimaging and cerebrospinal fluid (CSF) analysis are often necessary at least to exclude these treatable disorders.

Management

For an acute seizure, simple "first aid" measures usually suffice. For generalized convulsive seizures, the patient should be rolled onto their side and the mouth cleared of foreign material. This will reduce the possibility of aspiration. Lay persons should be dissuaded from placing an object between the teeth, a common practice in television dramas. The head should be protected from hitting hard objects. For nonconvulsive seizures with impaired consciousness, expectant watching and guidance without restraint is best. If seizures persist, the management for status epilepticus should be instituted (see below).

The diagnosis of a single seizure has a number of implications. The causes, of course, should be addressed. Prediction of subsequent attacks depends on a number of factors.[33,34] Most states, provinces, or countries have guidelines concerning the operation of motor vehicles after a seizure, as mentioned earlier, but if there is a significant risk of subsequent seizures, the physician has a social and usually a legal obligation to advise the patient not to drive for the specified time. The decision to use AEDs is based on both medical and social factors. Principles of AED therapy, including the use of newer agents, are contained in various excellent reviews.[35–44] Surgery is being increasingly utilized, with very favorable results being obtained for selected patients with disabling, refractory, partial seizures.[45]

STATUS EPILEPTICUS

Status epilepticus is defined as seizures that are continuous or recurrent for over 30 min, without either an improvement in clinical state or a return to a preictal EEG pattern between seizures.[46–51]

Classification and Clinical Features

There is not yet a standardized classification of status epilepticus. Any of the seizures listed in Table 17-1 may evolve into status epilepticus. Seizures are often clinically divided into convulsive status epilepticus (CSE) and nonconvulsive status epilepticus (NCSE) (Table 17-1). However, sometimes one blends into the other, e.g., NCSE after CSE is often mistaken for a prolonged "postictal state."

Simple Partial Status Epilepticus During focal status epilepticus from simple partial seizures, patients are usually not comatose, except for those who are unconscious from the event that precipitated the seizures. Others may show impairment of alertness, concentration, or other aspects of mental functioning, variously related to the seizure itself, coexisting metabolic derangements, large structural brain lesions, medications, or combinations of these. One variant of simple partial status epilepticus is "epilepsia partialis continua" (EPC, Kojewnikow syndrome).[52] These patients can be divided into two categories: those with acute focal lesions (e.g., ischemic or hemorrhagic lesions, tumor, severe trauma) or those with chronic focal conditions, including Rasmussen's encephalitis.[52–54] The EPC variant consists of continuous or nearly continuous focal clonic movements confined to one region of the body, often the upper limb. They remain segmental and do not "march" or evolve into either complex partial or secondarily generalized tonic-clonic seizures. Such seizures are notoriously difficult to control and it is usually counterproductive to attempt overtreatment with sedation-producing AEDs.

Convulsive Status Epilepticus These seizures are usually of the generalized tonic-clonic variety, either primarily or secondarily generalized. A CSE episode is often preceded by a premonitory stage of increasing frequency of isolated seizures with interictal recovery. As seizures increase in frequency and severity, patients become increasingly confused; postictal neurologic deficits may fail to clear before the next seizure. Patients with primary generalized epilepsy may develop progressive generalized myoclonic jerking leading up to convulsive status epilepticus. In most patients, loss of awareness occurs abruptly at the beginning of the attack. With secondary generalization of partial seizures (Table 17-1), the initial focal features may be apparent, although in seizures that progress to status epilepticus, the generalization is usually rapid. The initial tonic phase begins in the same manner as for short-duration tonic-clonic seizures. The clonic phase becomes shorter with each successive seizure and may disappear altogether. Biting of the tongue and buccal mucosa and incontinence of bowel and bladder are common. Marked augmentation of sympathetic nervous system activity separates status epilepticus from isolated seizures. Persistent tachycardia, hypersalivation (bloody, frothy saliva and increased risk of aspiration), and hypertension are characteristic of status epilepticus. Pupillary and corneal reflexes are commonly absent; the pupils are usually widely dilated. Patients may become pale or deeply cyanotic.

Following sequential convulsive seizures with incomplete interictal recovery, the level of consciousness may range from delirium to coma. Patients are usually pale and may show neurologic deficits, such as hemiparesis or aphasia. Babinski signs are the rule.

Myoclonic Status Epilepticus in Coma Myoclonic status epilepticus occurs most commonly in patients who are in coma from diffuse brain dysfunction. Shorvon recommends the term "myoclonic status epilepticus in coma."[55] The various conditions causing myoclonic status epilepticus are listed in Table 17-3. The most common condition, in the current authors' experience, has been the post anoxic-ischemic state after cardiac arrest. This is discussed in Chap. 15.

The myoclonus most commonly involves the face, eyes (extraocular eye muscles and orbicularis oculi), and axial muscles, such as the platysma

Table 17-3
Some causes of myoclonic status epilepticus in coma

Acute anoxic-ischemic cerebral damage
Cardiac arrest
Cardiopulmonary surgery
Acute intracranial vascular events
Carbon monoxide poisoning
Carbon dioxide narcosis

Metabolic/toxic encephalopathies
Renal failure
Hepatic failure
Hypoglycemia
Hyponatremia
Dialysis syndrome
Toxins (e.g., heavy metal, bismuth)
Drug intoxication: lithium, imipenim, tricyclics, anticonvulsants (especially carbamazepine), penicillin, haloperidol
Neonatal metabolic disorders
Nonketotic hyperglycemia
Thiamine and other cofactor deficiencies

Physical encephalopathies
Posttraumatic
Heat stroke
Electrical injury
Decompression injury

Degenerative conditions
Creutzfeldt-Jakob disease
Alzheimer disease
Other dementias

Acute viral or inflammatory encephalopathies
Herpes simplex encephalitis
Other viral and bacterial encephalitides
Subacute sclerosing panencephalitis
Acute disseminated encephalomyelitis
Hemorrhagic leukoencephalopathy
Infections in immunosuppressed patients (including HIV[a] infection)

[a] Human immunodeficiency virus.
Source: Adapted from Shorvon.[55]

and diaphragm. The limbs may also be involved. Rhythmic, small-amplitude, horizontal or vertical conjugate eye movement, as well as irregular, small facial twitches that are sometimes asynchronous on the two sides, have been emphasized.[56-58] Tonic-clonic, tonic or clonic seizures may be superimposed on the myoclonic status. Deeply

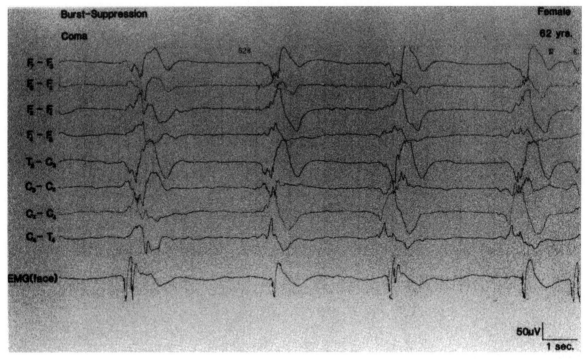

Figure 17-4

An EEG during myoclonic status epilepticus in a 62-year-old woman with severe anoxic-ischemic encephalopathy. Muscle twitches (EMG) occur during the bursts of a burst-suppression pattern. Note the variable relationship of the myoclonus to the bursts. (From Young et al,[59] with permission.)

comatose patients often have impaired cranial nerve reflexes.

The EEG is variable. One of the most common patterns is a generalized burst-suppression, commonly with epileptiform potentials within the bursts. Myoclonus often accompanies the EEG bursts, but the temporal relationship may be inconsistent (see Fig. 17-4). Other patterns include periodic complexes against a suppressed background; again, the relationship of the myoclonus to the complexes often fluctuates. Some EEGs may show no cortical spiking or complexes; in these situations, the myoclonus probably arises entirely from a subcortical structure, e.g., the brainstem reticular formation.

Other   Types   of   Convulsive   Seizures
Although a generalized atonic status epilepticus

is theoretically possible, truly continuous atonic seizures must be rare; sequential attacks with incomplete recovery in between are more likely.

Nonconvulsive Status Epilepticus   Nonconvulsive seizures are epileptic attacks without a tonic, clonic, or tonic-clonic component. The transition from a convulsive or nonconvulsive *seizure* (NCS) into NCSE is the change of a self-limited epileptic attack to a persistent or protracted epileptic state.

The term "generalized nonconvulsive status epilepticus" (generalized NCSE) is probably a better term than "absence status" for these seizures, but the latter term is entrenched. Generalized NSCE may not always be generalized from the onset, as some patients with focally originating seizures may develop the clinical and EEG appearance of generalized epileptiform activity.[60] Thus, generalized NCSE is heterogenous.

Some seizures cannot be easily classified by the International Classification of Epileptic Seizures (Table 17-1). Nevertheless, this system suffices if it is recognized that (1) persistently lateralized or localized seizures may be associated with loss of consciousness in the presence of a coma-producing illness; (2) "atypical absence" status epilepticus can include the following: (a) seizures that have arisen due to diffuse or multifocal brain disease, (b) seizures that have evolved from generalized convulsive seizure activity (in the advanced phase of generalized convulsions, whether primary or secondary generalized), (c) seizures that have a focal accentuation clinically or electrographically, or (d) seizures that respond to diazepam, phenytoin, or other agents.[61,62]

From a modification of the 1981 International Classification of Epileptic Seizures (Table 17-1), nonconvulsive seizures that are consistently associated with impairment of conscious activity principally include absence status epilepticus and complex partial status epilepticus.

In NCSE, mental obtundation varies from a subtle behavioral change, consisting of slowing of cognitive processing, to overt coma. Some patients display an acute confusional state with more profound behavioral change, e.g., aggressiveness or puerile behavior, as the prime manifestation. Many show considerable *fluctuation* in alertness and responsiveness. Such changes can occur abruptly, i.e., within a minute, with several changes over a few hours. Patients are amnestic for the seizures that involve the temporal lobes (most cases of complex partial status epilepticus), while those with true absence status epilepticus may recall a number of phenomena that occurred during the seizures.

Motor manifestations vary widely, from only a fixed stare and no adventitious movements; through repetitive blinking, swallowing, and chewing; to complex interactive automatisms, e.g., opening doors and taking a streetcar ride.[71] Andermann and Robb emphasize small myoclonic twitches in the face and extremities as a clue

for NCSE; nurses should be informed about the significance of this sign.[64]

Nonconvulsive status epilepticus should be considered especially in the following situations:[62,72]

1. An apparently prolonged "postictal state" following generalized convulsive seizures or with prolonged reduction of alertness from an operative procedure or acute lesion.

2. Acute confusion or other forms of impaired consciousness (including paranoia, agitation, or other inappropriate behavior that is out-of-character for the patient; and stupor or coma), or muteness without other obvious etiology, often fluctuating, with episodes of normal mentation.

3. Impaired mentation or consciousness *with* myoclonus of facial (especially periorbital) muscles, rhythmic blinking, or rapid, spontaneous nystagmoid eye movements in any plane, including nystagmus retractorius[63]; subtle limb myoclonus.

4. Episodic blank staring, aphasia, or automatisms (lick smacking, fumbling with fingers, or perseverative activity).

5. Acute aphasia without an acute structural lesion.

6. Acute catatonia.

Absence Status Epilepticus   About 3 percent of patients with typical absence seizures have absence status at some time.[64–65] Absence status almost never produces coma, but, instead, causes impairment in mental acuity and responsiveness.[64,66] In prolonged (more than several minutes) absence seizures, the rate of spike-and-wave often drops below 3 per second.

In contrast, "absence status" arising de novo (without a past history of primary generalized epilepsy), or "spike-and-wave stupor," often begins in older adults, and is often associated with a slower repetition rate of the electrographic discharges than in standard absence seizures.[64,67,68] Patients in absence status may show either slight clouding of consciousness, with defects in attention and concentration, impaired sequencing and planning or organization, and slowing ideation or cognition. Memory may not be seriously compromised, in contrast to complex partial status epilepticus (CPSE), and patients may later recall intraictal events. More severely affected patients show marked clouding to the point of akinetic mutism or marked abulia (see Chap. 2). Some appear to be in a trance-like state or show a puzzled expression. Occasionally, patients appear to be very lethargic or somnolent, suggesting more involvement of the reticular activating system, or, conceivably, spread to sleep centers. Memory may or may not be seriously compromised for the event. Automatisms of any type (see above) may occur. Unlike typical absence seizures is the gradual, rather than abrupt, transition to normality as the absence status ceases.

Complex Partial Status Epilepticus Complex partial status epilepticus has been divided into two main groups by Mayeux and Lüders.[75] The first has recurrent attacks with intervening periods of relative normality. There are florid psychomotor (automatisms), psychosensory (hallucinations, illusions), and psychoaffective (usually fear) symptoms. The EEG shows focal or lateralized abnormalities ictally and interictally. The second group has prolonged mental confusion or psychotic behavior, with or without automatisms. The EEG usually shows considerable involvement of one or both temporal lobes. Patients are amnestic for the attacks.

Epidemiology

The incidence of status epilepticus is not known with any precision, due to the following: difficulties in detection (seizures are infrequently timed or electroencephalographically confirmed); sample populations that vary for age, referral bias, location, and etiologies; and differing definitions, e.g., convulsive, nonconvulsive, or all types. Hauser estimates that 12 percent of patients with epilepsy (excluding those symptomatic of an acute brain lesion) present with status epilepticus, either convulsive or nonconvulsive.[69] Of those with established epilepsy, 0.5 to 1.0 percent will develop

status epilepticus.[69] Acute symptomatic (mainly convulsive) seizures annually affect 40 to 80 persons per million.[69]

Nonconvulsive seizures and NCSE are almost certainly underrecognized. Absence and complex partial status epilepticus likely account for most cases of NCSE outside of intensive care units (ICUs).[70] Celesia and Dunne et al found that NCSE constituted 19 to 25 percent of all cases of status epilepticus in their hospitals.[71,72] Tomson and colleagues reported an annual incidence of 1.5 per 100,000 patients in their district in Sweden.[73] This group found only a slight predominance of the generalized "absence status" type over complex partial seizures; other studies have shown a more striking predominance of generalized NCSE. These studies cannot be regarded as comprehensive, however, as a comprehensive survey was not executed, nor was there even a representative clinical-EEG–studied sample of patients with impaired consciousness, and continuous EEG monitoring was not used.

The EEG and clinical criteria for NCS are shown in Table 17-4; these are compatible with standard definitions.[74–76]

Pathophysiology

Mechanisms of Status Epilepticus Proposed mechanisms for the transformation of discrete seizures into status epilepticus have been extrapolated from studies in animal models and are surrounded by controversy. However, there are strong parallels with clinical-EEG features in humans. A potent precipitant, e.g., a strong electrical shock or severe injury, is more likely to cause continued seizures than a lesser one. Both "systemic" and cellular mechanisms are likely to be relevant. The involvement of the "area tempestas," a limbic epileptogenic region, may be important in the initiation and spread of seizures; the activation of reverberating circuits has been said to be important in focally originating status epilepticus, especially in CPSE.[77,78] Decreased inhibition [reduced gamma-aminobutyric acid (GABA) activity] and increased excitatory mechanisms (e.g., glutamate activity) in

Table 17-4

Criteria for the diagnosis of seizures on the electro-encephalogram

Guideline: To qualify, at least *one of* the primary criteria *and* one or more of the secondary criteria should be satisfied, with discharges $> 10\,s$

Primary criteria

1. Repetitive generalized or focal spikes, sharp waves, spike-and-wave, or sharp-and-low wave complexes at > 3 per second
2. Repetitive generalized or focal spikes, sharp waves, spike-and-wave, or sharp-and-slow wave complexes at < 3 per second *and* secondary criterion no. 4
3. Sequential rhythmic waves and secondary criteria 1, 2 *and* 3, ± 4

Secondary criteria

1. Incrementing onset: increase in voltage and/or increase or slowing of frequency
2. Decrementing offset: decrease in voltage or frequency
3. Postdischarge slowing or voltage attenuation
4. Significant improvement in clinical state or baseline EEG after AED administration

Source: From Young et al,[74] with permission.

cortical and cortical-subcortical neuronal systems have also been considered in various models of generalized epilepsy.[79,80]

The mechanisms of initiation of seizures in generalized status epilepticus may differ from that for partial seizures.[77] From a macroscopic electrophysiologic perspective, the discharges in generalized seizures spread over the cortex, eventually withdraw from the occipital regions, and evolve from synchronous spike-wave to rhythmic waves in CSE. Thalamic connections to the cortex foster synchronization of excitatory and inhibitory phenomena and allows for a more persistent generalized spike-wave pattern in generalized (absence) NCSE.

The EEG features of status epilepticus in an animal model have been explored by Treiman and colleagues, who showed parallels with protracted status epilepticus in humans.[81] In animals and human, convulsive seizures evolve into nonconvulsive status epilepticus over five stages (Figs. 17-5 to 17-9):

1. *Discrete seizures*: epileptiform activity occurs in discrete epochs separated by postictal slow-frequency waves.

2. *Merging seizures:* epileptiform activity persists throughout, but the discharges wax and wane in frequency and amplitude.

3. *Continuous seizures:* spikes and spike-waves are rhythmic and relatively constant throughout the seizure.

4. *Continuous with flat periods:* ongoing epileptiform activity is interrupted by generalized attenuation of voltage from 0.5 to 8 s.

5. *Periodic epileptiform discharges on a flat background:* high-voltage, repetitive epileptiform discharges occur regularly against a flat or suppressed background.

Although others have shown a similar evolution in experimental models, there is controversy regarding the clinical relevance of Treiman's stage 5.[82] It is rare in clinical experience, except in anoxic-ischemic encephalopathy, where it is usually associated with a poor prognosis.[83]

Periodic lateralized epileptiform discharges (PLEDs), especially "PLEDs plus" in which the epileptiform discharges are polyphasic and variable, are worthy of monitoring until they subside, as there is an imminent risk of seizures developing with this pattern.[84,85]

Periodic sinusoid paroxysmal activity (PSPA) is a recently described electrographic-clinical entity consisting of periodic bursts of sinusoidal waves at 7 to 9 Hz, followed by slow waves occurring in the posterior head and associated with mental status changes variably including confusion, aphasia, or stupor.[86] Several patients have had distal myoclonias. Clinical deficits cleared shortly after the PSPA disappeared. All patients were over 60 years of age and thought to be suffering from ischemia in the watershed regions, although this was not clearly substantiated. Most likely this is a variant of the "PLEDs plus" pattern discussed above. This illustrates the controversial border zone between

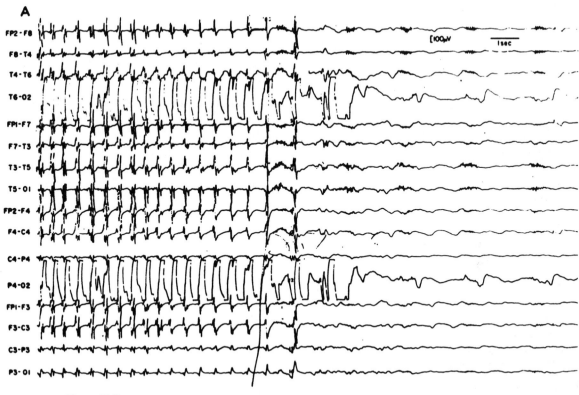

Figure 17-5
A discrete generalized seizure in a 39-year-old man. The recording shows the end of the clonic phase of the seizure and postictal slowing. (From Treiman et al,[81] with permission.)

interictal and ictal phenomena that is occupied by PLEDs.

Unresolved physiologic issues include the explanation for the changes in EEG patterns over time and a full explanation for the spontaneous termination of seizures. The roles of inhibitory mechanisms, such as increased extracellular adenosine and the increased activity of sodium-potassium ATPase activity, have been proposed for the latter.[87]

Neurochemical Aspects of Status Epilepticus As stated earlier, status epilepticus presumably results from a sustained imbalance of excitation and inhibition. There are, therefore, a number of receptor systems that may be differentially affected, either singly or in combination. Table 17-5 show chemicals and their receptors

that have been shown to either induce, perpetuate, or suppress seizures. These findings suggest that (1) an action of these substances on known brain receptors can produce, modify, or control status epilepticus; (2) similar chemicals are present in the nervous system; and (3) there is a possibility that these chemicals play a role in the initiation, enhancement, or cessation of status epilepticus.

Systemic Features of Convulsive Status Epilepticus Some general observations in CSE in nonhuman primates are probably relevant to the human condition, as described by Meldrum and Horton.[88] They describe two phases:

1. In phase 1, arterial and central venous pressure rise in humans and primates. Small

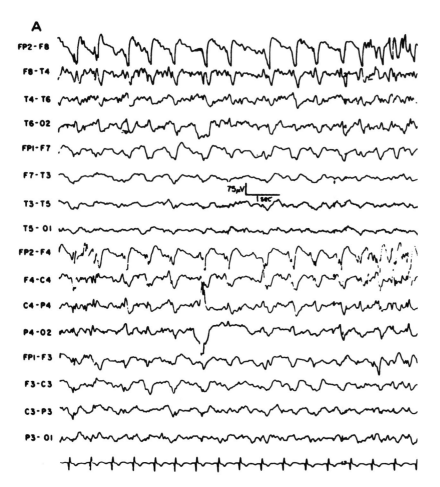

A

FP2-F8

F8-T4

T4-T6

T6-O2

FP1-F7

F7-T3

T3-T5

T5-O1

FP2-F4

F4-C4

C4-P4

P4-O2

FP1-F3

F3-C3

C3-P3

P3-O1

Figure 17-6

Merging of seizures in a 64-year-old man. Ictal discharges are continuous, but with waxing and waning of frequency and amplitude. (From Treiman et al,[81] with permission.)

subarachnoid hemorrhages occur. The Pa_{CO_2} rises and Pa_{O_2} falls; glucose and lactate serum concentrations rise.

2. Phase 2 begins about 20 to 30 min after the beginning of phase 1. Homeostatic mechanisms begin to fail. Hyperpyrexia becomes extreme. The Pa_{O_2} falls and Pa_{CO_2} rises further. Serum glucose concentration begins to fall, sometimes to severe hypoglycemic concentrations in the late stages. Hyperkalemia is a late event; electrolyte and pH changes may underlie the cardiac instability that leads to death, although autonomic effects on the heart are probably also important. Pulmonary edema or hemorrhages may occur. Energy failure (significant reduction in high-energy phosphate stores in the

mitochondria) of neuronal and other cells is a very late event.

Neuropathology of Status Epilepticus and the Pathophysiology of Brain Damage

Postmortem examinations of patients dying in status epilepticus often show no definite abnormalities on gross or light microscopic examination.[89] This is especially true in elderly patients in whom status epilepticus occurred without an obvious precipitant. Macroscopically, the brain is usually swollen and congested, with scattered petechial hemorrhages. The hippocampus is the most common site of microscopic pathology. Acutely,

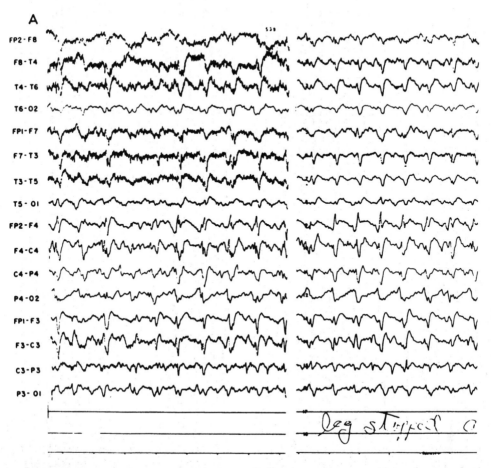

Figure 17-7

Continuous discharges recorded in a 68-year-old man. The two examples are 16 min apart. Continuous ictal activity persisted for 101 min, stopping only after phenytoin infusion was completed and 4 min after a lorazepam injection. (From Treiman et al,[81] with permission.)

"ischemic cell change" or, if the patient survives for several days, neuronal loss with gliosis, is found in the CA1, CA3, and end folium regions of the hippocampus. This creates the hippocampal sclerosis or mesial temporal sclerosis that is found in patients who have suffered many years of convulsive and nonconvulsive seizures.[90] In many patients with long-standing seizure disorders, it is difficult to know whether the hippocampal sclerosis is a result of previous bouts of status epilepticus or the cause (or a contributor) of the seizure disorder. In the older literature, with

freely convulsing patients, death of cerebellar Purkinje cells is also described. This finding is strongly associated with hyperpyrexia, as shown in controlled studies by Meldrum and colleagues.[91] When convulsions are prevented and systemic physiologic-biochemical (Pa_{O_2}, blood pressure, temperature, and serum glucose) security is assured, cerebellar and neocortical damage are prevented, but neurons die in the above-mentioned hippocampal regions. In animal models of status epilepticus, Auer and colleagues differentiated patterns of neuronal death in status

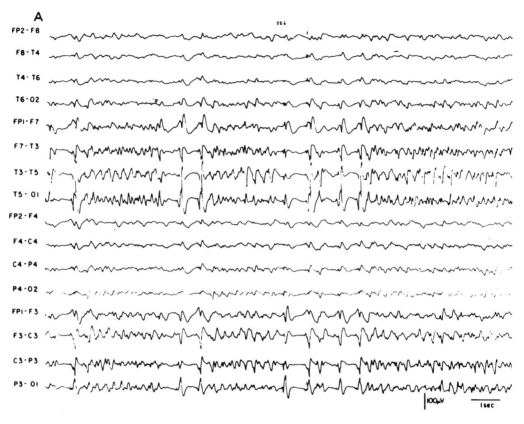

Figure 17-8

Continuous ictal discharges with flat periods recorded in a 68-year-old man. The seizure focus is clearly in the left hemisphere, but spread of ictal activity to the right hemisphere can be seen as well. (From Treiman et al,[81] with permission.)

epilepticus, anoxia-ischemia, and hypoglycemia (see Chap. 13).[92]

A final common pathway of neuronal death has been proposed for both status epilepticus and ischemic cell change. With seizures, as with other anoxia-ischemia, glutamate is thought to play a pivotal role. The activation of N-methyl-D-aspartate (NMDA) receptors has been emphasized, but their blockade does not completely prevent neuronal death in status epilepticus.[93,94] Activation of other non-NMDA receptors may also be important: early cell swelling may cause acute death of some neurons; the depolarization produced by their activation may be sufficient to activate the NMDA receptors. Delayed cell death is considered

to be due to NMDA receptor activation that leads to calcium influx, resulting in intracellular nitric oxide species generation, and proteolytic and lipolytic enzyme activation (see Chap. 15). Activation of other receptors and free-radical production probably contribute.[95–97] Much of this is speculative in clinical work. Apoptosis, or programmed cell death, may also be a mechanism for delayed neuronal necrosis: activation of intermediate early genes that code for endonucleases leads to destruction of nucleic acids.[98] Energy and substrate depletion are very late occurrences (Fig. 17-10).

The frequency of brain damage from NCSE has been debated. It is generally accepted that typical absence status epilepticus does not

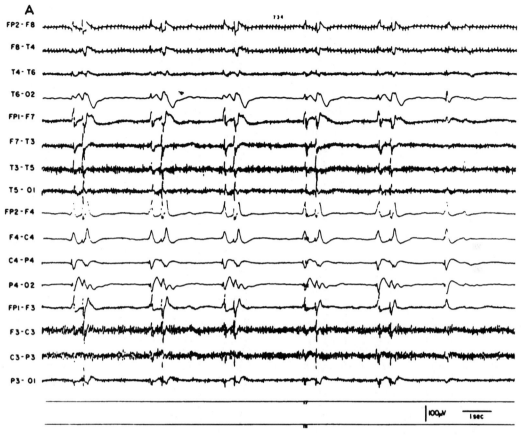

Figure 17-9
Periodic epileptiform discharges on a flat background recorded prior to treatment in a 64-year-old man. He was given 1000 mg of phenytoin and 5 mg lorazepam intravenously and the EEG was converted to a typical pattern of low-voltage slow waves. (From Treiman et al,[81] with permission.)

damage the brain. However, there is experimental and clinical evidence that other forms of NSCE may cause enduring memory problems, worsening of seizures in patients with previous epilepsy, the development of epilepsy in others, and risk of death during acute illnesses.

Experimental Evidence   In primates and rats, ongoing seizure activity can cause neuronal death, even without convulsive activity and its associated hypoxemia, acidosis, hyperthermia, and hypoglycemia.[99,100] Spontaneous seizure activity or NCSE is preceded by a reduction of

GABA-mediated inhibition, related to death of neurons that normally excite inhibitory neurons.[101–103]

Neuronal death, following NCSE confined to the limbic system (limbic status epilepticus), occurs at sites remote from local injections of neurotoxins or following the systemic injection of kainic acid, cholinergic drugs (with or without lithium), bicuculine, folic acid, or dipiperidinoethane.[104–108] Electrically or chemically induced limbic status epilepticus produces histopathologic changes that are identical to hippocampal sclerosis in humans.[109–112]

Table 17-5
Neurotransmitters, neuromodulators, receptor subtypes, and status epilepticus

Neurotransmitter or neuromodulator	Subclass of drugs	Specific examples
Glutamate	NMDA agonists	NMDA
	NMDA antagonists	MK801, ketamine
	Non-NMDA agonists	Kainate, quisqualate, demoic acid
	Non-NMDA antagonists	DNQZ, NBQX
GABA antagonism	GABA$_A$ antagonists	Pictrotoxin, bicuculine, PTZ, allyglycine
	GABA$_A$ agonists	Muscimol, benzodiazepines
	GABA$_B$ antagonists	Picrotoxin, bicuculine, PTZ, allylglycine
	GABA$_B$ agonists	Baclofen
Acetylcholine agonism	Muscarinic agonist	Pilocarpine + lithium
	Muscarinic antagonist	Scopolamine
Adenosine antagonism	A1 antagonists	Methylxanthines
	A1 agonists	N6-cyclohexyladenosine
Nitric oxide antagonism	NO synthetase inhibitors	L-Nitroarginine

Glutamate acts on N-methyl-D-aspartate (NMDA), kainate or quisqualate, or metabotropic (nonion channel, second messenger system) receptors. The effects are mainly excitatory, with the activation of voltage-dependent NMDA receptors, leading to neuronal depolarization and influx of calcium and sodium. Gamma aminobutyric acid type A (GABA$_A$) receptors enhance chloride conductance and decrease excitability by hyperpolarizing the neuron. The GABA$_B$ receptors are metabotropic. Adenosine acts as an intrinsic anticonvulsant, with neuromodulatory actions, inhibiting neurotransmitter release and interacting with the benzodiazepine receptor. Its antagonism produces a convulsant or excitability-enhancing action. More recently, nitric oxide acting *extracellularly* has some inhibitory effects.
Abbreviations: MK801 = an NMDA receptor blocker; DNQZ, NBQX = competitive blockers on glutamate non-NMDA receptors; PTZ = pentylenetetrazol; A1 = adenosine type-1 receptor; NO = nitric oxide.

Behavioral and electrophysiologic evidence of prolonged adverse changes in hippocampal function after partial kindling in animals (insufficient to produce convulsive seizures) include the following: long-lasting disruption of retention of spatial memory, increased paired pulse facilitation following Schaffer collateral stimulation, and enhanced long-term potentiation of population spikes after stimulation of the medial perforant path.[113–116]

Clinical Evidence   A similar series of changes occurs in the evolution of generalized CSE and NCSE.[117] Prolonged or repeated seizures without systemic effects can produce neuronal death in the vulnerable regions of the hippocampus.[12]

It is often difficult to assess the role of NCSE in producing brain damage in patients, because the underlying causes often injure the brain, or the patients may have been neurologically abnormal before NCSE occurred.[72,118] Proof necessitates an EEG to confirm NCS and NCSE (mimicked by numerous conditions), and continuous EEG recording to establish the duration of the seizure.[74,119] The precept that the brain insult must be separated from the effects of seizures is artificial, as the two probably act synergistically to produce brain damage, e.g., through augmented release of excitatory neurotransmitters.[120] In one study corroborated by the authors' experience, among a wide variety of patients admitted to a neuro-ICU, more than twice as many patients with NCS died or subsequently required custodial care than patients without seizures.[121] Seizures occur acutely in more than 20 percent of cases of fatal traumatic brain injuries, while they are uncommon

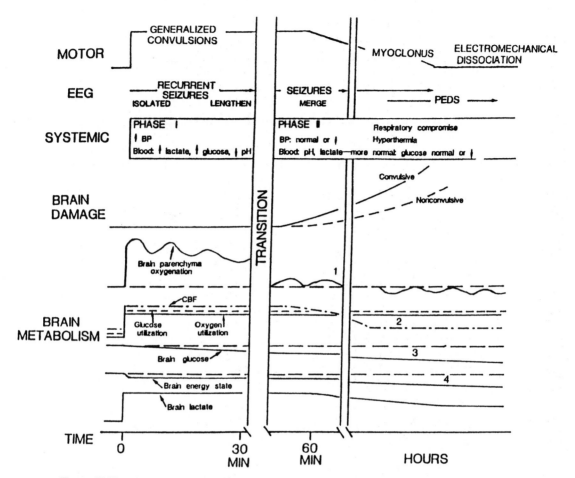

Figure 17-10

Summary of systemic alterations and brain metabolism in status epilepticus. Various events are aligned with respect to a time line. Note discontinuities in the time line and the designation of a critical transformation period over 30 min of status epilepticus. In the four lower traces depicting metabolic responses in the brain, information from several sources was combined. Included are the following: (1) findings of loss of "reactivity" of brain oxygen tension later in status epilepticus; (2) a mismatch between the sustained increase in oxygen and glucose and a fall in cerebral blood flow; (3) a depletion of brain glucose and glycogen (not labeled); and (4) a decline in the brain energy state. Note that brain damage begins before all but the first of these metabolic changes in both convulsive and nonconvulsive seizures. (From Lothman,[82] with permission.)

in less severe injuries.[122] Mortality is significantly higher when seizures accompany stroke than when stroke occurs without seizures.[123]

There are, however, some "pure cases" of NCSE without coincident derangements that would lead to brain damage. In these, there is

evidence of independent neuronal damage from the seizures alone. Among eight patients with NCS without additional acute neurologic conditions, the mean serum concentration of neuron-specific enolase, a marker for acute neuronal injury, was significantly elevated compared with that of epileptic controls.[124] Three of the eight patients had poor clinical outcomes (Glasgow Outcome Scores < 5). In another study, increases in enolase occurred in two patients with NCSE who had no coexistent cerebral injury.[125] Following methohexital-induced NCSE, enolase is elevated in both sera and CSF.[126,127]

Patients with NCSE but without other progressive disorders may have significant cognitive deficits after seizures.[128,129] Those with complex partial seizures sometimes develop persistent neurologic abnormalities.[130,131] Wasterlain and colleagues reported neuronal loss in the hippocampus and other brain regions after NCSE in three patients who did not have pre-existing seizures or systemic abnormalities.[132] Engel et al reported the case of a patient with recurrent complex partial seizures associated with reversible memory deficits who suffered an enduring memory loss after NCSE.[133] Treiman and colleagues reported cases of two similar patients, one of whom, besides having persistent memory problems, developed intractable complex partial seizures.[13] Within a large series, at least three epileptic patients, without other disorders, developed persistent cognitive (especially memory) deficits after bouts of CPSE.[134] Even though convulsive seizures occurred, they were brief. Similarly, Scholtes et al found the outcome following NCSE depended on both the underlying cause *and* the quality of treatment.[135] In three cases, inadequate treatment probably contributed to morbidity. For example, a 74-year-old woman with digoxin intoxication, who had CPSE lasting more than 24 h, had persistent word-finding problems and memory deficits.

Series of children with NCSE contain cases of dementia or progressive cognitive deficits that occurred without other progressive neurologic disorders.[136–138] In these cases, EEGs during NCS or NCSE often show irregular, generalized, slow spike and wave. The authors have also observed that some patients, without identifiable neurodegenerative or metabolic brain disease and with initially normal IQs, developed severe dementia after years of frequent NCSE. This occurred without convulsive seizures or with only infrequent, brief convulsions.

Statistical evidence suggests that the duration of NCSE correlates more closely with poor outcome than does etiology.[74] Of 49 cases of NCS studied with continuous EEG monitoring, multiple logistic regression analyses revealed that only duration of NCSE and delay to diagnosis were significantly related to mortality, confirming the conclusions of earlier studies.[139–141] Furthermore, several patients who died in coma or who left the hospital with increased neurologic disability had not had acute brain insults.

Etiologies of Status Epilepticus

Clinical Precipitants and Causes of Status Epilepticus
Besides clinical features and the EEG, other investigations, e.g., neuroimaging and CSF analysis, often are necessary to determine the cause of status epilepticus. Etiologies vary with age, seizure type, and mode of presentation. There are a number of problems with the literature: almost all series of cases of status epilepticus are selected from ICUs or specialized epilepsy centers. Most studies are retrospective and limited to certain age groups; the etiologies are often multifactorial but are seldom identified as such, in that only one cause is given for each patient.

Figure 17-11 shows the relative distribution of causes of CSE separated by the existence of prior epilepsy or status epilepticus as the first ictal manifestation. A consistent observation across various series is that an acute brain lesion or a metabolic stress is identifiable in most patients whose first seizure is status epilepticus. In contrast, for patients with established epilepsy who subsequently develop status epilepticus, an etiology is identified in no more than half. In the latter group, the most common *precipitant* of status epilepticus is a reduction in dose of AEDs. Additional contributory factors include fever, gastrointestinal upset, comedication with drugs that lower seizure threshold (e.g., tricyclic and tetracyclic antidepressants), and alcohol or drug abuse and withdrawal.

Among patients with head injury, the incidence of status epilepticus increases with the severity of the brain damage. With tumor, the

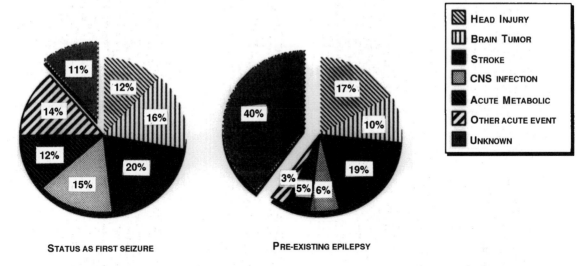

STATUS AS FIRST SEIZURE   PRE-EXISTING EPILEPSY

Figure 17-11

Relative distribution of causes of convulsive status epilepticus. The pie charts show the populations of patients who (left) *presented with status epilepticus as the first known seizure or* (right) *whose seizure occurred after previous epileptic seizures. The left figure is redrawn from a collection of 327 cases pooled from various published studies, while the right figure is from a group of 227 patients whose status epilepticus followed previously known discrete seizures.[207–211]*

frontal lobe cortex is the most common site; such patients freuquently present with status epilepticus. In the northern latitudes, most CNS infections associated with status epilepticus are viral encephalitides, while parasites, especially cysticercosis and malaria, predominate in the southern hemisphere. (Herpes simplex encephalitis, the most common sporadic encephalitis in adults, commonly causes seizures, but rarely produces status epilepticus.) Hemorrhagic strokes involving the cerebral cortex are more likely to cause seizures than are bland ischemic lesions, but the rate of status epilepticus in the first few weeks after the stroke is low. Venous infarction, i.e., cortical vein thrombosis (see Chap. 15), is especially epileptogenic. Metabolic causes, especially derangements of serum glucose concentration (either hypoglycemia or nonketotic hyperglycemia), electrolyte disturbances (especially hyponatremia, hypocalcemia, and hypomagnesemia), uremia, and advanced liver failure should be considered. Alcohol or drug withdrawal commonly contribute to, or independently cause,

status epilepticus. From time to time, status epilepticus results from multiple sclerosis, migraine, hypertensive encephalopathy, heat stroke, theophylline toxicity, imipenim therapy and, less commonly, other drugs such as penicillin or ceftazadime (espcially in the presence of renal failure), or boluses of lidocaine.[142–144] Abused drugs, including cocaine, amphetamines, and lysergic acid diethylamide (LSD) "laced" with strychnine are still commonly available. Deliberate overdoses with several drugs and accidental exposure to drugs or industrial agents sometimes may be causative. Infrequent causes include heat stroke or electrical shock, remote effect of cancer, acquired immunodeficiency syndrome (AIDS) encephalopathy, and early- or late-onset metabolic disorders including mitochondrial disorders (see pp. 373–375).[145,146] Some cases of NCSE have followed electroconvulsive therapy for psychoses.[147–149] Patients with this complication show fluctuating mutism, confusion, withdrawal, or other behavior that is atypical for the individual, sometimes associated with automatisms. The EEG, necessary to confirm the diagnosis, usually shows generalized epileptiform activity. Patients respond to AEDs.

In infants and very young children, congenital developmental and perinatal insults, metabolic disorders, and infections are most the frequent causes of status epileptics. A febrile seizure progressing to status epilepticus is one of the most common categories in children under 5 years of age, even though the number of febrile seizures that show this tendency is small.

Differential Diagnosis

The differential diagnosis of convulsive seizures includes pseudoseizures (Chap. 18) and some toxic conditions, such as organophosphate poisoning (Chap. 16), where the convulsive movements are not always due to cortically originating seizures. Some patients with decerebrate spasms, e.g., with basilar artery occlusion, are mistakenly thought to have convulsive seizures. The differentiation is not always easily made from observation alone and, indeed, there may be genuine synchronized electrical activity generated by the diencephalic centers. The context, the presence of other features, and the EEG recordings may help in the differentiation of decerebrate spasms from tonic or convulsive seizures.

The differential diagnosis of NCSE is essentially that of the acute confusional state and of fluctuating impairment of consciousness as discussed in Chap. 2. The main considerations are other causes of transient neurologic dysfunction, metabolic and toxic encephalopathies, migraine, and psychiatric disorders.[150,151] The diagnosis of NCSE is often delayed, often with unfortunate implications for increased morbidity and mortality (see below).[74,152] This underlines the confirmatory value of a prompt EEG, even in the emergency room.

As mentioned earlier, in patients with a previous history of seizures, the most common precipitant is a significant drop in the serum concentration of the maintenance AED. This should be measured. Besides poor compliance, alcohol intoxication or systemic infections may relate to drops in AED concentration.

Management

For the prevention of status epilepticus, prompt recognition and treatment of both convulsive and nonconvulsive seizures constitute the best measures. Regular follow-up and checks for AED compliance in patients with established epilepsy may help in preventing major relapses or the development of status epilepticus.

A rapid etiologic and diagnostic assessment should be considered us before deciding upon drug therapy for status epilepticus: (1) Are the seizures occurring in a patient with a pre-existing seizure disorder (raising the possibility of withdrawal from an AED)? (2) Are the seizures due to an acute condition affecting the brain—sometimes making them relatively resistant to conventional AEDs? (3) Does the patient have pseudoseizures/pseudostatus epilepticus (a frequent cause of therapy resistance—see Chap. 18)? A brief history and observation will usually allow such a classification; this has an enormous impact on the direction of investigation and treatment.

Both CSE and NCSE, excluding absence seizures, can damage the brain; thus, it is important to stop the seizures as soon as possible. A suitable regime for these urgent cases is given in the immediately following section. This is derived from several authoritative references, and their authors' collective experience with over 200 cases.[153–155] The management of absence status epilepticus will be discussed separately.

Prehospital Management   In San Francisco, paramedics have been trained to give AEDs as prehospital therapy to patients who collapse with recognized seizures.[156] This has reduced the incidence of such patients having subsequent seizures in the emergency room or requiring ICU admissions or endotracheal intubation.[156] The object is to shorten the duration of seizures and to lessen mortality and morbidity. Cost and resource savings are additional benefits. After obtaining intravenous access with a large-bore catheter, normal saline (NS) is infused. Usually, a benzodiazepine is given as first-line treatment: e.g., a single dose of lorazepam (2 to 4 mg in adults) or diazepam (5 to 10 mg in adults). The patient needs to be prevented from hitting the head or aspirating, as with any convulsive seizure. Oxygen should be delivered by mask for convulsive seizures. In general, this is sufficient for short trips until the patient is delivered to the emergency room.

In-hospital Management For discussion purposes, the various aspects are considered separately. In practice, however, the various steps are carried out concurrently.

Therapy and Monitoring If the patient has received multiple doses of benzodiazepines prior to arrival in the emergency room and is still convulsing, it is probably best to proceed with endotracheal intubation (see rapid sequence intubation in Chap. 20.)[157] This protects the unconscious patient's airway and adds a measure of safety, as the administration of more drugs may compromise ventilation. If the patient's airway can be adequately protected though positioning and suctioning, and if the patient is breathing adequately, it is reasonable to try to stop the seizures without endotracheal intubation.

A flow chart of AED therapy for status epilepticus is shown in Fig. 17-12. Lorazepam, 2 mg, is infused intravenously over 2 min, adding 1 to 2 mg increments every 2 min (the usual maximum is 8 mg, including that added in the prehospital phase.) Diazepam, 5 to 10 mg, administered intravenously at 2 mg/min, may also be used, but lorazepam is preferred because of its longer duration of action. The protocol for lorazepam or diazepam can be repeated in 10 to 15 min if seizures recur or if seizure control is not achieved initially. Since respiratory depression may occur with repeated doses, such treatment on the nonintubated patient is best used only when seizures are ongoing or recurring frequently.

Simultaneously with the first dose of lorazepam or diazepam, an infusion of phenytoin or fosphenytoin (see later) is begun, using a separate

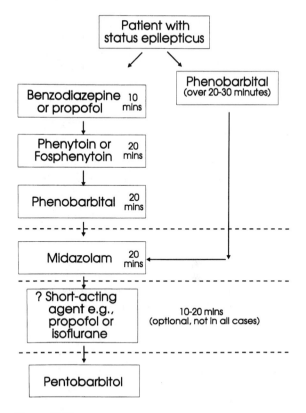

Figure 17-12

A flow chart of AED management for status epilepticus (see also text). Note that there is some flexibility, depending on the type and severity of the seizures and the patient's condition, and whether other short-acting agents are used before resorting to anesthetic barbiturates in refractory status epilepticus.

intravenous line with NS running (phenytoin precipitates in glucose solutions). Phenytoin or fosphenytoin, 15 to 20 mg/kg, diluted in NS, is given to achieve a concentration of about 4 mg/mL.[158–161] Phenytoin should be administered at ≤ 50 mg/min, while fosphenytoin is usually given at 100 to 150 mg/min. It should be noted that fosphenytoin is better tolerated by intravenous and intramuscular administration than phenytoin and it can be infused more rapidly. However, since the conversion of fosphenytoin to phenytoin takes several minutes, the dynamics of brain phenytoin concentrations achieved by the two formulations are approximately the same. Blood pressure should be monitored for hypotension and a continuous electrocardiogram (ECG) is recommended. (Phenytoin and fosphenytoin with cardiac conduction defects and should be used only very cautiously in the presence of shock or hypotension.) A maintenance dose of phenytoin can be commenced the next day.

If seizures fail to stop after administration of phenytoin or fosphenytoin, phenobarbital is given intravenously at ≤ 100 mg/min until seizures stop or until a maximum of 20 mg/kg is reached. Some neurologists use phenobarbital directly with status epilepticus, and avoid phenytoin. Careful observation is undertaken for cardiopulmonary depression, especially if the patient has received benzodiazepines earlier. Some units use midazolam (see below) directly after phenytoin, bypassing phenobarbital. It is a reasonable precaution to insert an endotracheal tube prior to the administration of phenobarbital or midazolam if the patient has received benzodiazepines earlier. Assisted ventilation may be required as well.

If these measures fail, as they do in about 20 percent of patients, the patient is considered to have refractory status epilepticus.[162] A qualified physician is then summoned for endotracheal intubation and assisted ventilation. Continuous EEG monitoring is recommended during further treatment. The authors favor midazolam as the second or third agent if status epilepticus persists beyond 10 min after the above therapies, beginning with a loading dose of 200 µg/kg as a slow intravenous infusion, followed by 0.75 to 10 µg/kg per minute. This dosage can be adjusted upwards or downwards, depending on the effect on EEG-recorded seizures. Midazolam infusion is commonly accompanied by hypotension; intravenous dopamine will usually counteract this complication. The administration of midazolam should be reviewed every hour and stopped when seizures are controlled. The authors have used midazolam for over 8 days with intermittent cessation to judge the clinical state and EEG.

If midazolam fails to stop continued seizures on the EEG over 30 to 60 min, pentobarbital is recommended, beginning with a loading dose of 5 to 20 mg/kg at ≤ 25 mg/min, followed by an infusion of 0.5 to 1.0 mg/kg per hour, increasing, if necessary, up to 1 to 3 mg/kg per hour. Additional boluses of 5 to 20 mg/kg can be given, intravenously for breakthrough seizures. The EEG should be monitored continuously or several times per hour at first, then every few hours. A burst-suppression pattern is usually sufficient, but complete suppression may be necessary if seizures fail to cease. Such therapy may be necessary for several days or more, especially in encephalitis.[163,164]

Thiopental, propofol, isoflurane, enflurane, paraldehyde, and xylocaine have also been used for refractory cases.[154]

Notes on Specific Drugs

Benzodiazepines Benzodiazepines act on the benzodiazepine receptor, which, in turn, enhances activation of GABA on the $GABA_A$ receptor. This enhances the conductance of chloride into neurons, hyperpolarizing the neurons and lowering excitability.[165] Lorazepam is generally preferred to diazepam, as its duration is longer. Although each drug acts fairly quickly and stops the seizure about 80 percent of the time, neither is suitable for sustaining a protective effect because their duration is only a few hours at best and they have sedative and respiratory depressant effects.[166]

Phenytoin Phenytoin approaches the ideal drug in achieving rapid penetration into the brain, high effectiveness, and production of minimal depression in respirations and alertness.[167] It does, however, have cardiovascular side effects. One of these, hypotension, is largely due to the propylene glycol in which the drug is suspended. This necessitates slow intravenous administration of the drug and an earlier injection of a benzodiazepine that can be delivered more quickly. The drug is also very alkaline and irritating to tissues if it extravasates from the vein. Phenytoin precipitates in tissues and in glucose solutions; as a corollary, it must be administered intravenously in saline solutions. Because of its half-life of 20 h and its nonlinear kinetics, a loading dose of 15 to 20 mg/kg will produce a serum concentration of 4 to 8 µg/mL (or 40 to 80 µmol/L).

Fosphenytoin Fosphenytoin,[168–170] the disodium phosphate ester of phenytoin (phenytoin prodrug), is converted into phenytoin by phosphatases in the liver, erythrocytes, and other tissues, with a conversion half-life of 8 to 15 min. A therapeutic serum concentration of phenytoin is obtained within 10 min of the completion of fosphenytoin infusion. Because fosphenytoin preparations do not contain propylene glycol, the drug can be infused more rapidly. This offsets the conversion time period in the body, but fosphenytoin has no advantage over phenytoin in the speed with which the seizure is stopped. Fosphenytoin is also rapidly absorbed from the intramuscular route. Advantages over phenytoin include the following: less hypotensive side effects, less local tissue irritation, and varied routes of administration—useful for certain emergency situations, e.g., with young children or for out-of-hospital administration. However, like phenytoin, it may precipitate complete heart block in predisposed patients.

Phenobarbital Phenobarbital has an action similar to the benzodiazepines in facilitating the binding of GABA to its receptor, among other actions.[171,172] Phenobarbital has theoretic disadvantages compared with phenytoin: it is not as lipid-soluble and causes more sedation and respiratory depression. However, in a comparative study, it proved to be equivalent to the phenytoin-diazepam regime in effectiveness and frequency of adverse effects.[173] Respiratory depression is seldom encountered at standard doses, unless the drug is preceded by a benzodiazepine. Very-high-dose phenobarbital [producing serum concentrations of about 100 μg/mL (650 μmol/L) or more] is sometimes used in refractory status epilepticus in children and occasionally in adults.[174] Comparative studies with pentobarbital have not been performed (see later).

Midazolam Midazolam is a very sedating benzodiazepine with a half-life of about 2 h. Its potency and short half-life make it a useful drug in cases of refractory status epilepticus. It can be given intramuscularly, but this is rarely necessary for status epilepticus, as the patient should be in an ICU with vascular lines in place by the time its use is indicated. Its method of administration is as described above, largely gleaned from the experience of several clinicians.[175,176]

Pentobarbital and Thiopental These two "anesthetic barbiturates," with GABA-ergic activity, are extremely potent when fully utilized and can stop virtually any seizure if given in sufficient quantity, as they can arrest electrocerebral activity, at least for a brief time. On their own, they render patients comatose and depress respirations. It is essential that the patient is intubated and on a ventilator when either drug is used. The drugs have profound effects on muscular relaxation; the authors have never required the use of skeletal muscle relaxants when these drugs are used. The drug is usually given to produce a burst-suppression pattern of 2 to 30 s on the EEG; this is usually necessary for successful arrest of the seizures.[163,177] The drugs have a cumulative effect if they are used for more than 2 days; patients often require endotracheal tubes, ventilation, and other ICU management for a week after the seizures are stopped. It has been suggested, at least for children, that initial tapering of pentobarbital is reasonable 12 h after an initial EEG burst-suppression pattern has been obtained.[178] Most patients do not relapse; those who do relapse have a greater chance of mortality or significant morbidity.[179] Other negative prognostic factors include the presence of hypotension or multiorgan failure during pentobarbital therapy.[180]

Other Agents Thiopental, propofol, isoflurane, enflurane, paraldehyde, and xylocaine have also been used for refractory cases. There are no comparative studies to evaluate their relative effectiveness. Like midazolam, they have advantages over the anesthetic barbiturates in having shorter sedative half-lives, and they are often worth trying before resorting to thiopental or pentobarbital. Such agents lessen the brain damage from status epilepticus in animal models.[181]

Propofol is especially promising. It has been used successfully in the prehospital phase of treatment of CSE.[182] In hospitalized patients, propofol may work after benzodiazepines have failed.[183] An initial bolus of 2 mg/kg or 100 mg followed by an infusion of 3 to 10 mg/kg per hour has been used, even for several days.[184-186] Potential problems include hypotension and the theoretic possibility that propofol may aggravate the seizures, as seizures have occasionally resulted from propofol anesthesia.[187]

Isoflurane is an inhalational agent that is rapidly absorbed and excreted, yet has little accumulation in the body. Induction of anesthesia requires minimum alveolar concentrations of 1.5 to 3.5% and maintenance of anesthesia requires 0.7 to 2.1%.[188] For status epilepticus, end tidal concentrations are about 0.8% initially, but this can be raised to about 2%.[189] Ropper and colleagues found isoflurane to be superior to halothane and nitrous oxide in a case of otherwise refractory status epilepticus.[190] Others have also found isoflurane to be effective in isolated cases.[191,192] Monitoring by EEG is essential. Disadvantages of isoflurane and other inhalational agents in the ICU include the need for scavenging the exhaled gas, the need for an anesthetic machine and availability of an anesthetist, and hypotension as a side effect.

Specific Agents and Circumstances Isoniazid-induced convulsions and pyridoxine deficiency or dependency in the neonate may respond to intravenous pyridoxine.[193,194] Adrenocorticotropic hormone (ACTH) is used to treat infantile spasms in young children; more recently, vigabatrin has been found to be effective.[195] Epilepsia partialis continua usually does not warrant AEDs in doses that produce anesthesia; the focal seizures are notoriously difficult to arrest and there is often more harm done by further compromising consciousness with the drugs than in treating the seizures more conservatively.

Clinical and Laboratory Evaluation While the patient is being treated and stabilized, others should obtain a history from witnesses, friends, or family and perform a neurologic and general physical examination. Blood is taken for determination of serum concentrations of AEDs,

glucose, urea, electrolytes, calcium, and magnesium, and the urine and blood are screened for drugs when appropriate. A serum theophylline concentration should be obtained if the patient has received this agent. Arterial or capillary blood gas determination is usually carried out. If the patient remains obtunded after initial treatment measures, an urgent EEG is advised to check for NCSE.

The principal test for seizures is the EEG. Because the clinical features of nonconvulsive epileptic attacks themselves blend with the postictal state, and since the clinical manifestations alone mimic many other conditions, the EEG plays a vital diagnostic role.

The EEG is diagnostically confirmatory and is of great value in guiding therapy. The authors suggest that the EEG be performed promptly, in the emergency room, on patients with a significant possibility of having NCSE (see above). This includes patients with prolonged unresponsiveness after a seizure or acute brain insult, or those with unexplained collapse. Continuous EEG monitoring provides the best opportunity for ongoing management, providing that the individual reading the EEG (usually the ICU nurse) is skilled in interpretation and acts on the findings.[196]

Seizures are not difficult to recognize on the standard "raw" EEG. Automated seizure-detection algorithms with commercial EEGs may assist, but well-trained nurses do as well or better.[74,196]

Patients with known seizure disorders should be checked for low serum concentrations of AEDs and for predisposing causes, such as underlying infections or use of the epileptogenic drugs mentioned earlier.

Patients who develop either CSE or NCSE de novo should be carefully investigated for acute structural or brain lesions, encephalitis, or metabolic disturbances, and for toxic or proconvulsant drugs, especially theophylline. Emergency determination of serum electrolytes, glucose, calcium, phosphate, magnesium, and urea should be obtained. Scanning by CT and, if negative, CSF analysis may be required. A caveat is the presence of postictal pleocytosis (usually < 12 white blood cells per cubic millimeter) in the CSF.[197] This phenomenon is found in about 11 percent of patients within 90 min to 72 h after either simple or complex partial seizures or following generalized convulsions.[197] The white blood cells are almost exclusively lymphocytes (< 2 percent polymorphs); CSF protein concentration was mildly increased in 16 percent of the total group.

Scanning by CT is often not sufficiently sensitive to detect very recent infarction or cortical vein thromboses, and a high index of clinical suspicion is required. Scanning by MRI is usually superior to CT, but is not as commonly available and is more difficult to perform on an intubated, unstable patient. It is usually deferred until the seizures are stopped and the patient is stabilized.

Convulsive status epilepticus is commonly associated with a combined metabolic and respiratory acidosis. The absence of an acidosis during or immediately following CSE raises suspicions of pseudoseizures. Muscle breakdown commonly causes elevation of serum creatine kinase and, if marked, this may be associated with myoglobinuria. If rhabdomyolysis is recognized, it should be treated with adequate hydration to ensure a good renal flow and to prevent renal failure. It is better to use normal saline than dextrose solutions to avoid aggravation of brain swelling.

Disseminated intravascular coagulation is a rare complication of status epilepticus. Reliable indicators include a prolonged prothrombin time [international normalized ratio (INR)], thrombocytopenia, and a positive D-dimer test.

Cardiac arrhythmias are often secondary to the physiologic sympathetic reaction. Electrocardiograms are appropriate, especially in older individuals; the authors have encountered elderly patients with underlying ischemic heart disease who suffered a myocardial infarction in association with convulsive seizures from a frontal lobe lesion.

General Measures For convulsive seizures, adequate padding should be used to prevent the patient from self-induced injury. A mouth guard may help prevent tooth fracture and tongue injury but should only be used only after the airway has been suctioned clean. Complications

of the seizure should be appropriately treated. Hypoglycemia, if significant, should be remedied, without producing hyperglycemia: administer 25 to 50 mL of 50% dextrose if the patient is hypoglycemia or if glucose measurement is not available. Concurrently or beforehand, thiamine, 100 mg, should be administered intravenously as a protective measure against iatrogenic Wernicke's encephalopathy (see Chap. 15), as hypoglycemic patients may be nutritionally deprived.

It is almost never necessary to give bicarbonate to treat the acidosis. The latter usually corrects itself with cessation of the convulsive movements and the re-establishment of effective ventilatory function or with assisted ventilation.

Treatment of the underlying disease process should proceed hand-in-hand with the management of the NCSE. Secondary worsening of either the neurologic or general state of the patient, after the status epilepticus has been successfully treated, always represents an emergency situation. This could indicate continued worsening of the condition that caused the status epilepticus (e.g., expanding hematoma, vasospasm, continued inflammation or ischemia, raised intracranial pressure) or a complication, such as sepsis or pulmonary edema. Intensive investigation, support, and definitive treatment are needed.

In some of the above acute symptomatic cases, NCSE convulsive or myoclonic status epilepticus may be an epiphenomenon of severe brain damage. This applies especially to NCSE and myoclonic status epilepticus from generalized anoxic-ischemic encephalopathy after cardiac arrest.[198] As discussed in Chap. 3, a burst-suppression pattern with epileptiform, discharges with bursts is usually associated with a poor outcome. This pattern may be quasiperiodic, resembling the potentially reversible stage 5 of Treiman (see earlier). Until the significance of the burst-suppression pattern or periodic complexes in anoxic-ischemic encephalopathy is resolved, it is best to treat the patient vigorously for the seizures with the regime for status epilepticus, unless there is strong evidence of irreversibility, e.g., absence of the N20 somatosensory evoked response. In such situations, assessment of the prognosis is assisted by other techniques, such as the demonstration of absent thalamocortical somatosensory evoked responses.[199] If the prognosis, based on clinical and electrophysiologic factors (see Chap. 3), is hopeless, it is reasonable to discuss the withdrawal of ICU support.

Absence Status Epilepticus: A Special Case

Typical absence seizures are not thought to damage the brain; therefore, treatment is not as urgent. Indeed, proceeding to the use of anesthetic agents sometimes resorted to in the control of CPSE and CSE is usually not necessary and is too hazardous. However, since some may evolve into generalized convulsive seizures, some efficiency of treatment is necessary. An intravenous benzodiazepine (e.g., lorazepam, 2 to 4 mg) is often effective in stopping the seizure. (Note that, occasionally, a paradoxical worsening in NCSE may occur in patients with atypical absence status epilepticus treated with benzodiazepines, especially clonazepam.[200]) Intravenous acetazolamide is sometimes promptly effective.[201] The patient can then be treated with valproate, ethosuximide, clonazepam, or clobazam; often, one of these drugs has been used earlier and the reinstitution of adequate maintenance is the best course. It is probably not justified to give anesthetic-type treatment, or neuromuscular paralysis, or artificial ventilation to such patients. On the other hand, patients require close observation in a special care unit for their safety and the prompt treatment of any progression to convulsive seizures.

Outcome

Risk factors for poor outcome include the presence of an active disease process causing the seizures, seizure duration, delay to diagnosis, and advanced age.[202–204] Many patients who remain in coma with difficult-to-control NCSE are later severely disabled, if they survive.

Conversely, the outcome is best for those patients who respond well to initial therapy and those with a prior history of epilepsy or with alcohol withdrawal seizures.[202,205,206]

References

1. Jackson JH: Investigation of the epilepsies, in Taylor J (ed): *Selected Writings of John Hughlings Jackson.* London, Hodder and Stoughton, 1931, p 99.
2. Hauser WA, Kurland LT: The epidemiology of epilepsy in Rochester, Minnesota, 1935 through 1967. *Epilepsia* 16:1, 1975.
3. Commission on Classification and Terminology, International League Against Epilepsy: Proposed revisions of clinical and electroencephalographic classification of epileptic seizures. *Epilepsia* 22:480, 1981.
4. Blume WT, Young GB, Lemieux JF: EEG morphology of partial epileptic seizures. *Electroenceph Clin Neurophysiol* 57:295, 1984.
5. Lerman P, Kivity S: Benign focal epilepsy of childhood. A follow-up study of 100 recovered patients. *Arch Neurol* 32:261, 1975.
6. Wieser HG: *Electroclinical Features of the Psychomotor Seizure.* Stuttgart-London, Gustav Fischer-Butterworth, 1983.
7. Williamson PD, Spencer DD, Spencer SS, et al: Complex partial status epilepticus: a depth electrode study. *Ann Neurol* 18:647, 1985.
8. Kivity S, Lennan P: Stormy onset with prolonged loss of consciousness in benign childhood epilepsy with occipital paroxysms. *J Neurol Neurosurg Psychiatry* 55:45, 1992.
9. Babb TL, Wilson CL, Isokawa-Akesson M: Firing patterns of human limbic neurons during stereoencephalography (SEEG) and clinical temporal lobe seizures. *Electroenceph Clin Neurophysiol* 66:467, 1987.
10. Weiser HG: Human limbic system seizures: EEG studies, origin, and patterns of spread, in Meldrum BS, Ferrendelli J, Wieser HG (eds): *The Anatomy of Epileptogenesis.* London, John Libbey, 1988, pp 127–138.
11. Escueta AV, Kunze U, Waddell A, et al: Lapse of consciousness and automatisms in temporal lobe epilepsy: a videotape analysis. *Neurology* 27:144, 1977.
12. Gloor P, Olivier A, Ives J: Loss of consciousness in temporal lobe seizures: observations obtained with stereotaxic depth electrode recordings and stimulations, in Canger R, Angeleri F, Penry JK (eds): *Advances in Epileptology: XI Epilepsy International Symposium.* New York, Raven Press, 1980, pp 349–353.

13. Treiman DM, Delgado-Escueta AV: Complex partial status epilepticus, in Delagado-Escueta AV, Wasterlain CG, Treiman DM, Porter RJ (eds): *Status Epilepticus: Mechanisms of Brain Damage and Treatment.* Advances in Neurology series, vol 34, New York, Raven Press, 1983, pp 69–81.

14. Spencer SS: Cortical and intercortical seizure spread, in Meldrum BS, Ferrendelli JA, Wieser HG: *Anatomy of Epileptogenesis.* London, John Libbey, 1988, pp 139–154.

15. Wieser HG: *Electroclinical Features of the Psychomotor seizure.* Stuttgart, Gustav Fischer,1983.

16. Kreinder A, Zucherman E, Steriade M, Chimion J: Electroclinical features of convulsions induced by stimulation of the brain stem. *J Neurophysiol* 21:430, 1958.

17. Browne TR, Penry JK, Porter RJ, et al: Responsiveness before, during and after spike-wave paroxysms. *Neurology* 24:659, 1974.

18. Penry JK, Dreifuss FE: Automatisms associated with the absence of petit mal epilepsy. *Arch Neurol* 21:142, 1969.

19. Mirsky AF, Duncan CC: Behavioral and electrophysiological studies of absence epilepsy, in Avoli M, Gloor P, Kostopoulos G, Naquet R (eds): *Generalized Epilepsy.* Boston, Birkhäuser, 1990, pp 254–269.

20. Gloor P: Neurophysiological mechanism of the generalized spike-and-wave, discharges and its implication for understanding absence seizures, in Myslobodsky MS, Mirsky AF (eds): *Elements of Petit Mal Epilepsy.* New York, Peter Lang, 1988, pp 159–209.

21. Porter RJ, Penry JK: Responsiveness at the onset of spike-wave bursts. *EEG Clin Neurophysiol* 34:239, 1973.

22. Howell DH: Unusual centrencephalic seizure patterns. *Brain* 78:199, 1955.

23. Jasper HH, Van Gelder NM (eds): *Basic Mechanisms of Neuronal Excitability.* New York, Allan R Liss, 1983.

24. Schwartzkroin PA, Wheal HV (eds): *Electrophysiology of Epilepsy.* London, Academic Press, 1984.

25. Meldrum BS, Ferendelli JA, Wieser HG: *Anatomy of Epileptogenesis.* London, John Libbey, 1988.

26. Jeffreys JGR: The pathophysiology of epilepsies, in Laidlaw J, Richens A, Chadwick D (eds): *A Textbook of Epilepsy.* Edinburgh, Churchill Livingstone, 1993, pp 241–276.

27. Reeves AL, Nollet KE, Klass DW, Sharbrough FW, So EL: The ictal bradycardia syndrome. *Epilepsia* 37:983, 1996.

28. Wilder-Smith E: Complete atrio-ventricular block during complex partial seizure. *J Neurol Neurosurg Psychiatry* 55:734, 1992.

29. Nashef L, Walker F, Allen P, Sander JWAS, Shorvon SD, Fish DR: Apnoea and bradycardia during epileptic seizures: relation to sudden death in epilepsy. *J Neurol Neurosurg Psychiatry* 60:297, 1996.

30. Laster DW, Penry JK, Moody DM, et al: Chronic seizure disorders: contributions of MR imaging when CT is normal. *Am J Neuroradiol* 6:177, 1985.

31. Theodore WH, Dorwart R, Holmes M, Porter RJ, DiChiro G: Neuroimaging in refractory partial seizures: comparison of PET, CT and MRI. *Neurology* 36:750, 1986.

32. Trimble MR: Serum prolactin in epilepsy and hysteria. *BMJ* 2:1682, 1978.

33. Hart YM, Sander JW, Johnson AL, Shorvon SD: National General Practice Study of Epilepsy: recurrence after a first seizure. *Lancet* 336:1271, 1990.

34. Hauser WA, Rich SS, Annegers JF, Anderson VE: Seizure recurrence after a 1st unprovoked seizure: an extended follow-up. *Neurology* 40:1163, 1990.

35. Levy RH, Dreifuss FE, Mattson RH, Meldrum BS, Penry JK: *Antiepileptic Drugs,* 3rd ed. New York: Raven Press, 1989.

36. Britton JW, So EL: Selection of antiepileptic drugs: a practical approach. *Mayo Clin Proc* 71:778, 1996.

37. Leach JP, Bordie MJ: New antiepileptic drugs: an explosion of activity. *Seizure* 4:5, 1995.

38. Overweg J: Withdrawal of anliepileptic drugs (AEDs) in seizure-free patients, risk factors for relapse with special attention for the EEG. *Seizure* 4:19, 1995.

39. Pellock JM: Antiepileptic drug therapy in the United States: a review of clinical studies and unmet needs. *Neurology* 45(3, suppl 2):S17, 1995.

40. Willmore LJ: The effect of age on the pharmacokinetics of antiepileptic drugs. *Epilepsia* 36(suppl 5):S14, 1995.

41. Bourgeois BF: Important pharmacokinetic properties of antiepileptic drugs. *Epilepsia* 36(suppl 5):S1, 1995.

42. Bruni J: Antiepileptic drug selection and adverse effects: an overview. *Can J Neurol Sci* 21:S3, 1994.

43. Chadwick D: Standard approach to antiepileptic drug treatment in the United Kingdom. *Epilepsia* 35(suppl 4):S3, 1994.

44. Ferrendelli JA: Relating pharmacology to clinical practice: the pharmacologic basis of rational polypharmacy. *Neurology* 45(3, suppl 2):S12, 1995.

45. Engel J Jr (ed): *Surgical Treatment of the Epilepsies.* New York, Raven Press, 1993.

46. Janz D: Status epilepticus and frontal lobe lesions. *J Neurol Sci* 1:446, 1964.

47. Sawyer GT, Webster DD, Schultz J: Treatment of uncontrolled seizure activity with diazepam. *JAMA* 203:913, 1968.

48. Rowan AJ, Scott DF: Major status epilepticus: a series of 42 patients. *Acta Neurol Scand* 46:573, 1970.

49. Gastaut H: Clinical and electroencephalographic classification of epileptic seizures. *Epilepsia* 11:102, 1970.

50. Commission on Classification and Terminology, International League Against Epilepsy: Proposed revisions of clinical and electroencephalographic classification of epileptic seizures. *Epilepsia* 22:480, 1981.

51. Working Group on Status Epilepticus: Treatment of convulsive status epilepticus. Recommendation of the Epilepsy Foundation of America's Working Group on Status Epilepticus. *JAMA* 270:854, 1993.

52. Bancaud J: Kojewnikow's syndrome (epilepsia partialis continua in children), in Roger J, Dravet C, Bureau M, Dreifuss FE, Wolf P (eds): *Epileptic Syndromes in Childhood and Adolescence.* London, John Libbey, 1985, pp 286–298.

53. Aguilar MJ, Rasmussen T: Role of encephalitis in the pathogenesis of epilepsy. *Arch Neurol* 2:663, 1960.

54. Li Y, Laxer KD, Jeong MC, et al: Local-clonal expansion of infiltrating T lymphocytes in chronic encephalitis of Rasmussen. *J Immunol* 58:1428, 1997.

55. Shorvon S: *Status Epilepticus: Its Clinical Features and Treatment in Children and Adults.* Cambridge, Cambridge University Press, 1994, pp 98–100.

56. Celesia GG, Grigg MM, Ross E: Generalized status myoclonicus in acute anoxic and toxic-metabolic encephalopathies. *Arch Neurol* 45:781, 1988.

57. Jumao-as A, Brenner RP: Myoclonic status epilepticus: a clinical and electrographic study. *Neurology* 40:1199, 1990.

58. Lowenstein DH, Aminoff MJ: Clinical and EEG features of status epilepticus in comatose patients. *Neurology* 42:100, 1992.

59. Young GB, Gilbert JJ, Zochodne D: The significance of post-anoxic myoclonic status epilepticus. *Neurology* 40:1843–1848, 1990.

60. Fagan KJ, Lee SI: Prolonged confusion following convulsions due to generalized nonconvulsive status epilepticus. *Neurology* 40:1689, 1990.

61. Granner MA, Lee SI: Nonconvulsive status epilepticus: EEG analysis of a large series. *Epilepsia* 35:42, 1994.

62. Jagoda A, Riggo S: Nonconvulsive status epilepticus in adults. *Am Emerg Med* 6:250, 1988.

63. Young GB, Brown JD, Bolton CF: PLEDs and nystagmus retractorius. *Ann Neurol* 1:61, 1977.

64. Andermann F, Robb JP: Absence status: a reappraisal following review of thirty-eight patients. *Epilepsia* 13:177, 1972.

65. Hauser WA: Status epilepticus: frequency, etiology and neurological sequelae, in Delgado-Escueta AV, Wasterlain CG, Treiman DM, Porter RJ (eds): *Status Epilepticus: Mechanisms of Brain Damage and Treatment.* Advances in Neurology series, vol 34. New York, Raven Press, 1983, p 3.

66. Browne TR, Penry JK, Porter RJ, et al: Responsiveness before, during and after spike-wave paroxysms. *Neurology* 24:659, 1974.

67. Porter RJ, Penry JK: Petit mal status, in Delgado-Escueta AV, Wasterlain CG, Treiman DM, Porter RJ (eds): *Status Epilepticus: Mechanisms of Brain Damage and Treatment.* Series, vol 34. New York, Raven Press, 1983, p 61.

68. Fujiwara T, Watanabe M, Nakamura H, et al: A comparative study of absence status epilepticus between children and adults. *Jpn J Psychiatry Neurol* 42:497, 1988.

69. Hauser WA: Status epilepticus: epidemiological considerations. *Neurology* 40(suppl 2):9, 1990.

70. Tomson T, Svanborg E, Wedlund JE: Nonconvulsive status epilepticus: high incidence of complex status epilepticus. *Epilepsia* 27:276, 1986.

71. Celesia GG: Modern concepts of status epilepticus. *JAMA* 235:1571, 1976.

72. Dunne JW, Summers QA, Stewart-Wynn EG: Non-convulsive status epilepticus: a prospective study in the adult general hospital. *QJM* 238:117, 1987.

73. Tomson T, Lindbom, Nilsson BY: Nonconvulsive status epilepticus in adults: thirty-two consecutive patients from a general hospital. *Epilepsia* 33:829, 1992.

74. Young GB, Jordan KG, Doig GS: An assessment of nonconvulsive seizures in the intensive care unit using continuous EEG monitoring: an investigation of variables associated with mortality. *Neurology* 46, 83, 1996.

75. Mayeux R, Lüders H: Complex partial status epilepticus: case report and proposal for diagnostic criteria. *Neurology* 28:957, 1978.

76. Treiman DM, Delgado-Eseueta AV: Complex partial status epilepticus, in Delgado-Escueta AV, Wasterlain CG, Treiman DM, Porter RJ (eds): *Status Epilepticus: Mechanisms of Brain Damage and Treatment.* Advances in Neurology series, vol 34. New York, Raven Press, 1983, p 69.

77. Gale K: Progression and generalization of seizure discharge: anatomical and neurochemical substrates. *Epilepsia* 29(suppl 2):S15, 1988.

78. VanLandringham AC, Magnus O: Self-sustaining limbic status epilepticus. II. Role of hippocampal commissures in metabolic responses. *Neurology* 41:1950, 1957.

79. Meldrum BS, Horton RW: Physiology of status epilepticus in primates. *Arch Neurol* 28:1, 1973.

80. Gloor P, Fariello RG: Generalized epilepsy: some of its cellular mechanisms differ from those of focal epilepsy. *Trends Neurosci* 11:63, 1988.

81. Treiman DM, Walton NY, Kendrick C: A prospective sequence of electroencephalographic changes during generalized convulsive status epilepticus. *Epilepsy Res* 5:49, 1990.

82. Lothman E: The biochemical basis and pathophysiology of status epilepticus. *Neurology* 40(Suppl 2):13, 1990.

83. Simon RP, Aminoff MJ: Electrographic status epilepticus in fatal anoxic coma. *Ann Neurol* 20:351, 1986.

84. Young GB, Goodenough P, Jacono V, Schieven JR: Periodic lateralized epileptiform discharges (PLEDs): electrographic and clinical features. *Am J EEG Technol* 28:1, 1988.

85. Reiher J, Grand'Maison F, Leduc CP: Partial status epilepticus: short-term prediction of seizure outcome from on-line EEG analysis. *Electroenceph Clin Neurophysiol* 82:17, 1992.

86. Beaumanoir A, André-Obadia N, Nahory A, Zerbi D: Special types of periodic lateralized discharges associated with confusional state in cerebral circulatory insufficiency. *Electroenceph Clin Neurophysiol* 99:287, 1996.

87. Heinemann U, Jones RSG: Neurophysiology, in Dam M, Cram L (eds): *Comprehensive Epileptology.* New York, Raven Press, 1990, pp 17–42.

88. Meldrum BS, Horton RW: Physiology of status epilepticus in primates. *Arch Neurol* 28:1, 1973.

89. Cosellis JAN, Bruton CJ: Neuropathology of status epilepticus in humans, in Delagado-Escueta AV, Wasteralin CG, Treiman DM, Porter RJ (eds): *Status Epilepticus: Mechanisms of Brain Damage and Treatment.* Advances in Neurology series, vol 34. New York, Raven Press, 1983, pp 129–139.

90. Marjerison JH, Cosellis JAN: Epilepsy and the temporal lobes: a clinical, electroencephalographic and neuropathological study of the brain with particular reference to the temporal lobes. *Brain* 89:499, 1966.

91. Meldrum BS, Brierley JB: Prolonged epileptic seizures in primates: ischemic cell change and its relation to ictal physiological events. *Arch Neurol* 28:10, 1973.

92. Auer RN, Siesjö BK: Biological differences between ischemia, hypoglycemia and epilepsy. *Ann Neurol* 24:699, 1988.

93. Jope RS, Johnson GVW, Baird MS: Seizure-induced protein tyrosine phosphorylation in rat brain regions. *Epilepsia* 32:755, 1991.

94. Bertram EH, Lothman EW: NMDA receptor antagonists and limbic status epilepticus: a comparison with standard anticonvulsants. *Epilepsy Res* 5:177, 1990.

95. Sloviter RS, Dempster DW: "Epileptic" brain damage is replicated qualitatively in the rat hippocampus by central injection of glutamate or aspartate but not GABA or acetylcholine. *Brain Res Bull* 15:39, 1985.

96. Meldrum BS: Cell damage in epilepsy and the role of calcium in cytotoxicity, in Delgado-Escueta AV, Ward AA, Woodbury DM, Porter RJ (eds): *Basic Mechanisms of the Epilepsies.* Advances in Neurology series, vol 44. New York, Raven Press, 1986, pp 849–855.

97. Siesjo BK, Ingvar M, Folbergova J, Chapman AG: Local cerebral circulation and metabolism in bicucidine-induced status epilepticus: relevance for development of cell damage, in Delgado-Escueta AV, Wasterlain CG, Treiman DM, Porter RJ (eds): *Status Epilepticus: Mechanisms of Brain Damage and Treatment.* Advances in Neurology series, vol 34. New York, Raven Press, 1983, pp 217–230.

98. Sakhi S, Bruce A, Sun N, et al: Kainic acid induces tumor suppressor p53 and apoptosis in the central nervous system. *Epilepsia* 35(suppl 8):5, 1994.

99. Meldrum BS, Brierley JB: Prolonged epileptic seizures in primates: ischemic cell change and its relation to ictal physiological events. *Arch Neurol* 28:10, 1973.

100. Nevander G Ingvar M, Auer RN, Siesjö BK: Status epilepticus in well-oxygenated rats causes neuronal necrosis. *Ann Neurol* 18:281, 1985.

101. Kapur J, Lothman EW: Loss of inhibition precedes delayed spontaneous seizures in the hippocampus after tetanic electrical stimulation. *J Neurophysiol* 61:427, 1989.

102. Sloviter RS: "Epileptic" brain damage in rats induced by sustained electrical stimulation of the perforant path. 1. Acute electrophysiological and light microscopic studies. *Brain Res Bull* 10:675, 1983.

103. Sloviter RS: Pemanently altered hippocampal structure, excitability and inhibition after experimental status epilepticus in the rat; the "dormant basket cell" hypothesis and its possible relevance to temporal lobe epilepsy. *Hippocampus* 1:41, 1991.

104. Ben-Ari Y: Limbic seizure and brain damage produced by kainic acid: mechanisms and relevance to human temporal lobe epilepsy. *Neuroscience* 14:375, 1985.

105. Shimosaka S, So YT, Simon RP: Distribution of HSP72 induction and neuronal death following limbic seizures. *Neurosci Lett* 138:202, 1992.

106. Corsellis JAN, Meldrum, BS: Epilepsy, in Blackwood W, Corsellis JAN (eds): *Greenfield's Neuropathology*, 3rd ed. London, Edward Arnold, 1976, pp 771–795.

107. McGeer PL, McGeer EG, Nagai T: GABAergic and cholinergic indices of rat brain after intracerebral injections of folic acid. *Brain Res* 260:107, 1983.

108. Olney JW, Fuller TA, Collins RC, deGubareff T: Systematic dipipidinoethane mimics the convulsant and neurotoxic actions of kainic acid. *Brain Res* 200:231, 1980.

109. Bertram EH, Lothman EW, Lenn NJ: The hippocampus in experimental chronic epilepsy: a morphometric analysis. *Ann Neurol* 27:43, 1990.

110. Collins RC, Lothman EQ, Olney JW: Status epilepticus in the limbic system—biochemical and pathological changes. In Delgado-Escueta AV, Wasterlain CG, Treiman DM, Porter RJ (eds): *Status Epilepticus: Mechanisms of Brain Damage and Treatment*. Advances in Neurology series, vol 34. New York, Raven Press, 1983, pp 277–288.

111. Menini C, Meldrum BS, Riche D, Silva-Comte, C, Stutzmann JM: Sustained limbic seizures induced by intraamygdaloid kainic acid in the baboon: symptomatology and neuropathological consequences. *Ann Neurol* 8:501, 1979.

112. Sloviter RS: Decreased hippocampal inhibition and a selective loss of interneurons in experimental epilepsy. *Science* 235:73, 1987.

113. Leung LS, Brzozowski D, Shen B: Partial hippocampal kindling affects retention but not acquisition and place but not cue tasks on the radial arm maze. *Behav Neurosci* 110:1017, 1996.

114. Dennison A, Teskey GC, Cain DP: Persistence of kindling: effect of partial kindling, retention interval, kindling site and stimulation parameters. *Epilepsy Res* 21:171, 1995.

115. Leung LS, Zhao DC, Shen BX: Long-lasting effects of partial hippocampal kindling on hippocampal physiology and function. *Hippocampus* 4:696, 1994.

116. Leung LS, Shen B, Sutherland R, Wu C, Wu K, Zhao D: Long-lasting behavioural and electrophysiological effects induced by partial hippocampal kindling, in Corcoran ME, Moshe SL (eds): *Kindling 5*, New York, Plenum Press, 1997.

117. Treiman DM: Electroclinical features of status epilepticus. *J Clin Neurophysiol* 12:343–362, 1995.

118. Cockerall OC, Walker MC, Sander JWAS, Shorvon SD: Complex partial status epilepticus. *Neurology* 47:308, 1996.

119. Hilkens PHE, de Weerd AW: Non-convulsive status epilepticus as cause for focal neurological deficit. *Acta Neurol Scand* 92:193, 1995.

120. Nilsson P, Ronne-Engstrom E, Flink R, et al: Epileptic seizure activity in the acute phase following cortical impact in the rat. *Brain Res* 637:227, 1994.

121. Jordan KG: Continuous EEG and evoked potential monitoring in the neuroscience intensive care unit. *J Clin Neurophysiol* 10:445, 1993.

122. Kotapka MJ, Graham DI, Adams JH, Doyle D, Gennarelli TA: Hippocampal damage in fatal paediatric head injury. *Neuropathol Appl Neurobiol* 19:128, 1993.

123. Waterhouse EJ, Sandoz G, Boggs JG, Towne AR: Mortality of status epilepticus and stroke. *Epilepsia* 36(suppl 4):46, 1996.

124. DeGiorgio CM, Gott PS, Rabinowiz AL, Heck CN, Smith TD, Correale JD: Neuron-specific enolase, a marker for acute neuronal injury, is increased in complex partial status epilepticus. *Epilepsia* 37:606, 1996.

125. Rabinowicz AL, Correale JD, Bracht KA, Smith TD, DeGeorgio CM: Neuron-specific enolase is increased after nonconvulsive status epilepticus. *Epilepsia* 36:475, 1995.

126. DeGeorgio CM, Correale JD, Ginsburg DL, et al: Serum neuron specific enolase in status epilepticus. *Neurology* 44(suppl 2):205, 1994.

127. Rabinowicz AL, Correale JD, Couldwell WT, DeGeorgio CM: CSF neuron specific enolase after methohexital activation during electrocorticography. *Neurology* 44:1167, 1994.

128. Dunne JW, Summers QA, Stewart-Wynne EG: Nonconvulsive status epilepticus: a prospective study in an adult general hospital. *QJM* 238:117, 1987.

129. Treiman DM, Delgado-Escueta AV, Clark MA: Impairment of memory following complex partial status epilepticus. *Neurology* 31:109, 1981.

130. Escueta AV, Boxley J, Stubbs N, Wadell G, Wilson WA: Prolonged twilight state and automatisms: a case report. *Neurology* 24:331, 1974.

131. Kitagawa T, Takashashi K, Matsushima K, Kawahara R: A case of prolonged confusion after temporal lobe psychomotor status. *Folia Psychiatrica et Neurologica* 33:279, 1989.

132. Wasterlain CG, Fugikawa DG, Penix LaRoy, Sankar R: Pathophysiological mechanisms of brain damage from status epilepticus. *Epilepsia* 34(suppl 1):37, 1993.

133. Engel J, Ludwig BI, Fetell M: Prolonged partial complex status epilepticus: EEG and behavioral observations. *Neurology* 28:863, 1978.

134. Krumholz A, Sung GY, Fisher RS, et al: Complex partial status epilepticus accompanied by serious morbidity and mortality. *Neurology* 45:1499, 1995.

135. Scholtes FB, Renier WO, Meinardi H: Nonconvulsive status epilepticus: causes, treatment and outcome in 65 patients. *J Neurol Neurosurg Psychiatry* 61:93, 1996.

136. Brett EM: Minor epileptic status. *J Neurol Sci* 3:52, 1966.

137. Doose H: Nonconvulsive status epilepticus in childhood: clinical aspects and classification, in Delgado-Escueta AV, Wasterlain CG, Treiman DM, Porter RJ (eds): *Status Epilepticus: Mechanisms of Brain Damage and Treatment*. Advances in Neurology series, vol 34. New York, Raven Press, 1983, pp 83–92.

138. Stores G, Zaiwalla Z, Styles E, Hoshika A: Nonconvulsive status epilepticus. *Arch Dis Child* 73:106, 1995.

139. Towne AR, Pellock JM, Ko D, DeLorenzo RJ: Determinants of mortality in status epilepticus. *Epilepsia* 35:27, 1994.

140. Drislane FW, Schomer DL: Clinical implications of generalized status epilepticus. *Epilepsy Res* 19:111, 1994.

141. Litt B, Dizon L, Ryan D: Fatal nonconvulsive status epilepticus in the elderly. *Epilepsia* 35(suppl 8):10, 1994.

142. Editorial: Penicillin, ceftazadime and the epilepsies. *Lancet* 340:400, 1992.

143. Klion AD, Kallsen J, Cowl CT, Nauseef WM: Ceftazidime-related nonconvulsive status epilepticus. *Arch Intern Med* 154:586, 1994.

144. Messing RO, Closson RG, Simon RP: Drug-induced seizures: a 10-year experience. *Neurology* 34:1582, 1984.

145. Drislane FW: Nonconvulsive status epilepticus in patients with cancer. *Clin Neurol Neurosurg* 96:314, 1994.

146. Wong MC, Suite NDA, Labar DR: Nonconvulsive generalized status epilepticus in AIDS. *Atm Intern Med* 116:171, 1992.

147. Grogan R, Wagner DR, Sullivan T, Labar D: Generalized nonconvulsive status epilepticus after electroconvulsive therapy. *Convuls Ther* 11:51, 1995.

148. Vanna NK, Lee SI: Nonconvulsive status epilepticus following electroconvulsive therapy. *Neurology* 42:263, 1992.

149. Hansen-Grant S, Trandon R, Maixner D, De Quardo JR, Mahapatra S: Subclinical status epilepticus following ECT. *Convuls Ther* 11:134, 1995.

150. Cascino GD: Nonconvulsive status epilepticus. *Epilepsia* 34(suppl 1):S21, 1993.

151. Louis ED, Pflaster NL: Catatonia mimicking nonconvulsive status epilepticus. *Epilepsia* 36:943, 1995.

152. Kaplan PW: Nonconvulsive status epilepticus in the emergency room. *Epilepsia* 37:643, 1996.

153. Lowenstein DH, Aminoff MJ, Simon RP: Barbiturate anesthesia in the treatment of status epilepticus: clinical experience of 14 patients. *Neurology* 38:395–400, 1988.

154. Shorvon S: *Status Epilepticus: Its Clinical Features and Treatment in Children and Adults*. Cambridge, Cambridge University Press, 1994.

155. Working Group on Status Epilepticus: Treatment of convulsive status epilepticus. Recommendation of the Epilepsy Foundation of America's Working Group on Status Epilepticus. *JAMA* 270:854–859, 1993.

156. Lowenstein DH: Update on status epilepticus. Course "Update on Critical Care" at 1996

American Academy of Neurology, syllabus 134, pp 134–15–134–28.

157. Runge JW, Allen FH: Emergency treatment of status epilepticus. *Neurology* 46(suppl 1):S20, 1996.

158. Levy R, Krall R: Treatment of status epilepticus with lorazepam. *Arch Neurol* 1:605, 1984.

159. Wallis W, Kutt H, McDowell F: Intravenous diphenylhydantoin treatment of acute repetitive seizures. *Neurology* 18:513, 1984.

160. Leppik I, Derivan A, Homan R, et al: Double-blind study of lorazepam and diazepam in status epilepticus. *JAMA* 249:1452, 1983.

161. Delgado-Escueta AV, Enrile-Bascal F: Combination therapy for status epilepticus: intravenous diazepam and phenytoin, in Delgado-Escueta AV, Wasterlain CG, Treiman DM, Porter RJ (eds): *Status Epilepticus: Mechanisms of Brain Damage and Treatment*. Advances in Neurology series, vol 34, 1983, pp 477–485.

162. Parent JM, Lowenstein DH: Treatment of refractory status epilepticus with continuous infusion of midazolam. *Neurology* 44:1837, 1994.

163. Young GB, Blume WT, Bolton CF, Warren KG: Anesthetic barbiturates in refractory status epilepticus. *Can J Neurol Sci* 7:291, 1989.

164. Lowenstein DH, Aminoff MJ, Simon RP: Barbiturate anesthesia in the treatment of status epilepticus: clinical experience with 14 patients. *Neurology* 38:395, 1988.

165. Biggio G, Costa E: *Benzodiazepine Recognition Site Ligands: Biochemistry and Pharmacology*. New York, Raven Press, 1983.

166. Treiman DM: The role of benzodiazepines in the management of status epilepticus. *Neurology* 40(suppl 2):32, 1990.

167. Wilder BJ, Rangel RJ: Phenytoin. Clinical use, in Levy R, Mattson R, Meldrum B, Penry JK, Dreifuss FE (eds): *Antiepileptic Drugs*, 3rd ed. New York, Raven Press, 1989, p 233.

168. Browne TR, Kugler AR, Eldon MA: Pharmacology and pharmacokinetics for fosphenytoin. *Neurology* 46(suppl 1):S3, 1996.

169. Ramsay RE DeToledo J: Intravenous administration of fosphenytoin: options for the management of seizures. *Neurology* 46(suppl 1):S17, 1996.

170. Uthman BM, Wilder BJ, Ramsay ER: Intramuscular use of phenytoin: an overview. *Neurology* 46(suppl 1):S24, 1996.

171. Olsen RW, Snowman AM: Chloride-dependent enhancement by barbiturates of gamma-aminobutyric acid binding. *J Neurosci* 2:1812, 1982.

172. Prichard JW, Ransom BR: Phenobarbital. Mechanisms of action, in Levy R, Mattson R, Meldrum B, Penry JK, Dreifuss FE (eds): *Antiepileptic Drugs*, 3rd ed. New York, Raven Press, 1989, p 267.

173. Shaner DM, McCurdy SA, Herring MO, Gabor AJ: Treatment of status epilepticus: a prospective comparison of diazepam and phenytoin versus phenobarbital and optional phenytoin. *Neurology* 38:202, 1988.

174. Crawford TO, Mitchell WG, Fishman LS, Snodgrass SR: Very high dose phenobarbital for refractory status epilepticus in children. *Neurology* 38:1035, 1988.

175. Kumar A, Bleck TP: Intravenous midazolam for the treatment of refractory status epilepticus. *Crit Care Med* 20:483, 1992.

176. Parent JM, Lowenstein DH: Treatment of refractory generalized status epilepticus with continuous infusion of midazolam. *Neurology* 44:1837, 1994.

177. Van Ness PC: Pentobarbital and EEG burst-suppression in treatment of status epilepticus refractory to benzodiazepines and phenytoin. *Epilepsia* 31:61, 1990.

178. Kinoshita H, Nakagawa E, Iwasaki Y, Hanaoka S, Sugai K: Pentobarbital therapy for status epilepticus in children. *Pediatr Neurol* 13:164, 1995.

179. Krishnamurthy KB, Drislane FW: Relapse and survival after barbiturate anesthetic treatment of refractory status epilepticus. *Epilepsia* 37:863, 1996.

180. Yaffe K, Lowenstein DH: Prognostic factors of pentobarbital therapy for refractory generalized status epilepticus. *Neurology* 43:895, 1993.

181. Kofke WA, Towfighi J, Garman RH et al: Effect of anesthetics on neuropathologic sequelae of status epilepticus in rats. *Anesth Analg* 77:330, 1993.

182. Kuisma M, Roine RO: Propofol in prehospital treatment of convulsive status epilepticus. *Epilepsia* 36:1241, 1995.

183. Campostrini R, Bati MB, Giorgi C, et al: Propofol in the treatment of convulsive status epilepticus: a report of four cases. *Rev Neurol* 61:176, 1991.

184. MacKenzie SJ, Kapadia F, Grant IS: Propofol infusion for control of status epilepticus. *Anaesthesia* 45:1043, 1990.

185. DeMaria G, Guanleri D Pasolini MP, Antonini L: Stato di male versivo trattato con propofol. *Bollitino di Lega Italiana Contro L'Epilepsia* 74:191, 1991.

186. Wood PR, Browne GPR, Pugh S: Propofol infusion for the treatment of status epilepticus. *Lancet* I:480, 1988.

187. Makela JP, Iivanainen M, Peininkeroinen IP, Waltimo O, Lahdensuu M: Seizures associated with propofol anesthesia. *Epilepsia* 34:832, 1993.

188. Cromwell TH, Eger EI, Stevens WC, Dolan WM: Forane uptake, excretion and blood solubility in man. *Anesthesiology* 35:401, 1971.

189. Kofke WA, Young RSK, Davis P, et al: Isoflurane for refractory status epilepticus: a clinical series. *Anesthesiology* 71:653, 1989.

190. Ropper AH, Kofke A, Bromfield EB, Kennedy SK: Comparison of isoflurane, halothane and nitrous oxide in status epilepticus. *Ann Neurol* 19:98, 1986.

191. Sakaki T, Ake K, Hosida T, et al: Isoflurane in the management of status epilepticus after surgery around the motor area. *Acta Neurochir* 116:38, 1992.

192. Hughes DR, Sharpe MD, McLachlan RS: Control of epilepsia partialis continua and secondary generalized status epilepticus with isoflurane. *J Neurol Neurosurg Psychiatry* 55:739, 1992.

193. Brent J, Vo N, Kulig K, Rumack BH: Reversal of prolonged isoniazid-induced coma by pyridoxine. *Arch Intern Med* 150:1751, 1990.

194. Swaiman KF, Milstein TM: Pyridoxine-dependency and penicillin. *Neurology* 20:78, 1970.

195. Chiron C, Dulac O, Beaumont D, et al: Therapeutic trial of vigabatrin in refractory infantile spasms. *J Child Neurol* 6(suppl 2):S52, 1991.

196. Jordan KG: Continuous EEG and evoked potential monitoring in the neuroscience intensive care unit. *J Clin Neurophysiol* 10:445, 1993.

197. Devinski O, Nadi S, Theodore WH, Porter RJ: Cerebrospinal fluid pleocytosis following simple, complex partial and generalized tonic-clonic seizures. *Ann Neurol* 23:402, 1988.

198. Young GB, Gilbert JJ, Zochodne D: The significance of post-anoxic myoclonic status epilepticus. *Neurology*, 40:1843–1848, 1990.

199. Chen R, Bolton CF, Young GB: Prediction of outcome in patients with anoxic coma: a clinical and electrophysiological study. *Crit Care Med* 24:672, 1996.

200. Livingston JH, Brown JK: Non-convulsive status epilepticus resistant to benzodiazepines. *Arch Dis Child* 62:41, 1987.

201. Browne TR, Mikati M: Status epilepticus, in Ropper AH, Kennedy SF (eds): *Neurological and Neurosurgical Intensive Care.* Rockville, MD, Aspen 1988, pp 83–92.

202. Lowenstein DH, Alldredge BK: Status epilepticus in an urban public hospital in the 1980s. *Neurology* 43:483, 1993.

203. Barois A, Estournet B, Baron S, Levy-Alcover M: Prognotic à long terme des états de mal convulsifs prolongés. *Annales de Pédiatrie* 32:621, 1985.

204. Sung C-Y, Chu N-S: Epileptic seizures in intracerebral hemorrhage. *J Neurol Neurosurg Psychiatry* 52:1273, 1989.

205. Krumholz A, Sung GV, Fisher RS, et al: Complex partial status epilepticus accompanied by serious mortality and moribidity. *Neurology* 45:1499, 1995.

206. Yager JY, Cheang M, Seshia SS: Status epilepticus in children. *Can J Neurol Sci* 15:402, 1988.

207. Janz D: Conditions and causes of status epilepticus. *Epilepsia* 2:170, 1961.

208. Oxbury JM, Whitty CWM: Causes and consequences of status epilepticus in adults: a study of 86 cases. *Brain* 94:733, 1971.

209. Aminoff MJ, Simon RP: Status epilepticus: causes, clinical features and consequences in 98 patients. *Am J Med* 69:657, 1980.

210. Goulon M, Lévy-Alcover MA, Nouailhat F: Etat de mal épileptique de l'adulte: etude épidémiologique et clinique en réanimation. *Revue d'Electroencéphalographie et de Neurophysiologie Clinique* 15:277, 1985.

211. Dunn DW: Status epilepticus in children: etiology, clinical features and outcome. *J Child Neurol* 3:167, 1988.

Chapter 18

OTHER CAUSES OF TRANSIENT OR REVERSIBLE IMPAIRMENT OF CONSCIOUSNESS

G. Bryan Young

Oh sleep, thou ape of death, lie dull upon her!
And be her sense but as a monument.
William Shakespeare, *Cymberline*

Brief loss of awareness may relate to dysfunction in the alerting system mediated by the ascending reticular activating system or to dysfunction of the higher functions carried out in the limbic system and neocortex (Table 18-1). These reversible lapses of function may be caused by syncope, epileptic seizures, transient ischemic attacks or migraine involving the vertebrobasilar system, concussion, metabolic derangements or intoxications, sleep-related disorders, and psychiatric disturbances. In addition, some patients have episodes of altered behavior or impairment of alertness that defy classification.

SYNCOPE

Definition

Syncope, or fainting, is defined as a temporary, completely reversible loss of consciousness due to a global reduction in blood flow to the brain. This traditional definition will be used throughout, although, in recent usage, the term "syncope" has been applied to any sudden, transient loss of consciousness.

Significance

The 26-year Framingham survey, which excluded persons with previously known cardiac disease, reported an occurrence of syncope in 3 percent of men and 3.5 percent of women.[1] More than 75 percent of subjects had only one attack. Syncope is more common in young adults and, to a lesser extent, the very old.[2,3] The causes and associated morbidity, and later mortality, depend on the patient population of the center.

Using clinical and commonly available investigative techniques, the cause can be determined in most cases. The etiological diagnosis is not often made with the first visit. Thus, further follow-up and investigations are necessary.

A major problem is that there have been no randomized, controlled studies that set a standard

Table 18-1

Classification of transient impairment of consciousness or memory function

Syncope: reflex fainting, cardiac or orthostatic hypotension

Seizures: especially complex partial, absence, and generalized convulsive

Transient vascular events and migraine

Transient global amnesia

Concussion and postconcussive confusional or amnestic states

Intoxications and metabolic derangements, including idiopathic recurring stupor

Sleep disorders, e.g., REM[a] behaviour disorder (RBD)

Psychiatric conditions and malingering

Transiently raised intracranial pressure

Cryptogenic (especially in the middle aged and elderly)

[a] Rapid-eye-movement sleep.

Table 18-2

Classification of syncope

Vasomotor instability
    Vasodepressor
    Situational
        Micturition
        Cough
        Swallowing
    Orthostasis (see Table 18-6 for a more detailed classification)
    Postprandial hypotension
    Drugs
    Neuralgias
Decreased venous return
    Hypovolemia: e.g., diuretics, bleeding
    Increased venous pooling
Decreased or limited cardiac output
    Aortic stenosis
    Bradycardia
    Mitral stenosis
    Atrial myxoma
    Cardiac failure
    Tamponade, dissection
    Arrhthymias: tachy- and bradyarrhythmias
Obstruction to right ventricular outflow
    Pulmonary stenosis
    Pulmonary embolism
    Pulmonary hypertension plus increased cardiac demand
    Myxoma

for the investigation, diagnosis, and management of syncope. This is compounded by its variable and unpredictable nature. Even though syncope is common, adequate clinical and electrophysiologic documentation of the events is infrequent.

Syncope related to significant heart disease has an associated 1 year mortality rate of 20 to 30 percent.[4] Mortality is higher in syncopal patients with left ventricular dysfunction or with inducible, sustained, monomorphic ventricular tachycardia on electrophysiologic testing.[5] These two variables may not be independent and have not been statistically separated for relative weighting.

Pathophysiologic Classification

There is either a transient loss of blood flow to the whole brain or to those parts involved in alertness, most commonly the former (Chap. 1). Mechanisms involve reduced blood flow to the heart, reduced or limited cardiac output, or reduced perfusion pressure (see Table 18-2).

The absence of brain blood flow causes loss of electroencephalogram (EEG) signal in 15 to 20 s. This occurs well before reduction in the energy charge potential, a measure of high-energy phosphate stores. Phosphocreatine becomes exhausted at about 1 min and adenosine triphosphate (ATP) and adenosine diphosphate (ADP) at 3 to 5 min, or there is a buildup of lactate (reaches maximal concentration at 3 min), after circulatory arrest at normal temperature.[6] The early, reversible failure in synaptic transmission responsible for EEG silence probably relates to the following:

1. Changes in postsynaptic excitability: Interruption of blood flow to the cortex results in an immediate neuronal hyperpolarization.[7] This probably relates to increased neuronal potassium conductance and increased carbon dioxide concentration.[8]

2. Failure of release of neurotransmitters from presynaptic terminals: Even a small decrease in ATP in axon terminals may be enough to block synaptic transmission.[9] This is a region of high metabolic activity as evidenced by abundant mitochondria in presynaptic regions. Also, there is a suppression of presynaptic calcium currents that leads to failure of neurotransmitter release.[8] Rising intracellular calcium has also been demonstrated and may contribute.[8]

If ischemia persists, there is an hypoxic depolarization resembling spreading depression across the neuronal population.[8] This begins minutes after oxygen withdrawal, after the failure of synaptic transmission. This "spreading depression," due to an increase in extracellular potassium, is a reversible phenomenon. However, it is followed by neuronal damage or death from a massive influx of cations—causing osmotic swelling and delayed calcium-mediated damage as a result of a large release of excitotoxic neurotransmitters.[10]

Clinical Features and Investigation

An overall approach begins with the history and physical examination but extends to various investigative strategies. This is shown in Fig. 18-1.

Figure 18-1

Flow diagram showing the approach to the evaluation of syncope. Abbreviations not used in the text: CPK-MB = creatine kinase, cardiac isoenzyme; CCU = critical care unit; MI = myocardial infarction. (From Kapoor,[173] with permission of the American Journal of Medicine.)

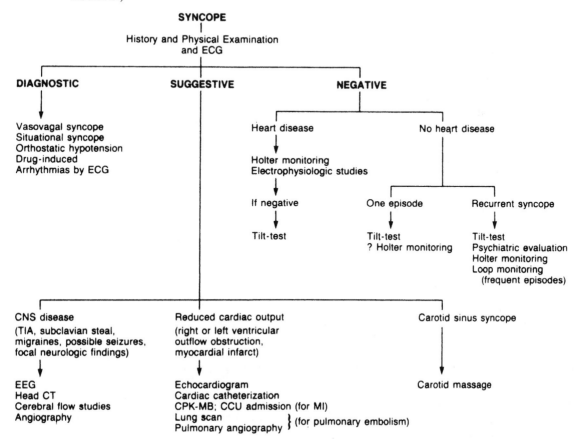

The main differential diagnosis is between syncope and epileptic seizures. Some symptoms, such as visual dimming and roaring in the ears, are more likely to be presyncopal than seizure-related. However, these and other symptoms, e.g., sweating, nausea, and light-headedness, are not as consistently reliable as differentiating premonitory features. Urinary incontinence also occurs with both syncope and seizures. Tongue-biting is suggestive of convulsive seizures, but it may occur accidentally in falls with syncope. In a study that compared the clinical symptoms of fits and faints, the best discriminatory symptom was disorientation and confusion after the event, which was much more common in seizures than syncope.[11]

The most careful study on syncope was performed by Lempert and colleagues.[12] Syncope was self-induced by a Valsalva maneuver in 42 healthy volunteers between 20 and 30 years of age. Because of the brief period of hypotension, their findings, although carefully documented, may not apply to all cases of syncope, e.g., cardiogenic cases, in which circulatory insufficiency is more intense and prolonged. Nonetheless, the observations are useful (see Table 18-3). This study underlines the overlap of syncopal phenomena with those experienced and witnessed in seizures.

Precipitating factors can be very helpful. Vasodepressor syncope is commonly brought on by unpleasant sights, sounds or smells, sudden unexpected pain, or other emotional shocks.

Table 18-3

Phenomena in induced syncope

Feature	Frequency	Comment
Visual and auditory hallucinations	60%	Visual: gray haze, colored or bright lights
		Auditory: rushing or roaring noises
Falling	80% fell backward 48% flexed at knees 52% extended lower limbs	Falling "like a tree" is not always due to a seizure
Myoclonus	90%; lasted 0.7–15.9 s (mean 6 s) 50% involved the face	Multifocal or mixed multifocal and generalized; only one with focal: all but one arrhythmic; none with only generalized bilaterally synchronous jerks
Vocalizations	40%	Simple, low-pitched, low-amplitude "growling" sounds
Head movement, with or without ipsiversive gaze deviation	Common	Head turning did not achieve "forced" quality found in seizures
Eye movements	Eyes open in 76% Blinks in 50% Change of eye position in 50%	Eye positions changed slowly, not like "epileptic nystagmus"
Other movements	Some patients	"Automatisms": lip smacking, chewing, fumbling—resembled epileptic automatisms
Overall subjective experience	83% had "positive" experience 17% had "negative" experience	Feelings of weightlessness, detachment, and peace were common

Table 18-4

Common drugs causing syncope

Vasodilators	*Psychoactive drugs*
Nitrates	Phenothiazines
Calcium channel blockers	Antidepressants (e.g., tricyclics, MAOIs)
ACE inhibitors	CNS depressants (e.g., barbiturates)
Other (prazocin, hydralazine)	
Drugs associated with torsades de pointes	*Other mechanisms*
Quinidine	Vincristine and other neuropathic drugs
Procainamide	Digoxin
Dispyramide	Insulin
Flecainide	Marijuana
Amiodarone	Alcohol
Sotalol	Cocaine
Diuretics	*Alpha₁-adrenergic blockers*
	Prazosin
	Doxazosin
	Terazosin

Abbreviations: ACE = angiotensin-converting enzyme; MAOIs = monoamine oxidase inhibitors.

Cough syncope, micturition syncope, and swallow syncope are reliably diagnosed clinically when loss of consciousness consistently follows these activities. Impending loss of consciousness that begins only with a standing posture, with light-headedness, sweating and visual dimming, and with arrest of the episode by promptly lying down, strongly favors syncope rather than seizures.

Cardiac syncope due to ischemic heart disease may or may not be accompanied by clinical angina. Loss of consciousness during or immediately after arm exercise raises the possibility of subclavian steal.[13] Recurrent loss of consciousness during excitement or exercise in a child should raise the possibility of prolonged QT syndrome.[14] The recent introduction of antihypertensives or other drugs that cause orthostatic hypotension or bradycardia (Table 18-4) suggests syncope.

On examination, a difference of more than 20 mmHg in blood pressure between the two arms raises the possibility of aortic dissection or (uncommonly) subclavian steal syndrome. The examination may lead to other diagnoses, including aortic stenosis, idiopathic subaortic stenosis, pulmonary hypertension, and other entities that may explain recurrent syncopal attacks on an exercise-induced or hemodynamic basis.

Neurocardiac Syncope (Vasovagal and Vasodepressor Syncope)

Neurocardiac, neurally mediated, neuroregulatory, reflex, vasovagal, and vagovagal and vasodepressor syncope are terms that refer to faints due to neurally mediated bradycardia and/or vasodilatation in discrete attacks (see Table 18-5). Pallid breath-holding spells of infants are probably similarly neurally mediated.

Attacks are sometimes precipitated by prolonged standing, sudden, powerful emotion—such as pain or fear, or the shock of seeing blood. There is usually a warning of light-headedness and feeling hot that lasts seconds to minutes. Pallor, yawning, and a rapid heart rate are followed by nausea, perspiration, and loss of consciousness with hypotension and bradycardia. Although these are common features, some patients have no warning. The limbic system, notably the insula, may initiate vasodepressor syncope when the precipitating factor has an emotional impact.

Table 18-5

Classification of neurally based syncope based on tilt table testing

Type 1: Mixed
Heart rate does not decrease to <40 beats per minute for >10 s, and no asystole lasts >3 s. Blood pressure decreases before heart rate at the time of syncope.

Type 2a: Cardioinhibitory
Heart rate decreases to <40 beats per minute for >10 s or asystole lasts >3 s. Blood pressure decreases before the heart rate.

Type 2b: Cardioinhibitory
Heart rate decreases to <40 beats per minute for >10 s or asystole lasts >3 s. Blood pressure decreases to hypotensive levels (<80 mmHg systolic) after the onset of heart rate decrease.

Type 3: Pure vasodepressor
Heart rate does not decrease >10% from its peak at the time of syncope, whereas blood pressure decreases during tilt to cause syncope.

Although bradycardia may accompany the faint, uncommonly is it the sole mechanism. Syncope is usually not prevented by atropine, which blocks the bradycardic component of fainting. The fall in blood pressure is mainly related to a reduction or loss in sympathetic tone to the vessels. The drop in blood pressure affects the arterial and arteriolar as well as the venous vessels. There is some evidence that patients with vasodepressor syncope have a hyperactive mechanoreceptor reflex. The sympatholysis may, in some cases, result from an overshoot baroreceptor response to an initial rise in blood pressure. Mechanoreceptors, located in the inferior and posterior walls of the left ventricle, are stimulated by increased left ventricular pressure. The left ventricle increases its contractility and transmural pressure if there is a drop in left ventricular blood volume or an increased systemic catecholamine release. In patients with a "hyperactive" mechanoreceptor reflex, this stimulation triggers the vasomotor centre in the medulla to reduce the sympathetic tone and to increase the vagal tone (Bezold-Jarish reflex). This then results in vasodepressor (with vasovagal) syncope. There is also a drop in

hormonal secretion, including epinephrine, angiotensin II, vasopressin, and endothelin 1. Recent studies also suggest that nitric acid synthesis increases, and this may contribute to the profound vasodilatation and resultant hypotension.[15]

Tests for Vasodepressor Syncope: The tilt table test is carried out with the patient strapped to a table that tilts to an upright position from the horizontal. Such tilting immediately reduces venous return to the right side of the heart. The resultant reduced left ventricular volume triggers an increase in left ventricular contractility and stimulates the left ventricular mechanoreceptors (see above). The tilt table test can be carried out passively or with the use of isoproteronol.[16] The isoproteronol is added, in some cases, as a provocative measure, but has a false positive rate of about 8 percent.[16] The tilt is usually to 60° to 80° for up to 45 min. The end point of a positive tilt table test is the development of syncope or presyncope with hypotension or bradycardia, or both. A positive tilt table test, however, does not prove that vasodepressor syncope is the mechanism for the loss of consciousness that precipitated the investigation. It does reveal, however, a "tendency" for vasodepressor fainting. A potential problem is that the test is often not consistent from one trial to the next on the same person. A somewhat useful classification system based on results of tilt table testing is presented in Table 18-5.[17]

For most patients, education and reassurance suffice. Young individuals may outgrow the tendency for fainting. Patients with mild and infrequent syncope may be able to avoid further attacks by avoiding precipitants and by lying or sitting down promptly with the first warning of an attack. Avoidance of stressors (including frightening situation), psychiatric intervention for phobias, the provision of adequate rest, and avoidance of excessive alcohol may serve as important measures in some individuals.

In some patients with recurrent vasodepressor syncope, e.g., children with an autonomic dysfunction in blood pressure control, the use of a salt-enriched diet may help. Other measures include fludrocortisone, and, in resistant cases, beta blockers, scopolamine, disopyramide, theophylline, or serotonin reuptake inhibitors such as fluoxetine have been suggested.[18] Beta blockers, such as metoprolol or propranolol, may help by decreasing myocardial contractility in patients with reflex fainting. Anticholinergic agents, such as transdermal scopolamine, may be useful in some patients with strong vasovagal as opposed to vasodepressor tendencies.

Cardiac (especially dual chamber) pacing may be useful in selected patients with predominant cardioinhibitory vasovagal as opposed to vasodepressor response, and similar cases of carotid sinus syncope.[19,20] Its usefulness will likely be limited to a small subpopulation with severe or malignant syncope who have been refractory to conservative management, and who have predominantly cardioinhibitory vasovagal bradycardia on tilt table testing (type 2b in Table 18-5).[20] The usefulness of this method has not been subjected to a controlled trial, however.

Postprandial Syncope

Postprandial hypotension is defined as a drop of 20 mmHg or more in systolic blood pressure (or when the postprandial systolic blood pressure is < 90 mmHg, when it had been > 100 mmHg beforehand) within 2 h, usually reaching a nadir at 30 to 60 min, from the start of a meal.[21] The relative roles of medication taken at mealtimes and the association of orthostatic drops in blood pressure have not been fully taken into account. The prevalence in the population is uncertain, but may approach 25 to 36 percent of patients in nursing homes.[22] The syndrome is probably more common than orthostatic hypotension. The following individuals may be most susceptible: healthy elderly persons, young and elderly with treated hypertension, the elderly in nursing homes, patients with diabetes mellitus, and other patients with autonomic insufficiency, anemia, Parkinson disease, cardiovascular disease, renal failure on hemodialysis, and adrenal impairment.

Carbohydrates, especially warm drinks containing glucose, have a strong association with postprandial syncope. The pathogenesis is uncertain. Hypotensive effects of insulin, splanchnic blood pooling, reduced peripheral vascular resistance, a blunted compensatory increase in heart rate, and an osmotic shift of vascular volume into the gut have all been proposed as mechanism.[21] The main factor may be a failure of vascular compensation for the physiologic vascular volume and vasomotor changes related to a meal.

Clinical symptoms are the expected symptoms of near-syncope or syncope: i.e., light-headedness, dizziness, weakness, falls, and visual changes. In patients with serious atherosclerotic vascular disease, angina pectoris or hemodynamic transient ischemic events may occur. Usually, the reduction of brain blood flow is gradual, allowing a protracted aura.

Management involves first identifying the underlying contributing, reversible causes and correcting them, e.g., discontinuing or reducing medications that contribute to orthostatic hypotension, and administering hypotensive medications between rather than during meals. In addition, it is best to caution susceptible patients of the risk of falling and syncope in the 90 min after meals. Ensuring an adequate vascular volume, including liberal use of salt, if tolerated, may help. Small, frequent meals with reduced carbohydrate content and avoidance of alcoholic beverages with meals may also help. Taking coffee or other caffeine beverages has some benefit. For more serious cases, consider fludrocortisone, indomethacin, octreocide, indomethacin, or alpha$_1$-adrenergic agonists such as midodrine.[21]

Swallowing Syncope

Syncope associated with swallowing is due to stimulation of the glossopharyngeal nerve that, through connections with the dorsal motor nucleus of the vagus and the medullary vasomotor depressor center, causes reflex bradycardia and hypotension.[23] The syndrome typically consists of pain on swallowing, variably associated with syncope, and often accompanied by bradycardia.[24] Neuralgic (brief, jabbing) pain is usually felt on one side of the oropharynx, tonsillar pillars, and root of the tongue and may radiate to the regional hemiface or the ipsilateral external ear.

Patients with heart block or sick sinus syndrome and those on digoxin may be susceptible to such reflexly induced physiologic degrees of vagal activity that trigger fainting.[25,26] Other cases may be due to esophageal dysfunction, such as spasm, excessively cold or hot foods, esophageal diverticulum, cancer, and inflammation.

Syncope may be due to glossophayngeal neuralgia or involvement of the glossopharyngeal nerve or root entry zone in the brainstem by intracranial vascular compression, head and neck cancers, parapharyngeal abscesses, trauma, and multiple sclerosis.[27–32] These need to be excluded. Other cases (a considerable component) are idiopathic.

Therapeutic modalities have not been subjected to controlled trials. Carbamazepine may be effective in the idiopathic cases and in some others, e.g., those in multiple sclerosis.[33] Cardiac pacing may be an option for some cases of syncope and marked bradycardia or aystole.[34] The most successful specific surgical procedure appears to be the sectioning of glossopharyngeal and upper vagal roots.[35]

Carotid Sinus Syncope

Carotid sinus syncope probably accounts for about 1 percent of cases of syncope and is mainly a disease of the elderly.[36] Carotid sinus hypersensitivity refers to a ventricular pause of ≥ 3 s and/or a drop in systolic blood pressure of ≥ 50 mmHg after massage of the carotid bulb.[37] Carotid sinus massage for carotid sinus syncope is performed with electrocardiogram (ECG) and blood pressure monitoring in either the supine or sitting position. Cardiac asystole for more than 3 s is taken as a positive cardioinhibitory response. A vasodepressor response is defined as the drop in systolic blood pressure of more than 50 mmHg, provided there is no bradycardia.

The hypersensitive carotid sinus is probably accentuated by atherosclerotic diseases in the walls of the carotid sinus. There may be a central nervous predisposition, however, as some patients have a history of vasodepressor syncope.[38] The most profound effects of carotid sinus stimulation are cardiac standstill and atrioventricular block, varying from first to third degree. Again, there is a problem with the specificity of the test. Although 5 to 25 percent of the population show carotid sinus sensitivity on testing, only 5 to 20 percent of these have clinical syncope. Furthermore, it is hard to prove, even in these cases, that carotid sinus syncope was the cause. A positive test does not necessarily require that treatment be instituted.

Among patients for whom there is no additional obvious cause, other than carotid sinus syndrome, some benefit may be gained from cardiac pacing or anticholinergics.[39] A recent controlled trial in Italy involved 32 patients randomly allocated to the paced group and 28 nonpaced controls.[40] Syncope occurred in 16 nonpaced (57 percent) and 3 paced (9 percent) patients over 3 years follow-up ($p = 0.002$). Some proposed predictors of success include: (1) the presence of multiple syncopal episodes before implantation of pacemaker; (2) episodes that occur when the patient is upright; (3) episodes preceded by a recognized trigger; and (4) episodes associated with marked bradycardia. An alternative therapy that may prove successful for some patients is denervation of the carotid sinus.[39]

Tussive (Cough), Micturition, and Defecation Syncopes

In tussive syncope, fainting episode occurs in the context of a bout of coughing. Syncope related to coughing may result from a sustained rise in the intrathoracic pressure that impedes venous return and reduces the cardiac output.[41] Chronic chest disease can further impair the venous return to the thorax, especially if the intrathoracic pressure rises to higher than normal values and is sustained during prolonged expiration.[42] Patients with idiopathic hypertropic subaortic stenosis may present with cough syncope, likely related to the combination of left ventricular obstruction in the heart and reduced venous return from raised intrathoracic pressure.[43] Some patients may have an intracranial rather than a pulmonary or cardiac predisposition.

Micturition syncope typically occurs in young and old men who lose consciousness while standing urinating. In older individuals with prostatic hypertrophy and urinary outlet obstruction, patients strain and increase intrathoracic pressure, reducing cardiac output. In younger individuals, the mechanism is likely to be a reflex vasodilatation near the end of micturition.

Defecation syncope is probably analogous to micturition syncope, with fainting occurring during or immediately after a bowel movement.[44]

Cardiac Syncope

The historical features, especially from an eyewitness, are valuable[45]:

> The patient with simple [vasodepressor] syncope is pale, with Stokes-Adams attack he looks dead. The quick recovery, usually short duration, and historical details from the patient are not seen with epilepsy. When the patient is recovered from an attack and attempts to get up with the return of the light-headed presyncopal feeling, the diagnosis is almost always orthostatic or vasovagal fainting and never a Stokes-Adams attack.

If cessation of brain blood flow is sudden, cardiac syncope may occur without warning. As a corollary, syncope without warning is almost always cardiac in origin.

Atrioventricular block, sick sinus syndrome, ventricular arrhythmias, and sinoatrial bradycardia are the main cardiac conditions that cause syncope. Less commonly, sinoatrial arrest is a cause. The prolonged QT interval is found predominantly in two hereditary disorders with considerable heterogeneity: the surdo(deafness)-cardiac (Jervell-Lange-Nielson) and Romano-Ward syndromes.[46] A new, autosomal-dominantly inherited syndrome with prolonged QT interval, atrioventricular block syndactyly, and patent ductus arteriosus has been described.[47] The loss of consciousness is typically abrupt, without presyncopal warnings, and precipitated by exertion or emotional excitement. Patients commonly have generalized clonic movements during attacks and are misdiagnosed as epileptics. Some may have presyncope without loss of consciousness and some may die during attacks. The QT interval is prolonged on ECG; patients develop ventricular fibrillation ventricular tachycardia, or *torsades des pointes* during attacks.

Syncope related to coronary artery disease may occur during exercise. Intermittent complete heart block or arrhythmias may produce syncope. Most cases occur in patients with structural heart disease, sometimes manifest in left bundle branch block.[48]

Other causes of cardiac syncope in young people include hypertrophic cardiomyopathy, aberrant coronary arteries, and aortic dissection secondary to Marfan syndrome.[49] Occasionally, toxic doses of drugs may produce cardiac arrhythmias, e.g., certain histamine receptor type-one antagonists.[50]

Syncope with hypertrophic obstructive cardiomyopathy has been related to a gradient between the left ventricular outflow tract and the aorta. This is caused by a sphincter-like action of the contracting septal musculature and the anterior mitral leaflet.[51] Indeed, there may be a variety of mechanisms, especially ventricular tachycardia.

Syncope after cardiac transplantation most commonly relates to bradyarrhythmias due to sinoatrial (SA) node dysfunction.[52] The etiology is uncertain, but it has been proposed that the SA node suffers ischemia in the transplantation procedure.

Investigations   The ECG may be abnormal, but this does not establish the cause of syncope in most cases. The following patterns offer important clues, however: the prolonged QT interval, recent myocardial infarction, and second- and third-degree heart block. Conversely, the absence of ECG abnormality does not rule out cardiogenic syncope.

More intensive noninvasive cardiac investigations have a low yield. Aggressive, prolonged cardiac monitoring over 6 months may yield only a 16 percent diagnostic rate.[53] When there is congruity of features of a recorded typical clinical attack and a diagnostic change on the 24 to 48 h continuous, ambulatory (Holter) ECG monitor, the test is very helpful. This is uncommon, however. Zeldis et al monitored 371 patients and found that 13 percent had abnormal rhythms at some time.[54] Thirty-four percent had typical symptoms with no change on the ECG and 86 percent of those with recorded tachycardias remained symptom free.[54]

A variation is the implantable loop recorder that can be used for long-term recording for months and years as opposed to days or weeks.[55] This should dramatically increase the yield of electrographically recorded events.

More invasive electrophysiologic tests may be necessary in some patients. These are reserved for patients with significant heart disease, such as those with known structural heart disease, including ischemic heart disease, congestive heart failure, valvular heart disease, and hypertrophic cardiomyopathies. Patients with ECG abnormalities associated with re-entry phenomena, such as the Wolff-Parkinson-White syndrome, also come into this category. Occasionally, patients with abnormalities detected on noninvasive cardiac monitoring will be candidates for this testing. Such tests include intracardiac recording, used to measure conduction time over the antrioventricular (AV) node and His bundle system.[56,57] Pacing can be used to stress the system and detect conduction blocks. Such intracardiac investigations can also be used to precipitate and diagnose re-entry phenomena, including AV node re-entry and recurrent monomorphic ventricular tachycardia.[58]

Management of Syncope from Cardiac Causes Treatment should be directed at the pathophysiologic mechanism for the syncope, usually a tachycardia or a bradycardia. Tachycardias require specific treatments depending on the type, while most bradyarrhythmias/bradycardias require pacing.

Beta blockers have been used with some success in the prolonged QT syndromes.[14] Overdrive pacing has been used with beneficial results in many patients; although some still have spells or die suddenly.[59] The combination of beta blockers and pacing provides the combined benefit of both for some patients.[59]

Implantable cardiac defibrillators have been used in some patients with recurrent cardiac arrest.[60] Cardiac pacing may be helpful in the prevention of recurrent atrial fibrillation, especially of the "bradycardia-dependent" type, although this is controversial.[61]

Beta blockers and calcium channel blockers have been used in hypertrophic obstructive cardiomyopathy to prevent or reduce the functional obstruction to left ventricular outflow. Cardiac pacing in patients with hypertrophic obstructive cardiomyopathy can reduce the gradient between the left ventricle and aorta.[62] Right ventricular pacing alters the activation sequence in the septum that contributes to the generation of the gradient. Pacing relieved presyncopal symptoms as well as angina in 42 of 44 patients in one series.[63] Apical septal activation may be pivotal in aiding such patients.[63]

Badyarrhythmias after cardiac transplantation tend to subside after about 3 weeks; it is probably best to wait until after this time before deciding on a permanent pacemaker. Until then, the patient can be managed, if necessary, with a temporary epicardial pacemaker.

Orthostatic Hypotension

Orthostatic hypotension is defined as a drop in blood pressure of more than 25 mmHg systolic and/or 10 mmHg diastolic upon arising.[64] A classification of causes of orthostatic hypotension is given in Table 18-6. The blood pressure should be taken after the patient has been supine for 10 to 15 min and then on standing. Usually, the patient should stand for at least 2 min, but it is sometimes worthwhile checking the blood pressure repeatedly while the patient is up and about, as it might fall to lower values. Since a modest drop in blood pressure is not uncommon in elderly patients, it is diagnostically helpful if presyncopal symptoms accompany the drop.

Idiopathic orthostatic hypotension, or the Bradbury-Eggleston syndrome, is an adult-onset, degenerative condition affecting the sympathetic nervous system and related to cell loss in the intermediolateral cell column in the gray matter

Table 18-6

Classification of orthostatic hypotension

Neurogenic	Miscellaneous
Primary autonomic failure	Increasing age
Central	Volume depletion (hemorrhage, gastrointestinal fluid
Multiple system atrophy	loss, diuresis)
Peripheral	Pooling of venous blood (pregnancy, varicose veins, vena
Idiopathic orthostatic hypotension	cava obstruction)
Central nervous system (CNS) of spinal cord disease	Vasodilatation (fever, heat exhaustion, intense exhaustion)
Ischemic, traumatic, inflammatory, neoplastic	Sympathicotonia (mitral valve prolapse)
or compressive C-cord lesion Parkinson disease	Medications (tricyclics, antihypertensives, major
	tranquillizers)
	Prolonged recumbancy or weightlessness

of the spinal cord. This aspect is similar to multiple system atrophy (MSA) or Shy-Drager syndrome, but in the latter there is also degeneration of other sites including the locus ceruleus, nucleus of the solitary tract, and preganglionic vagal neurons. In MSA, parkinsonian features are related to degeneration of the substantia nigra in the midbrain. In most cases of idiopathic orthostatic hypotension, plasma serum norepinephrine concentrations are low, suggesting also a postganglionic autonomic failure.

In the acquired immunodeficiency syndrome (AIDS), the autonomic nervous system may be involved, but probably less commonly than the brain. Plasma norepinephrine levels are low, suggesting a postganglionic mechanism.

The neurologic examination, if abnormal, may give clues for the mechanism of the orthostatic hypotension (e.g., parkinsonian features in MSA or the Shy-Drager syndrome, and sensory neuropathy in amyloidosis or diabetic peripheral neuropathy). If there are focal central neurologic signs, the possibility of epileptic seizures is strengthened.

For treatment, nonpharmacologic methods are preferred and should be tried first in mild cases.[65] These include increasing the sodium content in the diet, avoidance of suddenly rising to an upright posture, sleeping on an inclined plane with the head up (which helps to expand the blood volume), and wearing elastic stockings with a graded increase in tension from the foot to the upper thigh. If these measures are insufficient, or if the postural hypotension is marked and producing fainting, the drug of choice is fludrocortisone. Midodrine, an alpha$_1$-agonist drug used in a small randomized controlled trial in idiopathic orthostatic hypotension, helped 47 percent of patients in the treatment group, compared with 28 percent in the control group.[66] Other sympathomimetics, beta-adrenergic antagonists, monoamine oxidase inhibitors, and ergot alkaloids should only be administered to severely affected patients; these individuals must be closely monitored. Other agents include the following: prostaglandin synthetase inhibitors, clonidine, yohimbine, octretide, dopamine antagonists, desmopressin, and epoetin alfa.[67] Problems with these measures include the production of circulatory overload and congestive heart failure, as well as supine hypertension with its attendant complications.

SEIZURES

Seizures are finite events consisting of "an occasional, an excessive and a disorderly discharge of nerve tissue."[68] This "nerve tissue" is in the brain, with most discharges arising in the cerebral cortex. Epilepsy is a condition of recurring, unprovoked seizures.

Convulsive and nonconvulsive seizures are discussed in Chap. 17.

TRANSIENT VASCULAR EVENTS AND MIGRAINE

Vertebrobasilar ischemic events uncommonly are associated with loss of consciousness as a component.[69] Transient global amnesia may result from vertebrobasilar transient ischemic attacks (TIAs) of migraine.

Vertebrobasilar TIAs characteristically produce symptoms and signs of brainstem ischemia (e.g., diplopia, dysphagia, dysarthria vertigo, ataxia, circumoral numbness, bilateral limb weakness, or sensory loss) or symptoms related to ischemia in the cerebral distribution of the posterior cerebral arteries [binocular teichopsia (both visual fields or one hemifield), blindness, or transient memory disturbance]. Drop attacks are thought to be due to ischemia of the medullary pyramids, causing transient quadriplegia with preserved consciousness. The attacks are too brief to cause tissue infarction. Although, typically, the features completely resolve, sometimes this resolution may be incomplete and a partial stroke results. This is the case especially for events that last more than 24 h.[70]

Confusion, loss of consciousness, transient memory disturbance, or experiential phenomena including hallucinations have been described in migraine, mainly in young people.[71,72] Confusion may occur spontaneously or after a trivial head injury in acute confusional migraine. In patients with "Bickerstaff's migraine," consciousness is usually lost gradually; there are other symptoms or signs of vertebrobasilar ischemia (vertigo, tinnitus, diplopia, ataxia, dysarthria, bilateral or unilateral weakness, sensory symptoms or hemianopsia or complete loss of vision) and, characteristically," a nonspecific dream-like state from which they were temporarily arousable.[73-75] Patients awake without confusion, but usually have a severe headache and other features of migraine, e.g., nausea, vomiting, and photophobia. Rarely, basilar artery migraine may be associated with attacks of impaired consciousness that last for days or even several weeks.[76,77] During attacks of basilar migraine, Doppler studies show increased velocity through the basilar artery and the EEG

has generalized slowing but no epileptiform activity.[72,77,78,79]

Some migrainous patients may exhibit "hemispheric" signs, such as aphasia with hemiparesis, before losing consciousness. Some families have apparently dominantly inherited coma-associated migraine.[80,81] Some may be precipitated by minor blows to the head. Fever and cerebrospinal fluid (CSF) pleocytosis are common.[79] Cerebral edema on computed tomography (CT) is characteristically associated; the lateral shift may account for coma in affected patients (see Chap. 4).[79] Rarely the attack can be fatal.[82] Conventional cerebral angiography during the migrainous attack carries a greater than 40 percent risk of complications—worsening of edema with the threat of herniation—and is best avoided.[79,83] Magnetic resonance (MR) angiography is preferable. Most often, patients recover without evidence of cerebral infarction; the edema presumably represents an increase in blood-brain barrier permeability but not actual tissue necrosis. The majority of such patients are left with residual cerebellar ataxia, however; the mechanism for this is uncertain.[79] Patients may have multiple attacks.

The site of the initial disorder in migraine has been debated. The widespread EEG abnormalities in acute confusional and Biekerstaff's migraine point to a subcortical origin for many of the features, e.g., brainstem signs and widespread EEG abnormality. While it is presumed that the features of vertebrobasilar migraine are due to vasomotor disturbance in this arterial system, there are increased concentrations of gamma-aminobutyric acid (GABA) and cyclic adenosine monophosphate (cAMP) in the CSF in association with such ischemia.[77] A role for increased GABA-nergic activity in vertebrobasilar migraine is the worsening of impaired consciousness produced by benzodiazepines.[84] Other unconfirmed or unidentified metabolic factors may be at least contributory.

Patients with migrainous coma should be fully supported in the intensive care unit (ICU) with ventilatory support and antiepileptic drugs (AEDs), if necessary. Corticosteroids are sometimes used for those with cerebral edema, but their effectiveness has not been proven. Most patients make a good recovery, despite a swollen cerebral hemisphere and initial coma.

The differential diagnosis depends on the clinical picture, but may include thrombosis of the basilar artery, cerebellar infarction or hemorrhage, intoxications, metabolic disorders [including MELAS (mitochondrial myopathy, encephalopthy, lactic acidosis and stroke-like episodes)], encephalitis, hysteria, and temporal lobe epilepsy. These are usually excluded on clinical grounds, but some investigations, e.g., EEG, CT scan, and Doppler studies, may be necessary. The clinical picture, including a history of recurrent attacks and a positive family history of migraine, is strongly suggestive of the diagnosis.

For severe attacks preventive medication e.g., with a calcium channel blocker such as flunarizine, should be considered.

TRANSIENT GLOBAL AMNESIA

"Transient global amnesia" is a term coined by Fisher and Adams to describe a global memory defect that typically lasts several hours.[85] The patient, usually middle aged or elderly, has a profound defect for recent (weeks or years) memory and is unable to lay down memories during the attack. Alertness is intact, the patient knows his own identity and is able to interact with the environment. Procedural memory is normal and the patient can drive a vehicle or carry out other complex motor acts. Language function and praxis are intact. The patient typically appears confused, concerned, and bewildered and asks the same questions repeatedly. The mechanism has been debated. Some cases may be due to a limited type of temporal lobe seizure. Others may be vertebrobasilar ischemia, either embolic or hemodynamic; attacks have also been described in association with migraine.[86]

CONCLUSION

This syndrome of reversible alteration in consciousness, with or without a postconcussive confusional or amnestic state, is discussed in Chap. 6.

INTOXICATION

Intoxications or poisonings are discussed in Chap. 16. Alcoholic blackouts deserve emphasis. Although the syndrome has not been thoroughly researched, Goodwin et al found that 64 of 100 chronic alcoholics experienced lapses of memory.[87] Such episodes occur in the context of a bout of heavy drinking. Violent acts commonly accompany such blackouts, at least in a subgroup of alcoholics.[88] Tamerin et al studied patients during intoxication and found that short-term recall was impaired first, then amnesia occurred for the previous day.[89]

METABOLIC DERANGEMENTS

Intrinsic metabolic abnormalities sometimes cause transient alteration in alertness or functioning. Such intermittent abnormalities include the following: acute intermittent porphyria, hypoglycemia, chronic portal-caval hepatic disease, idiopathic recurring stupor, and various problems with fluids and electrolytes that may cause seizures (e.g., hyponatremia, uremia, hypocalcemia, hypomagnesemia). These often cause recurrent and fluctuating encephalopathies. Hepatic disease is especially likely to produce transient episodes of alteration in cognition or alertness.[90] Such attacks can be easily mistaken for transient ischemic attacks or nonconvulsive epileptic seizures.

Acute Intermittent Porphyria

Acute intermittent porphyria (AIP) may be associated with intermittent encephalopathy. In an attack, patients frequently have abdominal and/or lower extremity pain in association with increased sympathetic activity (i.e.., sweating and tachycardia). A polyneuropathy with autonomic and sensorimotor features that mimic Guillain-Barré syndrome may occur. Mental symptoms occur in about 30 percent of cases. The following features have been variably described: confusion, anxiety, psychotic, hallucinations, and depression. An acute confusional state is probably the underlying mental abnormality. Lethargy progressing to coma or generalized convulsions may occur.

Idiopathic Recurring Stupor

Idiopathic recurring stupor is a condition characterized by behavior resembling intoxication, with impaired alertness and mental acuity. In more severe attacks, patients may become comatose. Episodes usually come on gradually and may last for several days. The EEG typically shows increased beta ($> 13\,Hz$) activity with voltage of $> 3\,\mu V$, variably mixed with frequencies in the theta (> 4 but $< 8\,Hz$) or delta ($\leq 4\,Hz$) activity, diffusely. The impairment of alertness, higher functions and EEG features may be reversed by the benzodiazepine receptor antagonist, flumazenil.[91] Idiopathic recurring stupor is related to increased production of endogenous benzodiazepines, or endozepines, with increased concentrations in the plasma and CSF during attacks.[92] The source of these compounds is not known. The differential diagnosis includes the following: other metabolic encephalopathies or intoxications, narcolepsy, sleep apnea syndrome with excessive daytime somnolence, the idiopathic CNS hypersomnolence syndrome,[93] Kleine-Levin syndrome,[94] nonconvulsive status epilepticus, and bilateral subdural hematomas. Management consists of reversal of the stupor with flumazenil parenterally, confirmation of the diagnosis, and then maintenance flumazenil is given orally during the episode (usually a few days). Because the syndrome is intermittent, chronic use of flumazenil is unncessary and potentially problematic.

SLEEP-RELATED DISORDERS

Some cognitive and behavioral phenomena found in sleep disorders have limited clinical relevance to impaired consciousness and alertness. Excessive daytime somnolence may result from insomnia, specific sleep disorders (narcolepsy, sleep apnea

or periodic movements in sleep), or medical or neurologic problems that disturb sleep staging or sleep quality. Cognitive complaints include defects in attention, concentration, memory (spatial span and spatial working memory), cognitive processing speed, and learning.[95–98] Sleep-deprived patients sometimes experience feelings of unreality that may produce anxiety and further alter performance. In some insomniacs, other variables, such as affective disorders, contribute to alterations of attention, concentration, and memory.[99] Performance in patients may be improved in a dose-dependent fashion by sympathomimetics.[100]

Parasomnias occasionally cause diagnostic confusion with states of altered consciousness, but, in themselves, are odd behaviors in deep slow-wave or rapid-eye-movement (REM) sleep. Somnambulism (sleepwalking), peculiar to stage IV of slow-wave sleep, is a sequence of complex behaviors.[101] Patients may show perseveration of simple movements or get out of bed and walk about, even opening doors. Attempts at restraint usually lead to avoidance behavior. The patient is amnestic for such episodes. The REM sleep behavior disorder (RBD) is a somewhat similar phenomenon that happens in REM rather than non-REM sleep. In RBD, patients "act out their dreams" (normally movements are inhibited in REM sleep). They sometimes recall these actions after wakening, unlike patients with somnambulism. Occasionally, RBD is secondary to lesions in the brainstem tegmentum.[102–104] The locus ceruleus, which inhibits cholinergic centres in the brainstem involved in REM sleep, may be affected.[104] Drugs that reduce REM sleep, e.g., clonazepam, may be helpful.[102]

Some cases of transient unresponsiveness in the elderly may relate to problems in arousal from normal sleep (see "Transient Unresponsiveness of Uncertain Etiology" section later).

PSYCHIATRIC DISORDERS

Depressive illness and schizophrenia can alter cognitive function in various ways. In hyperventilation and panic attacks, normal cognitive function is blunted, although the patient remains awake. In episodic dyscontrol, the patient may perform violent, destructive acts that are associated with reduced responsiveness to others and amnesia for the event. Rage attacks are sometimes combined with intoxications, especially alcohol. Hysteria or conversion reactions may cause transient alterations in behavior for which the patient is later amnestic. In multiple personality disorders, patients assume different distinct identities without apparent recognition or memory of the other characters. In malingering, there is a deliberate feigning of various illnesses; in some cases, malingering and conversion reaction are combined in the same individual.

Depressive Illness

Depression or melancholia can be associated with a marked reduction in behavioral activity to a degree resembling stupor. Although this is usually regarded as a purely functional psychiatric disorder, imbalances in neurotransmitters may play a role, at least in some cases of endogenous depression. One patient who met *DSM*-III (*Diagnostic and Statistical Manual of Mental Disorders*) criteria for a major depressive illness with melancholia, associated with mutism and stupor, was completely relieved of symptoms when given lorazepam; relapse occurred promptly with a benzodiazepine receptor antagonist, the reverse of idiopathic recurring stupor.[105]

Schizophrenia

Schizophrenia, the most common psychosis, consists of two or more of the following: delusions, hallucinations, disorganized speech (frequent derailment or incoherence), grossly disorganized or catatonic behavior, or negative symptoms (i.e., affective flattening, alogia, or avolition).[106] If delusions are bizarre or hallucinations consist of a voice with a running commentary on the person's thoughts or behavior, or if two or more voices are conversing with each other, one criterion is sufficient.[106] In addition, social or occupational dysfunction should be present and the duration

of symptoms should be at least 6 months. There are exclusions including schizoaffective and mood disorders, drug abuse, autism, or a pervasive developmental disorder. Schizophrenia is associated with numerous behaviors, ranging from withdrawal and catatonic stupor, regression, infantilism, asocial and antisocial behavior, aberrant ideas (including paranoia), agitation, disorganized actions, and altered perceptions with delusions and hallucinations. The onset is usually in adolescence or early adulthood. Defects in the maintenance of selective attention and information processing have been shown.[107,108]

Catatonia

Catatonia refers to a motor sign (catalepsy, posturing, or waxy flexibility) in association with at least one sign of psychosocial withdrawal or excitement and/or bizarre repetitive movements (negativism, mutism, grimacing, stereotyped behavior, echolalia, echopraxia, automatisms, or verbiberation.)[109] The term is most commonly applied to schizophrenia and affective illnesses, but also occurs in a wide range of organic cerebral diseases including metabolic, drug-induced, and some degenerative conditions.[110] Although catatonic patients are usually not able to communicate effectively, some with psychiatric illnesses later recall their intense emotions, cognitive ambivalence and other subjective impressions.[111] Catatonia is especially common among elderly depressed patients who suffer major depression, severe cognitive impairment, and deficits in activities of daily living than in other depressed patients.[112] Malignant catatonia, in which patients are incapable of self-care, is a severe variant.[113]

Malignant catatonia must be distinguished from neuroleptic malignant syndrome (lethal catatonia), an extrapyramidal disorder due to the blockade of central dopamine receptors.[114] Intense muscular rigidity is associated with autonomic features (sweating, tachycardia, blood pressure elevation), delirium, and, often, oculogyric crisis. Shock, respiratory failure, myoglobinuria, and secondary renal failure may occur as complications in advanced cases.[115] In turn, this condition needs to be differentiated from malignant hyperthermia, a dominantly inherited disorder of the transport of calcium across the sarcoplasmic reticulum in muscle in which muscular rigidity and fever develop with exposure to various drugs, including inhalational anesthetics, muscle relaxants, tricyclic drug, and others.[116] Prophylaxis, definitive therapy for the acute attacks, and counseling are different in these various conditions.

Hyperventilation and Panic Disorder

Hyperventilation and panic disorder are linked, but can occur independently. Hyperventilation, or overbreathing, refers to an increased rate and/or depth of ventilation, beyond what is needed to adequately maintain blood gas or acid-base balance. It is characterized by a low Pa_{CO_2} and an increased pH. Attacks are usually precipitated by emotional stress and are associated with a feeling of panic or fear.

Symptoms due to the hyperventilation itself are related to the altered blood gases, which reduce total cerebral blood flow and ionized free calcium ions in the plasma. Table 18-7 lists the most common symptoms. Note that feelings of unreality and, occasionally, secondary (vasodepressor)

syncope may be associated with hyperventilation attacks. Such attacks last variable lengths of time, often tens of minutes. A syndrome of chronic hyperventilation has been described.[117] Often, but not invariably, there is a substrate of emotional depression, anxiety, phobias, or panic with mild chronic hypocapnea. Such patients complain of an inability to take a satisfying breath.[118] When such patients are further stressed, they readily experience the symptoms listed in Table 18-7.

Patients are observed to be overbreathing with increased use of intercostal muscles. They typically look anxious during acute hyperventilation attacks. Symptoms are relieved by having the patient rebreathe their expired air by using a paper bag.

In differential diagnosis, it is vital to exclude primary pulmonary or cardiac conditions, especially asthma, pulmonary embolism, congestive heart failure, pneumothorax, and pneumonia, as well as other conditions that may mimic acute anxiety, such as thyrotoxicosis, hypoglycemia, drug or alcohol withdrawal, and prolapsed mitral valve.[119–121]

In panic attack, sudden feelings of extreme anxiety or fear can be precipitated by a stressful situation, but they also occur when the patient is

Table 18-7

Major symptoms during hyperventilation

Neurologic features	*Cardiovascular*
Central nervous system	Palpitations, tachycardia
Dizziness/light-headedness	Precardiac pain
Sense of unreality	
Blurred vision	*Respiratory*
Anxiety/fear/panic	Shortness of breath
Secondary syncope	Chest pain
Peripheral nervous system	"Asthma"
Paresthesiae	
Tetany, carpal-pedal spasm	*Gastroenterologic*
	Heartburn, aerophagia
	Epigastric pain
	Nausea
	Musculoskeletal
	Muscle cramps
	Weakness and easy fatiguability

idle. Sometimes, the symptoms are attributed to medical problems, such as problems breathing or the problems with heart (e.g., chest pain) and are associated with a feeling of impending death. Agoraphobia, the pathologic fear of open spaces or crowds, is a common accompaniment with recurrent panic attacks.[122] The differential diagnosis is similar to that described above. The author has encountered a number of patients with mesial temporal-originating seizures who were misdiagnosed as having panic attacks.[123] The following features are helpful in differentiating such seizures from panic attacks:[124]

1. In seizures, the attacks of anxiety and fear are very brief, lasting only a few seconds. In contrast, panic attacks last minutes.

2. Seizures are more stereotyped in semiology than panic attacks.

3. Rapid shifts of symptoms are more typical of seizures than panic.

4. Focal seizures of mesial temporal origin often progress to complex partial seizures with stereotyped automatisms and impaired awareness.

5. Memory disturbances and other organic features such as aphasia are common with temporal lobe seizures.

6. Olfactory hallucinations are perceived as being external to the self in seizures, while they are more typically related to the self in depression.

Episodic Dyscontrol

The term "episodic dyscontrol syndrome" refers to behavioral disturbances in which (1) there have been several discrete episodes of loss of control or aggressive impulses resulting in serious assault or property damage; (2) the behavior is out of proportion to any psychosocial stressor; (3) there are no signs of generalized impulsivity or aggressiveness between the episodes; and (4) the phenomena are not due to underlying schizophrenia, antisocial personality disorder, or conduct disorder. The condition is not homogeneous. Some patients, however, have personality disorder or minimal brain dysfunction, especially related to previous head injury.[125,126] The aggression begins with a feeling of intense anger and the patient will act violently in a directed or nondirected manner. There is often evidence of increased sympathetic activity, such as tachycardia, flushing, and sweating. The patient may have a premonition that such an attack is likely to occur. Partial but not complete amnesia for the event is common.

Investigations are usually negative, but about one-third have nonspecific diffuse or focal slowing on EEG.[127] This indicates that many such patients have neurophysiologic evidence of brain dysfunction, possibly related to previous brain injury.

In differential diagnosis, aggressive behavior related to seizures is rare, is usually not directed specifically at target individuals or objects, and is stereotyped.[128] The author has not encountered such ictal or postictal aggression unless the confused patient is restrained. Aggressive behavior during intoxication with alcohol or drugs, during hypoglycemia, or during RBD should be considered.

Episodic dyscontrol has been treated with medications and psychotherapy. Carbamazepine, tranylcypromine, and trifluoperazine have all been used with some success in placebo-controlled trials.[129,130] Among these three drugs, carbamazepine was associated with the most improvement. The mechanism is probably a psychotropic one.

Dissociative Reactions

Pseudoseizures and Psychogenic Unresponsiveness Pseudoseizures, also known as psychogenic seizures, or nonepileptic or hysterical seizures, mimic epileptic attacks but are not due to epileptic phenomena or organic impairment of consciousness. Pseudoseizures are common: about 20 percent of patients referred to epilepsy centers (plus or minus genuine seizures), constituting at least several hundred thousand patients in the United States, have pseudoseizures.[131] They occur with female predominance, at ages from 4 to 77 years, with a mean age of onset in the twenties.[131,132] Several possibilities should be considered when a patient presents with pseudoseizures:

1. The symptoms are entirely related to a somatoform disorder, factitious disease, conversion reaction, or malingering.

2. The symptoms are part of another type of psychopathology (e.g., depression, panic attacks, posttraumatic stress disorder) unrelated to physical illness.

3. The symptoms are linked to an organic disorder.

4. The symptoms are an unusual manifestation of a physical disorder; especially noteworthy is the coexistence of pseudoseizures and epileptic seizures.

5. There may be a combination of the above factors.

The majority of patients with pseudoseizures have one or more psychiatric problems: somatoform, dissociative, affective, personality, anxiety, or posttraumatic stress disorders.[132] A history of sexual or physical abuse or other traumas, remote or shortly before the onset of pseudoseizures, is found in more than half the patients.[132] These often require exploration after the diagnosis of pseudoseizures is made.

Pseudoseizures may mimic generalized convulsive, nonconvulsive (absence or complex partial), focal motor or subjective seizures, or amnestic attacks.[133] There are some clinical clues that are helpful in differentiating pseudoseizures from genuine seizures.[131] These are summarized in Table 18-8 along with some caveats. It is more definitive to detect features that are physiologically improbable, such as the onset and termination of spells by suggestion, resistance to eye opening during convulsive-type spells, or eye deviation to the dependent side with repositioning of the patient.[134] (However, some cases of genuine stereotyped or nonstereotyped seizures can be precipitated by suggestion.[135,136]) If the features are bizarre and inconsistent from one attack to the next, pseudoseizures should be suspected, but no single feature reliably differentiates these from real seizures. The following are more typical of

pseudoseizures than real seizures: unresponsiveness without *any* motor manifestations (if one accepts this as simulating a nonconvulsive seizure), writhing limb and head movements, pelvic thrusting, arching of the back, alternating head deviation, grabbing the side rails of the bed and shaking them, asynchronous limb movements (e.g., flailing or bicycling), variable patterns of myoclonus in the same or different attacks for the same individual, atypical vocalization, and forced eyelid closure during generalized convulsive movements.[137–142] Tongue-biting is usually a sign of genuine seizures, while weeping after the attack is evidence for a pseudoseizure.[142] However, there are exceptions to these general rules. Misdiagnosis may also occur in the occasional patient with genuine seizures with these atypical features; frontal or, occasionally, lobe-originating seizures may show such atypical manifestations.[143,146]

In contrast to the above motor signs of a pseudoseizure, eyes are usually open during the motor phase of partial seizures. Eyes are not tonically closed, often leaving a rim of visible sclera.[142] The frontalis muscle is simultaneously contracted, causing elevation of the eyebrow. The mouth is typically opened in the tonic phase of a seizure, often assuming a triangular appearance with the base opposite of the hemisphere of origin.[142]

The following additional clinical features should raise suspicion of pseudoseizures: a consistent emotional trigger, prolonged seizures, or seizures that fail to respond to adequate AED therapy, and the lack of hard neurologic or significant interictal EEG abnormalities. Pseudoseizures tend to start and end gradually. Disorientation to self suggests a dissociative reaction. However, such features could also be found in patients with genuine seizures.

Pseudoseizures may simulate status epilepticus (psychogenic status or pseudostatus epilepticus).[144] These episodes may simulate generalized tonic-clonic or nonconvulsive seizures with apparently automatic behaviors or unresponsiveness without movements. "Slow, subtle writhing or in-phase limb movements" are also described.[145] The danger is in overtreatment. Patients may

Table 18-8

Features suggesting pseudoseizures

Clinical features	Caveats
Cause or precipitant: induced by environmental stress or emotional disturbance	Stress may precipitate epileptic seizures
Onset: often gradual, usually not during sleep	Occasionally, prolonged sensory aurae with genuine seizures; some pseudoseizures are abrupt in onset and may occur during the night after spontaneous arousal
Frequent seizure despite adequate AED levels	Refractory cases of epilepsy
Prompt recovery of consciousness	Absence, some seizures of frontal lobe origin
Bizarre features: hyperventilation syndrome, rigidity, flailing, asynchronous movements, complex or emotional vocalization, opisthotonus, pelvic thrusting, weeping, obscene gestures	Some seizures of frontal or temporal origin may have these features
Provoked by suggestion	Occasionally, genuine seizures may be provoked by strong suggestion
Responsiveness to environment: resistance to eye opening, rolling over when tickled	Some seizures of temporal or frontal origin
Lack of injury during seizures	Some genuine seizures may not lead to injury or tongue biting; some patients with pseudoseizures may injure themselves
Knowledge of epilepsy (model)	Does not preclude genuine epilepsy
Other functional features	Does not preclude genuine epilepsy
Psychiatric past history	Does not preclude genuine epilepsy
Positive family history of psychosocial problems	Does not preclude genuine epilepsy
Weeping after a seizure	Does not preclude genuine epilepsy
Lack of muscle soreness after convulsive seizure	May occur if seizure not prolonged
Nonstereotypic seizures	Some variability in frontal and temporal seizures
Grimacing, facial expressions	Does not preclude genuine epilepsy, e.g., some complex partial seizures
Gradual onset of ictus	Premonitory symptoms or aurae
Prolonged duration	Does not preclude genuine epilepsy
Bilateral motor activity and preserved consciousness	May occur in supplementary motor seizures
Clonic activity ends abruptly	In genuine seizures, clonic activity usually slows before ceasing, but not always
Myoclonic activity is variable and may subside with distraction or sleep	Nonepileptic (metabolic) myoclonus is often multifocal
Usually no defecation or urination	Both urination and defecation can occur in pseudoseizures and real seizures
Aggression during attack (especially directed)	May occur during or following real seizures if patient is restrained

receive sufficient antiepileptic medication to cause ventilatory suppression or unconsciousness, requiring intubation and ventilatory support, or to cause cardiovascular depression, especially hypotension. Some awake patients may even allow themselves to be intubated. Additional complications include infections (respiratory, urinary or "line" sepsis, or cellulitis), nerve pressure palsies, and venous thromboses.

The final diagnosis of pseudoseizures should not rest on any one single ictal feature, but should rest on a combination of data.[146] Clinical features of the attack are the most definitive, especially if there is no EEG change during attacks that resemble genuine seizures.[147] Capturing the attacks on video with simultaneous EEG recording is especially valuable. Clinicians should respect ethical principles in attempting to elicit pseudoseizures.[148] Honesty in the approach and considered differential diagnosis is the best policy (see Chap. 24). Home videotaping allows the physician to be an eyewitness to spontaneous attacks outside the hospital.[149] Witnessed and recorded episodes should be compared with the patient's usual attacks: it is common for patients to have both pseudoseizures and genuine epileptic seizures.

The coexistence of somatoform disorder, false sensory complaints and nongenuine weakness or sensory loss on examination, employment in a health profession, history of sexual or physical abuse, history of other "intractable" medical problems (e.g., headache), or hypochondriasis, "la belle indifference" (apparent unconcern or unusually "positive" attitude), presence of secondary gain, and positive family history of psychiatric problems add support to the diagnosis of pseudoseizures, but are not definitive in proving that the seizures are psychogenic. Indeed, errors can be made by biased physicians.[150] Patients with "pseudo complex partial seizures" commonly have primarily dissociative symptoms with guilt-laden bereavement as an important precursor.[151] Those with "pseudo grand mal" often have long-standing personality disorders.

Finding normal blood gases during apparent generalized convulsive seizures, or the lack of rise in serum prolactin taken within an hour of a convulsive or complex partial seizure, is supportive of pseudoseizures.[152,153] Genuine simple partial seizures typically do not cause a rise in prolactin.[154]

Approximately one-third of patients with pseudoseizures also have genuine epileptic seizures. This greatly complicates management if both types continue. Furthermore, they can sometimes arise in the context of serious, progressive neurologic disease. The author has observed pseudoseizures, with onset over age 50 years, in a patient with a right frontal-temporal astrocytoma.[155]

Management should be multidisciplinary, involving psychiatry and social services as well as the neurologist and nursing staff.[156] The presentation of the diagnosis to the patient should be tactful; confrontation should be avoided. It should be emphasized that the spells are not epileptic and do not require AEDs. A caring, nonjudgmental attitude should prevail on the ward. The prognosis is better if psychosocial intervention is instituted early, if genuine seizures do not coexist, and if the patient lives independently.[131] Psychosocial problems, especially abuse, should be inquired about and problems addressed.[157] Patients who continue for years with this behavior are often refractory. The use of behavior modification therapy may be helpful in such cases.[158]

Psychogenic Amnesia Including Hysterical Fugue States In amnesia due to a conversion or somatization disorder, patients typically do not know important personal information, sometimes their own identity.[159] However, they come to hospital or to a physician seeking help. Such individuals appear to have a total loss of memory for all past events up to the present. The onset is sudden and is only retrograde, lacking the anterograde component of genuine memory disturbance. Such patients are otherwise intact and are able to acquire new information and to interact meaningfully, promptly, and appropriately. This combination of features is not found in organic conditions associated with impaired memory, e.g., transient global amnesia, seizures, metabolic disturbances, intoxications, or postconcussive syndromes.

Fugue states consist of prolonged bouts of amnesia associated with wandering, which are related to various psychopathologies.[160] They are usually dissociative reactions. The fugue state is often preceded by an intense affective change that the patient finds overwhelming. The patient maintains contact with the environment in a meaningful way that would not be possible in a patient with ongoing memory impairment. Often, such patients lose their personal identity and manipulate the environment so as not to cast suspicion on themselves. Patients do not necessarily assume a new identity. Attacks may in early life, e.g., in adolescence.[161]

Differential diagnosis is that of transient global amnesia, temporal lobe seizures, metabolic causes including hypoglycemia, intoxications, rage attacks, concussions, and migraine.[162]

Effective management involves psychodynamic psychotherapy.[163]

Multiple Personality Disorder This disorder, in which patients assume various distinct "identities," is usually not difficult to recognize. The personalities are each intact, with responsiveness and behavior in keeping with that character. When appropriately documented, it is unlikely to be confused with an organic neurologic disorder such as seizures.

Malingering Malingering is the conscious, motivated simulation of disease to attain a desired goal. In the context of apparently impaired consciousness this can be simulated seizures, syncope, coma, or lesser degrees of obtundation. The diagnostic clues on examination during the attack are similar to those for conversion reaction. There are some differences, however: patients with conversion reactions are more susceptible to suggestion; attitudes differ in that the patient with conversion reaction seems more ill and invites support and investigation, while the malingerer may evade examination. The differences in management are obvious.

UNCONSCIOUSNESS FROM TRANSIENTLY RAISED INTRACRANIAL PRESSURE

Patients with Chiari malformations, associated with low-lying cerebellar tonsils and compromised CSF outflow from the fourth ventricle, may, with coughing, develop a sudden rise in intracranial pressure that reduces cerebral perfusion pressures and causes loss or near-loss of consciousness.[164] Similarly, patients with third ventricular tumors, especially colloid and other cysts and intraventricular masses, occasionally have episodes of transient coma.[165–168] These are sometimes preceded by severe bifrontal or generalized headache, suggesting transiently raised intracranial pressure. It has been assumed that this relates to transient obstruction of the foramina of Munro, allowing the intracranial pressure to rise abruptly. Indeed, this can be fatal in many cases. Another hypothesis is hypothalamic dysfunction, caused by pressure on the walls of the inferior aspect of the third ventricle.[169] The risk of death does not correlate strongly with the size of the cyst; cysts of more than 10 mm should probably be surgically removed.[169]

TRANSIENT UNRESPONSIVENESS OF UNCERTAIN ETIOLOGY

Haimovic and Beresford described five elderly patients who developed transient impairment of responsiveness with intact brainstem function.[170] The duration of the attacks was between 10 min and 6 h. The resting and ictal EEGs, which were nearly identical, showed diffuse background slowing. In one patient, the patterns resembled those of stages 1 and 2 of slow-wave sleep. There was no obvious metabolic, structural, convulsive, pharmacologic, or psychiatric explanation. Some cases recurred with similar features within days of the initial attack. Similar cases were described by Rao et al.[171]

The author of this chapter has encountered a similar syndrome in several middle-aged to elderly individuals with identical histories, and in another patient with chronic renal failure on thrice weekly hemodialysis. The EEGs, however, showed only nonspecific generalized slowing and the patients did not respond to flumazenil or naloxone. The uremic patient had recurrent attacks, while the others did not. Tinuper et al have suggested that previously undiagnosed recurring stupor in the elderly is due to endogenous benzodiazepine-like substances.[172] The EEGs and lack of response to flumazenil in the present authors's patients, however, does not support this hypothesis.

The syndrome remains unexplained. It appears to be a reversible metabolic encehalopathy that seems to be endogenous in its pathogenesis. Haimovic and Beresford[170] propose that, at least in some cases, the syndrome may be due to a defect in the arousal system, so that patients fail to arouse from physiologic drowsiness or sleep, of fail to maintain normal alertness.

REFERENCES

1. Savage DD, Corwin L, McGee DL, Kannell WB, Wolf PA: Epidemiologic features of isolated syncope: the Framingham study. *Stroke* 16:626, 1985.
2. Dermksian G, Lamb LE: Syncope in a population of healthy young adults. *JAMA* 168:1922, 1988.
3. Lipsitz LA, Pluchino FC, Wei JY, Rowe JW: Syncope in institutionalized elderly: the impact of multiple pathological conditions and situational stress. *J Chron Dis* 39:619, 1986.
4. Manolis AS: The clinical spectrum and diagnosis of syncope. *Herz* 18:143, 1993.
5. Klein GJ, Gersh BJ, Yee R: Electrophysiological testing. The final court of appeal for the diagnosis of syncope? *Circulation* 92:1332, 1995.
6. Siesjö BK, Johannsson H, Ljunggren B, Norberg K: Brain dysfunction in cerebral hypoxia and ischemia, Plum F (ed): Brain Dysfunction in Metabolic Disorders. *Res Publ Assoc Nerv Ment Dis* 53:75:112, 1974.
7. Glötzner F: Intracelluläre Potentiale, EEG und korticale Gleichspannung an der seonsorimotorischen Rinde der Katze bei akuter Hypoxie. *Arch Psychiatr Nervenkr* 210:274, 1967.
8. Somjen GG, Aitken PG, Czéh G, et al: Cellular physiology of hypoxia of the mammalian nervous system, in Waxman SG (ed): *Molecular and Cellular Approaches to the Treatment of Neurological Diseases,* Research Publication: Association for Research in Nervous and Mental Disease, vol. 71. New York, Raven Press, 1993, pp 51–65.
9. Somjen GG, Schiff SJ, Aitken PG, Balestrino M: Forms of suppression of neuronal function, in Chalazonitis N, Gola M (ed): *Inactivation of Hypersensitive Neurons.* New York, Allan R Liss, 1987, pp 137–145.
10. Cheung JY, Bonventre JV, Malis CD, Leaf A: Calcium and ischemic injury. *N Eng J Med* 314:1670, 1986.
11. Hoefnagels WAJ, Padberg GW, Overberg J, et al: Transient loss of consciousness: the value of the history for distinguishing seizures from syncope. *J Neurol* 238:39, 1982.
12. Lempert T, Bauer M, Schmidt D: Syncope: a videometric analysis of 56 episodes of transient cerebral hypoxia. *Ann Neurol* 36:233, 1994.
13. Luetmer PH, Miller GM: Right aortic arch syndrome with isolation of the left subclavian artery: case report and review of the literature. *Mayo Clin Proc* 65:407, 1990.
14. Hordt M, Haverkamp W, Oberwittler C, et al: The idiopathic QT syndrome as the cause of epileptic and nonepileptic seizures. *Nervenzart* 66:282, 1995.
15. Kaufmann H: Neurally mediated syncope: pathogenesis, diagnosis and treatment. *Neurology* 45(supp 5): S12-8, 1995.
16. Kapoor WN, Smith MA, Miller NL: Upright tilt table testing in evaluating syncope: a comprehensive review. *Am Med* 97:78, 1994.
17. Sutton R, Petersen M, Brignole M, et al: Proposed classification for tilt induced vasovagal syncope. *European Journal of Cardiac Pacing and Electrophysiology* 2:180, 1992.
18. Freed MD: Advances in the diagnosis and therapy of syncope: and palpitations in children. *Curr Opin Pediatr* 6:368, 1994.
19. Benditt DG, Petersen M, Lurie KG, Grubb BP, Sutton R: Cardiac pacing for prevention of recurrent vasovagal syncope. *Ann Intern Med* 122:204, 1995.
20. Maloney JD, Jaeger FJ, Rizo Patron C, Zhu DW: The role of pacing for the management of neurally mediated syncope: carotid sinus syndrome and vasovagal syncope. *Am J Heart* 127:1030, 1994.
21. Jansen RW, Lipsitz LA: Postprandial hypotension: epidemiology, pathophysiology and clinical management. *Ann Intern Med* 122:286, 1995.
22. Vaitkevicius PV, Esserwein DM, Maynaard AK, O'Connor FC, Fleg JL: Frequency and importance

of postprandial blood pressure reduction in elderly nursing home patients. *Ann Intern Med* 115:865, 1991.

23. Ferrante L, Artico M, Nardacci B, et al: Glossopharyngeal neuralgia with cardiac syncope. *Neurosurgery* 36:58, 1995.

24. Ferrante L, Artico M, Nardacci B, et al: Glossopharyngeal neuralgia with cardiac syncope. *Neurosurgery* 36:58, 1995.

25. Wik B, Hillestead L: Deglutition syncope. *BMJ* 3:747, 1975.

26. Guberman A, Catching J: Swallow syncope. *Can J Neurol Sci* 13:267, 1986.

27. Brihaye J, Perier O, Smulders, Franker L: Glossophayngeal neuralgia caused by compression of the nerve by an atheromatous vertebral artery. *J Neurosurg* 13:299, 1956.

28. Janetta PJ: Cranial nerve vascular compression syndromes (other than tic doloreux and hemifacial spasm). *Clin Neurosurg* 28:445, 1980.

29. Sobol SM, Wood BG, Conoyer JM: Glossopharyngeal neuralgia-asystole syndrome secondary to parapharyngeal space lesions. *Otolarngol Head Neck Surg* 90:16, 1982.

30. Waga S, Kojima T: Glossopharyngeal neuralgia of traumatic origin. *Surg Neurol* 17:77, 1982.

31. Macdonald DR, Strong E, Nielson S, Posner JB: Syncope from head and neck cancer. *J Neuro-Oncology* 1:257, 1983.

32. Kahana E, Leibowitz, Alter M: Brainstem and cranial nerve involvement in multiple sclerosis. *Acta Neurol Scand* 49:269, 1973.

33. Ekbom K, Westerberg CE: Carbamazepine in glossopharyngeal neuralgia. *Arch Neurol* 14:595, 1966.

34. Khero BA, Mullins CB: Cardiac syncope due to glossopharyngeal neuralgia. *Arch Intern Med* 128:806, 1971.

35. Rushton JC, Stevens JC, Miller RH: Glossopharyngeal (vagoglossopharyngeal) neuralgia: a study, of 217 cases. *Arch Neurol* 38:201, 1981.

36. Kapoor W: Evaluation and outcome of patients with syncope. *Medicine* 69:160, 1990.

37. Weiss, S, Baker JP: The carotid sinus reflex in health and disease. Its role in the causation of fainting and convulsion. *Medicine* 12:297, 1933.

38. Baig MW, Kaye GC, Perrins EJ: Can central neuropeptides be implicated in carotid sinus sensitivity? *Med Hypotheses* 28:255, 1989.

39. Maloney JD, Jaegar FJ, Rizo-Patron C, et al: The role of pacing for the management of neurally mediated syncope: carotid sinus syndrome and vasovagal syncope. *Am Heart J* 127:1030, 1994.

40. Brignole M, Oddone D, Cogorno S, et al: Long-term outcome in symptomatic carotid sinus hypersensitivity. *Am J Heart* 123:687, 1992.

41. Sharpey-Shafer EP: The mechanism of fainting after coughing. *BMJ* 2:860, 1953.

42. Corson WA: Cough syncope. *Minn Med* 53:43, 1970.

43. White CW, Zimmerman TJ, Ahmad M: Idiopathic hypertrophic subaortic stenosis presenting as cough syncope. *PACE* 3:332, 1975.

44. Pathy MS: Defaecation syncope. *Age Aging* 7:233, 1978.

45. Fisher CM: Syncope of obscure nature. *Can J Neurol Sci* 6:7, 1979.

46. Vincent GM: Heterogeneity in the inherited QT syndrome. *J Cardiovasc Electrophysiol* 6:137, 1995.

47. Marks ML, Whisler SL, Clericuzio C, Keating M: A new form of long QT syndrome associated with syndactyly. *J Am Coll Cardiol* 25:59, 1995.

48. Ninley C, Wharton JM: Ventricular tachycardias with left bundle branch block. *PACE* 18:334, 1995.

49. Williams CC, Bernhardt: Syncope in atheletes. *Sports Med* 19:223, 1995.

50. Rao KA, Adlakha A, Verma-Ansil B, Meloy TD, Stanton MS: Torsades de pointes ventricular arrhythmia associated with overdose of astemizole. *Mayo Clin Proc* 69:589, 1994.

51. Wynne J, Brauwald E: The cardiomyopathies and myocardiopathies: toxic, chemical, and physical damage to the heart, in Braumwald E (ed): *A Textbook of Cardiovascular Medicine,* 4th ed. Philadelphia, WB Saunder, 1992, pp 1394–1450.

52. Jacquet L, Ziady G, Stein K, et al: Cardiac rhythm disturbances early after orthotopic heart transplantation: prevalence and clinical importance of the observed abnormalities. *J Am Coll Cardiol* 16:832, 1990.

53. Kapoor WN: Diagnostic evaluation of syncope. *Am J Med* 90:91, 1991.

54. Zeldis SM, Levine BJ, Michelson E, et al: Cardiovascular complaints: correlation with cardiac arrhythmias on 24-hour electrocardiographic monitoring. *Chest* 78:456, 1980.

55. Murdock CJ, Klein GJ, Yee R, et al: Feasibility of long-term electrocardiographic monitoring with an implanted device for syncope diagnosis. *PACE* 13:1374, 1990.

56. Dhingra RC, Wyndham C, Bauerfeind R, et al: Significance of block distal to the His bundle

induced by atrial pacing in patients with bifascicular block. *Circulation* 60:1455, 1979.

57. Scheinman MM, Peters RW, Modin G, et al: Prognostic value of infranodal conduction time in patients with chronic bundle branch block. *Circulation* 56:240, 1979.

58. Prytowsky EN: Electrophysiologic-electropharmacologic testing in patients with ventricular arrythmias. *PACE* 11:225, 1988.

59. Glikson M, Espinosa RE, Hayes DL: Expanding indications for permanent pacemakers. *Ann Intern Med* 123:443, 1995.

60. Paz HL, MrCormick DL, Kutalek SP, Patchefsky A: The automatic implantable cardiac defibrillator. Prophylaxis in cardiac sarcoidosis. *Chest* 106:1603, 1994.

61. Sutton R: Pacing in atrial arrhythmias. *PACE* 13:1823, 1990.

62. Gilgenkrantz JM, Cherrier F, Pettier H, et al: Cardiomyiopathie obstructuve du ventricle gauche aver bloc auriculo-ventriculaire complet: considérations thérapcutiques. *Arch Mal Coeur Vaiss* 61:439, 1968.

63. Fananapazir L, Cannon RO III, Tripodi D, Panza JA: Impact of dual chamber permanent pacing in patients with obstructive hypertrophic cardiomyopathy with symptoms refractory to verapamil and beta adrenergic blocker therapy. *Circulation* 85:2149, 1992.

64. STASTSCAN, 1988 Census. Government of Canada Publication.

65. Stumpf JL, Mitrzyk B: Management of orthostatic hypotension. *Am J Hosp Pharm* 51:648, 1994.

66. Jankovic J, Gilden JL, Hiner BC, et al: Neurogenic orthostatic hypotension: a double-blind, placebo-controlled study with midrodrine. *Am J Med* 95:38, 1993.

67. Robertson D, Davis TL: Recent advances in the treatment of orthostatic hypotension. *Neurology* 45(Suppl 5):S26, 1995.

68. Taylor J (ed): Selected writings of John Hughlings Jackson, in *On Epilepsy and Epileptiform Convulsions*, vol 1. London, Hodder and Stoughton, 1931.

69. Pessin MS, Gorelick PB, Kwan ES, Caplan LR: Basilar artery stenosis: middle and distal segments. Neurology 37:1742, 1987.

70. Araki G: Small infarctions in the basal ganglia with special references to transient ischemic attacks. *Excerpta Medica Int Congr Ser* 469:161, 1979.

71. Bickerstaff ER: Impairment of consciousness in migraine. *Lancet* II:1057, 1961.

72. Haan J, Ferraru MD, Brouwer OF: Acute confusional migraine. *Clin Neurol Neurosurg* 90:275, 1988.

73. Bickerstaff ER: Basilar artery migraine. *Lancet* I:15, 1961.

74. Birkerstaff ER: Impairment of consciousness in migraine. *Lancet* II:1057, 1961.

75. Bickerstaff ER: Basilar artery migraine. *Megrim* 6:4, 1991.

76. Lees F, Watkins SM: Loss of consciousness in migraine. *Lancet* II:647, 1963.

77. Muellbacher W, Mamoli B: Prolonged impaired consciousness in basilar artery migraine. *Headache* 34:282, 1994.

78. Swanson JW, Vick NA: Basilar artery migraine. 12 patients, with an attack recorded electroencephalographically. *Neurology* 28:782, 1978.

79. Fitzsimons RB, Wolfenden WH: Migraine coma. Meningitic migraine with cerebral edema associated with a new form of autosomal dominant cerebellar ataxia. *Brain* 108:555, 1985.

80. Münte T-F, Müller-Vahl H: Familial migraine coma: a case study. *J Neurol* 237:59, 1990.

81. Marchioni E, Galimberti CA, Soragna D, et al: Familial hemiplegic migraine with prolonged aura: an uncertain diagnosis in a family report. *Neurology* 45:33, 1995.

82. Neligan P, Harriman DGF, Pearce J: Respiratory arrest familial hemiplegic migraine: a clinic and neuropathological study. *BMJ* 2:732, 1988.

83. Holtzer F, Wessely P, Zeiler K, Ehrmann L: Zerebrale Angiographie bei konplizierter Migraine-Reaktionnen. Zwischenfalle. *Klin Wochenschr* 63:116, 1985.

84. Rasmussen BK, Olesen J: Symptomatic and non-symptomatic headaches in a general population. *Neurology* 42:1225, 1995.

85. Fisher CM, Adams RD: Transient global amnesia. *Acta Neurol Scand* 40(suppl 9):7, 1964.

86. Frederiks JA: Transient global amnesia. *Clin Neurol Neurosurg* 95:265, 1993.

87. Goodwin DW, Crane JB, Guze SB: Alcoholic blackouts: a review and clinical study of alcoholics. *Am J Psychiatry* 126:191, 1969.

88. Virkkunen M, Kallio E, Rawlings R, et al: Personality profiles and state aggressiveness in Finnish alcoholics, violent firesetters, and healthy volunteers. *Arch Gen Psychiatry* 51:28, 1994.

89. Tamerin JS, Weiner S, Popper R, et al: Alcohol and memory: amnesia and short-term memory function

during experimentally induced intoxication. *Am J Psychiatry* 127:1659, 1971.

90. Abts H, Crois R, Marien P, et al: Paroxystic neuropsychological symptoms as the early expression of hepatic encephalopathy. *Acta Neurol* 15:268, 1993.

91. Tinuper P, Mortagna P, Plazzi G, et al: Idiopathic recurring stupor. *Neurology* 44:621, 1994.

92. Rothstein JD, Guidotti A, Tinuper P, et al: Endogenous benzodiazepine receptor ligands in idiopathic recurring stupor. *Lancet* 340:1002, 1992.

93. Guilleminault C, Faull KF: Sleepiness in non-narcoleptic non-sleep apneic EDS patients: the idiopathic CNS hypersomnolence. *Sleep* 5:S171, 1982.

94. Critchley M, Hoffman HL: The syndrome of periodic hypersomnolence and morbid hunger (Kleine-Levin syndrome). *BMJ* 1:137, 1942.

95. Jennum P, Sjol A: Self assessment cognitive function in snorers and sleep apneics. An epidemiological study of 1,504 females and males aged 30–60 years: the Dan-MONICA II Study. *Eur Neurol* 34:204, 1994.

96. Robbins J, Gottlieb F: Sleep deprivation and cognitive function testing in internal medicine housestaff. *West J Med* 162:82, 1990.

97. Joyce E, Blumenthal S, Wessely S: Memory, attention and executive function in chronic fatigue syndrome. *J Neurol Neurosurg Psychiatry* 60:495, 1996.

98. DeLuca J, Johnson SK, Beldowicz D, Natelson BH: Neuropsychological impairments in chronic fatigue syndrome, multiple sclerosis, and depression. *J Neurol Neurosur Psychiatry* 58:38, 1995.

99. Waters WF, Adams SG Jr, Binks P, Varnado P: Attention, stress and negative emotion in persistent sleep-maintenance insomnia. *Sleep* 16:128, 1993.

100. Newhouse PA, Belenky G, Thomas M, et al: The effects of d-amphetamine on arousal, cognition and mood after prolonged total sleep. *Neuropsychopharmacology* 2:153, 1989.

101. Rechtschaffen A, Kales A: *A Manual for Standardized Terminology. Techniques and Scoring for Sleep Stages of Human Subjects.* Washington, DC; Department of Health, Education and Welfare, 1968.Cu

102. Culebras A, Moore JT: Magnetic resonance findings in REM sleep behavior disorder. *Neurology* 39:1519, 1989.

103. Barros Ferreira DM, Chodkiewicz J, Lairy GC, Salzulo P: Disorganized relations of tonic and phasic events of REM sleep in a case of brain stem tumor. *Electroenceph Clin Neurophysiol* 38:203, 1975.

104. Uchiyama M, Isse K, Tanaka K, et al: Incidental Lewy body disease in a patient with REM sleep behavior disorder. *Neurology* 45:709, 1995.

105. Wetzel H, Heuser I, Beckert O: Stupor and affective state: alleviation of psychomotor disturbances by lorazepam and recurrence of symptoms after RO 15-1788. *J Nerv Ment Dis* 175:240, 1987.

106. Task Force on DSM-IV: *Diagnostic and Statistical Manual of Mental Disorders,* 4th ed (DSM-IV). Washington, American Psychiatric Association, 1994, pp 285–6.

107. Everett J, Laplante L, Thomas J: The selective attention deficit in schizophrenia. Limited resources or cognitive fatigue? *J Nerv Ment Dis* 177:735, 1989.

108. Spohn HE, Coyne L: The effect of attention/information processing impairment of tardive dyskinesia and neuroleptics in chronic schizophrenics. *Brain Cogn* 23:28, 1993.

109. Skinner HA: *The Origin of Medical Terms.* Baltimore, Williams and Wilkins 1949.

110. Dejoun HH: *Experimental Catatonia.* Baltimore, Williams and Wilkins, 1945.

111. Northoff G, Krill W, Wenke J, Travers H, Pflug B: Subjectives Weleben in der Katatonie: Systemische Untersuchung bei 24 katatonen Patienten. *Psychiatr Prax* 23:69, 1996.

112. Starkstein SE, Petraeca G, Teson A, et al: Catatonia in depression: prevalence, clinical correlates, and validation of a case. *J Neurol Psychiatry* 60:326, 1996.

113. Philbrick KL, Rummans TA: Malignant catatonia. *J Neuropsychiat Clin Neurosci* 6:1, 1994.

114. Guze BH, Baxter LR: Neuroleptic malignant syndrome. *N Eng J Med* 313:163, 1985.

115. Levenson JL: Neuroleptic malignant syndrome. *Am J Psychiatry* 55:16, 1985.

116. Lane RJM, Mastaglia FL: Malignant hyperthermia. *Lancet* 2:562, 1978.

117. Lewis BI: The chronic hyperventilation syndrome. *JAMA* 155:1204, 1954.

118. Bass C, Gardner WN: Respiratory and psychiatric abnormalities in chronic symptomatic hyperventilation. *BMJ* (Clin Res Ed) 290:1387, 1985.

119. Raj A, Sheehan DV: Medical evaluation of panic attacks. *J Clin Psychiatry* 48:309, 1987.

120. Mackenzie TB, Popkin MK: Organic anxiety syndrome. *Am J Psychiatry* 140:342, 1983.

121. Steel JM, Masterson G, Patrick AW, McGuire R: Hyperventilation or hypoglycemia? *Diabet Med* 6:820, 1989.

122. Eaton WW, Kessler RC, Wittchen HU, et al: Panic and panic disorder in the United States. *Am J Psychiatry* 151:413, 1994.

123. Young GB, Chandarana PC, Blume WT, et al: Mesial temporal lobe seizures presenting as anxiety disorders. *J Neuropsychiat Clin Neurosci* 7:352, 1995.

124. Pryse-Phillips W: An olfactory reference syndrome. *Acta Neurol Scand* 47:484, 1971.

125. Uomoto JM, Brockway JA: Anger management training for brain injured patients and their family members. *Arch Phys Med Rehabil* 73:674, 1992.

126. Woody S: Episodic dyscontrol syndrome and head injury: a case presentation. *J Neurosci Nursing* 20:180, 1988.

127. Drake ME Jr, Hietter SA, Pakalnis A: EEG and evoked potentials in episodic dyscontrol syndrome. *Neuropsychobiology* 26:125, 1992.

128. Delgado-Escueta AV, Mattson RH, King L, et al: Special report: the nature of aggression during epileptic seizures. *N Eng J Med* 305:711, 1981.

129. Cowdry RW, Gardner DL: Pharmacotherapy of borderline personality disorder. Alprazolam, carbamazepine, trifluoperazine and tranylcypromine. *Arch Gen Psychiatry* 45:111, 1988.

130. Rickler KC: Episodic dyscontrol, in Benson DF, Blumer D (eds): *Psychiatric Aspects of Neurological Disease*, vol II. Amsterdam, Elsevier/North Holland, 1978; pp 49–73.

131. Lesser RP: Psychogenic seizures. *Neurology* 46:1499, 1996.

132. Shen W, Bowman ES, Markand ON: Presenting the diagnosis of pseudoseizure. *Neurology* 40:756, 1990.

133. Rowan AJ: An introduction to current practice in the diagnosis of non-epileptic seizures, in Rowan AJ, Gates JR (ed). *Non-Epileptic Seizures*. Boston, Butterworth Heinemann, 1993, pp 1–8.

134. Henry JA, Woodruff GHA: A diagnostic sign in states of apparent unconsciousness. *Lancet* 2:920, 1978.

135. Persinger MA: Seizure suggestibility may not be an exclusive differential indicator between psychogenic and partial complex seizures: the presence of a third factor. *Seizure* 3:215, 1994.

136. Fenwick PB, Brown SW: Evoked and psychogenic seizures. I. Precipitation. *Acta Neurol Scand* 80:535, 1989.

137. Drake ME Jr, Pakalnis A, Phillips BB: Neuropsychological and psychiatric correlates of intractable pseudoseizures. *Seizure* 1:11, 1992.

138. Monday K, Jankovic J: Psychogenic myoclonus. *Neurology* 43:349, 1993.

139. Riley TL: Hysterical seizures. *Arch Neurol* 36:859, 1979.

140. Leis AA, Ross MA, Summers AK: Psychogenic attacks: ictal characteristics and diagnostic pitfalls. *Neurology* 42:95, 1992.

141. Tomb DA: Psychogenic seizures. *Neurology* 42:1848, 1992.

142. DeToledo JC, Ramsay RE: Patterns of involvement of facial muscles during epileptic and non-epileptic events: Review of 654 events. *Neurology* 47:621, 1996.

143. Sussman NM, Jackel RA, Kaplan LR, Harner RN: Bicycling movements as a manifestation of complex partial seizures of temporal lobe origin. *Epilepsia* 30:527, 1989.

144. Wilner AN, Bream PR: Status epilepticus and pseudostatus epilepticus. *Seizure* 2:257, 1993.

145. Leis AA, Ross MA, Summers AK: Psychogenic seizures: ictal characteristics and diagnostic pitfalls. *Neurology* 42:95, 1992

146. Boon PA, Williamson PD: The diagnosis of pseudoseizures. *Clin Neurol Neurosurg* 95:1, 1993.

147. Gates JR, Ramani V, Whalen S, Loewenson R: Ictal characteristics of pseudoseizures. *Arch Neurol* 42:1183, 1985.

148. Devinsky O, Fisher R: Ethical use of placebos and provocation in diagnosing nonepileptic seizures. *Neurology* 47:866, 1996.

149. Gumnit RJ: Behavior disorders related to epilepsy. *Electroencephalogr Clin Neurophysiol* 37(suppl):313, 1985.

150. Gould R, Miller BL, Goldberg MA, Benson DF: The validity of hysterical signs and symptoms. *J Nerv Mental Dis* 174–593, 1986.

151. Ramchandani D, Schindler B: Evaluation of pseudoseizures. A psychiatric perspective. *Psychosomatics* 34:70, 1993.

152. Anzola GP: Predictivity of plasma prolactin levels in differentiating epilepsy from pseudoseizures. *Epilepsia* 34:1044, 1993.

153. Laxer KD, Mullooly JP, Howell B: Prolactin changes after seizures classified by EEG monitoring. *Neurology* 35:31, 1985.

154. Meierkord H, Will B, Fish D, Shorvon S: The clinical features and prognosis of pseudoseizures

diagnosed using video-EEG telemetry. *Neurology* 41:1643, 1991.

155. Chandarana P, Young GB, Cairncross JD, Macdonald DR: Unusual neuropsychiatric symptoms of a fronto-temporal tumor. *Neuropsychiatr Neuropsychol Neurol* 5:53, 1992.

156. Riley TI, Roy A (eds): *Pseudoseizures*. Baltimore, Williams and Wilkins, 1982.

157. Shen W, Bowman ES, Markand ON: Presenting the diagnosis of pseudoseizure. *Neurology* 40:756, 1990.

158. Volow MR: Pseudoseizures: an overview. *South Med J* 79:600, 1986.

159. Mai FM: "Hysteria" in clinical neurology. *Can J Neurol Sci* 22:101, 1995.

160. Riether AM, Stoudemire A: Psychogenic fugue states: a review. *South Med J* 81:568, 1988.

161. Keller R, Shaywitz BA: Amnesia or fugue state: a diagnostic dilemma. *J Behav Pediatr* 7:131, 1986.

162. Kopelman MD, Panayiotopoulos CP, Lewis P: Transient epileptic amnesia differentiated from psychogenic "fugue": neuropsychological, EEG and PET findings. *J. Neurol Neurosurg Psychiatry* 57:1002, 1994.

163. Parfitt DN, Gall CM: Psychogenic amnesia: the refusal to remember. *J. Ment Sci* 90:511, 1944.

164. Larson SJ, Sances A, Baker JB, Reigal DH: Herniated cerebellar tonsils and cough syncope. *J Neurosurg* 40:524, 1974.

165. Cetinalp E, Ildan F, Boyar B, et al: Colloid cysts of the third ventricle. *Neurosurg Rev* 17:135, 1994.

166. Faris AA, Terrence CF: Limbic system symptomatology associated with colloid cyst of the third ventricle. *J Neurol* 236:60, 1989.

167. Tatter SB, Ogilvy CS, Golden JA, Ojemann RG, Louis DN: Third ventricular xanthogranulomas clinically and radiologically mimicking colloid cysts. Report of two cases. *J. Neurosurg* 81:605, 1994.

168. Couldwell WT, Chandrasoma P, Apuzzo ML, Zee CS: Third ventricular cysticercal cyst mimicking a colloid cyst: case report. *Neurosurgery* 37:1200, 1995.

169. von Haken MS, Aschoff AA: Acute obstructive hydrocephalus, in Hacke W (ed): *Neurocritical Care*. Berlin, Springer-verlag, 1994, pp 869–882.

170. Haimovic IC, Beresford HR: transient unresponsiveness in the elderly. *Arch Neurol* 49:34, 1992.

171. Rao TH, Schneider LB, Lupyan Y: Transient unresponsiveness in the elderly. *Arch Neurol* 51:644, 1994.

172. Tinuper P, Montagna P, Plazzi G, Lugaresi E: transient unresponsiveness in the elderly: possible episodes of idiopathic recurring stupor. *Arch Neurol* 52:232, 1995.

173. Kapoor WN: Diagnostic evaluation of syncope. *Am J Med* 90:91, 1991.

Part 6

IMPAIRED CONSCIOUSNESS IN CLINICAL CONTEXTS

Chapter 19

EMERGENCY MANAGEMENT OF THE COMATOSE PATIENT

Rocco V. Gerace
William A. McCauley
Eelco F. M. Wijdicks

Physicians are commonly called to the emergency department to manage patients with acutely impaired consciousness. The traditional approach to patient assessment, an initial history followed by physical examination and pertinent laboratory investigations, is, of course, not possible. The patient with impaired consciousness usually cannot give a reliable history, and others who can provide such information often are not present. The initial focus of management of such patients is the assessment and correction of those physiologic functions that threaten vital organs. Thus, the assessment of the patient with impaired consciousness therefore involves virtually simultaneous focused physical assessment, and initiation of therapeutic interventions and laboratory investigations, often without the completion of a thorough history and physical examination. This chapter will present an approach for patients with undifferentiated forms of impaired consciousness.

Case report

A 43-year-old woman was brought to the emergency department by ambulance. She had been found comatose at home by her 14-year-old child in the early afternoon. The patient had been well when the child went to school in the morning. She had no history of underlying medical problems except for emotional depression and apparently had been recently started on a new antidepressant found to be fluoxetine. There were no empty pill containers at the scene. The patient's son indicated that his parents had recently separated and that his mother had been a victim of an abusive relationship. En route, the patient was unresponsive to stimuli.

Vital signs in the emergency department were as follows: 105 beats per minute, blood pressure 150/90, respirations 18 per minute, and temperature 39.1°C. The patient continued to be unresponsive to deep painful stimuli. While the airway was clear, the gag reflex was absent. There was an odor of an alcoholic beverage on the breath. Auscultation of the chest revealed normal breath sounds and the cardiovascular examination was unremarkable. There was bruising of indeterminate age about her forehead and right eye. Within 4 to 5 min of presenting to the emergency department, while intravenous access was being established, the patient suffered a generalized tonic-clonic seizure.

In conjunction with airway management, the patient was administered anticonvulsant therapy and antimicrobial therapy. Computerized tomography (CT) was unremarkable, as was the lumbar puncture. A twelve-lead electrocardiogram (ECG) was suspicious for cyclic antidepressant intoxication. Screening blood work confirmed the presence of these agents. Following the initial seizure, the patient was admitted to the intensive care unit where she remained free of further seizures or arrhythmias. She ultimately awoke without further sequelae.

This case illustrates the importance of initiating resuscitative measures concurrently with the physical and laboratory assessment. This general rule is important, regardless of the complexity of the case.

INITIAL RESUSCITATION OF THE COMATOSE PATIENT

Airway

The initial attention must be directed to vital functions. The airway must be rapidly assessed and controlled. Indications for endotracheal or nasotracheal intubation include the loss of protective reflexes and respiratory failure [the latter indicated by hypoxemia ($Pa_{O_2} < 60$ mmHg) or hypercapnia ($Pa_{CO_2} > 60$ mmHg)]. In the patient with a potentially traumatic cause for depressed level of consciousness, consideration is given to stabilizing the cervical spine. In all cases, the cervical spine should be immobilized, e.g., by a collar (especially during intubation), until instability or malalignment is radiologically excluded.

The stimulation associated with intubation or tracheal suctioning causes a sympathetic response.[1] The resulting increase in heart rate and mean arterial pressure transiently raise the intracranial pressure (ICP).[2] This rise in ICP can be detrimental to patients with structural brain lesions,

intracranial hemorrhage of any type, central nervous system (CNS) infection, trauma, acute hydrocephalus, or cerebral edema. Lidocaine administration, either topically to the airway or intra-venously, blunts the cardiovascular response and diminishes the ICP rise due to intubation or endotracheal suctioning.[3-5]

The patient with a clenched jaw who is still breathing may be considered for blind nasotracheal intubation, accepting that increased ICP may be transiently worsened. Nasotracheal intubation is best avoided in the presence of extensive facial fracturing, severe skull base fractures, and with coagulopathies such as warfarin use (see Chap. 6.) Alternatively, combative, agitated patients should be considered for rapid sequence induction (RSI) to achieve endotracheal intubation. There are a number of important provisos for RSI. First, *the procedure should be performed by the most experienced physician who is immediately available*, such as an anesthesiologist, then an emergency physician, or intensivist. Second, since RSI involves the use of neuromuscular paralysis, *the physician must be prepared for, capable of, and willing to provide a surgical airway* if an airway cannot be secured or if it is impossible to ventilate the patient manually. Third, *all required equipment and drugs should be at the bedside before the administration of any drugs*.

In the procedure of RSI, the physician first assesses the patient's oropharyngeal anatomy to determine whether the intubation is likely to be difficult. A short thick neck, small mandible, oropharyngeal swelling or trauma, blunt anterior neck trauma, suspected cervical spine trauma, or arthritis of the spine are associated with difficult intubation and may preclude RSI. The patient should be preoxygenated with 100% oxygen by a nonrebreathing face mask. To reiterate, all equipment, and drugs necessary for surgical airway control, *must* be at the bedside before paralysis is induced. The following sequence of pharmacological administration is effective[6]:

- Approximately 3 min prior to intubation, lidocaine hydrochloride in a dose of 1.0 to 1.5 mg/kg may be given by bolus intravenous injection.

- Two minutes before intubation, sedation is accomplished by administration of sodium pentothal, 2 to 4 mg/kg, or fentanyl, 1.5 g/kg, with bolus intravenous injection. (Pentothal provides rapid sedation and suppression of respirations, but can cause profound hypotension in patients with limited cardiovascular reserve. In these patients, fentanyl would be a more prudent choice.)

- One minute before intubation, neuromuscular paralysis is attained by administration of succinylcholine, 1.0 to 1.5 mg/kg, by bolus intravenous injection.

As soon as breathing stops or neuromuscular paralysis is obtained (whichever comes first), an assistant applies gentle pressure on the cricoid cartilage (Sellick maneuver) to occlude the esophagus posteriorly, thus preventing aspiration. Once the patient is relaxed, the patient may be intubated, the cuff of the tube inflated, and the tube checked for position by listening to both lungs and the epigastrium. Additionally, one may check for carbon dioxide in the exhaled air by using an automated detector. Once tube placement has been confirmed clinically or radiographically, the cricoid pressure may be released.

Breathing

After control of the airway has been established, attention can be turned to assessing and supporting ventilation. The rate and depth of ventilation can provide an initial clue regarding the cause of the altered consciousness, on the basis of ventilatory patterns (see Chap. 3). Blood gases aid in establishing the presence of hyperventilation or hypoventilation (Chap. 3).

Ventilatory support is essential (especially in the case of hypoventilation) to ensure adequate oxygenation and carbon dioxide removal. Bedside monitoring of oxygen saturation ensures adequate oxygenation. Values above 90% are adequate, but it is ideal to achieve 99% with supplemented oxygen. Ventilation is assessed by measuring Pa_{CO_2}.

Therapeutic hyperventilation has been used to reduce ICP by causing vasoconstriction in cranial vessels, thereby decreasing intracranial blood volume.[7,8] However, deliberate mechanical hyperventilation also increases cerebrovascular resistance and reduces cerebral blood flow. There is, thus, a practical lower limit of hyperventilation (Pa_{CO_2} probably about 19 mmHg) that allows for both lowering of ICP and maintaining or improving cerebral blood flow (see also p. 168 in Chap. 6). The long-term or functional benefit of controlled hyperventilation in the patient with increased ICP, however, has yet to be demonstrated.[9] Since an abrupt increase in hyperventilation can be used to promptly reduce ICP, it is best to keep the maintenance ventilatory rate (or Pa_{CO_2}) as close to normal as possible without allowing an increase in ICP. Then, when peaks in ICP occur, the ventilatory rate can be temporarily increased to control such rises. When ICP is not being measured, but is likely to be significantly raised, hyperventilation can be continued with Pa_{CO_2} concentrations that will not produce ischemia (greater than 19 mmHg).

Care must be also taken to avoid inadvertent suppression of a helpful hyperventilatory response. For example, in salicylate intoxication, the primary respiratory alkalosis helps to prevent the crossing of salicylates into the cerebrospinal fluid (CSF), which would aggravate the CNS salicylism. The rate of assisted ventilation should take this protective mechanism into account.[10]

Circulation

Assessment of circulatory status should be coupled with ongoing stabilization of vital signs. Intravenous access with normal saline is accomplished early on in the resuscitation of all patients with impaired consciousness. *Hypotension*, while uncommonly the sole cause of impaired consciousness, is frequently an accompanying finding of the many causes of depressed level of consciousness, and should be treated aggressively if associated with impaired tissue perfusion (shock). The causes of hypotension are many but may be classified as hypovolemic, cardiogenic, or distributive—which includes hypotension of neurogenic, septic, and anaphylactic origin. The initial approach to the hypotensive patient with impaired consciousness usually involves a clinical assessment of intravascular volume and initial volume replacement with an isotonic crystalloid, such as normal saline or lactated Ringer's solution. Hypotension of cardiogenic origin must be carefully considered because cardiac failure may be precipitated by volume overload. A complete review of the cause and treatment of shock is beyond the scope of this chapter.

Marked *hypertension* can cause a decreased level of consciousness, with intracranial bleeding (intracerebral or subarachnoid) or hypertensive encephalopathy.[11] Hypertension associated with intracranial bleeding should only be controlled if the diastolic blood pressure is greater than 130 mmHg, and then should only be lowered such that the mean arterial blood pressure (MABP) is decreased by a maximum of one-third of the initial peak value. Hypertensive encephalopathy is a medical emergency that should be treated by immediate lowering of MABP using either intravenous sodium nitroprusside or labetolol.[12,13]

Temperature

Although extremes of temperature can, and do, cause an altered level of consciousness, the temperature change and the altered consciousness more often share a common etiology. While hyperpyrexia may require aggressive measures to restore normothermia, in all cases, a concurrent search for the cause of temperature alteration is necessary.

Hyperthermia   (see also Chap. 8) Environmental hyperthermia is a true emergency requiring prompt and aggressive treatment. Classically, heatstroke is associated with a triad of raised temperature > 40.5°C (105°F); warm, dry skin; and CNS dysfunction. With this syndrome, thermoregulatory control is lost. At 42°C, CNS dysfunction is universal.

Initial attention is directed at the stabilization of vital signs, in conjunction with rapid lowering of core body temperature to <40°C.[14] Following stabilization of the airway and intravenous

access, cooling is best achieved by using a modification of the so-called Body Cooling Unit.[15–17] This evaporation technique consists of a constant misting of the skin with water at 30 to 35°C while blowing air at room temperature over the patient's body with a fan. This method of cooling has been shown to be the most efficient, with rates of cooling of 0.3°C/min. Antipyretics are of little use in these patients. With treatment, the patient should be monitored for systemic complications.

Secondary hyperthermia can be caused by both intrinsic neurogenic processes and toxins. Examples of intrinsic causes of elevated temperature include stroke and seizures (see below). Toxic causes of elevated temperature are reviewed elsewhere (see Chap. 16) and include malignant hyperthermia, neuroleptic malignant syndrome, and serotonin syndrome, as well as individual agents that increase heat production, e.g., amphetamines or cocaine, or that decrease heat loss, e.g., anticholinergics.

Special mention must be made of CNS infection as a cause of elevated temperature and an altered level of consciousness. Given the rapidly progressive nature of meningitis or herpes simplex encephalitis, if these conditions are distinct possibilities, the administration of antimicrobial or antiviral agents should precede investigations (see Chap. 11.) The selection of antimicrobial agents should be based on the locus of infection and the prevalent strains in the geographic area.

Hypothermia   (see also Chap. 8) Hypothermia is defined as a core temperature below 35°C. As temperature falls, the level of consciousness decreases to coma. There are multiple potential etiologies for hypothermia, including environmental, metabolic (myxedema coma), structural, drug-induced, and numerous others. Patients at the extremes of age and those with an altered sensorium are especially vulnerable to hypothermia.

Environmental hypothermia, while often readily evident, can be subtle in presentation. With severe hypothermia, the usual resuscitative modalities are employed with further attention to rewarming the patient. In the *severely hypothermic* patient (core temperature $< 30°C$), there is risk of cardiovascular instability, especially ventricular tachycardia, and rewarming should be controlled with active internal rewarming techniques.[18] These are discussed in more detail in Chap. 8.

INITIAL ASSESSMENT OF THE COMATOSE PATIENT

The general approach is discussed in detail in Chap. 3. The discussion that follows is focused on the emergency room presentation.

Several causes of coma are fairly obvious: massive head injury, subarachnoid hemorrhage, carbon monoxide intoxication from a house fire, and environmental hypothermic exposure. However, determining the cause of coma in the emergency room can be a major challenge when there is little information and the patient does not have localizing signs. Furthermore, multiple causes are often simultaneously implicated, e.g., cocaine or alcohol intoxication and trauma. Some causes, e.g., infection or traumatic lesions, are obscured by intoxications; or a "pure" neurologic disorder may not be appreciated, e.g., subarachnoid hemorrhage or nonconvulsive status epilepticus, with profoundly altered behavior. The neurologic and general physical assessments are relatively straightforward (see Chap. 3). However, the differential diagnosis, priorities, tests performed, and the administration of antidotes and nutrients or vitamins are highly variable, depending on the situation.

Some clues give direction to the investigation and management strategies. For example, fever limits the number of diagnostic possibilities (see Table 12-1 in Chap. 12). See Fig. 19-1 for a general approach to coma in the emergency room. If the reason for coma is not obvious, drug intoxication should be high on the list of possibilities. There are some clues as to the type of toxin, based on simple aspects of the clinical presentation (see Table 19-1). Also, see Chap. 16 for a more extensive discussion of intoxications.

The performance of tests for arterial blood gases often narrows the number of possibilities and gives direction to investigations. In patients with an increased anion gap acidosis (see Fig. 19-1), one should look for a bitten tongue (convulsive seizures), retinal edema (methanol poisoning), calcium oxylate crystals in the urine (ethylene glycol intoxication), and serum salicylates or a positive ferric chloride test (aspirin). A check for ketones (diabetes mellitus, alcoholism, and salicylate poisoning) in the urine and blood is simple. A disturbance in respiratory acid-base balance is associated with many potential toxins (Fig. 19-1). An increased osmolar gap usually indicates intoxication with one of the alcohols. The absence of ketones with anion gap acidosis further favors methanol or ethylene glycol poisoning. Normal acid-base balance in a comatose patient excludes many disorders. Fluorescein is added to many antifreeze preparations; a Wood's lamp can show the fluorescence in the urine.

Additional Investigative and Management Steps

Other tests are usually necessary. Computed tomographic scanning is often necessary if there is not an adequate metabolic, toxic, or systemic infectious cause for the coma. Localizing signs on neurologic examination should prompt a scan; in the absence of focal signs, CT is often necessary to exclude subarachnoid hemorrhage (SAH), symmetric hemispheric lesions, or a diencephalic disorder that may mimic a metabolic encephalopathy. Some conditions may be missed or overlooked by nonradiologists: e.g., isodense subdural hematomas, small amounts of blood in the CSF spaces with SAH and cerebellar or brainstem ischemic lesions, and cerebral shear injuries.

Some metabolic and toxic conditions may be associated with abnormal CT scans. Adolescent and young adults with pronounced cerebral or cerebellar atrophy may have long-term alcohol or intravenous drug abuse, human immunodeficiency virus (HIV) infection, or other substance abuse (glue sniffing). Magnetic resonance imaging (MRI) scanning may be impractical in the acute

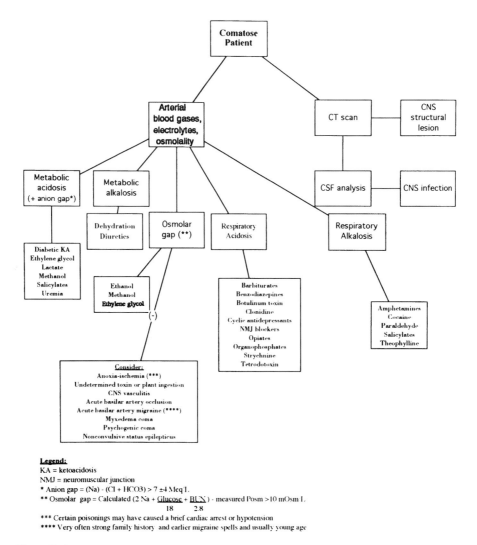

Figure 19-1

Flow chart depicting the sequence of diagnostic steps for the comatose patient. In osmolar gap calculation, BUN= blood urea nitrogen.

setting, but later, elective scans will often show characteristic changes. Normal findings on neuroimaging should prompt examination of the CSF to search for a CNS infection (meningitis or encephalitis) or SAH. The risks of CSF examination are negligible if contraindications are considered (see Chaps. 3 and 11). The failure to exclude a treatable cause may have devastating consequences.

Abdominal radiographs are helpful in establishing whether the patient has ingested tablets or foreign materials. Examples of radiopaque pills include chloral hydrate, trifluoperazine, amitriptyline, and enteric-coated tablets, but sometimes the tablets have all dissolved before the patient comes to the emergency room.

An ECG should be obtained as soon as is coveniently possible for diagnostic and

Table 19-1

Some neurologic findings in intoxications and poisonings that cause coma

Finding	Agent
Mydriasis	Anticholinergics
	Carbon monoxide (anoxia)
	Lysergic acid diethylamide (LSD)
	Cyanide
	Ergot preparations
	Insulin
	Monamine oxidase inhibitors
	Cocaine, amphetamines, tricyclic antidepressants
Miosis	Opioids
	Organophosphates
	Cholinergics (excluding eyedrops)
	Clonidine
Papilledema	Arsenic
	Lead
	Vitamin A
Trismus	Phenothiazines
	Ingestion of water hemlock
Neck stiffness	Cocaine
	Phenothiazines
	Nonsteroidal anti-inflammatory drugs (ibuprofen)
Ophthalmoplegia	Botulism
	Ethylene glycol
	Curare
	Ergot preparations
	Lead
	Thallium

Table 19-2

Investigations in the assessment of a patient with altered consciousness

Routine
Complete blood count (CBC)
Electrolytes
Glucose
Urea nitrogen and creatinine
Calcium, magnesium
Liver function studies
Arterial blood gases
Osmolality (by freezing point depression)
Electrocardiogram (ECG)
Routine urinalysis

Specialized (as needed)
Acetaminophen screen
Limited toxicologic testing (per clinical suspicion)
Serum ethanol
Thyroid-stimulating hormone (TSH)
Blood cultures
Lumbar puncture (see Chaps. 3 and 11)
Magnetic resonance imaging (MRI)

management purposes. Changes on ECG may give a clue to the etiology of the altered consciousness. The many and varied toxicologic causes of coma may have significant and sometimes pathognomonic ECG findings (see Chap. 16). Hypothermic patients may have various ECG findings, but elevation of the J point, the so-called Osborn wave, may be present. Increased ICP of acute origin may cause ECG abnormalities. These include large, wide, inverted precordial T waves that may be continuous with large U waves, giving the effect of a long drawn-out TU complex. Myxedema coma has typical ECG findings of low or inverted T waves in the majority of leads, low voltage, and bradycardia. The patient should have ongoing cardiographic monitoring in conjunction with monitoring of blood pressure (either by cuff or arterial line). Simultaneous continuous pulse oximetry should be considered mandatory in all patients, allowing timely intervention when life-threatening alterations occur.

Investigations can be divided into routine and special. These investigations should be directed towards those conditions that are potentially immediately reversible. Some of the tests used commonly in the emergency room are listed in Table 19-2.

Resuscitative Measures

In the resuscitation of the coma patient, a number of therapies have evolved and are generally considered routine at this stage. Many of these have not undergone critical evaluation. They will be discussed independently.

Management of Herniation Syndromes Herniation syndromes are discussed in detail in Chap. 4. Obtunded patients with hemiplegia, marked anisocoria, or one or more poorly reactive pupils, should be given a bolus of mannitol before undergoing CT scanning. It may be necessary to ventilate the patient to a Pa_{CO_2} of 25 mmHg if herniation is strongly suspected.

Thiamine Patients who are malnourished may suffer from thiamine deficiency; Wernicke's encephalopathy can be precipitated or aggravated by glucose administration if unaccompanied or preceded by thiamine administration (see Chap. 15). In North America, thiamine deficiency is most commonly seen in the alcoholic population. There are few significant side effects of thiamine (100 mg intravenously); its administration should be considered routine in at-risk patients.[19]

Glucose Hypoglycemia can lead to permanent neurologic injury if left uncorrected. This had prompted the recommendation that hypertonic glucose be used routinely in the management of the poisoned patient.[20] However, it is now recognized that administration of glucose can be associated with increased neurologic injury, e.g., in ischemia.[21] With the widespread availability of bedside glucose testing, the need to administer glucose empirically is no longer necessary. During the resuscitation, a rapid screen for hypoglycemia is conducted and glucose is administered only for documented hypoglycemia.

Naloxone Naloxone is a pure opioid antagonist (lacking agonist action) that acts at the mu, kappa, and sigma opiate receptors. It is extremely effective in rapidly reversing the effects of opiates. While it has been recommended as a routine agent in the coma patient, this view has been appropriately challenged.[22] While some patient populations have a high incidence of opiate abuse leading to coma, this is not prevalent. Further, it has been shown that opiate intoxication as a cause of coma is clinically predictable. When accompanied by all or some of the following

three criteria—hypoventilation (< 12 breaths per minute), miosis, and evidence of drug abuse, e.g., track marks or drug paraphernalia—the likelihood of opiate use is much higher.[23] It has long been believed that, while uncomfortable, opiate withdrawal is not associated with life-threatening complications. However, a recent critical evaluation of complications has demonstrated the potential for serious complications, including arrhythmias and seizures when naloxone is given to heroin users.[24] Therefore, while useful both as a diagnostic agent and treatment modality, caution should be exercised in its use.

The usual dose of naloxone is 0.4 to 2.0 mg intravenously. It can also be given through the endotracheal tube. The dose should be titrated to response, initially giving 0.4 mg and raising the dose to 2.0 mg in increments. If the patient remains unresponsive following the 2.0-mg dosage, this can be repeated every 2 min to a total of 8 mg. Synthetic opioids, e.g., propoxyphene, may require doses in this higher range to achieve reversal. The half-life of naloxone is shorter that of most opioids. Therefore, the wakened patient can relapse into coma and respiratory depression following a single dose of naloxone. This becomes problematic in the patient wanting to leave hospital. To avoid this scenario, naloxone can be administered as a continuous infusion in doses sufficient to maintain respirations and airway protection but not causing full arousal.

Flumazenil Flumazenil is an effective competitive antagonist of benzodiazepines, acting at the benzodiazepine receptor.[25] It has a limited role in treatment of benzodiazepine overdose, idiopathic recurring stupor, and, possibly, hepatic encephalopathy. Its use as a routine agent in the undifferentiated coma patient cannot be supported. Like naloxone, flumazenil is capable of producing an acute withdrawal syndrome associated with seizures and arrhythmias.[26,27] Flumazenil is especially dangerous in patients who have coingested arrhythmogenic (chloral hydrate) or epileptogenic (cyclic antidepressants) agents, because the abrupt loss of inhibition may precipitate cardiac arrhythmias or seizures.

The recommended administration of fluma-zenil is by slow intravenous infusion of 0.1 mg/min to a total dose of 1.0 mg. It has been argued that benzodiazepine overdose is seldom life-threatening and that patients can be effectively managed with supportive care alone.

DRUG AND CHEMICAL INTOXICATION

The most common cause of altered level of consciousness presenting to the emergency department is intoxication with pharmaceuticals or other agents.[28] While this topic is discussed in detail in Chap. 16, the initial management of this problem is addressed here. Following the stabilization of vital signs (as has been outlined), attention is directed to preventing further absorption of the substance and then enhancing its elimination. Finally, when available, antidotal therapy may be used.

Prevention of Absorption

Dermal Exposure Agents such as organophosphate insecticides are readily absorbed by the dermal route. With agents such as these, it is important to consider dermal decontamination as an essential component of treatment. Generally, copious skin irrigation is sufficient. In so doing, care must be taken to prevent staff exposure and if possible, environmental contamination.

Oral exposure The majority of intoxications occur by the oral route. Therefore, consideration must be given to decontamination of the gastrointestinal tract. Traditionally, this has involved a three-pronged approach of gastric emptying, administration of activated charcoal to bind toxin in the gut, and, finally, a cathartic to hasten elimination. More recently, these modalities have come under more rigorous scrutiny, leading to changes in this traditional management.

Enhanced gastric emptying has been a mainstay of gastrointestinal decontamination. The stomach can be emptied by syrup of ipecac-induced emesis or gastric lavage. However, with critical assessment of efficacy, both human studies and clinical trials have failed to demonstrate significant benefit with these modalities.[29] While ipecac continues to be used in the management of pediatric minor poisonings in the home environment, its use in the hospital setting has been largely abandoned. Gastric lavage in the emergency department is similarly falling into disuse. As mentioned, critical evaluation of this technique in the clinical setting has failed to demonstrate any improvement in outcome.[30,31] In fact, the employment of either gastric-emptying techniques will delay the administration of activated charcoal and thereby delay a potentially effective technique. Exceptions to this practice involve the exposure to toxins not adsorbed by activated charcoal.

The use of activated charcoal is the principal step in gastric decontamination in the poisoned patient. While its efficacy has been clearly demonstrated in controlled human trials, its effect in the clinical setting has never been studied. In the poisoned patient, the optimal dose of activated charcoal is a gram amount multiplied by 10 times the weight of the ingested toxin. In ingestions of unknown type, 50 to 100 g are given orally. Activated charcoal can cause constipation or obstipation in the gastrointestinal tract and is highly toxic when aspirated into the pulmonary tree. Therefore, airway protection must be afforded to the obtunded patient. It is important to be aware of toxins that are not well bound to activated charcoal.[32] These include the following: corrosives (both alkali and mineral acids), ethanol and other alcohols, ethylene glycol, iron, lithium, potassium, fluoride, and cyanide. Given that most exposures involve two or more substances, even if exposure with one of the above is suspected, activated charcoal is still utilized (with the exception of corrosive poisoning). However, one must consider other decontamination techniques in this patient population.

Bowel emptying continues to be commonly used despite the lack of clear evidence for its effectiveness. Generally, either a saline cathartic, e.g., magnesium sulfate, or a sorbitol is given with the first dose of charcoal. Whole bowel irrigation is the term used for complete emptying of the gastrointestinal tract using a polyethylene glycol electrolyte solution. A preparation such as GoLytely® is administered orally, either by nasogastric tube or having the patient drink it, at the rate of 2 L/h (500 mL/h in children) until the rectal effluent is clear. This modality is recommended in the patient exposed to large amounts of iron or lithium, or sustained-release preparations.[33–35]

Enhanced Elimination

With the completion of gastrointestinal decontamination, or when patients present long after the exposure when decontamination techniques are no longer efficacious, attention can be directed to the removal of agents already absorbed.

Multidose activated charcoal has been shown to reduce effectively the half-life of a number of absorbed substances.[36] With certain substances, binding in the gastrointestinal tract is felt to establish a concentration gradient across the bowel wall, enhancing secretion and subsequent binding in the gastrointestinal tract. This is commonly referred to as gastrointestinal (or GI) dialysis. There are a number of substances known to be effectively removed by this technique (see Table 19-3). In this technique, activated charcoal, 0.5 to 1.0 g/kg, is given every 2 to 3 h, either orally or through a nasogastric tube. One must ensure that sorbitol or other cathartics are not given concurrently. Multiple doses of cathartics can be associated with electrolyte abnormalities and life-threatening dehydration, and must therefore be avoided.

Urinary alkalinization in the absence of diuresis will enhance renal excretion of salicylates,

phenobarbital, chlorpropamide, and chlorphenoxy herbicides. Complications include fluid overload, cerebral edema, adult respiratory distress syndrome (ARDS) (with salicylates), fluid and electrolyte imbalances, and acid-base abnormalities.

Extracorporeal techniques of detoxification include the use of hemodialysis and hemoperfusion. Peritoneal dialysis has no role in the management of the patient with toxicosis. Generally, agents amenable to removal must have a low molecular weight, a low volume of distribution (< 1 L/kg), and, in the case of hemodialysis, be water soluble and poorly protein-bound. The decision to employ these techniques is based on the type of intoxicant coupled with the degree of current or potential toxicity.

Antidotes

Antidotes, when available, may attenuate toxicity. Unfortunately, many toxins do not have effective antidotes, or, in the case where antidotal efficacy has been demonstrated, their availability may be limited. A list of effective antidotes is shown in Table 19-4.

EMERGENCY ASPECTS OF METABOLIC COMA

Metabolic encephalopathies are discussed in detail in Chap. 13. The metabolic causes for coma that need to be considered in the emergency management of the comatose patient include myxedema coma, hypoglycemia (see above), coma associated with hyperglycemia [diabetic ketoacidosis and hyperglycemic hyperosmolar nonketotic coma (HHNKC)], hypercalcemia, hyponatremia, and the many and varied toxic causes of coma. The emergency considerations in each of these conditions will be discussed in turn.

Diabetes

The patient who presents with depressed level of consciousness and who is found to be hyperglycemic may be suffering from diabetic ketoacidosis or from hyperglycemic hyperosmolar nonketotic

Table 19-3
Agents effectively removed with multidose activated charcoal

Carbamazepine
Dapsone
Digitoxin
Meprobamate
Phenobarbital
Phenytoin
Salicylate
Theophylline

Table 19-4

Specific antidotes for the toxic patient

Antidotes	Toxin(s) treated	Other toxins that may benefit
Acetylcysteine	Acetaminophen	Carbon tetrachloride, methyl bromide, ethylene dibromide
Antivenims	Rattlesnake, coral snake, black widow spider, botulinus toxin	
Atropine	Cholinergic agents, organophosphate and carbamate insecticides	
Dimercaprol (BAL)	Lead, arsenic, mercury	Selected other heavy metals
Calcium salts	Calcium antagonists, fluoride, hydrofluoric acid	
Sodium thiosulfate	Cyanide	
Deferoxamine	Iron	
Diazepam	Chloroquine	
Diazoxide	Oral hypoglycemics	
Digoxin-specific F_{ab} antibody fragments	Digoxin	Selected plant cardiac glycosides (e.g., oleander)
Dimercaptosuccinic acid (DMSA)	Lead	Arsenic, mercury
Ethanol	Methanol, ethylene glycol	
Flumazenil	Benzodiazepines	
Folic acid (leucovorin)	Methanol, ethylene glycol	
Glucagon	Beta blockers	Calcium channel blockers
Methylene blue	Methemoglobinemia	
Naloxone	Opiates	
Oxygen	Carbon monoxide	
Pralidoxime	Organophosphate insecticides	
Pyridoxine	Isoniazid	Ethylene glycol
Sodium nitrite	Cyanide	
Sodium thiosulfate	Cyanide	
Vitamin K_1	Oral anticoagulants	

coma (HHNKC). These two conditions, while pathophysiologically quite different, share some common clinical findings, especially severe dehydration due to hyperglycemia-induced osmotic diuresis. These patients often present with a negative fluid balance of several liters. Both conditions also present with profound electrolyte abnormalities, with significant deficiencies in total body sodium, potassium, magnesium, and phosphate.

Initial management of both conditions includes aggressive fluid resuscitation with central venous pressure monitoring and close monitoring of urine output. Intravenous insulin is indicated in both conditions, with a recommended initial dose of 0.1 units of regular insulin per kilogram of body weight followed by an infusion of 0.05 units/per hour. Close monitoring of serum glucose and electrolytes is essential as overly rapid lowering of serum glucose has been associated with the development of cerebral edema due to intracellular water shift.

Hyponatremia

Severe hyponatremia may present with altered sensorium or refractory seizures. The causes of hyponatremia may be divided grossly into those causes that represent pseudohyponatremia, dilutional effects of excess body water, or depletion of total body sodium. The presentation depends to a certain degree on the rapidity with which the hyponatremia develops, as well as the level of hyponatremia. A slow development of hyponatremia generally results in less profound clinical manifestations than a more acutely lowered serum sodium. A serum sodium level of greater that 120 mmol/L is generally associated with mild symptoms, whereas levels less than 120 mmol/L are associated with increasing irritability and depressed level of consciousness.

The urgency of treatment of hyponatremia depends on the degree of hyponatremia and the severity of symptoms. Mild symptoms are treated with conservative replacement of sodium or restriction of fluid intake. More severe symptoms require active sodium replacement. Care must be taken not to replace sodium too quickly in patients without life-threatening symptoms as overly rapid correction has been associated with the development of the catastrophic complication of central pontine myelinolysis.[37]

Hypercalcemia

Hypercalcemia as a cause of coma is a difficult clinical diagnosis. The patient often presents with severe dehydration, and depressed level of consciousness or confusion on the background of a condition that puts the patient at risk for the development of hypercalcemia. This would include malignancy, endocrine disorders, granulomatous disease, renal dysfunction, or the effects of a large number of medications.[38] As serum calcium is a routine laboratory assay performed in the patient with undifferentiated coma, it is often not until the laboratory test results are available that the diagnosis of hypercalcemia is apparent.

Emergency measures include the administration of large quantities of intravenous isotonic crystalloid to obtain a urinary diuresis of 500 mL/h or above. Intravenous furosemide may be added to achieve this diuresis, so long as it has been ascertained that the intravascular space has been completely replenished. Other therapies aimed directly at acutely lowering serum calcium include diphosphonates and intravenous corticosteroids. Therapy, recommended in the emergency setting only in the severe and refractory case, includes intravenous phosphate, mithramycin, and calcitonin.

Myxedema

Myxedema coma is a rare condition that occurs in approximately 0.1 percent of patients with underlying hypothyroidism.[39] It is defined as coma that exists either due to hypothyroidism alone or more commonly as a result of a physiologic stress that occurs on a background of hypothyroidism. Various factors that may precipitate coma in the hypothyroid patient include cold exposure infection, sedating drugs, hypoglycemia, and hyponatremia. The clinical presentation of depressed level of consciousness, hypothermia, and bradycardia in an elderly woman should trigger the concern for myxedema coma.

Diagnosis of myxedema coma is readily apparent in the patient presenting with the above triad who is known to be hypothyroid, but it may be more of a challenge in the patient not previously recognized as being hypothyroid. The diagnostic test for hypothyroidism, the thyroid-stimulating hormone (TSH) level is often not available on a "stat" basis; thus, treatment of the condition is often initiated on an empiric basis. Therapy includes acute thyroid hormone replacement, a search for and correction of underlying precipitants, and supportive care.

Thyroid hormone replacement is accomplished by administration of intravenous levothyroxine (T_4) at a dose of 300 to 500 g. The patient must be closely monitored because of the

Table 19-5

Poisonings reported to cause seizures

Acetone cyanohydrin	Chlorprothixine	Ibuprofen	Phenol
Acetonitrile	Cocaine	Imipramine	Phenothiazines
Alfentanil	Colistin	Iopamidol	Phenylenetetrazole
Aliphatic thiocyanates	Creosote	Isoniazid	Phenylhydrazine
Allyglycine	Cresols		Phenylpropanolamine
Amantadine	Crimidine	Kerosene	Phenytoin (toxic concentrations)
Aminocaproic acid	Cyanide		
Aminopyridine	Cyanogen cyanides	Lead	Phosphine
Amitriptyline	Cyclonite	Lidocaine	Phosphorus
Ammonium alum	Cyslosporine	Lindane	Picrotoxin
Amphetamines	Cyclotrimethylene-	Lithium	Pilocarpine
Aniline	trinitramine		Polymyxin B
Anticholinergics		Maprotiline	Potassium chlorate
Antidepressants, cyclic	1,2-Dichloroethane	Mefenamic acid	Probenicid
Antihistamines	Diethylaniline	Mercaptans	Propafenone
Aspartame (?)	*N,N*-Diethyltoluamide	Methaldehyde	Propofol
	Dimethylaniline	Methoxypyridoxine	Propranolol
Baclofen	Dimethyl sulfate	Methyl alcohol	Propylene glycol
Barbiturate withdrawal	Dinitrophenol	Methyl bromide	Pyrethrins
Barium and compounds	Diquat	Methyl chloride	Pyridines
Benzene	Disulfiram	Methyl formate	
Bucuculine		Methylprednisolone	Ramantidine
Borate	Endrin	Metrizimide	Rauwolfia alkaloids
Boric acid	Ethchlorvinol withdrawal	Moxalactam	Resorcinol
Boron hydrides			Rotenone
Bromochloromethane	Ethylene chlorohydrin	Naloxone	
Bromoform	Ethylene glycol	Naphthol	Salicylic acid
Buprion		Nickel carbonyl	Sodium fluoroacetate
Busulfan	Fentanyl	Nicotine	Sodium pentachlorophenate
Butyrophenones	Flecainide	Nitrobenzene	Strychnine
	Fluorides	Nitrogen dioxide	Sufentanil
Cadmium and compounds	Fluoxetine	Nitrophenols	Sulfuryl fluoride
	Formaldehyde		
Camphor		Organochlorine pesticides	Tetrachloroethylene
Captopril	Gasoline	Organophosphates	Tetraethyl lead
Carbamate insecticides	Glutethimide withdrawal	Organotin compounds	Thallium and compounds
Carbamazepine (massive overdose)	Glycerol	Oxalic acid	Theophylline
		Oxamiquine	Toluidine
Carbon monoxide	Halogenated pesticides		Trazodone
Cefazolin	Heroin	Pefloxacin	Trichloroethylene
Cefonizid	Hexachlorophene	Penicillin (massive overdose/renal failure)	Turpentine
Chlorambucil	Hydrogen cyanide		
Cholorophenoxy herbicides	Hydrogen peroxide (ingestion)	Pentachlorophenol	Verapamil
		Pentazocine	
	Hydroquinone	Phencyclidine	Zinc phosphide

possibility of dysrhythmias occurring with acute thyroid hormone replacement.[40]

SEIZURE DISORDERS

Coma is commonly associated with generalized tonic-clonic seizures, but nonconvulsive seizures (usually absence seizures or complex partial status epilepticus) also produce various degrees of obtundation. This topic is discussed in detail within Chap. 17. While most seizures are self-limiting, with spontaneous arousal following a postictal state, status epilepticus is associated with prolonged coma, with or without tonic-clonic movement. Status epilepticus is defined as more than 30 min either of either (1) continuous seizure activity or (2) two or more sequential seizures without full recovery of consciousness between the seizures.[41] The presence of status epilepticus represents a true emergency with immediate therapy required to end the seizures. Prolonged seizure activity leads to neurologic damage, with the extent of damage dependent on the length of seizure activity. With attention paid to airway control, breathing, and circulation, antiseizure drug therapy is indicated acutely. Seizures secondary to drug intoxication (see Table 19-5) may have treatments that differ somewhat from the usual standard. Examples of this are pyridoxine for isoniazid-induced seizures and the lack of efficacy of phenytoin in theophylline-induced seizures.

SUMMARY

The emergency management of the patient with an altered level of consciousness consists of stabilization of vital signs with specific treatment modalities while concurrent assessment is taking place. Hesitation in treatment while searching for an etiologic agent can increase morbidity and mortality.

REFERENCES

1. Fox EJ, Sklar GS, Hill CH, et al: Complications related to the pressor response to endotracheal intubation. *Anesthesiology* 47:524, 1977.

2. Gildenberg P, Frost EZ: Respiratory care in head trauma, in Becker D, Povlishock JT, (eds): *Central Nervous System Trauma Status Report*. Bethesda, National Institutes of Health, 1985, p 161–17.

3. Denlinger JK, Ellison N, Ominsky A: Effects of intratracheal lidocaine on circulatory responses to tracheal intubation. *Anesthesiology* 41:409, 1974.

4. Bedford RF, Winn HR, Tuson G, et al: Lidocaine prevents increased ICP after endotracheal intubation, in Shulman K, Mamarou A, Miller JD, et al (eds): *Intracranial Pressure* 4:595, 1980.

5. Hamill JF, Bedford RF, Weaver DC, et al: Lidocaine before intubation: intravenous or laryngotracheal. *Anesthesiology* 55:578, 1981.

6. Morris IR: Airway management, in Rosen P, Barkin RM (eds): *Emergency Medicine: Concepts and Clinical Practice*, 3rd ed. St. Louis, Mosby, 1992, pp 79–105.

7. Crockard HA, Coppel DL, Morrow WF: Evaluation of hyperventilation in treatment of head injuries. *BMJ* 4:634, 1973.

8. Paul RL, Polanco O, Turney SZ, McAsland TC, Cowley RA: Intracranial pressure responses to alterations in arterial carbon dioxide pressure in patients with head injuries. *J Neurosurg* 36:714, 1972.

9. Muizelaar JP, Marmarou A, Ward JD: Adverse effects of prolonged hyperventilation in patients with severe head injury: a randomized clinical trial. *J Neurosurg* 75:731, 1991.

10. Yip L, Dart RC, Gabow PA: Concepts and controversies in salicylate toxicity. *Emerg Med Clin N Am* 12:351, 1994.

11. Ferguson RK, Vlasses PH: Hypertensive emergencies and urgencies. *JAMA* 255:1607, 1986.

12. Lebel M, Langlois S, Bellean LJ, Grose JH: Labetolol infusion in hypertensive emergencies. *Clin Pharmacol* 37:615, 1985.

13. Cressman MD: Intravenous labetalol in the management of severe hypertension and hypertensive emergencies. *Am Heart J* 108:980, 1984.

14. Sprung CL: Heat stroke: modern approaches to an ancient disease. *Chest* 77:461, 1980.

15. Weiner JS, Khogali MA: A physiological body-cooling unit for treatment of heat stroke. *Lancet* 1:507, 1980.

16. Khogali M, Weiner JS: Heat stroke: report on 18 cases. *Lancet* 1:276, 1980.

17. Khogali M: The Makkah Body Cooling Unit, in Khogali M, Hales JRS, (eds): *Heat Stroke and*

Temperature Regulation. Sydney, Academic Press, 1983, pp 116–121.

18. Moss JF: A model for the treatment of accidental severe hypothermia. *J Trauma* 26:68, 1986.

19. Doyon S, Roberts JR: Reappraisal of the "Coma Cocktail". *Emerg Med Clin N Am* 12:301, 1994.

20. Plum F, Posner JB: Approach to the unconscious patient. In: Plum F, Posner JB (eds). *The Diagnosis of Stupor and Coma,* 3rd ed. Philadelphia, FA Davis, 1980, pp 345–364.

21. Browning RG, Olson DW, Stueven HA, Mateer JR: 50% Dextrose: antidote or toxin? *Ann Emerg Med* 19:683, 1990.

22. Hoffman JR, Schriger DC, Luo JS: The empiric use of naloxone in patients with altered mental status: a reappraisal. *Ann Emerg Med* 20:246, 1991.

23. Hoffman JR Schriger DC, Luo JS: The empiric use of naloxone in patients with altered mental status: a reappraisal. *Ann Emer Med* 20:246, 1991.

24. Osterwalder JJ: Naloxone—for intoxications with intravenous heroin and heroin mixtures—harmless or hazardous? A prospective clinical study. *J Toxicol Clin Toxicol* 34:409, 1996.

25. Brogden RN, Goa KL: Flumazenil. A preliminary review of its benzodiazepine antagonist properties, intrinsic activity and therapeutic use. *Drugs* 35:44, 1988.

26. Short TG, Maling T, Galletly DC: Ventricular arrhythmia precipitated by flumazenil. *BMJ* 296:1070, 1988.

27. Burr W, Sandham P: Death after flumazenil. *BMJ* 298:713, 1989.

28. Plum F, Posner JB: The pathologic physiology of signs and symptoms of coma, in Plum F, Posner JB (ed): *The Diagnosis of Stupor and Coma,* 3rd ed. Philadelphia, FA Davis, 1980, pp 1–86.

29. Tenenbein M, Cohen S, Sitar DS: Efficacy of ipecac induced emesis orogastric lavage and activated char-

coal for acute drug overdose. *Ann Emerg Med* 16:838, 1987.

30. Kulig K, Bar-Or D, Cantrill SV, Rosen P, Rumack BH: Management of acutely poisoned patients without gastric emptying. *Ann Emerg Med* 14:562, 1985.

31. Pond SM, Lewis-Driver DJ, Williams GM, et al: Gastric emptying in acute overdose: a prospective randomized controlled trial. *Med J Aust* 163:345, 1995.

32. Neuvonen PJ, Olkkola KT: Oral activated charcoal in the treatment of intoxications: role of single and repeated doses. *Med Toxicol* 3:33, 1988.

33. Tenenbein M: Whole bowel irrigation in iron poisoning. *J Pediatr* 111:142, 1987.

34. Smith SW, Ling LJ, Halstenson CE: Whole-bowel irrigation as a treatment for acute lithium overdose. *Ann Emerg Med* 20:536, 1991.

35. Kirshenbaum LA, Mathews C, Sitar DS, Tenenbein M: Whole-bowel irrigation versus activated charcoal in sorbitol for the ingestion of modified-release pharmaceuticals. *Clin Pharmacol Ther* 46:264, 1989.

36. Tenenbein M: Multiple doses of activated charcoal: time for reappraisal? *Ann Emerg Med* 20:529, 1991.

37. Ayus JC, Krothapalli RK, Arieff AI: Changing concepts in treatment of severe symptoznatic hyponatremia: rapid correction and possible relation to central pontine myelinolysis. *Am J Med* 78:897, 1985.

38. Janson CL, Marx JA: Fluid and electrolyte balance, in Rosen P, Barkin RM (eds): *Emergency Medicine: Concepts and Clinical Practice,* 3rd ed. St. Louis, Mosby, 1992, pp 132–2175.

39. Meek JC: Myxedema coma. *Crit Care Q* 3:131, 1980.

40. Urbanic RC, Mazzaferri EL: Thyrotoxic crisis and myxedema coma. *Heart Lung* 7:435, 1978.

41. Working Group on Status Epilepticus: Treatment of convulsive status epilepticus. *JAMA* 270:854, 1993.

Chapter 20

COMA IN MEDICAL AND SURGICAL INTENSIVE CARE UNITS

Eelco F. M. Wijdicks

Neurologic complications are prevalent in intensive care units (ICUs) and are a significant determinant for the patients' outcome.[1] The nature of neurologic complications depends on the population of patients in the ICU. The length of stay in the ICU is twice as long for patients in whom neurologic complications develop during the critical illness, and such patients are twice as likely to die as patients without neurologic complications.[2] Patients who have pulmonary disease and acute hypoxemic respiratory failure, sepsis syndrome, hypovolemic shock caused by gastrointestinal tract bleeding, or hemoptysis are often admitted to medical ICUs. The number of admissions for management of opportunistic pulmonary infections (particularly *Pneumocystis carinii* infection) has increased since the arrival of the acquired immunodeficiency syndrome (AIDS) epidemic, and this has been accompanied by an increase in the number of patients with neurologic manifestations. Drug overdose or poisoning is a common reason for monitoring and treating patients in an ICU. In addition, when neurologic or neurosurgical ICUs are not organized as separate units, often a high percentage of patients with primary disorders of the central nervous system are admitted directly to medical ICUs.

This chapter discusses the reasons for patients in medical or surgical ICUs to either fail to awaken or to become comatose. (Patients with primary disorders of the central nervous system and those with drug poisoning are considered in Chaps. 11, 12, and 16).

FAILURE TO AWAKEN IN THE MEDICAL INTENSIVE CARE UNIT

The most common reason that patients fail to awaken is that they have been given a combination of sedative agents and narcotics. The clearance of benzodiazepines is a problem in critically ill patients. Despite the use of new short-acting pharmacologic agents, a common cause of altered consciousness in critically ill patients is that, over several days, sedative drugs accumulate because of diminished clearance or pharmacologic interaction. This is particularly evident in patients who have been given several low doses of opioids or barbiturates for bedside surgical procedures.

Midazolam is the drug used most commonly for intravenous infusion in patients requiring mechanical ventilation or sedation. These infusions are used increasingly in medical and surgical ICUs and have two major advantages. First, the elimination half-life is 1 to 4 h after a single injection, which is remarkable for a benzodiazepine twice as potent as diazepam. However, midazolam may accumulate in significant amounts in critically ill patients. After continuous infusion of midazolam (10 mg in an hourly infusion, or more) for several days, awakening takes much longer, up to several days.[3,4] Also, multiorgan failure, associated liver disease, or concomitant use of barbiturates may significantly prolong the clearance of midazolam. Second, the effects can be reversed with flumazenil. A small dose of flumazenil (0.4 to 1.0 mg) completely antagonizes the sedative action of midazolam for a brief period. The reversal effect is apparent within 3 min, but resedation may occur within 2 h.

Narcotic agents may contribute to a decrease in the level of consciousness, and these agents should be suspected when the patient's pupils are small. Naloxone, titrated in 0.05-mg increment, is helpful in determining the contribution of opioids to impaired consciousness, and is without major side effects.

Other medications should be excluded as a cause of impaired consciousness. Antibiotics can be implicated only occasionally, and when renal failure is pronounced.

A sudden decrease in the level of consciousness in patients in an ICU, whether they have significant localizing signs or not, often indicates development of an ischemic or hemorrhagic stroke. Ischemic strokes are common causes of coma or impaired consciousness in patients in medical ICUs. These strokes may involve the territory of a single major cerebral artery (e.g., the middle cerebral artery or basilar artery) or, more often, the territories of multiple arteries. Ischemic strokes in a medical ICU may be caused by discontinuation of warfarin. Oral anticoagulation therapy is often discontinued before an invasive procedure (e.g., bronchoscopic biopsy, placement of a chest tube, or diagnostic pleural puncture) is performed. Transesophageal echocardiography (TEE) may demonstrate mural thrombus and should be considered before anticoagulation therapy is discontinued. The risk may be higher in patients with chronic atrial fibrillation.

Cardioversion may produce a major ischemic stroke and, thus, impaired consciousness and coma, but the risk in a patient with a fairly recent cardiac arrhythmia is very low.

Hemorrhagic stroke is usually a direct manifestation of marked thrombocytopenia or a complication of an acute hematologic oncologic disorder. The use of fibrinolytic agents in disorders such as acute myocardial infarction, massive pulmonary embolism, and acute arterial occlusion may have increased the frequency of intracerebral hematoma, particularly among the elderly, but its occurrence remains rare. Fibrinolysis-associated hemorrhages are significant and often located in several compartments, e.g., the subarachnoid space, subdural space, and parenchymal compartment. Many of these hemorrhages are severe enough to produce brain death or extreme neurologic disability.[5,6]

The differential diagnosis of intracranial hemorrhage in critically ill patients includes excessive anticoagulation, intravascular coagulation, coagulopathy of any type, and, in immunosuppressed patients, overwhelming toxoplasmosis or aspergillosis.[1,7]

Failure to awaken often occurs in association with sepsis.[8,9] The condition of some of these patients has been diagnosed as "toxic-metabolic encephalopathy," but only because the pathogenesis is a mystery. If acute confusional episodes or other significant cognitive abnormality develops during septicemia, the diagnosis has been "septic encephalopathy." If cofounders are excluded, it is not known whether a distinct metabolic encephalopathy of sepsis exists. Coma associated with septic shock or sepsis syndrome is a poor sign.[10] It is difficult to ascertain why some patients with sepsis remain unresponsive after the associated life-threatening insults are controlled. In patients who remain comatose, it seems reasonable to conclude that marked hypotension that requires increasing doses of inotropic medication may contribute to the development of ischemic damage in both cerebral hemispheres.

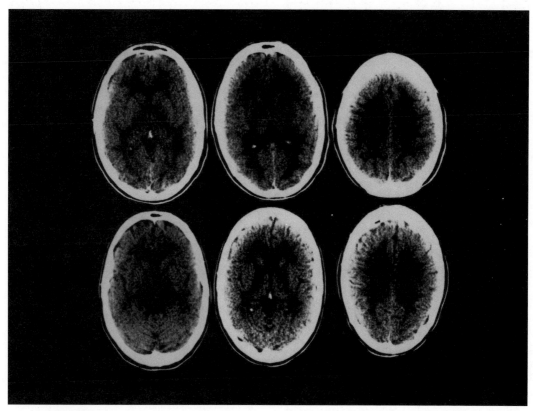

Figure 20-1
Scanning by CT in a patient with cerebral edema due to fulminant hepatic failure. Top, *disappearance of sulci;* bottom, *sulci reappear after orthotopic liver transplantation.*

Acute hepatic failure often occurs in patients with pre-existing liver disease. Many patients with long-standing cirrhosis have an episode of acute bleeding of the gastrointestinal tract that further develops into acute hepatic encephalopathy.

A more specific and challenging disorder is fulminant hepatic failure, which is triggered by acetaminophen overdose, hepatitis (A, B, or C), or hepatic vein occlusion. The patients lapse rapidly into coma and have spontaneous extensor motor responses. Patients in coma caused by fulminant hepatic necrosis have diffuse cerebral edema. Immediately, their intracranial pressure (ICP) needs to be monitored with an epidural device, while they await emergent liver transplantation[11,12]. Although the sensitivity of computed tomography (CT) in cerebral edema is low,

the edema can be demonstrated and quantified by examining the disappearance of sulci, the sylvian fissure, and white and gray matter differentiation.[11] The cerebral sulci reappear after liver transplantation (Fig. 20-1).

Coma in a medical ICU results from various disorders. The most common disorder remains global ischemic encephalopathy or ischemic stroke. Many other causes can be considered and these are summarized in Table 20-1.

FAILURE TO AWAKEN IN SURGICAL INTENSIVE CARE UNITS

In postoperatively critically ill patients, two clinical scenarios are likely: failure to awaken after a

Table 20-1
Major causes of coma in patients in medical intensive care units

Cause	Clues
Prolonged sedation	<ul><li>Combination of benzodiazepines and opioids</li><li>Previous use of barbiturates</li><li>Multiorgan failure</li><li>Intravenous infusion of benzodiazepines</li></ul>
Drug intoxication (e.g., penicillin derivatives, amphotericin B, immunosuppressive agents)	<ul><li>Renal failure</li><li>Liver failure</li></ul>
Hypoxic-ischemic encephalopathy	<ul><li>Hypotension supported by inotropic medication</li><li>Documented circulatory arrest</li><li>Asphyxia, laryngeal edema</li></ul>
Intracerebral hematoma, subarachnoid hemorrhage	<ul><li>Anticoagulation</li><li>Thrombolytic agents</li><li>Endocarditis</li><li>Thrombocytopenia</li><li>Disseminated intravascular coagulation</li></ul>
Acute bihemispheric or brainstem ischemic stroke	<ul><li>Atrial fibrillation[a]</li><li>Endocarditis</li><li>Thrombocytopenic thrombotic purpura</li><li>Acute myocardial infarction</li><li>Cardioversion</li><li>Collagen vascular disorder</li></ul>
Acute metabolic or endocrine crises	<ul><li>Severe hypoglycemia</li><li>Diabetic ketoacidosis[b]</li><li>Severe hyponatremia[c]</li><li>Acute uremia</li></ul>

[a] May be associated with brief discontinuation of anticoagulation therapy before an invasive procedure or biopsy.

[b] May be related to parenteral nutrition.

[c] May cause central pontine myelinolysis (CPM) or extra CPM.

surgical procedure performed with the patient under general anesthesia, and loss of consciousness after a documented asymptomatic interval. Although it may be difficult to appreciate an asymptomatic interval in some patients, the distinction is important.

Neurologic complications after anesthesia are infrequent and, according to one study, occur in about 0.04% percent of patients.[13] Failure of a patient to awaken postoperatively is an ominous sign if mundane causes, such as delayed anesthetic emergence (up to 10 percent of patients are difficult to arouse for several hours postoperatively), administration of high doses of opioids (frequently used in major cardiovascular repairs), and severe electrolyte abnormalities (severe postoperative hyponatremia, as in transurethral resection of the prostate), are excluded.

The risk of postoperative stroke is low, reported to occur in 19 of 24,641 patients (0.08 percent) after noncardiac or carotid artery operations,[14] but in surgical ICUs, a devastating ischemic stroke is a more frequent cause of a patient's failure to awaken. Postoperative stroke is most common after cardiac surgery or major vascular repairs. Patients with postoperative ischemic strokes often have had a significant event perioperatively. Pronounced hypotension, especially during unclamping of the aorta, can be implicated only if it persists for a certain period or

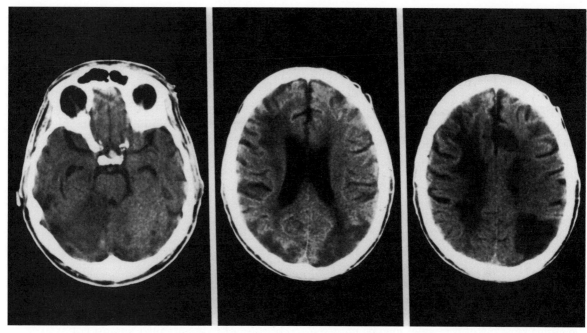

Figure 20-2

CT scans from a patient with multiple ischemic strokes after coronary artery bypass grafting. Note the hypodensities in the territories of both the anterior and middle cerebral arteries.

is associated with cardiac arrhythmia.[15] (Hypotension usually is anticipated by anesthesiologists and quickly remedied.)

The CT findings are often abnormal in patients who fail to awaken after cardiovascular repairs; typical findings are multiple territorial infarcts in watershed distributions (Fig. 20-2). If CT is performed soon after the event, the findings may be normal, and magnetic resonance imaging (MRI) or repeat CT is helpful in delineating cerebral infarction. In addition to perioperative hypotension and cardiac resuscitation during surgery, multiple embolic events are possible reasons for multiple cerebral infarction. The risk is significant in patients with severe atherosclerotic disease of the aorta and infarction, and almost certainly occurs at the time of clamping.[16] Ideally, the diagnosis of a "shaggy aorta" should be made preoperatively with TEE. However, circumferential atherosclerotic involvement of the aorta and protruding atheroma usually are detected during palpation or

insertion of extracorporeal circulation cannulae. When this condition is recognized, the cardiovascular surgeon may decide to use alternative surgical techniques to prevent intimal damage caused by clamping.

Air embolism may occur during orthopedic operations. Air entrapment in open veins or bone can occur when patients are in Trendelenburg's position (e.g., pelvic operations) or when the patient's hip is elevated above the level of the heart during hip operations.[17] Cardiac collapse, acute bronchospasm, and pulmonary edema usually occur in association with air embolism. A patent foramen ovale may be present, but air emboli can squeeze through pulmonary capillaries, especially during conditions of sudden excessive exposure to large volumes of air.

If failure to awaken occurs after trauma and the patient has been admitted directly to the operating room from the emergency department, intracranial contusion or extraparenchymal hematoma should be considered. Patients taken directly to the operating room after experiencing a life-threatening blunt abdominal trauma may have head injury, subdural hematoma, or epidural hematoma that was not detected on initial examination. One study suggested that correction of shock may produce increased perfusion and enlargement of an intracranial hematoma.[18] A unilateral fixed pupil, or, worse, bilaterally fixed pupils, may become evident during surgical repair. (In these patients, pupillary light reflexes are the only brainstem reflexes that can be monitored during general anesthesia.)

New-onset coma after an asymptomatic interval rarely occurs in critically ill postoperative patients. Acute electrolyte imbalance is a relatively frequent cause of postoperative confusion, progressive drowsiness, or coma. Increased levels of antidiuretic hormone associated with decreased serum osmolality and hyperosmolar urine are typical during the first five postoperative days.[19] Postoperative handling of free water may be impaired. "Third spacing" occurs in the immediate postoperative period, and replacement of this fluid, lost from the extracellular space, is important. Isotonic or hypertonic solutions (3% sodium chloride or Ringer's solution) are used to correct fluid loss. However, hyponatremia can occur rapidly. When free water is used, renal handling of free water is impaired because renal function is decreased after the use of inhalational anesthetics, barbiturates, and opioids. Severe hyponatremia is a life-threatening condition that may result in seizures, progressive coma, and apnea and cardiac arrhythmias.[20]

Common causes of acute postoperative hyponatremia are (1) administration of large doses of hypotonic fluid to patients with impaired ability to excrete water after transurethral prostatectomy, and (2) administration of oxytocin to patients during obstetric procedures. Hyponatremia may be associated with progressive impairment of consciousness, often at levels below 125 meq/L. Seizures emerge if the plasma level of sodium continues to decrease.[1,21]

A group of investigators has claimed that healthy young females are susceptible to pronounced hyponatremia postoperatively.[20] In this extremely rare catastrophic syndrome,[22,23] respiratory arrest and seizures suddenly develop and the pupils remain dilated and fixed after resuscitation Massive brain swelling and extensive demyelination have been reported at autopsy.[20]

The correction of severe hyponatremia, rather than the hyponatremia itself, may contribute to the gradual deterioration in consciousness after hyponatremia and to the myelinolysis found in the pons and deep layers of the cerebral cortex. Central pontine myelinolysis (CPM) is the more frequent finding, but lesions may be scattered in the hemispheric white matter and globus pallidus bilaterally. Rapid correction (more than 24 mmol/L per 24 hours) or correction of hyponatremia to values greater than 140 meq/L is a major factor in causing CPM.[24–26]

Central pontine myelinolysis can cause stupor. Magnetic resonance imaging is an essential diagnostic study when patients become comatose because of hyponatremia, and do not awaken, or when pseudobulbar palsy and facial weakness develop and the patient is unable to swallow or speak but has normal extraocular eye movements.

Hyponatremia occurs in about 4 percent of patients after transurethral resection of the prostate; however, only a small proportion (~1 percent) of them become comatose.[27] The main cause of hyponatremia in these patients is the absorption of large amounts of prostate irrigants, many of which are composed of sorbitol, glycine, urea, and mannitol. Mannitol and sorbitol may increase the extracellular volume, resulting in cerebral edema. However, after glycine is absorbed and metabolized, it may cause hyperammonemia—thus, contributing to coma. Therefore, glycine alone may cause progressive drowsiness during the first postoperative day.[22,27]

A frequent cause of coma in surgical ICUs is acute renal failure that results in acute uremic encephalopathy. Acute uremia occurs in about 20 percent of critically ill patients in surgical ICUs and 20 percent of patients who are critically ill postoperatively. In hospitals, acute dialysis is frequently initiated because of perioperative acute renal failure.[28–30] Valvular heart repair, coronary artery bypass grafting, and aortic aneurysm repair typically are associated with postoperative acute renal failure; however, the incidence is also high when major surgical repair is complicated by sepsis or involves considerable abdominal gastrointestinal repair. The development of acute uremia in surgically ill patients markedly increases the risk of postoperative mortality, which approaches 100 percent if mechanical ventilation is needed.[28]

The common causes of acute renal failure in surgically ill patients are renal hypoperfusion or nephrotoxic insults. As expected, patients with pre-existing renal dysfunction, left ventricular dysfunction, and diabetes mellitus, or those who have been given nephrotoxic antibiotics, are at risk.

Coma due to uremic encephalopathy usually develops gradually, with the patient progressing from drowsiness, asterixis, and myoclonus to an unresponsive state with virtually no motor response to pain. Frontal release signs may be elicited, such as marked snout response, grasp reflexes, or a brief jerk of retroflexion of the neck after glabellar tapping.[31] Cranial nerve function remains intact, as it does in many metabolic encephalopathies. Uremic encephalopathy can usually be implicated as a cause of coma when the values for blood urea nitrogen (BUN) and creatinine are twice their normal value. However, in a patient with multiorgan failure, severe hypoxemia caused by acute respiratory distress syndrome (ARDS) or increased bilirubin due to liver failure may be contributory factors. Improvement after dialysis is critical. Failure to awaken after dialysis may indicate that hypoxemic or hypotensive events have occurred; occasionally, bilateral subdural hematomas are implicated.[20] The clinical signs of uremic encephalopathy may resolve almost completely after dialysis.

Cholesterol embolization is an uncommon cause for coma in surgically ill patients, despite autopsy studies indicating a high incidence of these emboli in patients who died after vascular catheterization (25 percent incidence overall, with 5 percent incidence of emboli to the brain).[32,33] This condition is difficult to diagnose antemortem. The syndrome is not well delineated, and the argument for a distinct clinical entity rests largely on the results of meticulous pathologic studies. An intra-arterial procedure precipitates cholesterol embolization. Dislodgement of cholesterol crystals can produce massive showers in any organ as well as the brain. New-onset renal failure, hypertension, and livido reticularis are clues to cholesterol embolization, but are not very specific.[32,33] Renal biopsy specimens, showing the needle-shaped crystals, are necessary for making the diagnosis. Funduscopy is essential, and a cholesterol embolus may be diagnostic by funduscopy in a patient with otherwise unexplained multiorgan involvement and coma.

Fat embolization to the brain must be considered, at least theoretically, in patients who have had major orthopedic procedures or have experienced multitrauma.[34] Coma is uncommon in these patients, who more often have generalized tonic-clonic seizures, a confusional state, axillary petechia, pulmonary edema, and significant hypoxemia.

Fat embolism may occur 12 to 72 h after the initial traumatic impact and is usually indicated by sudden tachypnea and tachycardia. Although CT may demonstrate multiple hypodensities in the white matter of the frontal lobe, MRI is usually needed to demonstrate these scattered lesions.[35] Fat in the urine or sputum (e.g., bronchoalveolar lavage) is pathognomonic of this condition. Outcome is generally satisfactory if the patient survives the initial catastrophic presentation.

The common causes of coma in patients in surgical ICUs are summarized in Table 20-2.

LABORATORY TESTS

The decision to perform additional diagnostic tests in patients who are critically ill and comatose depends on the underlying condition. Routinely performing CT cerebrospinal fluid (CSF) examinations of comatose patients in the ICU is unnecessary. Transporting patients to the CT scanner may be difficult because of mechanical ventilation. Some modes of ventilation [e.g., positive end expiratory pressure (PEEP), inverse ratio] cannot be maintained during transport and may cause significant problems if discontinued. Lumbar puncture may be dangerous in patients with labile blood pressure or coagulopathy.

Table 20-2

Major causes of coma in patients in surgical intensive care units

Cause	Clues
Cholesterol embolization syndrome	• Arteriographic findings • Major vascular repair
Fat embolism Multiterritorial ischemic stroke	• Multitrauma with long-bone fractures • Shaggy aorta on TEE or palpation with surgery • Hypotension during aortic declamping
Hypoxic-ischemic encephalopathy	• Cardiac tamponade after aortic valve repair • Hemorrhagic shock postoperatively
Diffuse axonal shear injury Traumatic subdural hematoma Acute metabolic derangements	• Multitrauma • Fall or deceleration trauma • Severe postoperative hyponatremia • Acute uremia

The cause of coma may be obvious after careful review of the patient's medical record. Particular attention should be paid to acute changes in laboratory values (e.g., major shifts in plasma osmolality or sodium concentration), recent invasive procedures, documented hypoxemic periods, cardiac arrhythmias documented with rhythm strips, and any recent change in medication. The laboratory tests that need to be

Table 20-3

Laboratory tests to review comatose patients in intensive care units

• CT (plus repeat CT scan 3 days after ictus) or MRI of head
• EEG
• SSEPs
• CSF examination
• Transesophageal echocardiography (ECG)
• Recent cardiac rhythm strips
• Arterial blood gas measurement
• Plasma concentration of sodium for preceding 3 days
• Creatinine, BUN, arterial ammonia
• Blood smear, platelet counts
• Prothrombin time, fibrinogen, split products, D-dimer test
• Blood cultures
• Serum osmolarity
• Thyroid and adrenal function

reviewed are listed in Table 20-3. The "one metabolic trigger–one cause of coma" model may not apply to every case, but an overriding laboratory derangement is often found. A CT scan of the brain is important, and the findings may explain the origin of the coma, which may not be apparent after meticulous neurologic examination. Examination of the CSF and repeat CT, or preferably MRI, should be performed in patients with unexplained coma (Fig. 20-3).

In the authors' experience, the yield of CSF examination in comatose patients in an ICU is low, and the examination should be performed only if there is strong clinical evidence of infection. This generalization has two exceptions. First, patients with long-standing immunosuppression may harbor opportunistic infections that can be diagnosed only with appropriate CSF cultures (cryptococcidiosis, candidiasis, aspergillosis, and toxoplasmosis), and, second, patients with underlying cancer may have carcinomatous meningitis. A less likely cause of coma is paraneoplastic encephalitis in patients with small-cell carcinoma of the lung.[36]

Coma occurring in association with undiagnosed systemic illnesses may have its origin in cerebral vasculitis (particularly systemic lupus erythematosus). Cerebral angiography is indicated if multiple cortical infarcts are seen.

The value of performing electrodiagnostic studies in an ICU varies. Their value in predicting outcome is probably more important than in ferreting out a possible cause of coma. Nonconvulsive status epilepticus is often considered, but seldom diagnosed, in patients in medical ICUs. Electroencephalography can be helpful: dominance of beta activity indicates benzodiazepine accumulation; triphasic waves indicate hepatic failure; and burst-suppression pattern indicates anoxic damage or barbiturate overdose. (See Chaps. 3, 12, 14, and 16.)

If the electroencephalogram (EEG) is normal in a patient with unexplained coma, one should suspect a psychogenic origin.[37] (One of the authors has diagnosed psychogenic coma in a patient in the ICU.)

Somatosensory evoked potential (SSEP) recording can be useful. The absence of these evoked scalp potentials indicates significant brain injury. Whether the source of the injury is traumatic, metabolic, or anoxic, those patients with absent SSEPs do not recover beyond a persistent vegetative state.

OUTCOME OF COMA IN INTENSIVE CARE UNITS

Prognostic factors for comatose critically ill patients seen in medical or surgical ICUs have not been consistently identified. In most patients, individual categories of coma are assessed without much attention being paid to an associated medical illness. Mortality is increased significantly in patients who remain comatose during a critical illness after possible confounders have been excluded, metabolic derangements have been corrected, or appropriate neurosurgical intervention has been performed. The management plan is often reassessed when coma develops during critical illness. Often, an acute neurologic event is a final complication of a severe illness: seldom is it only a temporary setback.

A simple prognostic scoring system has been developed for patients with coma due to a nontraumatic (but including cerebral infarction and cerebral hematoma) or unknown cause.[38] Many metabolic causes of coma were excluded. According to this scoring system, the outcome is poor (defined as a 5 percent probability of survival at 2 months) if coma persisting for 3 days was associated with four or five risk factors. These risk factors included the following: (1) abnormal brainstem response (at least an abnormal pupillary or corneal reflex or abnormal eye movement); (2) no motor withdrawal to pain; (3) no verbal response; (4) creatinine levels greater than or equal to and 132.6 µmol/L (1.5 mg/dL); and (5) age 70 years or older.[38]

The outcome of coma due to metabolic causes can be predicted only after the underlying metabolic trigger has been reversed and the patient's condition has been observed for several days. It is well known that after hyponatremia, hyperglycemia, or hypoglycemia has been corrected, the impact of the disorder may linger for several days.[39,40]

Predicting outcome of the different types of metabolic coma is discussed in the relevant chapters, but several important differences exist. Using Levy's criteria the outcome of hypoxic ischemic encephalopathy can be predicted without difficulty if the patient had a circulatory arrest during the critical illness or had been markedly hypotensive and hypoxemic for a prolonged period of time.[41]

Coma in a patient with hepatic encephalopathy is a poor clinical sign. However, recovery is possible in patients with acute fulminant hepatic failure after successful liver transplantation and ICP control. Without liver transplantation, only one-third of these patients regain independent function; the other two-thirds die without regaining consciousness. Many patients who recover from coma-associated severe hepatic encephalopathy, but not from acute liver necrosis, remain cognitively impaired.

The outcome of septic encephalopathy is a poor if motor responses are absent (neuromuscular blockers must be excluded as confounders). Progressively severe EEG rhythm abnormalities in patients with septic encephalopathy are associated with an increased rate of mortality. The mortality

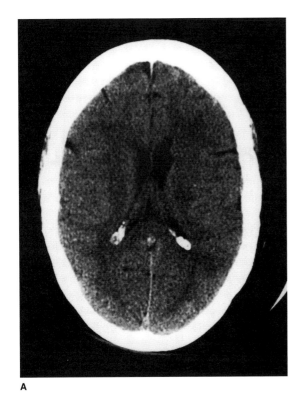

A

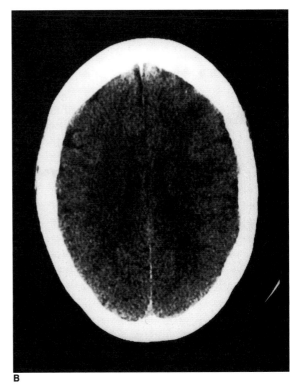

B

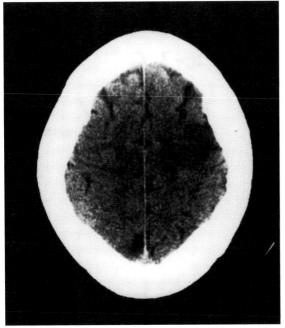

C

Figure 20-3

(A–C) *Normal CT scan (with a hint of hypodensity) in a comatose patient with nonlocalizing neurologic signs and symptoms (Glasgow Coma Scale: GCS = 6).* (D–F) *Abnormal MRI findings on the same day indicate bilateral infarction in the territories of the anterior and middle cerebral arteries. G. Bilateral infarction is caused by acquired occlusion of the right carotid artery and likely embolus to the left carotid, supplying the territories of both the anterior cerebral and middle cerebral arteries.*

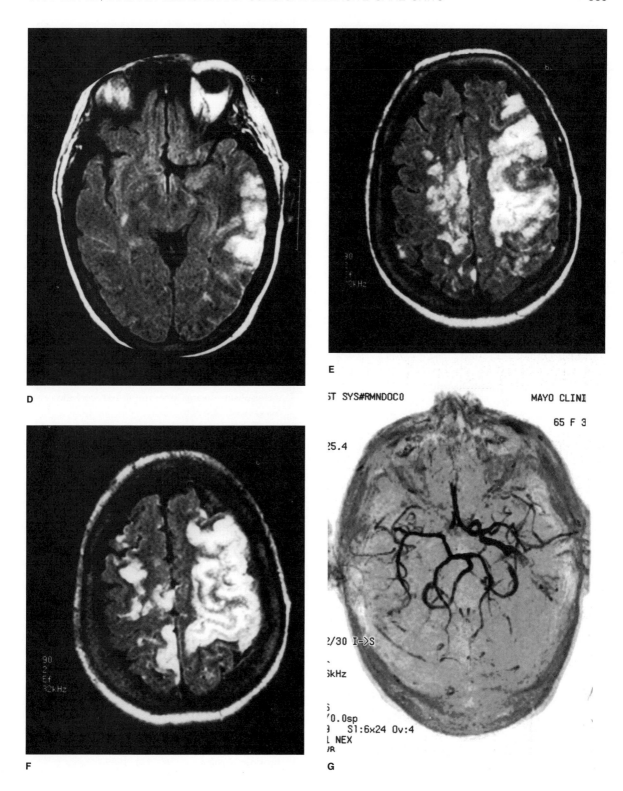

E

D

F

G

rate associated with theta activity is 19 percent; that with delta activity 36 percent, with triphasic wave, 50 percent, and with burst-suppression pattern, 67 percent.

REFERENCES

1. Wijdicks EFM: *Neurology of Critical Illness*. Contemporary Neurology series. Philadelphia, FA Davis, 1995.
2. Bleck TP, Smith MC, Pierre-Louis SJ, et al: Neurologic complications of critical medical illnesses. *Crit Care Med* 21:98–103, 1993.
3. Carrasco G, Molina R, Costa J, et al: Propofol versus midazolam in short-, medium-, and long-term sedation of critically ill patients. A cost-benefit analysis. *Chest* 103:557-564, 1993.
4. Pohlman AS, Simpson KP, Hall JB: Continuous intravenous infusions of lorazepam versus midazolam for sedation during mechanical ventilating support: a prospective, randomized study. *Crit Care Med* 22:1241–1247, 1994.
5. Wijdicks EFM, Jack CR Jr: Intracerebral hemorrhage after fibrinolytic therapy for acute myocardial infarction. *Stroke* 24:554–557, 1993.
6. Sloan MA, Price TR, Petito CK, et al: Clinical features and pathogenesis of intracerebral hemorrhage after rt-PA and heparin therapy for acute myocardial infarction: the thrombolysis in myocardial infarction (TIMI) II pilot and randomized clinical trial combined experience. *Neurology* 45:649–658, 1995.
7. Wijdicks EFM, Silbert PL, Jack CR, Parisi JE: Subcortical hemorrhage in disseminated intravascular coagulation associated with sepsis. *AJNR* 15:763–765, 1994.
8. Young GB, Bolton CF, Austin TW, et al: The encephalopathy associated with septic illness. *Clin Invest Med* 13:297–304, 1990.
9. Sprung CL, Peduzzi PN, Shatney CH, et al: Impact of encephalopathy on mortality in the sepsis syndrome. *Crit Care Med* 18:801–806, 1990.
10. Wijdicks EFM, Stevens M: The role of hypotension in septic encephalopathy following surgical procedures. *Arch Neurol* 49:653–656, 1992.
11. Wijdicks EFM, Plevak DJ, Rakela J, Wiesner RH: Clinical and radiologic features of cerebral edema in fulminant hepatic failure. *Mayo Clin Proc* 70:119–124, 1995.
12. Lee WM: Acute liver failure. *N Engl J Med* 329:1862–1872, 1993.
13. Zelcer J, Wells DG: Anesthetic-related recovery room complications. *Anesthetic Intensive Care* 15:168–174, 1987.
14. Parikh S, Cohen JR: Perioperative stroke following general surgical procedures. *NY State J Med* 93:162–165, 1993.
15. Wijdicks EFM, Jack C: Coronary artery bypass grafting associated ischemic stroke: a clinical and neuroradiologic study. *J Neuroimaging* 6:20, 1996.
16. Wareing TH, Davila-Roman VG, Daily BB, et al: Strategy for the reduction of stroke incidence in cardiac surgical patients. *Ann Thorac Surg* 55:1400–1408, 1993.
17. Liu S, Holley HS, Stulberg SD, et al: Failure to awaken after general anesthesia secondary to paradoxical venous embolus. *Can J Anaesth* 38:335–337, 1991.
18. Bucci MN, Phillips TW, McGillicuddy JE: Delayed epidural hemorrhage in hypotensive multiple trauma patients. *Neurosurgery* 19:65–68, 1986.
19. Hayes MA, Williamson RJ, Heidenreich WF: Endocrine mechanisms involved in water and sodium metabolism during operation and convalescence. *Surgery* 41:353–386, 1957.
20. Arieff AI: Hyponatremia, convulsions, respiratory arrest, and permanent brain damage after elective surgery in healthy women. *N Engl J Med* 314:1529–1535, 1986.
21. Arieff AI, Llack F, Massry SG: Neurological manifestations and morbidity of hyponatremia: correlation with brain, water, and electrolytes. *Medicine* 55:121–129, 1976.
22. Jensen V: The TURP syndrome. *Can J Anaesth* 38:90-96, 1991.
23. Wijdicks EFM, Larson TS: Absence of postoperative hyponatremia syndrome in young, healthy females. *Ann Neurol* 35:626–628, 1994.
24. Berl T: Treating hyponatremia. Damned if we do and damned if we don't. *Kidney Int* 37:1006–1018, 1990.
25. Laureno R: Central pontine myelinolysis following rapid connection of hyponatremia. *Ann Neurol* 232–242, 1983.
26. Wright DG, Laureno R, Victor M: Pontine and extrapontine myelinolysis. *Brain* 102:361–385, 1979.
27. Henderson DJ, Middleton RG: Coma from hyponatremia following transurethral resection of the prostate. *Urology* 15:267–271, 1980.

28. Spregel DM, Ullian ME, Xerbe GO, Berl T: Determinants of survival and recovery in acute renal failure patients dialyzed in intensive care units. *Am J Nephrol* 11:44–47, 1991.

29. Pascual E, Gómez-Arnau J, Pensado C, et al: Incidence and risk factors of early acute renal failure in liver transplant patients. *Transplant Proc* 25:1837, 1993.

30. Hou SH, Bushinsky DA, Wish JB, Cohen JJ, et al: Hospital-acquired renal insufficiency: a prospective study. *Am J Med* 74:243–248, 1983.

31. Bolton CF, Young GB: *Neurological Complications of Renal Disease*. Boston, Butterworth, 1990.

32. Colt HG, Begg RJ, Saporito JJ, et al: Cholesterol emboli after cardiac catheterization: eight cases and a review of the literature. *Medicine* (Baltimore) 67:389–400, 1988.

33. Fine MJ, Kapoor W, Falanga V: Cholesterol crystal embolization: a review of 221 cases in the English literature. *Angiology* 38:769–784, 1987.

34. Levy D: The fat embolization syndrome. A review. *Clin Orthop* 261:281–286, 1990.

35. Saito A, Mequro K, Matsumura A, et al: Magnetic resonance imaging of a fat embolism of the brain—case report. *Neurosurgery* 26:882–885, 1990.

36. Glantz MJ, Biran H, Myers ME: The radiographic diagnosis and treatment of paraneoplastic central nervous system disease. *Cancer* 73:168–175, 1994.

37. Plum F, Pomer J: *The Diagnosis of Stupor and Coma*. Contemporary Neurology series. Philadelphia, FA Davis, 1980.

38. Hamel MB, Goldman L, Teno J, Lynn J, Davis RB, Harrell FE, Connors AF, Califf R, Kussin P, Bellamy P, Vidaillet H, Phillips RS: Identification of comatose patients at high risk for death or severe disability. *JAMA* 273:1842–1848, 1995.

39. Guisado R, Arieff AI: Neurologic manifestations of diabetic comas: correlation with biochemical alterations in the brain. *Metabolism* 24:665–679, 1975.

40. Malouf R, Brust JC: Hypoglycemia: causes, neurological manifestations, and outcome. *Ann Neurol* 17:421–430, 1985.

41. Levy DE, Caronna JJ, Singer BH, et al: Predicting outcome from hypoxic-ischemic coma. *JAMA* 253:1420–1426, 1985.

Chapter 21

COMA IN THE TRANSPLANT INTENSIVE CARE UNIT

Eelco F. M. Wijdicks

Transplantation surgery is often followed by complex postoperative critical care management. Vigilance is often impaired in patients who have just returned from a major transplant procedure. After heart (or heart/lung) or liver transplantation, patients are not fully alert for at least 12 to 24 h because of the high doses of narcotic agents and benzodiazepines administered during the lengthy procedure. Although patients often awake soon after heart transplantation, their postoperative alertness is markedly impaired. In addition, awakening after liver transplantation is often a sign of graft *function*. However, there is less reason for patients to be drowsy in the postoperative phase after renal, pancreas, or bone marrow transplantation, and the length of their stay in the intensive care transplant unit may be relatively short.

This chapter emphasizes the differential diagnosis and management of failure to awaken or of worsening coma after organ transplantation. The chapter is organized by type of transplantation, so that a physician can quickly refer to the appropriate section when called to evaluate a patient in the transplant intensive care unit. As would be expected, neurotoxicity due to immunosuppressive agents is a frequent cause of impaired consciousness after any type of transplantation.

HEART TRANSPLANTATION

With the exponential growth in the number of heart transplantations, the number of requests for consultations for serious neurologic complications can also be expected to increase. A major proportion of neurologic complications is associated with impairment of consciousness and involves the entire spectrum from failure to awaken postoperatively to worsening coma. In evaluating patients who have impaired consciousness, the postoperative period can be arbitrarily divided into two phases. The early postoperative phase is the first 2 days after transplantation, and the late postoperative phase extends from day 3 to 2 weeks (Table 21-1).

Early Postoperative Phase: Causes of Impaired Consciousness and Coma

During the early postoperative phase, induction immunosuppression is initiated.[1] Thus, if the level of consciousness deteriorates markedly, immunosuppressive agents are implicated.

Failure for a patient to awaken after heart transplantation is rarely due to a structural lesion in the central nervous system. In the absence of localizing neurologic findings, the most common cause of unresponsiveness is medication-induced

Table 21-1

Causes of coma in heart transplant recipients

Early postoperative phase (0 to 2 days)	• Postanoxic-ischemic encephalopathy • Multiple cerebral infarcts • Drug-induced toxic encephalopathy • Acute renal failure
Late postoperative phase (3 days to 2 weeks)	• OKT3 toxicity • Cyclosporine toxicity • Steroid psychosis associated with therapy to counter rejection • Cerebral infarcts and hemorrhage • Seizures, nonconvulsive status

coma. Narcotic agents are often used liberally to decrease pain and to overcome postoperative hypertension. These agents (usually morphine and fentanyl) may cause significant sedation, but only when intermittent doses are given. The elimination half-life of most narcotic agents is 3 to 4 h. Typically, high doses of narcotic agents are given intraoperatively, and the operative anesthesiology list should be scrutinized carefully. Many anesthesiologists use fentanyl (with diazepam) or sufentanil (with lorazepam). Naloxone (0.04 to 0.08 mg) reverses the effects of narcotic agents. Volatile anesthetic agents should not influence the level of consciousness, because they wash out within several minutes of being administered. These agents can be measured in end tidal volume if sufficient concern about their contribution to level of consciousness remains.

An important cause for the failure of a patient to awaken immediately after transplantation is the administration of benzodiazepines. The preferred benzodiazepine is midazolam, but even with moderate intravenous infusions (doses of $\geq 10\,\text{mg/kg}$ per hour), recovery time is prolonged (benzodiazepines are preferred because they induce amnesia). Contrary to the belief that midazolam is short-acting, it may take several days for patients to recover from its effects. Flumazenil should seriously be considered for countering overmedication with benzodiazepines.

It is crucial to exclude the possible effects of lingering neuromuscular blockade. In most cases, neuromuscular blockade can be adequately reversed, e.g., with neostigmine. Persistent neuromuscular blockade may produce a virtually locked-in syndrome that may be difficult to detect in heavily sedated patients. By using a peripheral nerve stimulator to demonstrate four equal twitches (train of four), neuromuscular blockade can be excluded. Occasionally, drug interaction with neuromuscular blocking agents may be implicated in prolonging the neuromuscular blocking effect; potent drugs are aminoglycosides, polymyxin, and cyclosporine in susceptible patients.

Failure of patients to awaken may originate with the marked hypotension that occurs intraoperatively, episodes of significant hypoxemia, or, more often, cardiac resuscitation for asystole or ventricular fibrillation. Cardiac arrest can occur in the immediate postoperative phase and can be devastating. The most common clinical problems associated with perioperative cardiac arrest are hypovolemia, tamponade, and overdose of potent vasodilators.

Neurologic complications in the early postoperative phase have decreased in recent years.[2] Much of this decrease has been due to meticulous care in removing all residual atrial tissue or thrombus. Also, the use of more precise everting anastomosis may have decreased intracardiac thrombus formation on the suture interface that may have resulted in massive embolic showers and cerebral infarcts. Air embolism generally occurs early after transplantation and, despite a dramatic presentation with a flurry of seizures and coma, it usually resolves without neurologic sequelae. Techniques such as continuous intra-arterial irrigation of the left side of the heart have made this complication uncommon. In one recent series of 113 consecutive patients who had heart transplantation, only two had a neurologic complication in the early postoperative phase (one of these patients had a seizure induced by lidocaine toxicity and the other had a transient ischemic attack).[3]

Late Postoperative Phase: Causes of Impaired Consciousness and Coma

In many cardiac transplant units, immunosuppression is initiated with OKT3. Neurotoxicity due to OKT3 is rare because induction protocols have been careful to monitor the concentration of CD3+ cells in peripheral blood rather than blood levels.[4,5] Often, after the second dose (the first dose is usually administered in the operating suite), nonspecific chills and a flu-like uncomfortable malaise with myalgia may occur, but it subsides spontaneously. Usually, within the first 2 weeks (as early as 5 days) after transplantation, these side effects may occur. After the use of OKT3 is discontinued, these symptoms resolve in 2 days. Many patients complain of a headache that may reflect a mild aseptic meningitis.[5]

Because aseptic meningitis due to OKT3 is mild, it should not influence the level of consciousness, despite fever and nuchal rigidity, unless a significant OKT3-related pulmonary edema with respiratory acidosis develops (OKT3 encephalopathy is usually seen in association with these systemic manifestations).

A rare complication is OKT3 encephalopathy.[4] This has not been observed in the Mayo Clinic Heart Transplant series in which patients are treated initially with OKT3. This type of encephalopathy is characterized by psychosis, multifocal myoclonus, or seizures progressing to deep coma with extensor posturing if not recognized as such. The computed tomography (CT) scanning of cases of OKT3 encephalopathy has shown cerebral edema, which was reversed after the use of the drug was discontinued. Resolution of this severe encephalopathy may take 2 to 3 weeks, but the outcome can be quite favorable.

If a heart transplant recipient has worsening coma after an asymptomatic interval in the intensive care unit, cyclosporine toxicity should be suspected (see "Liver Transplantation" for details on cyclosporine toxicity). Holding the dose of cyclosporine or switching to the use of FK506, which has an identical immunosuppressive effect, is recommended.

Patients with worsening coma after heart transplantation may have had an ischemic stroke involving the territory of a large cerebral artery, resulting in brain swelling. Risk factors for heart transplant–associated ischemic stroke are retained thrombi in the graft and complications of the placement of catheters during cardiopulmonary bypass. Intracerebral hemorrhages are not common during the late postoperative phase, but they have been linked to aspergillosis and severe coagulopathy, as in liver transplantation. Intracerebral hematomas that occur after heart transplantation have not been carefully characterized; they may be lobar or ganglionic. It is not likely that acute hypertension due to significantly improved ventricular function is a contributory factor unless inotropes have been used in excessive doses.

Convulsive or nonconvulsive status epilepticus is an unusual explanation for impaired consciousness after heart transplantation, and, when it does occur, it often signals an ischemic or hemorrhagic stroke. A 10 to 15 percent incidence of seizures has been found in a series of heart transplant recipients, but, in the author's experience, the incidence is much lower. The use of high doses of methyl prednisolone is another cause of confusion and impaired consciousness during the late postoperative phase. High doses of this drug induce a corticosteroid psychosis characterized by major mood swings, hallucinations, and agitation. However, progression to coma is not expected.[6]

LUNG TRANSPLANTATION

The number of lung transplantations performed since the procedure was introduced in 1983 has increased remarkably. Donors are scarce, and only 5 to 15 percent of organ donors provide suitable lungs. Reasons for rejection of donor lungs include pulmonary contusion, significant aspiration pneumonitis, and high incidence of development of neurogenic pulmonary edema in brain-death patients. Transplantation can be with a single lung, double lung, or heart-lung combination.[7,8] Experience with the neurologic complications that occur after lung transplantation is limited and prevalence is difficult to estimate.[9]

Early Postoperative Phase: Causes of Impaired Consciousness and Coma

Neurologic evaluation in the first days after transplantation is extremely difficult because most patients are sedated, paralyzed, and mechanically ventilated. Some programs dictate continuing mechanical ventilation to decrease stress on the critical trachea anastomosis, but most patients are rapidly weaned within 36 h.[10]

Hemorrhage and marked pulmonary infection may dominate the early postoperative course, and impaired consciousness may reflect the hypoxemia associated with pulmonary edema from capillary injury due to ischemia and subsequent reperfusion (Table 21-2).[10,11] Multiple embolic strokes may occur as a consequence of thrombus formation at the atrial cuff, but this is rare.

Late Postoperative Phase: Causes of Impaired Consciousness and Coma

Cyclosporine neurotoxicity is the most common cause of neurologic complications and impaired consciousness (Table 21-2). Rejection of the transplanted lung may occur in the late postoperative phase and is associated with significant hypoxemia produced by obliterative bronchiolitis. Mortality in lung transplant recipients is frequently caused by

overwhelming cytomegalovirus infection (which does not necessarily result in cytomegalovirus encephalitis). Although bacterial pneumonia is common, bacterial meningitis has not been reported. Any infectious complication can occur and is a major cause of mortality.

LIVER TRANSPLANTATION

Liver transplant recipients do have a propensity to develop central nervous system manifestations. This can be explained by a direct effect of liver failure on brain functioning, but also because the postoperative course is often complicated by significant coagulopathy, sepsis, and often dramatic electrolyte shifts. Neurologic complications occur in approximately 10 percent of the patients with liver transplantation.

Early Postoperative Phase: Causes of Impaired Consciousness and Coma

An important subset of patients who almost invariably are drowsy after liver transplantation are those with fulminant hepatic failure (Table 21-3). Patients with fulminent hepatic failure are prone to increased intracranial pressure (ICP) because of brain edema. Recovery from cerebral edema (i.e., return of consciousness to baseline level) takes days. In extreme cases, brain death is diagnosed postoperatively. Many patients have cerebral edema that can be visualized on CT scan when hepatic encephalopathy grade 3 is approached. These patients typically have a more prolonged postoperative course, with a possible increase in ICP prior to and during transplantation.

Table 21-2

Causes of coma in lung transplant recipients

Early postoperative phase (0 to 2 days)	• Iatrogenic (sedation and neuromuscular blockade) • Significant hypoxemia from pulmonary edema • Multiple cerebral infarcts from retained atrial cuff
Late postoperative phase (3 days to 2 weeks)	• Cyclosporine toxicity • Hypoxic-ischemic encephalopathy associated with acute rejection • Overwhelming cytomegalovirus infection

Table 21-3
Causes of coma in liver transplant recipients

Early postoperative phase (0 to 2 days)	• Cerebral edema associated with fulminant hepatic failure • Central pontine myelinolysis • Anoxic-ischemic encephalopathy • Hyperglycemia
Late postoperative phase (3 days to 2 weeks)	• Cyclosporine neurotoxicity • FK506 (tacrolimus) neurotoxicity • Intracranial hematoma • Recurrent seizures • Septic encephalopathy • Hepatic encephalopathy associated with graft failure • Hypoglycemia • Acute renal failure

Treatment of refractory-increased ICP results in brain death, and this very unfortunate outcome has been observed in virtually every program of liver transplantation. In other patients, the effects of cerebral edema may linger for 7 to 10 days before the patient recovers. In the author's patients with fulminant hepatic failure, barbiturate coma was indicated to control ICP. Therefore, the use of barbiturates perioperatively may contribute substantially to postoperative altered consciousness.

Central pontine myelinolysis should be considered in patients who fail to awaken[12,13] Impaired consciousness can be explained by damage to the thalamus as an extrapontine manifestation of osmotic demyelination. Extension of demyelination to the pontine tegmentum may be the pathologic substrate in other patients. Central pontine myelinolysis usually is associated with marked fluctuations in the serum levels of sodium; also, it is typical of patients who were alcoholics. The CT findings are normal, but the magnetic resonance imaging (MRI) scans may show the characteristic trident or bat-shaped abnormality in the pons. The cause of central pontine myelinolysis after liver transplantation has not been defined completely. Marked shifts in osmolality and the plasma concentration of sodium are observed in many transplant recipients, but, despite these shifts, the incidence of central pontine myelinolysis (by autopsy criteria) is low. In the author's series of patients with central pontine myelinolysis

(Fig. 21-1), it was difficult to implicate sodium and osmolality changes as the main factors.[12] The outcome is good for survivors of central pontine myelinosis.

Another cause of the failure of patients to awaken after transplantation is anoxic-ischemic encephalopathy, which produces severe cortical laminar necrosis and watershed infarctions. Anoxic-ischemic changes in the brain have been described in 20 to 40 percent of the liver transplant recipients who came to autopsy.[14] Hypoxemic-ischemic encephalopathy could result from marked hypotension occuring during reperfusion of the transplanted liver or from massive bleeding intraoperatively. Hypoxemic-ischemic encephalopathy may progress to deep coma, and the presence of fixed pupils or myoclonus status epilepticus indicates a poor prognosis. It is possible, but unproven, that hypoxemic-ischemic encephalopathy in liver transplant recipients may be more important in impairing the level of consciousness than was previously thought. After the initial insult has passed, many patients may continue to be less alert while recovering from hypoxemic-ischemic encephalopathy.

Late Postoperative Phase: Causes of Impaired Consciousness and Coma

The most common cause of the reduced level of consciousness in liver transplant recipients, and of

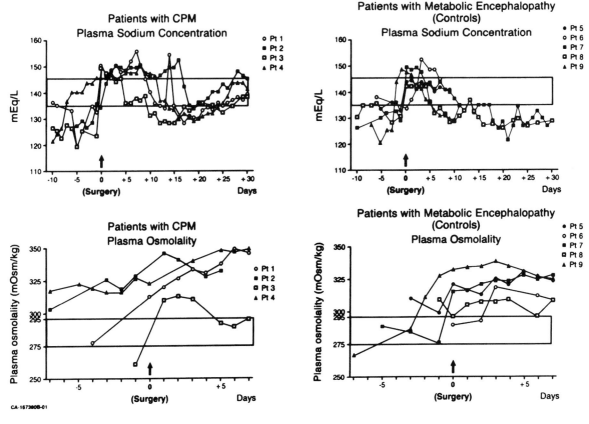

Figure 21-1

Perioperative changes in serum concentration of sodium (top panels) and plasma osmolality (bottom panels) in four patients with central pontine myelinolysis (left panels) and five control subjects with metabolic encephalopathy (right panels). Boxes show normal range. (From Wijdicks et al,[12] with permission.)

their difficulty with remaining awake during examination, is sedation produced by drugs that have accumulated over 24 h because of diminished clearance or pharmacologic interactions (Table 21-3). Cyclosporine neurotoxicity remains a comparatively frequent cause of unresponsiveness.[15–19] Typically, cyclosporine neurotoxicity produces an acute confusional state characterized by tremulousness and restlessness; it is associated with psychosis in one-half of the patients. Other manifestations of cyclosporine toxicity, such as seizures, speech apraxia or mutism, or cortical blindness, occur in only a small number of patients, but this presentation is seen occasionally during intravenous

loading. Cyclosporine neurotoxicity can be recognized when visual hallucinations, typically associated with bright colors, are reported. Cyclosporine neurotoxicity occurs in about 10 percent of liver transplant recipients.[16] The incidence of cyclosporine neurotoxicity may be increased in patients who have previously had hepatic encephalopathy. (See Figs. 21-2 and 21-3.)

In a large proportion of patients, impaired consciousness is attributed to a transient metabolic encephalopathy for which no obvious cause can be found.[20] Typically, many metabolic abnormalities are present, but none of them contribute to the diminished alertness of the patients. The use of the

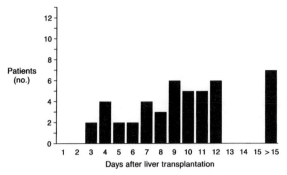

Figure 21-2

Cyclosporine neurotoxicity: time from OLT liver transplant. (From Wijdicks et al,[16] with permission.)

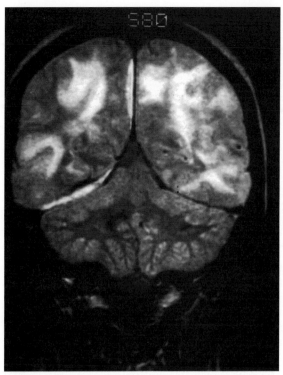

Figure 21-3

Abnormalities of the MRI consistent with cyclosporine toxicity. (From Wijdicks et al,[16] with permission.)

term "multifactorial" in this setting is unsatisfactory (and may not be correct). In the Mayo Clinic transplant series, a large proportion of these patients had been alcoholics. It is well known that delirium occurs in patients who were alcoholics before undergoing liver transplantation; however, the circumstances that cause the delirium are not well known. In many patients, the metabolic encephalopathy is transient and the outcome is good; however, intensive care unit stay can be prolonged.

Impaired consciousness due to metabolic encephalopathy may be associated with primary nonfunction of the transplanted graft.[21] Laboratory evidence of graft nonfunction is usually present: i.e., a marked increase in liver enzymes, prothrombin time, and arterial concentration of ammonia. Hepatic encephalopathy can also be caused by hepatic artery thrombosis or portal vein thrombosis. Acute renal failure may contribute, as well, in this phase of postoperative care. Uremic encephalopathy is encountered more often in patients who had renal dysfunction preoperatively. Acute renal failure may be associated with cyclosporine use, and the correction of cyclosporine infusion sometimes improves this metabolic abnormality.[21]

Another cause of diffuse brain dysfunction is septic encephalopathy. The initial clinical manifestations are nonspecific. Patients are confused, disoriented, and restless, and many of them are tachypneic and hyperventilate, which may be the result of early lung injury or the effect of circulating immunologic mediators on respiratory drive. Hypoxemia in combination with hypercarbia may result in early central nervous system manifestations of encephalopathy. However, after these acute respiratory problems have been corrected, consciousness often remains impaired. Marked hypotension may be a contributing factor.[22]

An acute clinical deterioration may occur in the condition of some patients after initial postoperative awakening and uncomplicated course. Sudden coma is often associated with intracranial hematomas. Virtually all patients with intracranial hematomas seen at the Mayo Clinic had acute deterioration and showed massive lobar hemorrhage on CT scan.[23] Intracranial hematomas following orthotopic liver transplantation may be caused by coagulopathy or by a ruptured mycotic aneurysm (e.g., aspergillosis).

Other causes of sudden neurologic deterioration after liver transplantation include seizures (occasionally resulting in nonconvulsive status epilepticus)[24] and acute metabolic change (e.g., severe hypoglycemia).[25]

BONE MARROW TRANSPLANTATION

The indications for bone marrow transplantation have broadened. Leukemia is still the most common indication, but lymphoma, aplastic anemia, and, more recently, thalassemia and sickle cell disease have been accepted as hematologic disorders that can be cured with transplantation.[26,27]

The pretransplant procedures include conditioning regimens and infection prophylaxis. A large number of potentially neurotoxic agents is used, and each agent should be considered as a possible cause when seizures occur or consciousness is impaired. In addition, a previous course of chemotherapy may have a delayed effect on the central nervous system. The possible effects of preparative drugs are listed in Table 21-4. Most frequently, neurotoxicity is observed with the use of high doses of cytarabine (36 g/m^2)[28]; its manifestation can be impressive. Recovery is expected, but persistent neurologic sequelae are possible in the most severe cases.

Carmustine (BiCNU) at high doses produces a diffuse encephalopathy immediately after administration. Ifosfamide may cause neurotoxicity when administered in oral doses, and its toxic effect may be potentiated by cisplatin therapy. (Other neoplastic agents are discussed in more detail in Chap. 7.)

Early Postoperative Phase: Causes of Impaired Consciousness and Coma

Neurologic complications involving the level of consciousness rarely occur during the early postoperative phase after bone marrow transplantation. Most often, generalized tonic-clonic seizures are observed, frequently implicating busulfan, high doses of corticosteroids, and cyclosporine.

Cerebrovascular complications may occur and may be related to nonbacterial thrombolic endocarditis. The prevalence of this disorder is greater in bone marrow transplant recipients and is triggered by fibrin deposition associated with a deficiency in circulating anticoagulant protein C. Multiple cerebral infarctions are common, and the mortality rate is high.[29] During the neutropenic period, septicemia, due to both gram-positive and gram-negative bacteria, is present in as many as 50 percent of the patients. These bacteremias, particularly gram-positive (*Staphylococcus aureus*), may cause a life-threatening illness with shock, and the patients may become unresponsive. Severe sepsis in these patients may also produce acute hepatic failure with encephalopathy.

Toxicity due to changes in renal function should be considered strongly in patients who received bone marrow transplants for multiple myeloma, which may be associated with pre-existing kidney involvement. However, nephrotoxicity may be caused by cyclosporine and conditioning drugs, and may result in drug toxicity, particularly for penicillin derivatives. Penicillin intoxication can significantly decrease the level of consciousness and can produce characteristic multifocal myoclonus (Table 21-5).

Table 21-4
Neurologic side effects of drugs used in preconditioning regimens

Agent	Features
Cytarabine	Drowsy, frontal release signs, cogwheel rigidity, mute, cerebellar signs, tremor
Methotrexate	Fluctuating aphasia, hemiparesis, drowsiness
Busulfan	Seizures,[a] drowsiness, Wernicke-like syndrome, confusional state, ataxia, ophthalmoplegia
Etoposide	Drowsiness, seizure, hemiparesis
Ifosfamide	Confusional state, seizures

[a] May virtually be eliminated with prophylactic phenytoin loading.
See also Refs. 9, 28–34.

Table 21-5
Causes of coma in bone marrow transplant recipients

Early postoperative phase (0 to 2 days)	• Preconditioning drugs (see Table 21-4) • Cyclosporine toxicity • Sepsis • Ischemic stroke with endocarditis
Late postoperative phase (3 days to 2 weeks)	• Subdural hematoma • Cytomegalovirus encephalitis • Disseminated toxoplasmosis • Meningitis in chronic graft-versus-host syndrome

Late Postoperative Phase: Causes of Impaired Consciousness and Coma

If patients recover from the early postoperative phase, complications are rare. However, during the late postoperative phase, a fairly high proportion of patients have cerebrovascular complications, although the incidence is less than 2 to 4 percent of all patients. Subdural hematomas and multiple small parenchymal hematomas are observed in many patients when the level of consciousness suddenly decreases. In a large percentage of patients, these hemorrhages occur at the time of overwhelming sepsis and thrombocytopenia[30] One autopsy series claimed nearly a 40 percent incidence in intracranial hemorrhages, but this series included small petechial hemorrhages and subarachnoid hemorrhage.[31]

Infectious causes for worsening coma after bone marrow transplantation have been traced to cytomegalovirus (CMV) encephalitis, but the diagnosis was made only at autopsy (Table 21-5).[9] Many months may elapse before serious central nervous system infections occur. Varicella-zoster encephalitis may occur but only in patients with disseminated varicella-zoster virus. Overwhelming toxoplasmosis may occur as early as 9 days after bone marrow transplantation in all patients with positive results on serologic testing for *Toxoplasma gondii* preoperatively.[35,36] In one reported series, none of the patients recovered, and mortality and morbidity were extremely high.[36] The presence of characteristic brain lesions, fever, and confusion suggested the diagnosis in all the patients.

Patients with chronic graft-versus-host syndrome are at increased risk for infection, and fulminant bacterial meningitis may cause coma.[37-39] The cerebrospinal fluid should be examined in these patients. No specific fungal infection has been linked with bone marrow transplantation; thus, any opportunistic infection should be suspected.

RENAL TRANSPLANTATION

The enormous benefit of renal transplantation has been established. The overall success rate for this type of transplantation is excellent. Neurologic complications during the postoperative phase are uncommon, but postoperative management remains challenging.

In the immediate postoperative period, colloids need to be administered to maintain an increased intravascular volume to promote renal perfusion and to induce diuresis. Other aspects of care include initial immunosuppression and management of general surgical complications. Neurologic complications may occur in association with each of these.

Early Postoperative Phase: Causes of Impaired Consciousness and Coma

A major early problem after renal transplantation is allograft failure, in which acute allograft rejection, vascular complications (e.g., renal artery or vein thrombosis), cyclosporine nephrotoxicity, and decreased intravascular volume may be implicated

Table 21-6
Causes of coma in renal transplant recipients

Early postoperative phase (0 to 2 days)	• Acute uremia from allograft rejection
	• OKT3 neurotoxicity from countering acute rejection
	• Watershed infarction from postoperative hypovolemic shock
Late postoperative phase (3 days to 2 week)	• Seizures
	• Cyclosporine neurotoxicity
	• FK506 neurotoxicity
	• Any overwhelming opportunistic infection

(Table 21-6). The serum level of creatinine continues to increase when acute rejection causes acute renal failure. Fever and hypertension may emerge. Prompt management with OKT3 or antithrombocyte globulin may salvage the allograft.

Acute renal failure can usually be recognized by gradually progressive drowsiness, multifocal myoclonus, and, most commonly, asterixis. Patients may become restless and have disorganized and rambling speech and hallucinations. Without dialysis, patients progress to coma, without motor response to pain or extensor posturing. (A confounding factor at this juncture is the use of OKT3 and corticosteroids to counter acute rejection, because both agents may produce hallucinations and acute psychosis.)

Postoperative bleeding from arterial branches that were not ligated properly or disruption of vascular anastomosis may cause shock, which places the patient at risk for cerebral infarcts in the watershed zones. Cerebral infarcts in these zones may become hemorrhagic initiall, before hypodensities are identified on CT scan and MRI is needed.

Late Postoperative Phase: Causes of Impaired Consciousness and Coma

The most common cause of coma is cyclosporine or FK506 neurotoxicity (Fig. 21-4); however, viral infections are potentially serious, especially cytomegalovirus infections. Central nervous system infections may occur as early as the first month after a successful renal transplant (Table 21-6), but they more often develop many months after engraftment. Patients given high doses of immunosuppressive agents are at higher risk for these infections, as are patients with chronic allograft rejection. The infectious disorders most commonly described in association with renal transplants are listed in Table 21-7.

Seizures are the main cause of sudden loss of consciousness in patients who recently received a renal transplant. Often, a single tonic-clonic seizure with a postictal state is seen. The differential diagnosis of the origin of seizures in renal transplant should include antibiotic toxicity (imipenem-cilastatin, ciprofloxacin, (β-lactam antibiotics, and penicillin), subdural hematoma, and recent ischemic stroke.[40,41]

APPROACH TO PATIENTS WITH IMPAIRED LEVEL OF CONSCIOUSNES AFTER ORGAN TRANSPLANTATION

The evaluation of patients with impaired level of consciousness after liver transplantation includes CT scan, MRI (if transport is possible), measurement of blood levels of immunosuppressive agents, determination of arterial ammonia, creatinine and blood urea nitrogen (BUN), and determination of sodium concentration and osmolarity of plasma. Cerebrospinal fluid examination can be considered, but patients rarely are susceptible to systemic infection within the first month of immunosuppression. *Cryptococcus neoformans* and *Aspergillus* spp. are the fungal infections most frequently involved in the patients with fungal meningitis, but this is an unusual development during the perioperative phase. If no explanation can be found on the basis of these tests, one

Figure 21-4
*Abnormalities of the MRI
consistent with FK506 toxicity.*

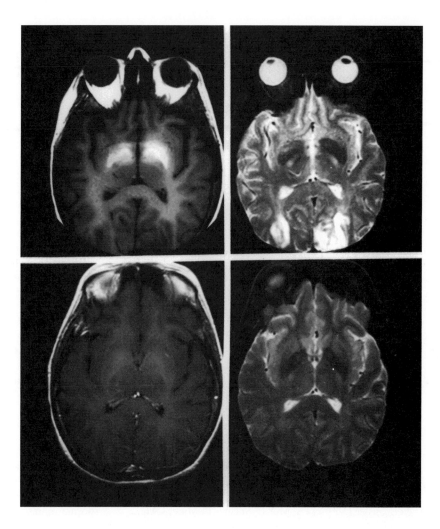

Table 21-7
Central nervous system infections in renal transplant recipients

Clinical syndrome	Microbial agent
Acute meningitis	*Listeria monocytogenes*
Subacute or chronic meningitis	*Cryptococcus neoformans, Mycobacterium tuberculosis, Listeria monocytogenes, Strongyloides stercoralis, Coccidiodes immitis, Histoplasma capsulatum*
Encephalitis or meningoencephalitis	*Listeria monocytogenes, Toxoplasma gondii*
Localized mass lesion (brain abscess)	*Aspergillus* spp., *Nocardia asteroides, Toxoplasma gondii*

Source: From Patchell,[9] with permission.

may consider administering flumazenil (for patients previously given benzodiazepines) or naloxone (for patients previously given narcotic agents). Use of the electroencephalogram (EEG) in this setting is debated, although the presence of epileptiform changes on EEG in patients following liver transplantation indicate a poor prognosis. The value of performing EEG in patients with normal results on CT and MRI is not known. The EEG usually shows nonspecific mild-to-moderate generalized slowing. Occasionally, it may show epileptiform abnormalities that may or may not have been associated with seizure. The finding of nonconvulsive status epilepticus in the setting of liver transplantation is unexpected and most unusual, but it may occur in patients with a history of exposure to high doses of benzodiazepine and sudden withdrawal.[42]

The outcome for patients with impaired levels of consciousness is good for those who survive the critical illness. However, long-term studies on intellectual function have not been performed in this subset of patients.

REFERENCES

1. Bolman RM III, Saffitz J: Early postoperative care of the cardiac transplantation patient: routine considerations and immunosuppressive therapy (review). *Prog Cardiovasc Dis* 33:137–148, 1990.
2. Bronster DJ, Emre S, Mor E, Sheiner P, Miller CM, Schwartz ME: Neurologic complications of orthotopic liver transplantation (review). *Mt Sinai J Med* 61:63–69,1994.
3. Jessen ME, Meyer DM, Moncrief CL, Wait MA, Melamed NB, Ring WS: Reducing neurological complications after cardiac transplantation: technical considerations. *J Cardiac Sur* 8:546–553, 1993.
4. Thislethwaite JR Jr, Stuart JK, Mayes JL, et al: Complications and monitoring of OKT3 therapy. *Am J Kidney Dis* 11:112–119, 1988.
5. Adair JC, Woodley SL, O'Connell JB, et al: Aseptic meningitis following cardiac transplantation: clinical characteristics and relationship to immunosuppressive regimen. *Neurology* 41:249–252, 1991.
6. Lewis DA, Smith RE: Steroid-induced psychiatric syndromes: a report of 14 cases and a review of the literature. *J Affective Disord* 5:319–332, 1983.
7. Judson MA: Clinical aspects of lung transplantation (review). *Clin Chest Med* 14:335–357, 1993.
8. Gayes JM, Giron L, Nissen MD, Plut D: Anesthetic considerations for patients undergoing double-lung transplantation (review). *J Cardiothoracic Anesth* 4:486–498, 1990.
9. Patchell RA: Neurological complications of organ transplantation. *Ann Neurol* 36:688–703, 1994.
10. Todd TR: Early postoperative management following lung transplantation (review). *Clin Chest Med* 11:259–267, 1990.
11. Héritier F, Madden B, Hodson ME, Yacoub M: Lung allograft transplantation: indications, preoperative assessment and postoperative management. *Eur Respir J* 5:1262–1278, 1992.
12. Wijdicks EFM, Blue P, Wiesner R, Steers J: Central pontine myelinolysis after liver transplantation presenting with stupor alone. *Liver Transplant Surg* (in press).
13. Wszolek ZK, McComb, Pfeiffer RF, Ste RE, et al: Pontine and extrapontine myelinolysis following liver transplantation. *Transplantation* 48:1006–1012, 1989.
14. Adams DH, Gunson B, Honigsberger L, et al: Neurological complications following liver transplantation. *Lancet* 1:94–951, 1987.
15. de Groen PC, Aksamit AJ, Rakela J, et al: Central nervous system toxicity after liver translantation: the role of cyclosporine and cholesterol. *N Engl J Med* 317:861–866, 1987.
16. Wijdicks EFM, Wiesner RH, Krom RAF: Neurotoxicity in liver transplant recipients with cyclosporine immunosuppression. *Neurology* 45:1962–1964, 1995.
17. Stein DP, Lederman RJ, Vogt DP, et al: Neurological complications following liver transplantation. *Ann Neurol* 31:644–649, 1992.
18. Rowley HA, Kaku DA, Ascher NL, et al: Neurologic findings in 100 consecutive liver transplant recipients. *Neurology* 40:181, 1990.
19. Bronster DJ, Emre S, Mor E, Sheiner P, Miller CM, Schwartz ME: Neurologic complications of orthotopic liver transplantation. *Mt Sinai J Med* 61:63–69, 1994.
20. Singh N, Yu VL, Gayowski T: Central nervous system lesions in adult liver transplant recipients: clinical review with implications for management. *Medicine* 73:110–118, 1994.
21. Carton EG, Plevak DJ, Kranner PW, Rettke SR, Geiger HJ, Coursin DB: Perioperative care of the

liver transplant patient: part 2. *Anesth Analg* 78:382–399, 1994.

22. Wijdicks EFM, Stevens M: The role of hypotension in septic encephalopathy following surgical procedures. *Arch Neurol* 49:653–656, 1992.

23. Wijdicks EFM, de Groen PC, Wiesner RH, Krom RAF: Intracranial hemorrhage after liver transplantation. *Mayo Clin Proc* 70:443–446, 1995.

24. Wszolek ZK, Aksamit AJ, Ellingson RJ, Sharbrough FW, Westmoreland BF, Pfeiffer RF, Steg RE, de Groen PC: Epileptiform electroencephalographic abnormalities in liver transplant recipients. *Ann Neurol* 30:37–41, 1991.

25. Wijdicks EFM: Impaired consciousness after liver transplantation. *Liver Transplant Surg* 1:329–334, 1995.

26. Walters MC, Sullivan KM, Bernaudin F, Souillet G, Vannier J-P, Johnson FL, Lenarsky C, Powars D, Bunin N, Ohene-Frempong K, et al: Neurologic complications after allogeneic marrow transplantation for sickle cell anemia. *Blood* 85:879–884, 1995.

27. Reece DE, Frie-Lahr DA, Shepherd JD, Dorovini-Zis K, Gascoyne RD, Graeb DA, Spinelli JJ, Barnett MJ, Klingemann H-G, Herzig GP, Phillips GL: Neurologic complications in allogeneic bone marrow transplant patients receiving cyclosporine. *Bone Marrow Transpl* 8:393–401, 1991.

28. Lopez TA, Agarwal RF: Acute cerebellar toxicity after high-dose cytarabine associated with central nervous system assimilation of its metabolite uracil arabinoside. *Cancer Treatment Reports* 68:1309, 1984.

29. Gordon BG, Savings KL, McCallister TA, et al: Cerebral infarction associated with protein C deficiency following allogenic bone marrow transplantation. *Bone Marrow Transpl* 8:323–325, 1991.

30. Meanwell CA, Blade AE, Kelley KA: Prediction of ifosfamide/mesna associated encephalopathy. *Eur J Clin Oncol* 22:81–819, 1986.

31. Pomeranz S, Naparstek E, Ashkenazi E, Nagler A, Lossos A, Slavin S, Or R: Intracranial haematomas following bone marrow transplantation. *J Neurol* 241:252–256, 1994,

32. Zalupski M, Baker LH: Ifosfamide. *J Nat Cancer Inst* 80:556–566, 1988.

33. Goren MP, Wright RK, Pratt CB, et al: Potentiation of ifosfamide neurotoxicity by prior cis-diamine dichroroplatinum therapy. *Cancer Res* 47:1457–1460, 1987.

34. Mohrmann RL, Mah V, Vinters HV: Neuropathologic findings after bone marrow transplantation: an autopsy study. *Hum Pathol* 21:630–639, 1990.

35. Grigg AP, Shepard JD, Phillips GL: Busulfan and phenytoin. *Ann Intern Med* 111:1049–1050, 1989.

36. Derouin F, Devergie A, Auber P, Gluckman E, Beauvais B, Garin YJF, Lariviere M: Toxoplasmosis in bone marrow-transplant recipients: report of seven cases and review. *Clin Infect Dis* 15:267–270, 1992.

37. D'Antonio D, Di Bartolomeo P, Iacone A, Olioso P, Di Girolamo G, Angrilli F, Papalinetti G, Fioritoni G, Betti S, Torlontano G: Meningitis due to penicillin-resistant *Streptococcus pneumoniae* in patients with chronic graft-versus-host disease. *Bone Marrow Transpl* 9:299–300, 1992.

38. Long SG, Leyland MJ, Milligan DW: Listeria meningitis after bone marrow transplantation. *Bone Marrow Transpl* 12:537–539, 1993.

39. Marosi C, Budka H, Grimm G, Zeitlhofer J, Sluga E, Brunner C, Schneeweiss B, Volc B, Bettelheim P, Panzer S, Kier P, Graninger W, Haas OA, Hinterberger W: Fatal encephalitis in a patient with chronic graft-versus-host disease. *Bone Marrow Transpl* 6:53–57, 1990.

40. Adams HP, Dawson G, Coffman TJ, Corry RJ: Stroke in renal transplant recipients. *Arch Neurol* 43:113–115, 1986.

41. Bergen DC, Ristanovic R, Gorelick PB, Kathpalia S: Seizures and renal failures. *Int J Artif Organs* 17:247–251, 1994.

42. Thomas P, Mantik B, Genton A, et al: "De novo" absence status of late onset: report of 11 cases. *Neurology* 42:104–110, 1992.

Chapter 22

THE MATERNITY WARD

G. Bryan Young

Also there is great perill in labouring...
Thomas Raynalde, 1540[1]

Pregnancy is associated with a number of neurologic and systemic conditions that impair consciousness. These include eclampsia, worsening of pre-existing epilepsy, ischemic stroke, ruptured berry aneurysm or vascular malformations, intracranial venous thrombosis, brain tumor complications, systemic illnesses (coagulopathies, systemic infections, exacerbations of diabetes mellitus, renal disease, liver disease, and nutritional deficiency), amniotic fluid embolism, and psychiatric disorders.

Symptoms, observations of eyewitnesses, neurologic examination, and general physical evaluation, including blood pressure measurement, will usually allow localization of the problem and offer clues as to the pathogenesis and etiology. Investigative tests are then implemented.

Management of the pregnant patient needs to consider the health of the unborn baby as well as that of the mother. In the postpartum or puerperal patient, management, is, of course, specific to the mother.

ECLAMPSIA

Definition

Eclampsia is defined as the occurrence of one or more seizures in a patient with earlier pre-eclampsia (toxemia), providing that the seizures are not due to a coincidental neurologic disorder such as idiopathic epilepsy.[2] Pre-eclampsia is a multisystem disorder of pregnancy primarily consisting of recently elevated arterial blood pressure (systolic >140 mmHg or a rise of >30 mmHg; diastolic >90 mmHg or a rise of >15 mmHg), proteinuria (>300 mg in 24 h), and limb edema. Thrombocytopenia and elevation of serum aspartate transaminase are common accompaniments.

Despite official definitions, a strict separation of eclampsia from severe pre-eclampsia is probably artificial. Patients with severe hypertensive pre-eclampsia may develop deficits, e.g., blindness, hemiplegia from ischemic or hemorrhagic strokes, or coma from multifocal brain disease, without suffering a convulsion. This concept has practical importance as it is best to treat vigorousy those patients at serious risk of developing vascular complications of any type, without using convulsions as the defining point for a qualitatively different disorder.

The HELLP (hemolysis, elevated liver enzymes, and low platelet count) syndrome, often with further seizures and intracerebral hemorrhage, together with renal failure probably represents an extreme variant of eclampsia.[3]

Epidemiology and Significance

In the United Kingdom, eclampsia occurs at a rate of 4.9 cases per 10,000 pregnancies, and arises in 2 percent of pre-eclamptic patients.[4,5] The incidence of eclampsia has declined over the past several decades in developed countries. Forty-four percent of eclamptic seizures occur in the early postpartum period, 38 percent are antepartum, usually after 28 weeks of gestation, and 18 percent appear during delivery. Antepartum convulsions are associated with multiple seizures, a higher complication rate, and small-for-date babies and a higher neonatal mortality than intrapartum or postpartum eclampsia.

There are marked differences in the prevalence of pre-eclampsia in various countries, with China having over 5 times the rate of cases in Viet Nam.[6] The explanation is uncertain. Pre-eclampsia may, however, be underrecognized. This is an important health issue in that effective management of pre-eclampsia may prevent eclampsia.

Clinical Features

The principal symptoms and signs of pre-eclampsia are those related to proteinuria (edema of the extremities and periorbital edema in the morning) and hypertension. Patients commonly complain of "spots" or holes in their vision. This reflects dysfunction of either the retina or the visual cortex. Funduscopic changes include segmental arteriolar narrowing (the initial change), retinal edema, flame-shaped retinal nerve fiber layer hemorrhages, papilledema, signs from occlusion of the central retinal artery, or spontaneously reversible serous retinal detachment.

Patients sometimes develop cortical blindness due to ischemic lesions in the visual cortex. Pupillary reflexes are preserved, but the opticokinetic response is lost.

Danger signals of impeding eclampsia, stroke, or coma include the following: impaired alertness, attention, and orientation (confusional state); stupor; throbbing headache; photophobia; visual disturbances; epigastric pain; increased briskness of deep tendon reflexes; and focal or generalized myoclonic twitching. Findings include funduscopic changes of malignant or accelerated hypertension, a rapid increase in blood pressure, acute peripheral edema, and decreased urine volume.

Eclamptic seizures are typically of the generalized convulsive type. These are, of course, always associated with loss of consciousness followed by a postictal period of drowsiness and confusion. If the latter is prolonged, the possibility of nonconvulsive status epilepticus (see Chap. 17) or a complication (e.g., ischemic stroke or intracranial hemorrhage) should be considered.

Differential Diagnosis

A number of conditions should be considered, depending on the clinical presentation and timing with respect to delivery:

1. Epilepsy associated with or aggravated by pregnancy.

2. Cortical venous thrombosis (see later).

3. Hyponatremia (see later).

4. Thrombotic thrombocytopenic purpura (TTP): the initial attack or relapses may occur in association with pregnancy; this is discussed in Chap. 14.

5. Ischemic strokes in pregnancy (see later).

6. Drug use: illicit drugs that may cause hypertension and seizures include cocaine, amphetamines, and other sympathomimetics.

7. Complications of connective tissue diseases; these are discussed in Chap. 12.

8. Anxiety hyperventilation, conversion reactions and depression (especially postpartum).

Investigations

The following investigations are indicated to confirm the suspicion of eclampsia and to rule out other conditions: complete blood count (CBC), platelet count, electrolytes (especially serum sodium concentration), liver function tests, serum urea and creatinine, urinalysis, and a drug or toxicology screen. In selected cases, e.g., when cortical venous thrombosis is considered to coexist, screens for hypercoagulable states might be conducted, including a blood smear, protein C, protein S, antithrombin III, and factor V (Leiden mutation).[7] A blood smear is performed when

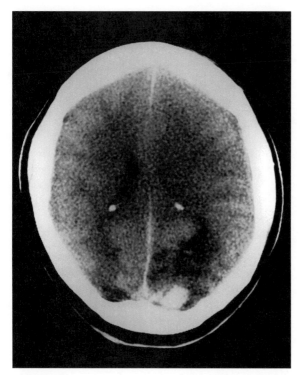

Figure 22-1

A CT scan showing an area of hemorrhage in the left occipital region surrounded by a region of attenuation. There is a smaller region of diminished density in the opposite occipital lobe. There is diffuse cerebral edema, indicated by the ventricular compression and reduced gray-white matter differentiation. The patient presented with eclampsia and features of the HELLP syndrome and died of progressive brain edema.

TTP is considered. Computed tomography (CT) and magnetic resonance imaging (MRI) scanning may reveal cerebral edema, infarcts, or hemorrhages (see Fig. 22-1).

Pathology

Neuropathologic findings in fatal cases of eclampsia include multiple cortical petechial hemorrhages in the cortex (ring hemorrhages around small vessels, with or without intraluminal thromboses) and larger hypertensive-type hemorrhages in deep gray structures; subarachnoid hemorrhages may also occur.[8] Multifocal areas of ischemic infarction

and small hemorrhages most commonly affect the watershed areas in the posterior cerebrum, including the occipital lobes (Fig. 22-2). Brainstem structures can also be affected. Diffuse cerebral edema is often associated with increased intracranial pressure (ICP) and papilledema.[9,10] Microscopically, the vessel arteriolar walls commonly show splitting of elastic fibers, edema, or necrosis of the vessel wall (see Fig. 22-3).

Pathophysiology

The pathogenesis of pre-eclampsia is not completely understood, but it is likely to be multifactorial: the failure of trophoblastic inactivation of autonomic control of the endometrial spiral arteries indirectly leads to decreased local nitric oxide and prostacyclin production; uteroplacental angiotensin II (increases placental perfusion pressure) is enhanced; and increased serotonin release (from platelets) leads to further vasoconstriction and platelet aggregation.[11-15] The prostacyclin-thromboxane A2 and renin-angiotensin-aldosterone systems are both likely to be involved, resulting in increased blood pressure and coagulability of the blood.

A unifying hypothesis for eclampsia is that the brain loses its autoregulation to relative hypertension.[16] The neuropathology of eclampsia shares many of the features of hypertensive encephalopathy. As a consequence of severe hypertension, regulatory arterioles allow increased regional blood flow, damaging the walls of capillaries and small arterioles, and producing vasogenic edema and pericapillary hemorrhages.[17] This causes tissue edema, multifocal ischemia, and seizures in eclampsia. "Watershed areas," the sites of anastomotic channels between the territories of the major cerebral arteries, are the most vulnerable regions to develop these complications, as the greatest changes in arteriolar caliber occur in these vessels.[18] This explains the occipital lesions that cause phosphenes, visual field defects, and cortical blindness as early features of severe toxemia.

Additionally, in eclampsia, coagulability of the blood is increased beyond that usual for

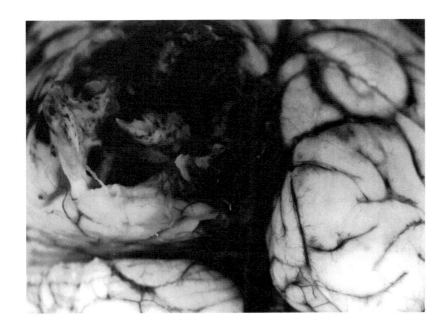

Figure 22-2
Formalin-fixed brain of the patient whose CT is shown in Fig. 22-1. At postmortem, the gyri were flattened; the occipital pole had ruptured from the hemorrhage. The photomicrograph shows the clot cavity surrounded by hemorrhagic, necrotic brain tissue.

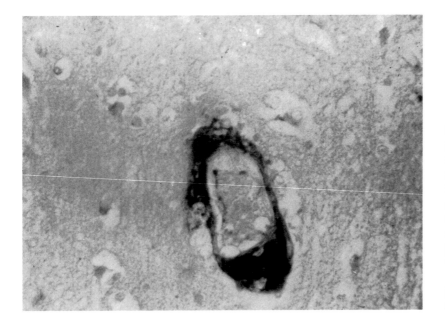

Figure 22-3
Photomicrograph of a small intracerebral arteriole showing fibrinoid necrosis of the vascular wall and surrounding edematous cortical tissue with some viable and some ischemic neurons [Mallory's phosphotungstic acid–hematoxylin (PTAH) stain, 100×]. This is from the same patient as depicted in Figs. 22-1 and 22-2.

pregnancy, with increased fibrin production and decreased fibrinolytic activity resulting in increased fibrin and platelet deposition on placental arteries. With intravascular coagulation, fibrin degradation products are increased and thrombocytopenia is found. The related HELLP syndromes comprises hemolysis, elevated liver enzymes, and a low platelet count.

Management

Prevention of Seizures in Pre-eclamptic Patients
Lucas and colleagues have shown

that magnesium sulfate ($MgSO_4$) given to pregnant women with hypertension that was noted upon their admission for delivery was superior to phenytoin in preventing seizures.[19] Of 1049 women randomly assigned $MgSO_4$, none had seizures, while 10 of 1089 who received phenytoin had convulsions.

General measures to reduce stimulation include darkening the room, reducing noise, and light sedation. Monitoring of blood pressure and urine output, hematology, and fetal status, well as the neurologics examination—especially mental status, funduscopic examination, and status of reflexes—are important.

Patients should be monitored neurologically. Serial ophthalmologic examinations are important as funduscopic changes reflect cerebral events and visual symptoms often precede seizures.

Neuroradiologic investigation is often difficult and impractical if the patient is in labor or about to deliver, or is to have a cesarean section.

Treatment of Eclampsia A recent multinational study for eclamptic seizures was designed to compare $MgSO_4$ with diazepam (bolus plus infusion) as well as $MgSO_4$ with phenytoin.[20] In the $MgSO_4$ versus diazepam comparison, recurrence of seizures and maternal mortality were significantly lower in the former group. In the following aspects, the $MgSO_4$-treated eclamptic patients also did better than those who received phenytoin: reduced recurrence of seizures, lower rate of maternal need for assisted ventilation and lower incidence of pneumonia, and fewer babies requiring intubation or special care units.

Thus, $MgSO_4$ has been re-established as the optimal treatment for pre-eclamptic and eclamptic patients. These well-designed studies are instructive that unconfirmed hypotheses, uncontrolled studies, and common practice patterns can be misleading: there was a strong bias of neurologists and others against the use of $MgSO_4$ for eclampsia.

The explanation for the success of $MgSO_4$ is uncertain. Hypotheses include the following:

1. Blockade of *N*-methyl-D-aspartate (NMDA) channels preventing calcium influx into neurons, thus offering neuroprotection as well as antiepileptic activity.

2. Reduced vasospasm: cerebral blood flow increases in pre-eclamptic women who receive $MgSO_4$.[21] The $MgSO_4$ has a relaxant effect on cerebrovascular smooth muscle, probably due to increased release of prostacyclin, a potent vasodilator, by the vascular endothelium.[22]

3. Reduced vascular endothelial damage: $MgSO_4$ protects against free radical damage.[23]

Magnesium sulfate can be administered by either the intramuscular or intravenous routes. The latter may be advisable in emergency situations, e.g., with active convulsions or severe hypertension, although one route was not found to be superior to the other in the Eclampsia Trial.[20] The dosage is 4 to 5 g given intravenously, followed by an infusion of 1 g/h for 24 h. Alternatively, 10 g are given intramuscularly, then 5 g intramuscularly every 4 h. Patients should be monitored for magnesium toxicity or the risk of this developing. In particular, respirations should be more than 12 per minute, urine output more than 100 mL every 4 h, and knee jerk reflexes should be preserved.[2] After delivery, the baby should be monitored for signs of hypermagnesemia: i.e., weak or absent cry, flaccidity, absent deep tendon reflexes, and respiratory failure. However, this is unlikely if the mother is not suffering from magnesium toxicity.

In the management of eclampsia, there is no proven value of adding traditional antiepileptic drugs (AEDs), although these would appear to be indicated if the patient continues to have seizures. Phenytoin, phenobarbital, benzodiazepine, and chlormethiazole have been used. Rapid control of seizures can usually be achieved with diazepam or lorazepam (see Chap. 17). One theoretic concern that cannot be dismissed is that the phenytoin-treated group from the Eclampsia Trial may have done worse than those mothers and babies who received $MgSO_4$ because of adverse effects of phenytoin.[20] In the patient who has not delivered, it is probably best to avoid benzodiazepines if possible (administration of $MgSO_4$ alone may stop the patient's seizures), because of possible depression of the baby's respirations.[24]

Electroencephalograms (EEGs) are often impractical in the acute setting, but are helpful in monitoring for seizure activity in comatose patients and in guiding drug administration in refractory status epilepticus (see Chap. 17). Continuous EEG monitoring may prove useful in assessing brain function in patients with cerebral edema and increased ICP who are being treated with anti-hypertensive drugs.

Systemic Aspects   Severe hypertension in pre-eclampsia or eclampsia is characterized by blood pressure of >160/110, 3+ proteinuria, visual changes, and abdominal pain. Intravenous hydralazine is a good drug choice as it relaxes smooth muscle and may increase renal blood flow. Excessive tachycardia, a common side effect, can be offset by a beta blocker such as propranolol. If severe hypertension fails to respond to hydralazine, the blood pressure can be reduced by administration of pentolinium, trimethaphan, diazoxide, or nitroprusside.[25] Care should be taken that acute hypotension does not develop as this may seriously compromise cerebral blood flow, or perfusion of other organs and the placenta.

In eclampsia, it is generally advisable to terminate the pregnancy as soon as possible, using appropriate monitoring. In pre-eclampsia, if the pregnancy is over 36 weeks gestation, immediate delivery is advised if blood pressure is >150/100, with significant proteinuria. If the pregnancy is under 36 weeks, factors that argue for delivery include the following: failing placental function as judged by reduced fetal growth, oligo-hydramnios, reduced fetal movements, abnormal fetal heart rhythms, or biochemical signs of placental failure; also, maternal deterioration with conservative treatment (blood pressure >180/100 or proteinuria of >5 g in 24 h).

Postpartum vasculopathy and hypertension may respond well to calcium channel blockers (Kaplan, L., personal communication).

Differential Diagnosis of Toxemia and Eclampsia

Rarely, other conditions can mimic toxemia. Pheochromocytoma should be suspected if hypertension is combined with orthostatic hypotension, pounding headaches, sweating, and nasal congestion.[26] Pheochromocytoma can be diagnosed by ultra-sonography, CT or MRI of the abdomen, and elevated metanephrines or vanillylmandelic acid in the urine and dopamine β-hydoxylase in the serum.[8] After diagnosis, management of the pregnancy should be planned with the internist. Alpha-adrenergic blocking can be accomplished with phenoxybenzamine, to prevent accelerated hypertension.

Thrombotic thrombocytopenic purpura, discussed in Chap. 15, occasionally complicates pregnancy. Neurologic complications, including strokes and seizures, and renal impairment with hypertension may mimic eclampsia.

Water intoxication, related to excessive water intake or excessive oxytocin administration, may produce hyponatremia, cerebral edema, and convulsions. Usually, the serum sodium concentration is <120 meq/L (120 mmol/L). When any of these factors is found, the oxytocin infusion should be stopped and fluid intake restricted. Hypertonic saline, used very judiciously, may be necessary in extreme cases (see Chap. 13).

Systemic absorption of local anesthetics used for perineal blocks, producing toxic serum concentrations, may cause seizures.[27] Patients develop confusion, drowsiness, circumoral or generalized paresthesiae, dysarthria, blurred vision, euphoria, tachycardia, and elevated blood pressures with the administration of lidocaine.[28] Convulsions or myoclonic seizures may supervene. Intravenous benzodiazepines may help acutely. Patients should be watched carefully for cardiac arrest, and a bolus of 50% dextrose should be given intravenously along with oxygen by mask. Pentobarbital or thiopental is sometimes necessary to arrest refractory status epilepticus.[8]

PREGNANCY IN PATIENTS WITH EPILEPSY

Significance

In patients with known epilepsy (see Chap. 17), seizures can occur any time during the pregnancy.

Seizures are increased during pregnancy in about one-third of epileptic patients, possibly due to the following: plasma concentrations of AEDs decrease during pregnancy, especially in the third trimester; serum concentrations of estrogens (considered to be epileptogenic) are increased; other aggregating factors, such as stress and sleep deprivation, may be increased during pregnancy.[29] Monitoring of serum AED concentrations and subsequent AED dosage adjustments are usually adequate measures to keep seizures under control.

Patients may have noneclamptic seizures only during pregnancy (gestational epilepsy). The likelihood of recurrence in subsequent pregnancies is uncertain, but only 2 of 12 multiparous patients with gestational epilepsy had recurrences in one reported series.[30]

Clinical Features

The appearance of a seizure-like event in pregnancy or during delivery should be considered carefully before concluding that it is a true seizure. The author of this chapter has observed psychogenic episodes with agitated behavior and hyperventilation in some patients during delivery of their first child.

Seizures should be classified using the International Classification of Epileptic Seizures (see Chap. 17).[31]

Management

Antiepileptic drugs are usually well tolerated by the fetus beyond the first trimester, i.e., past the time of organogenesis. The principles of AED use in pregnancy include the following: the use of monotherapy (single drug therapy) whenever possible; multiple daily doses to avoid large fluctuations in serum AED concentrations; the use of the lowest effective dose; the administration of folate unless contraindicated, at least before pregnancy and throughout the first trimester; and the administration of vitamin K, 10 mg, to the mother 2 weeks before delivery and to the baby upon delivery.[32,33] The serum concentration of AEDs should be monitored monthly; upward dosage adjustment is

sometimes necessary, especially in the third trimester. Because protein binding of phenytoin is reduced in pregnancy, it is recommended that the free fraction be monitored. These measures are usually sufficient to control seizures and to allow for a normal baby in the vast majority of cases.[34]

ISCHEMIC STROKE

Ischemic stroke is discussed in detail in Chap. 15. Pregnancy increases the likelihood of arterial occlusive stroke by 10 to 13-fold that of nonpregnant, aged-matched women, or to about 1 stroke in every 3000 pregnancies.[35,36]

Clinical Features

Basilar artery occlusions and large middle cerebral artery territory infarctions with edema are the most likely single-vessel strokes to compromise alertness (see Chap. 15).[37] Most strokes in pregnancy are in the anterior circulation. Most occur *during pregnancy*, but a disproportionately greater number happen in the puerperium, considering that this period is only the 42 days postdelivery.[38] Multiple strokes in various cerebral regions may produce diffuse or multifocal brain dysfunction.

Etiology of Stroke in Pregnancy

Behind the various immediate mechanisms of most strokes in pregnancy, there is an increased coagulability of the blood. The relative weighting of the various hematologic change of pregnancy is unclear, but an increase in procoagulant factors (except factors XI and XII), enhanced thrombin activity, reduced inhibitors of coagulation (proteins C and S), and lowered fibrinolytic activity of the blood are among these changes.[39] Patients with circulating antiphospholipid antibodies are especially at risk for stroke and miscarriage.[40,41]

Cardiac Causes As with other young persons suffering ischemic stroke, cardiogenic emboli constitute the most common cause during pregnancy.[42] Atrial septal defects and patent foramen ovale with transient right-to-left shunts, e.g., with pulmonary embolism (increased risk in pregnancy, and with leg or pelvic deep venous thromboses) or Valsalva maneuvers, are among the most common conditions.[43]

Peripartum cardiomyopathy affects mainly black women over 30 years of age in the last 2 months of pregnancy.[44] Patients usually present with heart failure and dilated cardiac chambers; cerebral emboli may result. There is a significant risk of hypotension during delivery; this may produce bilateral watershed cerebral infarctions as well as loss of the baby.[45]

Emboli from mitral valve prolapse, atrial fibrillation, and infectious endocarditis are other cardiogenic causes of embolic stroke in pregnancy.[43] Bacterial endocarditis in pregnancy is usually caused by *Streptococcus viridans* and *Staphylococcus aureus*, but enterococci cause endocarditis in some patients after cesarean section or uterine curettage.[46,47]

Arterial Disease Arterial disease includes premature atherosclerosis, arterial dissection, vasculitis, emboli from aneurysms, and moya-moya disease.[43]

Premature atherosclerosis causes 15 to 25 percent of the cerebral infarctions during pregnancy.[8] Diabetes mellitus, cigarette smoking, hypertension, and hyperlipidemia are major risk factors. The hypercoagulable state of pregnancy may contribute. Heterozygosity for homocystinuria is occasionally an underlying cause.[48]

Arterial dissection of carotid or vertebral arteries occasionally occurs after delivery.[49,50] This may be due to arterial damage caused by vigorous neck movements during delivery. Fibromuscular hyperplasia is a predisposing cause.

Berry aneurysms often have intraluminal thrombus that may become dislodged and cause a more distal embolic infarction.[51]

Systemic lupus erythematosus (SLE) is the most common vasculitis of pregnancy.[8] The puerperal period may be the most common time for exacerbations of the condition. Encephalopathy and seizures are the most common manifestations, followed by cranial nerve palsies and hyperemesis gravidarum. Patients with active cerebral lupus usually have a decreased C3 component of complement (see Chap. 12).[8] Takayasu disease occurs in women of childbearing age; stroke is a late manifestation. Because circulation to the limbs is seriously compromised, it may be difficult to monitor the patient's blood pressure. Primary or isolated (granulomatous) angiitis of the central nervous system (PACNS) (see Chap. 12) has been reported in pregnancy.[52] Although syphilis is an uncommon cause of stroke, it should be considered. Moyamoya disease is common in Japan and patients with this disease may present with ischemic stroke or intracerebral or subarachnoid hemorrhage.[53] Drug-induced vasculitis is another cause in large centers.

Hematologic Conditions Hematologic conditions [including TTP, sickle cell disease, and disseminated intravascular coagulation (DIC)] in systemically ill patients are less common causes.

Thrombotic thrombocytopenic purpura (see above and Chap. 15) has an increased tendency to occur during pregnancy and the puerperium and to recur in subsequent pregnancies.[54]

Patients with sickle cell anemia or sickle cell trait may have large arterial strokes, multiple small ischemic strokes, or subarachnoid hemorrhage.[55] The vasa vasorum of larger arteries can become occluded, causing thromboses or rupture of the parent vessel. Fat embolism can follow bone marrow infarction in sickle cell disease.[56]

Disseminated intravascular coagulation may result from activation of the clotting system with, or following, parturition.[57] This may affect the GS brain as part of a general DIC or as a more limited form, causing ischemic or hemorrhagic strokes. Sometimes, DIC follows amniotic fluid embolism or occurs in conjunction with systemic infections, e.g., streptococcal group A infections, during pregnancy or the puerperium.[58,59]

Investigations

A thorough investigation, including cardiac investigations (e.g., transesophageal echocardiography), cerebral angiography (magnetic resonance angiography may suffice for most cases and is safest in patients with sickle cell disease), and tests for vasculitis and coagulopathies are indicated. Management is dependent on the underlying cause, as discussed in Chap. 15.

CORTICAL VENOUS THROMBOSIS

Incidence and Significance

Cerebral venous thrombosis (CVT), contrary to popular concepts, is much less common than arterial occlusive disease as a cause of stroke in pregnancy or the puerperium.[43] The incidence is estimated to be less than 1 in 10,000 deliveries.[60] This subject is reviewed in Chap. 14.

Cortical venous thrombosis is the only form of intracranial thrombosis of venous channels that commonly affects consciousness in pregnancy or the puerperium.[8] Cavernous sinus thrombosis is not related to pregnancy.[8] Thromboses of lateral or superior sagittal sinuses do not usually compromise consciousness. Cortical venous thrombosis is more likely in the early postpartum period; 80 percent of cases occur in the second or third week after delivery.[8]

Clinical Features

The constellation of severe headache followed by multifocal deficits, e.g., aphasia and focal weakness, focal seizures arising independently from each hemisphere, progressive obtundation with reduced alertness, and papilledema forms the complete picture. Some elements, e.g., papilledema or multifocal seizures, may be lacking.

Fever may be present. Leg and visceral veins may be simultaneously affected, especially in hypercoagulable states.

Pathogenesis

The impairment of consciousness with cortical vein thrombosis relates to multifocal brain dysfunction caused by seizures or ischemic changes in the cerebral cortex. Massive brain swelling or hemorrhage with mass effect and herniation are other mechanisms.

Investigations

An MRI scan of the head is the diagnostic procedure of choice (see Chap. 15). The CT scan is less sensitive. In equivocal cases, a lumbar puncture may be necessary to help exclude meningitis or encephalitis. An EEG is useful in determining the relative contribution of nonconvulsive seizures to obtundation.

Patients with CVT should be screened for hypercoagulable states that predispose to venous clotting: antiphospholipid antibodies, and deficiencies of protein S and C and antithrombin III.

Prognosis

The prognosis is dependent on the extent of the venous infarction, edema, brain herniation, and compromise of the intracranial circulation.[8] This is related to the degree of impairment of alertness, the CT or MRI appearance, and complications such as status epilepticus or superimposed infections.

Treatment

Anticoagulants are effective, but their use increases the possibility of hemorrhagic complications for the mother during delivery and for the baby. When possible, it is best to give anticoagulants after delivery or to use heparin, which can be stopped or reversed for the delivery. Coumadin should be avoided while the patient is still pregnant.[61] Antiepileptic drugs are often necessary to control seizures acutely (see Chap. 17). Antibiotics are sometimes necessary if there is an underlying infection that preceded or followed the acute illness produced by the CVT.

INTRACRANIAL HEMORRHAGE

Most cases of intracranial hemorrhage in pregnancy usually result from ruptured aneurysms and vascular malformations. (See Chap. 5 for a complete discussion of intracranial hemorrhage.) Complications of pregnancy, including eclampsia, cortical vein thromboses, and coagulopathies are discussed earlier in this chapter. Hemorrhages related to leukemia, metastatic tumors, trauma, hemorrhagic stroke, and therapies are additional causes. The incidence of intracranial hemorrhage in pregnancy is about 1 in 10,000 cases, five times higher than in age-matched nonpregnant women.[61]

Clinical and Pathologic Features

Bleeding from berry aneurysms (three-quarters of cases) and arteriovenous malformations (AVMs) (one quarter of cases) is more common after the end of the second trimester when the blood volume has peaked.[62] Such patients present with sudden severe headache and variable deficits. Patients may have reversible loss of consciousness with the ictus. Subsequent impairment of consciousness usually reflects multifocal ischemia from vasospasm, ischemia in the posterior circulation, hydrocephalus, seizures, or metabolic or systemic disturbances such as hyponatremia. Berry aneurysms usually rupture into the subarachnoid space, but commonly also affect the parenchyma with hemorrhage or ischemia due to vasospasm. With intraparenchymal bleeding, focal deficits are the rule. Patients with AVMs fare worse in pregnancy than those in the nongravid state: in the large review of Dias and Sekhar, 58 percent were stuporous or comatose at presentation.[63]

Prognosis

In a large literature review, the overall mortality was 35 percent for aneurysmal and 28 percent for AVM rupture; both these figures are higher than for the nongravid population.[63] Risk of recurrent bleeding from an untreated aneurysm or AVM in pregnancy is between 33 percent and 50 percent, with a mortality rate of between 50 percent and 68 percent.[63]

There is a strong tendency for AVMs to rebleed during the same pregnancy; there is also a higher mortality rate following such bleeding.[63]

Management

Surgical clipping of unruptured berry aneurysms is advised before the patient becomes pregnant. Since mortality and morbidity of patients with AVMs in pregnancy is so high, neurosurgeons should seriously consider obliterating the malformation, if feasible without causing deficit, before pregnancy occurs.

Scanning by CT and cerebral angiography is recommended with intracranial hemorrhage. Appropriate shielding of the fetus from radiation is feasible.

Surgical clipping of berry aneurysms that rupture in pregnancy is associated with a lower maternal and fetal mortality than when surgery was not performed.[63] This held true with logistic regression analysis, weighing various factors. Nimodepine is sometimes used, but care should be taken to avoid hypotension and fetal ischemia. (Nimodepine is teratogenic in animals.) Ventricular drains or shunts are sometimes necessary for those with hydrocephalus or a ventricular clot; these can improve the conscious level considerably. Management of arteriovenous malformations is more controversial; acute surgical therapy was not found to reduce mortality in collected series.[63] Clot evacuation is probably worthwhile in selected cases with marked mass effect. One should be aware of the effects of mannitol (fetal dehydration) or barbiturates (sedation) if given just before delivery of the baby.

Management of the pregnancy should be conducted using obstetric not neurosurgical, criteria. The fetus should be monitored. If persisting distress occurs in the viable fetus, immediate cesarean section should be performed.[63] When the aneurysm or arteriovenous malformation has been clipped, ligated, or removed, the baby can be delivered vaginally. When there remains a risk of rupture, or if the rupture occurs after 35 weeks gestation and the fetus is viable, cesarean section is recommended.[64]

BRAIN TUMORS IN PREGNANCY

Epidemiology and Significance

The association of brain tumors and impaired consciousness is discussed in detail in Chap. 7. Although brain tumors are probably not more common during pregnancy, they tend to enlarge more than expected during this period.[65] This may be due to estrogen receptors present in meningiomas and other tumors, a reduced immune response to "new growths," and facilitation of "vascular growths" such as meningiomas and high-grade gliomas.[65,66] One-third of patients with brain tumors die from herniation during the pregnancy, especially those with gliomas, choroid plexus papillomas, and infratentorial tumors; brain tumors account for 10 percent of maternal deaths.[67] Enlargement of pituitary tumors is common, but this is significant to management only when the initial tumor is large and subsequently causes mass effect, or in the event of pituitary apoplexy (see Chap. 13).[68]

Metastatic tumors are also problematic, but, overall, their incidence during pregnancy is probably not significantly increased above that for nongravid, aged-matched patients.[65] Metastatic choriocarcinoma occasionally occurs, especially in those with hydatidiform moles, after the termination of the pregnancy.[65] Such metastases are often multiple and hemorrhagic. Thyroid cancer is the most common malignancy in the childbearing years, but the probability of a woman of childbearing years developing cerebral metastases is about 0.008 percent.[65]

Clinical Presentation

The relevant neurologic manifestations of neoplasms are discussed in detail in Chap. 7.

Diagnosis

With appropriate shielding, CT scanning of the brain should be feasible without endangering the fetus. Magnetic resonance imaging is probably safer. Biopsies can be performed if necessary.

Management

The management of brain tumors in pregnancy should be individualized to the particular patient. Individual factors include the grade, type, size, and location of the tumor; the stage of the pregnancy; the neurologic state of the patient; the patient's

wishes; and the projected outcomes for the mother and fetus.

Surgical treatment of the tumor during pregnancy is sometimes necessary. For some patients in the first trimester with large malignant tumors, termination of the pregnancy is advisable. Even then, modern neurosurgical techniques may allow debulking during pregnancy. Hormonal or drug therapy, e.g., corticosteroids for tumors with edema or bromocriptine for enlarging prolactinomas, is sometimes necessary.

Radiation treatment and chemotherapy put the fetus at greater risk than surgery. Corticosteroids, e.g., dexamethasone, are often necessary to control cerebral edema. This is usually possible without causing serious harm to the fetus.

The principles for management of the epileptic patient who becomes pregnant were discussed earlier in this chapter.

Pituitary apoplexy, with hemorrhage or necrosis into pituitary adenomas, is discussed in Chap. 13.

AMNIOTIC FLUID EMBOLISM

Amniotic fluid embolism is an acute complication of pregnancy characterized by features of pulmonary embolism (acute dyspnea, hypoxemia, and hypotension).[69] This is followed by left ventricular failure, pulmonary edema, and, if the patient lives long enough, DIC.[70] The condition is due to the forceful introduction of amniotic fluid, containing fetal meconium, squame, and other debris, into the maternal circulation. This is most likely to happen during or immediately following vaginal delivery (uterine, cervical, or vaginal tears are portals of entry), cesarean section, or amniocentesis.

Amniotic fluid in the systemic circulation can plug capillaries and initiate DIC. Paradoxical embolism of amniotic material to the brain occurs in some cases.

Clinical Features

The condition is acutely fatal in probably at least 85 percent of cases.[70] Patients develop dyspnea, cyanosis, shock, and coma. Ten percent of patients develop convulsive seizures within minutes, probably on an ischemic basis.

Diagnosis

Diagnosis is mainly dependent on finding the above-described clinical picture, followed by DIC in those who survive the immediate collapse. The diagnosis can be confirmed by looking for fetal epithelial squamous cells above the buffy coat in blood taken from the right atrium if a central venous pressure catheter is so placed.

Management

Resuscitative measures include cardiopulmonary resuscitation and administration of oxygen. Packed red blood cells, fresh-frozen plasma, and crystalloids are often needed to maintain perfusion pressure and blood volume. Cryoprecipitate and exchange transfusion as acute therapies used independently in single cases were associated with favorable outcomes.[71,72] Those who ultimately survive would be at risk for the neurologic sequelae of severe arterial hypotension, cardiac arrest, or DIC.

AIR EMBOLISM

Air emboli can occur during pregnancy or the puerperium and account for 1 percent of maternal deaths.[8] Criminal abortion is the most common cause but accidental air embolism may complicate cesarean section or vaginal delivery, or may occur during knee-chest exercises carried out in the puerperium.[73] Such patients feel faint, collapse, convulse, and frequently die. Air embolism is discussed in detail in Chap. 15.

PITUITARY INSUFFICIENCY

Postpartum pituitary insufficiency, or Sheehan syndrome, refers to acute hypopituitarism occurring in the early postpartum period.[74] Early epidemiologic estimates are 1.25 per 100 women who lost more than 100 mL of blood with delivery.

Clinical Syndrome

Peripartum pituitary insufficiency can also be the result of lymphocytic adenohypophysitis, an autoimmune destruction of the anterior pituitary gland.[75,76] This can present before or after labor and delivery. These patients are listless and weak. Impaired consciousness usually relates to systemic metabolic problems or circulatory collapse, rather than to hypothalamic compression as in cases of pituitary apoplexy (see Chap. 13). There are overlap features with panhypopituitarism, however, including lactation failure and more extensive deficiencies realized with time. Some patients have an inflammatory mass that compresses the lower part of the optic nerves or chiasm, causing a bitemporal hemianopsia. About one-third of patients have concurrent autoimmune disease, such as thryoiditis, rheumatoid arthritis, SLE.[75]

In chronic hypopituitarism, the sequel of Sheehan syndrome, the patient is vulnerable to stress. This may cause collapse, coma, or death. Chronically, the patient may be apathetic, forgetful, and depressed, related to panhypopituitarism. Hyponatremic or hypoglycemic convulsions can occur.[77]

Pathology

Sheehan studied the pituitary glands of 18 women with postpartum hypopituitarism, most of whom died years after childbirth, while under therapy for their pituitary insufficiency. Most of the anterior pituitary gland of these women had atrophied to 2 to 5 percent of its normal size.

In lymphocytic adenohypophysitis, there is diffuse infiltration of the anterior and intermediate lobes of the pituitary gland with lymphocytes and plasma cells. With time, the gland atrophies and becomes fibrotic. Residual chronic inflammatory changes may persist.[78]

Pathogenesis

In Sheehan's series, patients had a drop in blood pressure at or following delivery; the severity (degree and duration) of the hypotension, commonly associated with excessive hemorrhage, correlated with the subsequent severity of the pituitary insufficiency. Sheehan attributed the pituitary insufficiency to hypotension-induced vasospasm, causing ischemia of the anterior pituitary gland supplied by the hypophyseal artery.[79] Postpartum pituitary necrosis is thus considered to be secondary to necrosis of, or hemorrhage into, the anterior pituitary gland. In most cases, this is *not* due to infarction or hemorrhage into a pituitary adenoma (see later), but such can occur as well. Blindness may occur due to infarction of the optic nerves or chiasm due to ischemia, as these are supplied, in some cases, by twigs from the superior hypophyseal artery.[80]

While the cause may be vascular in most cases, inflammatory disease of the anterior pituitary gland has recently been increasingly recognized as a complication of late pregnancy or the early postpartum period.[75,76,81] The autoimmune disorder presents as an expanding pituitary mass, sometimes with compression of the optic chiasm, or as acute pituitary failure, similar to a subacute form of "pituitary apoplexy" when the gland is destroyed by inflammation and replaced by fibrotic tissue.[82] Surgical intervention is not always necessary. If the gland is not totally destroyed, it may recover function.[81] It is quite likely that some patients diagnosed with Sheehan syndrome actually had lymphocytic adenohypophysitis; the presentations can be very similar. Furthermore, 18 percent of patients with Sheehan syndrome have antipituitary antibodies.[83]

Management

The most important aspects of care include the prompt institution of corticosteroid coverage to prevent "adrenal crisis" and to correct fluid imbalance electrolyte imbalance, and hypoglycemia. Emergency decompressive operations are probably only necessary in cases of hemorrhage or mass effect from infarction or inflammation that threaten vision and hypothalamic function.

Long-term management includes hormone replacement for panhypopituitarism, including special provision with corticosteroid enhancement at times of stress.

SYSTEMIC COMPLICATIONS

Sepsis, often related to premature rupture of the membranes, develops either before delivery or in the puerperal period. Some patients develop urinary tract infections because of the effect on the ureters and bladder. Severe noneclamptic hypertension may occur in some previously hypertensive patients.

Hyperemesis gravidarum can lead to vitamin deficiency syndromes, including Wernicke's encephalopathy (see Chap. 15).

Worsening of organ (e.g., renal, hepatic and cardiac) failures and diabetes mellitus can secondarily affect brain function (see Chap. 13), as can systemic infections (see Chaps. 11 and 12).

Hyponatremia sometimes arises from water intoxication due to excessive administration of fluids, with or without Syntocinon, especially in patients with impaired renal function.

Although the frequency of neurologic complications of connective tissue disorders is not increased during pregnancy, exacerbations of disease occasionally occur.[84] Termination of pregnancy is considered only in severe vasculitic disease, e.g., periarteritis nodosa or Wegener's granulomatosis, in patients with cardiac or renal failure, or when treatment of severe systemic, including neurologic, disease is ineffective.

PSYCHIATRIC CONDITIONS

Psychoses (see Chap. 18), e.g., schizophrenia or endogenous depression, are sometimes aggravated during pregnancy. This relates, at least in some cases, to the reduction or discontinuation of antipsychotic drugs.[85] Some psychiatric illness are activated or reactivated by the pregnancy itself.[86] Postpartum depression can mimic disturbances in alertness or content of consciousness, but its incidence and predictive factors are uncertain.

MANAGEMENT

Prior to pregnancy, physicians should discuss the risks of pregnancy on pre-existing neurologic disease, the potential risks to the fetus, and the implications for therapy modification imposed by the pregnancy.[87] One should bear in mind the condition of both the mother and the fetus when dealing with the pregnant woman. A team approach, which includes the patient or substitute decision maker, is usually required.[88]

REFERENCES

1. Raynalde T: *The Byrthe of Mankynde. Book II* (Translation of *Rosengarten* by Eucharius Rösllin). London, 1540. As cited in Morton LT: *A Medical Bibliography*, 4th ed. London, Frome and Tanner, 1983, p 828.

2. Committee on Terminology of the American College of Obstetricians and Gynecologists: *ACOG Technical Bulletin: The Management of Pre-eclampsia.* Washington, DC, February, 1986.

3. Weinstein L: Syndrome of hemolysis, elevated liver enzymes and low platelet count. A severe consequence of hypertension in pregnancy. *Am J Obstet Gynecol* 142:159, 1982.

4. Douglas KA, Redman CWG: Eclampsia in the United Kingdom. *Lancet* 309:1395, 1995.

5. Sibai BM, McCubbin JH, Anderson GD, Lipshitz J, Dilts PV: Eclampsia: observations from 67 recent cases. *Obstet Gynecol* 58:609, 1981.

6. World Health Organization International Collaborative Study of Hypertensive Disorders of Pregnancy: Geographic variation in the incidence of hypertension in pregnancy. *Am J Obstet Gynecol* 158:80, 1988.

7. Brey RL, Coull BM: Cerebral venous thrombosis. Role of activated protein C resistance and factor V gene mutation. *Stroke* 27:1719, 1996.

8. Donaldson JO: *Neurology of Pregnancy.* 2nd ed. London, WB Saunders, 1989.

9. Richards A, Graham D, Bullock R: Clinicopathological study of neurological complications due to hypertensive disorders of pregnancy. *J Neurol Neurosurg Psychiatry* 51:416, 1088.

10. Hallum AV: Eye changes in hypertensive toxemia of pregnancy. *JAMA* 106:1649, 1936.

11. Brosens J, Robertson WB, Dixon HG: The physiological response of the vessels of the placental bed to normal pregnancy. *J Pathol Bacteriol* 93:569, 1967.

12. Pijnenborg R, Bland JM, Robertson WB, et al: Utero-placental arterial changes related to interstitial trophoblast migration in early human pregnancy. *Placenta* 4:387, 1983.

13. Zeeman GG, Dexter GA: Pathogenesis of pre-eclampsia: a hypothesis, in Brooks PG, Sibai BH, Pitkin RM, Scott JR (eds): *Clinical Obstetrics and Gynecology. Pathogenesis of Preeclampsia: A Hypothesis,* vol 35. Philadelphia, Lippincott, 1992, pp 317–337.

14. Friedman SA: Preeclampsia: a review of the role of prostaglandins. *Obstet Gynecol* 71:122, 1988.

15. Friedman SA Taylor RM Roberts JM: Pathophysiology of preeclampsia. *Clin Perinatol* 18:661, 1991.

16. Donaldson JO: Eclamptic hypertensive encephalopathy. *Semin Neurol* 8:230, 1988.

17. Johansson BB: The blood-brain barrier and cerebral blood flow in acute hypertension. *Acta Med Scand Suppl* 678:107, 1983.

18. Johansson B: Regional changes of cerebral blood flow in acute hypertension in cats. *Acta Neurol Scand* 50:366, 1974.

19. Lucas MJ, Leveno KJ, Cunningham FG: A comparison of magnesium sulfate with phenytoin for the prevention of eclampsia. *N Eng J Med* 333:201, 1995.

20. The Eclampsia Trial Collaborative Group: Which anticonvulsant for women with eclampsia? Evidence from the Collaborative Eclampsia Trial. *Lancet* 345:1455, 1995.

21. Belfort MA, Moise KJ Jr: Effect of magnesium sulfate on maternal brain blood flow in preeclampsia: a randomized, placebo-controlled study. *Am J Obstet Gynecol* 167:661, 1992.

22. Sipes SL, Weiner CP, Gellhaus TM, Goodspeed JD: Effects of magnesium sulfate infusion upon plasma prostaglandins in preeclampsia and preterm labor. *Hypertens Pregnancy* 13:293, 1994.

23. Dickens BF, Weglicki Y, Li S, Mak IT: Magnesium deficiency in vitro enhances free radical-induced intracellular oxidation and cytotoxicity in endothelial cells. *FEBS Lett* 311:187, 1992.

24. Crowther C: Magnesium sulfate versus diazepam in the management of eclampsia: a randomized controlled trial. *Br Obstet Gynecol* 97:110, 1990.

25. Kaplan PW, Repke JT: Eclampsia, in Yerby MS, Devinsky O (eds): *Neurologic Clinics: Neurologic Complications of Pregnancy* 12(3):565–582, 1994.

26. Schenker JG, Chowers I: Pheochromocytoma and pregnancy: review of 89 cases. *Obstet Gynecol Surg* 26:740, 1971.

27. Berger GS, Tyler CW, Harrod EK: Maternal deaths associated with paracervical block anesthesia. *Am J Obstet Gynecol* 118:1142, 1974.

28. Wagman IH, deJong RH, Prince DA: Effects of lidocaine on the central nervous system. *Anesthesiology* 28:155, 1967.

29. Yerby MS: Pregnancy and epilepsy. *Epilepsia* 32(suppl 6):S51, 1991.

30. Knight AH, Rhind EG: Epilepsy and pregnancy: a study of 153 pregnancies in 59 patients. *Epilepsia* 16:99, 1975.

31. Commission on Classification and Terminology, International League Against Epilepsy: Proposed revisions of clinical and electroeneephalographic classification of epileptic seizures. *Epilepsia* 22:480, 1981.

32. Yerby MS: Problems and management of the pregnant woman with epilepsy. *Epilepsia* 28(suppl 3):S29, 1987.

33. Yerby MS: Pregnancy and epilepsy. *Epilepsia* 32(suppl 6):S51, 1991.

34. Yerby MS: Epilepsy and pregnancy. New issues for an old disorder. *Neurol Clin* 11:777, 1993.

35. Weibers DO, Whisnant JP: The incidence of stroke among pregnant women in Rochester, Minnesota, 1955 through 1979. *JAMA* 254:3055, 1985.

36. Fox MW, Harms RW, Davis DH: Selected neurologic complications of pregnancy. *Mayo Clin Proc* 65:1595, 1990.

37. Cross JN, Castro PO, Jennett WB: Cerebral strokes associated with pregnancy and the puerperium. *BMJ* 3:214, 1968.

38. Cross JN, Castro PO, Jennett WB: Cerebral strokes associated with pregnancy and the puerperium. *BMJ* 3:214, 1968.

39. Finley BE: Acute coagulopathy of pregnancy. *Med Clin North Am* 73:723, 1989.

40. Levine SR, Welch KMA: Antiphospholipid antibodies. *Ann Neurol* 26:368, 1989.

41. Branch DW: Antiphospholipid antibodies and pregnancy: maternal complications. *Semin Perinatol* 14:139, 1990.

42. Bogousslavsky J, Pierre P: Ischemic stroke in patients under age 45. *Neurol Clin* 10:113, 1992.

43. Donaldson JO, Lee NS: Arterial and venous stroke associated with pregnancy, in Yerby MS, Devinsk O (eds): *Neurologic Clinics: Neurologic Complications of Pregnancy* 12(3):583, 1994.

44. Hodgman MT, Pessin MS, Homans DC, et al: Cerebral embolism as the initial manifestation of peripartum cardiomyopathy. *Neurology* 32:668, 1982.

45. Connor RCR, Adams JH: Importance of cardiomyopathy and cerebral ischaemia in the diagnosis of fatal coma in pregnancy. *J Clin Pathol* 19:244, 1966.

46. Cox SM, Hankins GD, Leveno KJ, et al: Bacterial endocarditis, a serious pregnancy complication. *J Reprod Med* 33:671, 1988.

47. Lein JN, Stander RW: Subacute bacterial endocarditis following obstetric and gynecologic procedures. *Obstet Gynecol* 13:568, 1959.

48. Constantine G, Greene A: Untreated homocystinuria: a maternal death in a woman with four pregnancies. *Br J Obstet Gynaecol* 94:803, 1987.

49. Weibers DO, Mokri B: Internal carotid artery dissection after childbirth. *Stroke* 16:956, 1985.

50. Mas JL, Bousser MG, Corone P, et al: Anéurusme disséquant des artères, vertébrales extracraniennes et grossesse. *Rev Neurol* 143:761, 1987.

51. Brownlee RD, Tranmer BI, Sevick RJ, Larmy G, Curry BJ: Spontaneous thrombosis of an unruptured anterior communicating aneurysm. An unusual cause of ischemic stroke. *Stroke* 26:1945, 1995.

52. Farine D, Andreyko J, Lysikiewcz A, et al: Isolated angiitis of the brain in pregnancy and puerperium. *Obstet Gynecol* 63:586, 1984.

53. Enomoto H, Goto H: Moyamoya disease presenting as intracerebral hemorrhage during pregnancy: case report and review of the literature. *Neurosurgery* 20:33, 1987.

54. Pinette MG, Vinttzileos AM, Ingardia CJ: Thrombotic thrombocytopenic purpura as a cause of thrombocytopenia in pregnancy: literature review. *Am J Perinatol* 6:55, 1989.

55. Powars DR, Sandu M, Niland-Weiss J, et al: Pregnancy in sickle cell disease. *Obstet Gynecol* 67:217, 1986.

56. Milner PF, Jones BR, Döbler J: Outcome of pregnancy in sickle cell anemia and sickle cell-hemoglobin C disease. *Am J Obstet Gynecol* 138:239, 1980.

57. Letsky EA: Disseminated intravascular coagulation, in Morgan B (ed): *Problems in Obstetrical Anaesthesia*. Chichester, John Wiley and Son, 1987, pp 69–87.

58. Sharshar T, Lamy C, Mas JL.: Incidence and causes of strokes associated with pregnancy and puerperium. A study in public hospitals of Ile de France. *Stroke* 26:930, 1995.

59. Swingler GR, Bigrigg MA, Hewitt BG, McNulty CA: Disseminated intravascular coagulation associated with group A streptococcal infection in pregnancy. *Lancet* 1(8600):1456, 1988.

60. Cross JN, Castro PO, Jennett WB: Cerebral strokes associated with pregnancy and the puerperium. *BMJ* 3:214, 1968.

61. Fox MW, Harms RW, Davis DH: Selected neurologic complications of pregnancy. *Mayo Clin Proc* 65:1595, 1990.

62. Hytten F: Blood volume changes in normal pregnancy, in Letsky EA (ed): Haematological disorders in pregnancy. *Clin Haematol* 14:601, 1985.

63. Dias MS, Sekhar LN: Intracranial hemorrhage from aneurysms and arteriovenous malformations during pregnancy and the puerperium. *Neurosurgery* 27:855, 1990.

64. Wiebers DO: Subarachnoid hemorrhage in pregnancy. *Semin Neurol* 8:226, 1988.

65. Simon RH: Brain tumors in pregnancy. *Semin Neurol* 8:214, 1988.

66. Cahill DW, Bashirelahi N, Solomon LW, et al: Estrogen and progesterone acceptors in meningiomas. *J Neurosurg* 60:985, 1984.

67. Chaudhuri P, Wallenburg NCS: Brain tumors and pregnancy. *Eur J Obstet Gynecol Reprod Biol* 11:109, 1980.

68. Reidl RL, Quigley ME, Yen SSC: Pituitary apoplexy: A review. *Arch Neurol* 42:712, 1985.

69. Steiner PE, Lushbaugh CC: Maternal pulmonary fluid embolism by amniotic fluid as a cause of obstetric shock and unexpected deaths in obstetrics. *JAMA* 255:2187, 1986. (Landmark article reprinted from *JAMA* 117:1245 and 1341, 1941.)

70. Hardin L, Fox LS, O'Quinn AG: Amniotic fluid embolism. *South Med J* 84:1046, 1991.

71. Dodson J, Martin J, Boswell J, Goodall HB, Smith R: Probable amniotic fluid embolism precipitated by amniocentesis and treated by exchange transfusion. *BMJ* (Clin Res Ed) 294:1322, 1987.

72. Rodgers GP, Heymach GJ III: Cryoprecipitate therapy in amniotic fluid embolism. *Am J Med* 76:916, 1984.

73. Nelson PK: Pulmonary gas embolism in pregnancy and the puerperium. *Obstet Gynecol Surg* 15:449, 1960.

74. Sheehan HL: The frequency of postpartum hypopituitarism. *J Obstet Gynecol Br Comm* 72:103, 1965.

75. McDermott MW, Griesdale DE, Berry K, Wilkins GE: Lymphocytic adenohypophisitis. *Can J Neurol Sci* 15:38, 1988.

76. Hashimoto M, Yanaki T, Nakahara N: Lymphocytic adenohypophysitis: an immunohistochemical study. *Surg Neurol* 36:137, 1991.

77. Farmer TW, Flowers CA: Neurologic manifestations of postpartum pituitary insufficiency. *Neurology* 5:212, 1955.

78. Asa SL, Bilbao JM, Kovacks K, et al: Lymphocytic adenohypophysitis of pregnancy resulting in hypopituitarism: a distinct clinical–pathological entity. *Ann Intern Med* 95:166, 1981.

79. Sheehan HL., Stanfield JP: The pathogenesis of postpartum necrosis of the anterior lobe of the pituitary gland. *Acta Endocrinologica* 37:479, 1961.

80. Stewart A: A case of Simmond's disease. *Lancet* II:1391, 1936.

81. Cosman F, Post KD, Wardlaw SL: Lymphocytic hypophysitis. Report of 3 cases and a review of the literature. *Medicine* 68:240, 1989.

82. Castle D, deVilliers JC, Melvill R: Lymphocytic adenohypophysitis. Report of a case with demonstration of spontaneous tumor regression and a review of the literature. *Br J Neurosurg* 2:401, 1988.

83. Engelberth O, Jezkova Z: Auto antibodies in Sheehan's syndrome. *Lancet* 1:1075, 1965.

84. Futrell N, Millikan C: Neurologic complications of pregnancy. *Neurol Clin* 12:527, 1994.

85. Altshuler LL, Szuba MP: Course of psychiatric disorders in pregnancy, in Yerby MS, Devinsky O (eds): *Neurologic Clinics: Neurologic Complications of Pregnancy* 12(3):613, 1994.

86. Altshuler LL, Szuba MP: Course of psychiatric disorders in pregnancy, in Yerby MS, Devinsky O (eds): *Neurologic Clinics: Neurologic Complications of Pregnancy* **12**(3):613–635, 1994.

87. Finucane AK: Legal issues in neurology and pregnancy. The physician's duty of care. *Neurol Clin* 12:637, 1994.

88. Raps EC, Galetta SL, Flamm ES: Neuro-intensive care of the pregnant woman. *Neurol Clin* 12:601, 1994.

Chapter 23

IMPAIRED CONSCIOUSNESS IN NEURODEGENERATIVE DISORDERS

G. Bryan Young

Last scene of all, that ends this strange eventful history, is second childishness and mere oblivion, sans teeth, sans eyes, sans taste, sans everything.

William Shakespeare, *As You Like It*

The neurodegenerative disorders constitute a group of diseases that cause a pathologic, chronic, progressive loss of neurons, synaptic connections or tracts, with associated clinical dysfunction. Those relevant to consciousness usually cause a dementia, or a significant decline in cognitive function or "content of consciousnes." These may progress to a persistent vegetative state (see Chap. 2). Disorders of alertness (stupor or coma) may never occur, except in the terminal stages or with complications, e.g. seizures, or septic or metabolic encephalopathy, or as adverse effects of drug therapy.

In the subsequent discussion, dementia of the Alzheimer type (DAT) will be used as the main example. Other disorders also have an insidious onset and gradual, inexorable progression, although there are variations in tempo and associated features, such as various motor phenomena, that reflect the distribution of the neuropathology.

CLASSIFICATION

The neurodegenerative disorders that impair higher functions can be divided, somewhat imprecisely, into major categories: cortical dementias, subcortical dementias, combined cortical and subcortical dementias, vascular dementias, white matter disease, and a miscellaneous group (Table 23-1).[1] Their differentiating clinical features are discussed subsequently.

PREVALENCE

Dementia of the Alzheimer type is by far the most common dementing illness, accounting for about 70 percent of dementias in combined series.[2] The incidence and prevalence of dementia increase with age: between 2 and 4 percent of persons over 65 years of age are demented; this rises to 20 percent after age 80 years.

Table 23-1
Dementias

Cortical dementias	*Vascular dementias*
Dementia of the Alzheimer type (DAT)	Multiple lacunes
Pick disease	Binswanger disease (?)
Frontal lobe dementia	Multiple cerebral infarctions
Creutzfeldt-Jakob disease (some cases)	Watershed (boundary zone) infarctions
Subcortical dementias	*White matter disorders*
Huntington disease	Multiple sclerosis (extreme/advanced cases)
Progressive supranuclear palsy	Leukodystrophies (adrenoleukodystrophy, metachromatic
Dementia in Parkinson disease	leukodystrophy)
Hallervorden-Spatz disease	Anoxia and carbon monoxide poisoning
Paraneoplastic syndromes	
Spinocerebellar degeneration	*Miscellaneous disorders*
ALS-Parkinson-dementia complex	Trauma
Wilson disease	Neoplasms—direct, indirect, and remote effects
	HIV
Combined cortical-subcortical dementias	Toxins
Creutzfeldt-Jakob disease	Other metabolic diseases
Subacute sclerosing panencephalitis	Other infections
Cortical-basal degneration	Miscellaneous hereditary disorders
Lewy body disease	Hydrocephalus
Fatal familial insomnia	Dementia in epilepsy (?)

The dementias that make up other groups are uncommon, with the possible exception of vascular or multi-infarct dementia.

DIAGNOSIS

The essential clinical criteria for dementia include memory impairment and at least one of the following: aphasia, apraxia, agnosia, or a disturbance in executive functioning.[1] The impairment must be sufficient to produce occupational or social dysfunction; there must, of course, also be a *decline* from a previously higher level of function.

CLINICAL FEATURES

Dementia of the Alzheimer Type

Cognitive (Content of Consciousness) Deficits   Cortical dementia is typified by DAT and consists of impaired memory storage and retrieval, and defects in the other cognitive functions mentioned above, usually without motor problems apart from gait disorders.

The evolutionary changes in DAT can be divided into three stages. These are summarized in Table 23-2, which considers the cognitive, behavioral and neurologic features. The speed of such progression or deterioration is highly variable; there are no reliable predictors of the tempo of decline, although the early onset of aphasia appears to be associated with more rapid worsening.[3]

Amnesia is an essential and early component in cortical dementia, a feature that underlines the importance of valid assessment of memory. Executive, primarily frontal lobe, functions are also affected early, often indicated by difficulty in planning. Inflexibility in mental "set," with fixed attitudes, coexists with distractibility and difficulty in performing tasks that require the attention to be divided between a number of near-simultaneous activities. Personality changes include angry outbursts, paranoia, passivity, delusions, hallucinations, and self-centeredness.[4] These often begin

Table 23-2

Clinical features of dementia of the Alzheimer type by stage

Feature	Early	Intermediate	Late
Cognitive			
Memory	Poor recall of new information, remote memory relatively preserved	Remote memory affected	Untestable
Language	Dysnomia, mild loss of fluency	Nonfluent, poor comprehension, impaired repetition	Near-mutism
Visuospatial	Misplacing objects, difficulty driving	Getting lost, difficulty copying figures	Untestable
Behavioral	Delusions, depression, insomnia	Delusions, depression, agitation, insomnia	Agitation, wandering
Neurologic	Minimal abnormality	Abnormal face-hand test, nonspecific gait disorder	Mutism, incontinence, rigidity ± myoclonus

Source: Modified from Corey-Bloom J, Galasko D, Thal LJ: Clinical features and natural history of Alzheimer's disease, in Calne DB (ed): *Neurodegenerative Diseases*. Philadelphia, WB Saunders, 1994, p 632.

early in the dementing process. Delusions are usually poorly systematized persecutory impressions involving the immediate environment and family or close friends. Some patients become disinhibited, e.g., sexual improprieties appear. Depression also appears early and probably affects at least 40 percent of patients.[5] Patients often show motor restlessness, including pacing and fidgeting. Dysfunctions in language, praxis, and visuospatial function are usually the next to arise. Aphasia begins with word-finding problems, followed by deficiencies in comprehension. Visuospatial disturbances include dressing apraxia, getting lost easily, and difficulty recognizing places, drawn figures, and people. Motor deficits are uncommon in the early stages, but gait abnormalities, especially gait apraxia or postural instability, do occur; paratonic or extrapyramidal rigidity and myoclonus are even less frequent. Myoclonus is more common in cases with early onset and more rapid progression.[6,7]

In the last phase of cortical dementias, the patient is unable to feed themself and is doubly incontinent. Significant weight loss is common. Speech is lost or becomes limited to palilalia or echolalia. Patients become rigid and bradykinetic and adopt a fetal posture—"paraplegia in flexio."[8]

Patients may remain alert with sleep and wake cycles (often disturbed, however) and normal arousability.

Alertness Abnormalities

Seizures (see Chap. 17) Dementia of the Alzheimer type and other dementias, especially those with cerebral cortical involvement, are associated with a greater than sixfold increased risk of generalized or partial epileptic seizures, and account for about 7 percent of adult-onset seizures.[9,10] The occurrence of generalized convulsive seizures correlates with a reduced number of pyramidal cells in layers 3 through 4 of the parietal cortex (area 7) and in the parahippocampal gyrus (area 28).[11] The dementia is usually advanced when seizures develop.[12] Seizures occur in over 80 percent of patients with Down syndrome with Alzheimer disease.[13] As mentioned above, myoclonus is also common in DAT patients, in one study occurring in 46 percent of DAT patients followed until death and in none of the controls.[14] Myoclonus has a strong association with seizures and with increased risk for early mortality in patients with early-onset Alzheimer disease.[15] Patients with familial, early-onset Alzheimer disease, due to a chromosome 21 locus, have a higher than expected incidence of both myoclonus and seizures.[16] Although most seizures are convulsive, non-convulsive seizures, including nonconvulsive status epilepticus, occasionally occur in cortical dementias.[17]

Systemic Complications Sepsis (see Chap. 12), especially from pneumonia and urinary tract infections, is common when patients become debilitated from dementia.[18] With these complications, alertness is compromised along the spectrum from a confusional state to coma. Even mildly disordered cardiac, pulmonary, hepatic, or renal function predisposes the elderly demented patient to superimposed encephalopathy—a "beclouded dementia."[19] Sepsis in this context often leads to death, but septic encephalopathy is usually reversible if the patient recovers systemically; however, the author has seen some patients who are left with permanent added cognitive and motor deficits.[20,21]

Pulmonary embolism is often unrecognized in debilitated, bedridden patients.[22] This may produce transient loss of consciousness or a more protracted, acute confusional state, stupor, or coma, depending on the severity of hypoxemia, hypocarbia, and hemodynamic effects. Clinical clues include sudden dyspnea, tachycardia, low-grade fever, and signs of deep venous thrombosis in the leg veins. Arterial or capillary blood gases usually show hypoxemia and hypocapnia with respiratory alkalosis. The diagnosis can be confirmed by pulmonary perfusion radionuclide scans or pulmonary angiography.

Fluid, electrolyte, and nutritional disorders are common when patients are bedridden and unable to feed themselves or satisfy thirst. Dehydration, hyperosmolality, and hypophosphatemia may escape detection unless fluids, serum electrolytes, and nutritional intake are monitored and actively managed. The author has found Wernicke's encephalopathy at autopsy in some severely demented patients from chronic care facilities who, while in a prolonged, terminal vegetative state, were given intravenous glucose solutions without vitamins.

Traumatic Complications The demented elderly who fall are more susceptible to complications that increase morbidity, mortality, and length of hospital stay.[23] These include direct trauma to the head, cervical spinal cord injury, bone fractures (with fat embolism), and the complications of immobilization and sensory deprivation.[24–26] The author of this chapter would emphasize subdural hematoma.

Patients with DAT are usually elderly, have atrophic brains and coagulopathies (sometimes iatrogenic), and are prone to falls. These factors predispose to subacute or chronic subdural hematomas.[27] Hematomas usually arise because of tears in veins that drain into the superior sagittal sinus. Because of the association with congophilic angiopathy, with amyloid deposition in arterial and arteriolar walls, DAT patients may develop acute, spontaneous subdural hematomas without trauma.[28,29] Subdural hematomas are treatable, potentially fatal complications that are commonly missed clinically. Patients usually have impaired alertness and focal signs.[30] However, bilateral subdural hematomas, which are more common in the elderly, may not produce lateralized signs. Bilateral subdural hematomas are associated with gait apraxia, and they aggravate cognitive dysfunction or alertness, mimic a metabolic encephalopathy, or, terminally, cause raised intracranial pressure and central herniation.[31] Simple surgical drainage is usually adequate to allow complete recovery, providing that the patient is treated promptly.[32,33] Patients with atrophic brains or coagulopathies are prone to postoperative recurrence of the subdural hematoma.[34]

Other Complications in Dementia of the Alzheimer Type Drugs, hospitalization, operations, nosocomial infections, and other factors may combine to produce a multifactorial delirium or stupor in the elderly demented patient. The primacy of drug side effects and the exclusion of this circumstance are detailed later in this chapter and in Chap. 16. Frequently, there is more than one determinant.

Vascular (Multi-infarct) Dementias

Although vascular dementias are not truly "neuro-degenerative," they are briefly reviewed here, as they are commonly mistaken for DAT, are common in our population, and share management issues with degenerative diseases. Vascular dementias are related to tissue destruction, usually from ischemia due to vascular occlusions. Vascular dementias produce a varied clinical picture, but features that differentiate these from other demential conditions are are follows: abrupt onset, step-wise (as opposed to gradual) deterioration, a history of previous transient ischemic attacks (or transient focal neurologic dysfunction), a history of hypertension and other risk factors for vascular disease, and evidence of multifocal disease on neurologic examination. The latter include asymmetric spasticity, rigidity, extensor plantar responses, pseudobulbar palsy, upper motor neuron distribution of weakness, sensory loss, aphasia, visual-spatial dysfunction, visual field defects, and lateralized neglect. Focal or asymmetric deficits are found on and neuropsychologic testing, including acalculia and language problems, as well as disorientation, dysmemory, and disorders in abstraction.

Vascular dementias can be divided into cortical and subcortical disorders. The latter is more common with multiple lacunar strokes and is associated with extrapyramidal features and pseudobulbar palsies. Binswanger disease, or a diffuse white matter disease in association with hypertensive vascular disease, is a controversial entity, but cumulative, subcortical infarcts are well described.[35,36] These affect the white matter and subcortical gray structures. Cortical infarcts are commonly multifocal and embolic, and are more likely to produce aphasias, agnosias, and apraxias, as well as various sensory and motor deficits.

The pathogenesis of vascular dementia consists of either embolic strokes, multiple small vessel occlusive disease from hypertension, or, uncommonly, bilateral watershed or borderzone infarction in association with hypotension and hypoperfusion in the terminal portions of major arteries.[37,38] Appropriate investigation for stroke is discussed in Chap. 14.

Although it is not possible to reverse the damage that has been done, if the pathogenetic mechanism can be addressed, e.g., control of hypertension and prevention of cardiogenic emboli by anticoagulation, further strokes may be prevented.

Subcortical Dementias

"Subcortical dementia" is characterized by mental slowness, inertia, abulia, forgetfulness, mood disturbances, and usually some motor problems such as extrapyramidal syndromes (parkinsonism, myoclonus, tremor, chorea, or dystonia). Representative diseases include Huntington disease, progressive supranuclear palsy, fatal familial insomnia, Hallervorden-Spatz syndrome, Wilson disease, some cases of Parkinson disease, and the amyotrophic-parkinsonism-dementia complex.

Fatal familial insomnia may be one of the best examples of a subcortical disorder. This disease begins with insomnia, due to diencephalic damage. A progressive disorder of attention and vigilance is accompanied by a memory deficit, including working memory, and frontal lobe dysfunction with impaired planning.[39] There is typically autonomic and endocrinologic dysfunction, due to the hypothalamic disease. The progression of the disorder varies from patient to patient. The clinical presentation reflects the involvement of various structures, including the cerebral cortex, the basal ganglia, and the cerebellum. In other cases, the disease may be more restricted to the thalamus.[40] Patients ultimately become demented with impairment of memory and other cognitive functions. They can also show extrapyramidal features, such as dystonia, spasticity, hypotonia, febrile episodes, ventilatory failure, myoclonus, and hypersomnia alternating with insomnia.

Cortical-Subcortical Combined Dementias

Patients with cortical-basal ganglionic degeneration (CBGD) display prominent extrapyramidal rigidity as well as dementia. The disorder usually presents with rigidity and ideomotor apraxia, an asymmetric onset of motor symptoms and any of the following abnormal saccadic eye movements, alien limb phenomenon, postural instability, myoclonus, cortical sensory loss, or tremor. Cognitive problems include memory impairment, aphasia, apraxia, impaired judgement, and disordered frontal executive functions. In one study, in contrast with patients with dementia of the Alzheimer type, those with CBGD were more depressed emotionally and their memory functions were relatively better preserved.[41] They may show the "alien limb" phenomenon, in which the person does not realize the limb, which behaves in an apparently autonomous manner, is his own.[42]

Patients with Pick disease usually closely resemble those with DAT, although some demonstrate gait and extrapyramidal features early in the course of the disorder.[43] In some patients, the frontal lobes alone appear to be affected initially, with impaired executive functions and behavioral disorder, but with relatively preserved memory and other "posterior" functions.

CLINICAL EVALUATION

Investigation of Dementia

The major treatable causes of the dementia syndrome are as follows: depression, drugs, metabolic disorders, normal pressure hydrocephalus, and neoplasms, in approximate descending order of their frequency according to clinical practice.[54] Treatable causes are more likely to be acute or subacute in onset and usually show more clinical fluctuation than degenerative diseases. Depression can be difficult to differentiate from dementia, but, as in delirium, depressed patients often have problems in concentrating or attending and show vegetative features commonly found in depression, such as insomnia, anorexia, weight loss, and anhedonia. The depression inventories of Beck and Hamilton are helpful in this regard.[44,45]

Dementia must also be differentiated from confusional (delirious) states that interfere with cognitive function. Delirium, characterized by abnormal attention, typically shows striking fluctuations. The onset of delirium is more sudden than a demential illness; the duration is shorter. Delirium is often accompanied by postural tremor, asterixis, or multifocal myoclonus. Delirium may also be associated with agitation, increased sympathetic nervous system activity, hallucinations, and delusions. The problem of delirium superimposed upon a pre-existing mild dementia has been mentioned earlier.

To confirm the diagnosis of dementia, a history of vocational and social deterioration is necessary. This can be obtained by questioning the patient and their family, but more formal assessments are available, e.g., Scales of Independent Behavior, the Vineland Adaptive Behavioral Scale and the Disability Assessment Schedule.[46–48] These and others, e.g., the Clinical Dementia Rating or Global Deterioration Scales, are used in serial assessments as a powerful method of demonstrating deterioration.[49,50] A history of incontinence, epileptic seizures, change in gait, or myoclonus gives support to an organic mental process. Serial testing or historical evidence of decline (from persons who know the patient well) is especially necessary in patients with a background of mental retardation.[51] The validity of such retrospective historical information is dependent on the reliability of the observer. Even professionally trained care givers may be too subjective if a deterioration is "anticipated," e.g., in middle-aged patients with Down syndrome. Bedside tests of memory function (memorizing the names of objects, recalling recent activities, meals, etc.) and neuropsychologic testing can provide a useful baseline. The recruitment of a neuropsychologist is strongly advised for early and follow-up assessments of the above functions. There are formal dementia scales that are useful for initially normal adults as well as for those with intellectual disabilities.[51]

Mental status testing can utilize the Mini-Mental State exam at the bedside.[52] In addition, for tests of praxis (ability to perform motor tasks in the absence of defects of motor or sensory function, and comprehension of instructions), the patient is asked to mime certain motor tasks, e.g., brushing the teeth or combing the hair, or to perform common motor tasks, such as using a pencil or waving good-bye. One checks for visual agnosia by having the patient identify common objects. Executive functions assess judgment, e.g., noting similarities or differences in lists or groups of pictures. Tests of language function, including reading and writing, are performed in a standard clinical fashion.

Certain abnormalities of the neurologic examination, apart from mental status evaluation, provide important support for neurodegenerative conditions. While a declining memory predominates in most cases of Alzheimer disease, some patients also have gait abnormalities or myoclonus, as well as focal abnormalities such as aphasia. The presence of pathologic reflexes (palmomental, grasp, rooting, sucking, and tonic foot reflexes), especially in younger individuals, gives further support to a dementing process. Some of these so-called "primitive reflexes," e.g., the palmomental reflex, are present in a small number of normal aged individuals and in younger individuals with intellectual disability.[53] Therefore, they alone are not necessarily indicative of a neurodegenerative process. A Babinski reflex is always abnormal, but is quite rare in DAT. The development of extrapyramidal dysfunction raises the possibility of a number of disorders, e.g., Huntington Wilson, and Creutzfeldt-Jakob diseases, that can often be sorted out if one considers the age of onset, family history, and other abnormalities on the examination or laboratory investigation.

Investigations Tests are conducted to determine the underlying cause of dementia; with special consideration for treatable causes (estimated to be about 15 percent of cases), and to establish the prognosis with as much certainty as is possible.[54] Furthermore, in patients with established, untreatable neurodegenerative disorders, reversible complications may be found.

In the early phases of dementia, neuropsychologic testing is helpful in establishing a baseline, differentiating dementias from conditions that mimic dementia, and determining the types of cognitive deficits and their localization. Some neurodegenerative disorders, e.g., Pick disease, may have a prominent frontal or executive dysfunction, e.g., impaired judgment, planning, and ability to change the mental "set," associated with behavioral disturbance. These may require special tests of frontal lobe dysfunction.

Human immunodeficiency virus (HIV) testing is advised in patients at risk for such infection or those with clinical or laboratory features compatible with the acquired immunodeficiency syndrome (AIDS), e.g., opportunistic infections or lymphopenia.[55] Neurosyphilis should be excluded by using the Venereal Diseases Research Laboratory (VDRL) test and the *Treponema pallidum* antibody absorption test if there is a strong suspicion of syphilis and in AIDS patients. Thyroid function and serum vitamin B_{12} or cobalamin testing are usually worthwhile.

Neuroimaging with computer tomography (CT) or magnetic resonance imaging (MRI) scanning excludes neoplasms, strokes, white matter disease, and hydrocephalus. Cerebral atrophy in dementia, unless marked and accentuated in the mesial temporal lobes, shows too much overlap with normal brain shrinkage to be useful in the elderly.[56] Periventricular white matter changes, termed leukoaraiosis, are common in DAT, AIDS, and vascular dementia.[57] Specific distributions of atrophic changes in deeper structures are helpful in the diagnosis of Huntington disease and progressive supranuclear palsy.

The electroencepalogram (EEG) can be useful, but it is rarely specific. An exception is the pattern of generalized periodic sharp-wave complexes at about 1 per second against a suppressed background, a finding that strongly supports the diagnosis of Creutzfeldt-Jakob disease.[58] Cortical disease, e.g., DAT, is characterized by mild generalized slowing, sometimes associated with interictal epileptiform discharges or spikes.[58] White matter disease usually produces marked slowing in the delta (≤ 4 Hz) range.[58] This may be focal, multifocal, or diffuse, depending on the distribution of the white matter pathology.

Investigation of Impaired Consciousness in the Demented Patient

The patient with established dementia who develops an impairment of alertness and arousal must, of course, have dysfunction of the ascending reticular activating system (ARAS) (see Chaps. 1 and 2). In most dementias, as mentioned, stupor or coma occur as superimposed complications. Whether they should be investigated and treated depends on the autonomy of the patient and the stage of the dementia (see "Management" below and Chap. 24).

In our experience, the adverse effects of drugs (especially those with anticholinergic activity), either singly or in combination, and underlying infection are the most common causes of altered alertness in the demented elderly. A careful review of medications, chest film and urinalysis will capture most of these. Subdural hematomas are underrecognized in this population; a CT scan is often warranted.[27] Metabolic complications, including unrecognized myxedema, and fluid and electrolyte imbalance (especially in patients in acute-care hospitals), are worthy of consideration. Some elderly patients develop a delirium-like state as a result of urinary retention or constipation.[59] Less commonly, other systemic disease or organ failure may be the main cause of deterioration in alertness.

PATHOGENESIS

The centers for alertness are spared, at least in the early phases, for most demential illnesses, as they primarily involve the cerebral cortex, rather than deeper structures. Furthermore, the processes usually begin in restricted regions and progress regionally, and then gradually spread to involve other regions. The cognitive problems worsen over time, to the point that most patients are incapable of self-care. They lose continence, become more withdrawn, and eventually become vegetative.

The pathogenesis of the neuronal loss in neurodegenerative disorders is likely to be due to a combination of excitotoxic damage and oxidative stress, with varied roles played by apoptosis and other mechanisms.[60] Some specific diseases have other mechanisms. For example, fatal familial insomnia is due to a mutation in the prion protein gene.[61,62]

MANAGEMENT

Management can be divided into specific and symptomatic therapies. Specific or definitive treatment is designed to reverse the underlying disease process and to prevent further progression. Examples include thyroid replacement for myxedema, antibiotic treatment of neurosyphilis, anticoagulation for the antiphospholipid antibody syndrome, ventriculoperitoneal shunting of patients with hydrocephalus, and removal of meningiomas.

Unfortunately, most cases of dementia are not curable, reversible, or preventable. Despite some progress in the treatment of DAT, there have been, thus far, no major advances in controlling the disease process. There are often reversible complications, such as seizures, metabolic disorders, adverse effects of drugs, underlying infections, and complications of trauma. The decision is whether to treat these reversible conditions in the presence of an inexorably progressive, ultimately fatal neurodegenerative process. The wishes of the patient, when competent, and the substitute decision-maker, when the patient is incompetent, must be given primacy (see Chap. 24). In the early phases of the disease, the patient may have "something to live for," and it seems reasonable to reverse treatable complications. When the patient has deteriorated to an irreversible persistent vegetative state, few would argue that such a life is worth preserving by treating reversible complications. The management of these complications and the intermediate levels of deterioration are best considered using the principles discussed in Chap. 24.

In the management of disturbing behaviors, it is best to consider the putative pathogenesis. For example, agitation may reflect anxiety but may be symptomatic of an acute confusional state due to a treatable complication, e.g., urinary tract infection, pain, or severe constipation. It is best to start with a nonpharmacologic approach. Drugs may compound problems and precipitate institutionalization, while many patients can live in their homes for extended times if adequate support of psychologic, social, and environmental factors is given.[63] This requires effective assessment of the patient's profile and the elimination of factors, e.g., some drugs, that may aggravate confusion and memory problems.[64,65] Specific drug therapy, dependent on the behavioral abnormality, is discussed under the acute confusional state in Chaps. 2 and 3. One should be aware of the altered pharmacodynamics and drug interactions in the elderly when prescribing any medication.[66]

REFERENCES

1. Task Force on DSM-IV: *Diagnostic and Statistical Manual of Mental Disorders,* 4th ed: DSM-IV. Washington American Psychiatric Association, 1994, pp 133–155.
2. Cummings JL, Benson DF: *Dementia: A Clinical Approach* 2nd ed. Boston, Butterworth, 1992.
3. Drachman DA, O'Donnell BF, Lew, RA, Swearer JM: The prognosis in Alzheimer's disease: "How far" rather than "how fast" best predicts the course. *Arch Neurol* 47:851, 1990.
4. Rubin EH, Morris JC, Berg L: The progression of personality changes in senile dementia of the Alzheimer type. *J Am Geriatr Soc* 35:721, 1987.
5. Sim M, Sussman I: Alzheimer's disease: its natural history and differential diagnosis. *J Nerv Mental Dis* 135:489, 1962.
6. Chui HC, Teng EL, Henderson VW, Moy AC: Clinical subtypes of dementia of the Alzheimer type. *Neurology* 35:1544, 1985.
7. Mayeux R, Stern Y, Spanton S: Heterogeny of dementia of the Alzheimer type. *Neurology* 35:453, 1985.
8. Yakovlev P: Paraplegia in flexion of cerebral origin. *J Neuropath Exp Neurol* 13:267, 1954.
9. Hersdorffer DC, Hauser WA, Annegers JF, Kokmen E, Rocca WA: Dementia and adult-onset unprovoked seizures. *Neurology* 46:727, 1996.
10. Forsgren L, Bucht GM, Eriksson S, Bergmark L: Incidence and clinical characterization of unprovoked seizures in adults: a prospective population-based study. *Epilepsia* 37:224, 1996.
11. Forstl H, Burns A, Levy R, et al: Neurologic signs in Alzheimer's disease. Results of a prospective clinical and neuropathological study. *Arch Neurol* 49:1038, 1992.
12. Romanelli MF, Morris JC, Ashkin K, Coben LA: Advanced Alzheimer's disease is a risk factor for late-onset seizures. *Arch Neurol* 47:847, 1990.
13. Lai F, Williams RS: A prospective study of Alzheimer's disease in Down syndrome. *Arch Neurol* 46:849, 1989.
14. Risse SC, Lampe TH, Bird TD, et al: Myoclonus, seizures and paratonia in Alzheimer's disease. *Alzheimer Dis Assoc Disord* 44:217, 1990.
15. Samson WN, van Dujin CM, Hop WC, Hofman A: Clinical features and mortality in patients with early-onset Alzheimer's disease. *Eur Neurol* 36:103, 1996.
16. Bergamini L, Pinessi L, Rainero I, et al: Familial Alzheimer's disease. Evidences for clinical and genetic heterogeneitv. *Acta Neurol* 13:534, 1991.
17. Sung CY, Chu NS: Status epilepticus in the elderly: etiology, seizure type and outcome. *Acta Neurol Scand* 80:51, 1989.
18. Nicolle LE, Henderson E, Bjornson J, et al: The association of bacteriuria with resident characteristics and survival in elderly institutionalized men. *Ann Intern Med* 106:682, 1987.
19. Adams RD, Victor M, Ropper AH: *Principles of Neurology.* New York, McGraw-Hill, 1997.
20. Katzman R: The prevalence and malignancy of Alzheimer disease. *Arch Neurol* 33:217, 1976.
21. Bolton CF, Young GB, Zochodne DW: The neurological complications of sepsis. *Ann Neurol* 33:94, 1993.
22. Goldhaber SZ: *Pulmonary Embolism and Deep Venous Thrombosis.* Philadelphia, Saunders, 1985.
23. Smith DP, Enderson BL, Maull KI: Trauma in the elderly: determinants of outcome. *South Med J* 83:171, 1990.
24. Ryan MD, Taylor TK: Odontoid fractures in the elderly. *J Spinal Disord* 6:397, 1993.
25. Creditor MC: Hazards of hospitalization in the elderly. *Ann Intern Med* 118:219, 1993.
26. Jarrett PG, Rockwood K, Cancer D, Stolee P, Cosway S: Illness presentation in elderly patients. *Arch Intern Med* 155:1060, 1995.
27. Velasco J, Head M, Farlin E, Lippmann S: Unsuspected subdural hematoma as a differential diagnosis in elderly patients. *South Med J* 88:977, 1995.
28. Leblanc R, Preul M, Robitaille Y, Villemure JG, Pokrupa R: Surgical considerations in cerebral amyloid angiopathy. *Neurosurgery* 29:712, 1991.

29. Borzone M, Altomonte M, Baldini M, Rivano C: Pure subdural haematomas of arteriolar origin. *Acta Neurochir* 121:109, 1993.

30. Barzone M, Altomonte M, Baldini M, Rivano C: Typical interhemispheric subdural hematomas and falx syndrome: four eases and a review of the literature. *Zentral Neurochir* 56:51, 1995.

31. Spallone A, Giuffre R, Gagliardi FM, Vagnozzi R: Chronic subdural hematoma in extremely elderly patients. *Eur Neurol* 29:18, 1989.

32. Rychlicki F, Recchioni MA, Burchianti M, et al: Percutaneous twist-drill craniotomy for the treatment of chronic subdural haematoma. *Acta Neurochir* 113:38, 1991.

33. Kotwica Z, Brzezinski J: Chronic subdural haematoma treated by burr holes and closed system drainage: personal experience in 131 patients. *Br J Neurosurg* 5:461, 1991.

34. Stroobandt G, Fransen P, Thauvoy C, Menard E: Pathogenetic factors in chronic subdural hematoma and causes of recurrence after drainage. *Acta Neurochir* 137:6, 1995.

35. Babikian V, Ropper AH: Binswanger's disease: a review. *Stroke* 18:2, 1987.

36. Hachinski V: Binswanger's disease: Neither Binswanger's nor a disease. *J Neurol Sci* 103:1, 1991.

37. Romanul FCA, Abramowicz A: Changes in brain and pial vessels in arterial border zones. *Arch Neurol* 11:40, 1964.

38. Torvik A: The pathogenesis of watershed infarcts in the brain. *Stroke* 15:221, 1984.

39. Medori R, Montagna P, Tritschler HJ, Le Blanc A, et al: Fatal familial insomnia: a second kindred with a mutation at prion protein at codon 178. *Neurology* 42:669, 1992.

40. Perani D, Cortelli P, Lucignani G, et al: [18F]FDG PET of fatal familial insomnia: the functional effects of thalamic lesions. *Neurology* 43:2565, 1993.

41. Massman PJ, Kreiter KT, Jankovic J, Doody RS: Neuropsychological functioning in cortical-basal ganglionic degeneration: differentiation from Alzheimer's disease. *Neurology* 46:720, 1996.

42. Banks G, Short P, Martinez AJ, et al: The alien hand syndrome. *Arch Neurol* 46:456, 1989.

43. Neary D, Snowden JS, Northen B, Goulding P: Dementia of the frontal lobe type. *J Neurol Neurosurg Psychiatry* 51:353, 1988.

44. Beck AT, Ward CH, Mendelson M, et al: An inventory for measuring depression. *Arch Gen Psychiatry* 4:561, 1961.

45. Hamilton M: Development of a rating scale for primary depressive illness. *Br J Soc Clin Psychol* 6:278, 1967.

46. Bruininks RH, Woodcock RW, Weatherman RF, et al: *Woodcock-Johnson Psycho-Educational Battery/ Part Four: Scales of Independent Behavior*. Chicago, Riverside Publishing, 1985.

47. Sparrow SS, Balla DA, Cicchetti DV: *Vineland Adaptive Behavioral Scales*. Circle Pines, Minn., American Guideline Service, 1984.

48. Holmes N, Shah A, Wing L: The Disability Assessment Schedule: a brief screening device for use with the mentally retarded. *Psychol Med* 12:879, 1982.

49. Hughes CP, Berg L, Danziger WL, et al: A new clinical scale for the staging of dementia. *Br J Psychiatry* 140:1982.

50. Reisberg B, Ferris SH, de Leon MJ, Crook T: The Global Deterioration Scale (GDS): an instrument for the assessment of primary degenerative dementia (PDD). *Am J Psychiatry* 139:1139, 1982.

51. AAMR-IASSID Working Group for the Establishment of Criteria for the Diagnosis of Dementia in Individuals with Intellectual Disability: *Diagnosis of Dementia in Individuals with Intellectual Disability*. Washington, American Association on Mental Retardation ATTN: Alzheimer Disease Workgroup, 1995.

52. Folstein ME, Folstein SE, McHugh PR: "Mini-Mental State." A practical guide for grading the cognitive state of patients for the clinician. *J Psychiatr Res* 12:189, 1975.

53. Orefice G, Modafferi N, Selvaggio M, et al: Archaic reflexes in normal elderly people. *Acta Neurol* 13:19, 1991.

54. Nadeau S: Multi-infarct dementia, subcortical dementia and hydrocephalus. *South Med J* 84(suppl 1):1S–41, 1991.

55. Rubin RH, Young LS: *The Clinical Approach to Infection in the Immunocompromised Host,* 2nd ed. New York, Plenum Press, 1988,

56. Faulstich ME: Brain imaging in dementia of the Alzheimer type. *Int J Neurosci* 57:39, 1991.

57. Hachinski VC, Potter P, Merskey H: Leuko-araiosis. *Arch Neurol* 44:21, 1987.

58. Gloor P, Kalabay O, Giard N: The electroencephalogram in diffuse encephalopathies: eleetroencephalographic correlates of gray and white matter lesions. *Brain* 91:779, 1968.

59. Blackburn T, Dunn M: Cystocerebral syndrome. Acute urinary retention presenting as confusion

in elderly patients. *Arch Intern Med* 151:2557, 1990.

60. Coyle JT, Puttfarcken P: Oxidative stress, glutamate and neurodegenerative disorders. *Science* 262:689, 1993.

61. Medori R, Tritschler H-J, LeBlanc A, et al: Fatal familial insomnia, a prion disease with a mutation at codon 178 of the prion protein gene. *N Eng J Med* 326:444, 1992.

62. Reder AT, Mednick AS, Brown P, et al: Clinical and genetic studies of fatal familial insomnia. *Neurology* 45:1068, 1995.

63. Carlson DL, Fleming KC, Smith GE, Evans JM: Management of dementia-related disturbances: a nonpharmacologic approach. *Mayo Clin Proc* 70:1108, 1995.

64. Fleming KC, Adams AC, Petersen RC: Dementia: diagnosis and evaluation. *Mayo Clin Proc* 71:821, 1996.

65. Flint AJ: Delusions in dementia: a review. *J Neuropsychiatry Clin Neurosci* 3:121, 1991.

66. Fleming KC, Evans JM: Pharmacologic therapies in dementia. *Mayo Clin Proc* 70:1116, 1995.

Chapter 24
ETHICS

G. Bryan Young
Paul R. Steacy

No man is good enough to govern another man without that other's consent.
    Abraham Lincoln, Lincoln-Douglas debate

PRINCIPLES OF ETHICAL BEHAVIOR

Physicians are often required to make management decisions on comatose patients. These decisions based on an understanding of the disease process and the prognosis for the particular patient, involve ethical and legal values and principles.

Ethics are "a group of moral principles or set of rules . . . governing the behavior of an individual or a profession."[1] Such principles do not endorse the tenets of any single religion, but, in practice, the religious beliefs of the patient should be respected. Ethical principles include the perspectives of both utilitarianism (the greatest good for the greatest number) as well as deontology (the basic moral duties of physicians).[2] The "principles" that are traditionally cited for ethical behavior in health care are:

1. *Autonomy*: This is the respect for personal choice and self-rule. This principle is derived from a respect of the rights of the individual in society, as reflected in the statements, "Whose life is this, anyway?"[3] and "Whose death is it, anyway?"[4] The patient with impaired consciousness has reduced autonomy in the usual sense, but his wishes from an earlier time may be known. The choice should be one that is fully informed, rational, and freely made.[5] This has implications for physicians, who must remember to listen to patients and to establish what their wishes are before they become incapacitated.

2. *Beneficence*: This is the moral duty to promote goodness or benefit to the patient and their family. It is not merely the flip-side of nonmaleficence or not doing bad, but implies *preventing* evils from occurring.[6] It has been argued that, for physicians, this ethical principle should have primacy over all others. Thus, the physician should take an active role in directing decision-making to do what is best to help the patient. Also, we should keep in mind the aphorism that the physician's role is "to cure sometimes, to relieve often and to comfort always."

3. *Nonmaleficence*: This principle requires that we do no harm to the patient; i.e., that we do not kill, cause pain or disability, or detract from quality of life. It is embodied in the Latin motto: *Primum, non nocere* (above all, do no harm).

4. *Justice*: This is the most controversial of principles, in that there is debate among the utilitarian, libertarian, and egalitarian schools of philosophy. For practical purposes, the physician should respect fairness for individuals as well as resources, including the costs and availability of diagnostic and therapeutic modalities. In general, however, this principle should be secondary to that of beneficence if doctors function as physicians rather than hospital administrators or societal

gate-keepers. Justice for the individual may, it seems, be in conflict with justice for society.

INFORMED CONSENT

It is essential that physicians obtain consent from the patient whenever possible. This respects the ethical principle of autonomy and allows the patient to make a choice regarding the level of care. In obtaining the consent, the following should be observed: (1) physicians must convey adequate information to their patients; (2) consent must be made without coercion; and (3) the patient must be competent to consent or refuse.[2] When patients are not competent, either on a lasting basis or, in the case of an emergency, on a short-term basis, then consent from a proxy should be obtained.

If, in an emergency, there is not time to obtain consent from a proxy in the case of a patient who cannot communicate, the doctor must act in the best interest of the patient, respecting the second principle of beneficence. The physician should document the circumstances and the reasons for the action.

Each of the principles mentioned above are especially put to the test in clinical research.[7] Adequacy of information should follow the rules of the Declaration of Helsinki. Any study should explicitly state that voluntary withdrawal of the patient can occur and will not further bias care in any way, i.e., there should be no coercion.

WITHDRAWAL OF CARE

Patients should be aware that they have the *right* to refuse treatment, i.e., that the proposed treatment is an option. Better communication of this right, with clear descriptions of the likely outcome of different courses of management will allow for better, informed decision-making. This will help diffuse the fear of meddlesome management. Whatever the patient's decision, it is important always to provide comfort and relief. Physicians should recognize that to prolong the dying process is unkind and unethical.

Patients sometimes wish not to receive medical treatment if they cannot enjoy what they perceive as a reasonable quality of life in the future. This is exemplified by the case of Georgia Hansot as related by her daughter.[8] The patient had left an advance directive that she did not want to live in a dependent, disabled state. Yet after suffering a stroke at age 87 years, she received vigorous treatment in an intensive care unit (ICU), with the plan to send her to a nursing home with a tracheostomy. The competent patient has the right to decide whether or not to accept the level or type of care offered. It should be assured that the patient is or was competent at the time of decision-making and that the planned refusal of therapy was made optimally.[9] To proceed with treatment against his/her well-considered wishes is, in essence, a battery or assault, even if those wishes are contrary to a medical plan of management.

Every case of withdrawal of care has the potential to be unique. Plans need to be made with the collective input of care givers and the patient or his representative; orders need to be individualized.

Levels of Care

Treatment can be stratified into four levels:

- Level 1: High technology, high expense, high invasive care involving respirators, ICUs, cardiopulmonary resuscitation, dialysis, and pacemakers.

- Level 2: None of above-mentioned level 1 measures, but does include drugs such as vasopressors and antibiotics.

- Level 3: Nutrition and hydration are provided but other level 1 and 2 measures are not.

- Level 4: None of above-mentioned level 1, 2, or 3 measures, but nursing care necessary to achieve hygiene and dignity, and medical care to treat pain and to comfort the patient and their family.

In practice, the withdrawal of care in the ICU setting usually begins with level 1 and progresses to other levels sequentially.[10] The stages of withdrawal can be made in small, frequent, sequential steps so the patient can be observed for suffering or discomfort. Some aspects of care can be maintained for preservation of comfort. Sometimes, all but level 4 care are eliminated simultaneously; level 4 care is always provided. More specifically, the following are usually withdrawn (in this order): cardiopulmonary resuscitation (CPR), vasopressors, ventilators, oxygen therapy, blood transfusions, antibiotics, antiarrhythmic drugs, dialysis, neurosurgical intervention, total parenteral nutrition, intravenous fluids, enteral nutrition and hydration.[2]

Physicians show a bias towards withdrawing the following: (1) support for organs that fail due to natural rather than iatrogenic causes; (2) recently instituted rather than long-sustained treatments; (3) forms of therapy that, when withdrawn, result in immediate rather than delayed death.[11]

"No code," "No CPR," "Do not resuscitate," "DNR," or "DNAR" (do not attempt resuscitation) orders are written on patient charts to prevent efforts at CPR in the event of cardiovascular or respiratory arrest.[12] Such decisions should be made based on the severity and reversibility of the illness and the wishes of the patient. When possible, physicians should discuss CPR with the terminally ill patient while he/she is still able to make decisions. Discussions among the patient (if possible), the family, physicians, and nurses should be documented in the chart, along with the rationale for the decision. Involvement of the hospital ethics committee is sometimes valuable.[13] The local hospital policies for CPR orders should be understood and respected. Decisions should be communicated to all the patient's care givers in addition to family members and significant others.

"Do not resuscitate" orders are more difficult in patients with an acute, unexpected, incapacitating illness, e.g., stroke, than in others with slowly progressive illnesses, such as a brain tumor. Unless advance directives are given, decision-making is dependent mainly on the prognosis and discussion with family members. Landi has cautioned against DNR criteria based *solely* on physician-determined prognosis.[14,15] Although scales with reasonable predictive value exist,[16] such decision-making is as much a social as a medical issue. What is the acceptable threshold for considering further treatment as futile? Severe disability is not equivalent to death; some patients and families may be willing to accept severe disability rather than death as the outcome. This applies especially to outcomes better than persistent vegetative state (PVS), e.g., severe motor disability or dementia.

Brain Death

Brain death was discussed in Chap. 2. Most states, provinces, or countries have legislation that recognizes brain death as equivalent to death of the person. Brain death must be declared in accordance with established standards and laws. Transplantation of organs can then take place, if appropriate consents are completed. Withdrawal of care should not be an issue when brain death is declared in a valid manner. It is advisable to obtain the full agreement of family members whenever possible, but families should not be made to feel that they are making the decision of whether or not to withdraw care.

Incompetency

Further discussion involves patients who are not brain dead, but who are incompetent at the time of their severe illness. Withdrawal of care is a reasonable and generally accepted course of action if certain conditions (discussed below) prevail. Decision-making in such cases must respect the ethical principles of autonomy, beneficence, nonmaleficence, and justice. The patient's wishes, if known and if legal, should always prevail, and are most valid if written in a legal document often called a "living will."[17] It is very important that care givers are knowledgeable of the legal requirements for their jurisdiction. Other transmitted advance directives or the establishment of power of attorney for personal care are also valid methods. It is wise for physicians to urge their patients, while competent, to consider their values and to clarify in a legal document their preferences for management in the event of incapacity, including naming a proxy, attorney, or surrogate. Such directives should not demand care that would be deemed futile or unreasonable when there is no hope of recovery.

Where questions arise about the initial or ongoing validity of the legal will, a competent legal opinion or the direction of the courts must be obtained.[18] Before a proxy can use such a document in decision-making for the patient, it must be understood that the patient at such time must be incapable of making his/her own decisions. If this becomes disputed, an independent determination may have to be made in accordance with the legislation.

In the event that there is no living will or a proxy is not specified, the legal order in such jurisdiction for selection of substitute decision-maker should be known by the care givers, e. g., legally appointed guardian of the patient, then spouse, child, parent, sibling, or other relative in descending order of preference. Where there is no living will, the substitute decision-maker's previous oral communications with the patient, in which the patient stated his/her treatment preferences, should be considered. If there are no written or oral advance directives, beneficence, nonmaleficence, and justice become the predominant ethical principles.

Decision-making must involve discussions with families, and ideally should include other care givers, such as nurses and allied health professionals. It is essential to keep the health care objectives for the patient in mind when considering and discussing the level of care. Ethics committees or optimum care committees in some hospitals play a helpful role in advising re the level of care for critically ill patients.[19]

The risk-benefit ratio is also a useful concept. The benefit is the prolongation of the patient's life. If, for example, the diagnosis of a PVS is determined with certainty (e.g., patients who have advanced degenerative or developmental disorders or patients who meet the guidelines of the American Academy of Neurology), the benefits of prolonging such a low-quality life are usually less than the burdens created to society and the family. In general, unless advance directives to the contrary are in place, it is best not to treat such patients with vigorous, intensive management.

The issue of whether or not to provide level 3 care, hydration and nutrition, is the most controversial. Some regard these as basic provisions rather than medical therapies. The physician should consider that the administration of nutrition and hydration sometimes requires invasive management, such as the placement of gastrostomy tubes and central lines, and considerable technology for administration as well as professional surveillance.[20–22] The withholding of food and nutrition in hopeless cases is in keeping with the position statement of the American Medical Association.[23] In a questionnaire survey (58 percent response rate), most internists favoured withdrawing nasogastric feeds from patients who were in a PVS for a year.[24]

The Issue of Advance Directives and Medical Futility

Even in the face of medical futility, the wishes of the patient should be respected. This was exemplified by the case of Helga Wanglie in Minneapolis in 1991. Mrs Wanglie, an 85-year-old woman in a PVS for several months from hypoxic-ischemic encephalopathy from a cardiac arrest, had left an advance directive that "she did not want anything to prematurely shorten or prematurely take her life."[25] In this case, the patient's relatives wished to maintain a high level of care on a ventilator; her attending physicians regarded such treatment as futile and recommended discontinuation of the ventilator, in view of her poor prognosis. The court named her husband as her custodian. Consequently, the hospital maintained treatment with the ventilator until she died many months later. This decision respected the patient's advance directive. If, however, such treatment would deny a patient with a more favorable prognosis the access to a ventilator, it would be reasonable to reverse this decision, in accordance with the position of the Society of Critical Care Medicine.[26]

Such decision-making involves the management of patients with a hopeless prognosis in the face of societal responsibilities and limited resources.

Persistent Vegetative State

The clinical syndrome is discussed in Chap. 2.

As a prerequisite to decision-making, accuracy in diagnosis and prognosis must be assured.[27] Prognosis is largely determined by etiology, duration, and patient age.[28] To ensure accuracy, clinical assessment alone usually requires 3 months for metabolic encephalopathy and 12 months for cases of traumatic head injury.[29–31] Electrophysiologic testing may allow an earlier prognosis when such findings are definitive (see Chaps. 2 and 3).

Obviously, the acute brain disorder category is the most problematic, as the outcome is often not as clear; there is no reversibility in PVS patients with chronic degenerative disorders and neurodevelopmental conditions. The issues therefore, apply to acute brain disorders. Prognostic determination in this group is problematic because (1) most studies are retrospective, and therefore, biased; (2) outcome measures in some studies in some patients are often not clearly defined, e.g., "poor outcome" refers to PVS as well as patients with various degrees of disability who are not vegetative; and (3) there is an effect of perceived prognosis on quality of care, i.e., the care is less vigorous in patients who are perceived to have a poor outcome.[32,33]

The value of adherence to valid guidelines in arriving at a prognosis in PVS was emphasized in a recent survey in London's Royal Hospital for Neurodisability. Of 40 patients deemed to be in PVS, 17 were, in fact, aware.[34]

Management issues hinge on an accurate diagnosis and prognosis. After this is established, the management of the "whole person" needs to include both science and considerations of the individual case.[35]

The Quality Standards Subcommittee of the American Academy of Neurology has made the following recommendations for the managment of patients with PVS:

1. The physician has the responsibility of discussing with the family or surrogates the probabilities of the person's attaining the various stages of recovery or remaining in a PVS.

2. Patients in PVS should receive appropriate medical, nursing or home care to maintain their personal dignity and hygiene.

3. Physicians and the family must determine appropriate levels of treatment relative to the administration or withdrawal of:

   a. medications and other commonly ordered treatments;
   b. supplemental oxygen and use of antibiotics;
   c. complex organ-sustaining treatments such as dialysis;
   d. administration of blood products;
   e. artificial hydration and nutrition.

4. Once PVS is considered to be permanent, a DNR order is appropriate. A DNR order includes no ventilation or cardiopulmonary resuscitation. The decision to implement a DNR order, however, may be made earlier in the course of the patient's illness if there is an advance directive or agreement of the patient and the physician (or physicians) responsible for the care of the patient.

The Issue of Refusal of Medical Therapy

The cases of Karen Ann Quinlan in New Jersey and Nancy Beth Cruzan in Missouri were among the first to raise before the courts the legal issue of the right of patients or their proxies to refuse medical therapy. Both were young women in PVS for months from anoxic-ischemic encephalopathy. Although neither had given written advance directives, their families stated that the patients, when well, had each expressed the wish not to be maintained with medical therapy in the event of PVS. Quinlan's family successfully brought legal action to have her removed from a ventilator. The Cruzans' attempt to have tube feeds discontinued, based on their daughter's earlier-expressed oral wishes, was unsuccessful because the court was unwilling to accept the proxy testimony and insisted on a *written* advance directive. These cases, however, appear to establish that patients have a right to refuse any medical treatment providing that an adequate standard of documentation is met. However, the outcome in all legal cases is dependent upon the legislation of the jurisdiction in which they arise and also the facts as they are revealed in court. A competent legal opinion may be required where there is no consensus.

A recent British survey showed that only 39 percent of consultants considered that an advance directive would have a decisive influence in a decision to withdraw nutrition or hydration.[36] It appears many physicians do not recognize the validity of advance directives.

There are gray areas for patients with PVS, e.g., those cases with verbal but no written advance directives re feeding, and cases of children or patients of any age who never expressed a preference. Many courts have ruled that properly appointed proxies or surrogates can make decisions for the incompetent patient. Some states, e.g., New York and Missouri, will not accept surrogate or proxy representation. However, there is a general move towards accepting proxy opinion. Doctors should overrule properly appointed proxies only if there is clear evidence that these individuals are not acting in the patient's best interest.[37]

Legal Issues

Most courts in North America recognize the right of competent patients to refuse treatment. With incompetent patients, a written advance directive in the form of a "living will" or power of attorney for personal care is usually recognized. Failing the availability of these, verbal discussions with family, cohabitants, or close friends are at least regarded seriously. Every reasonable attempt should be made to give autonomy primacy over other considerations and ethical principles.

The terminal patient who was *never* competent, for whom there is no way of knowing the person's preferences for management, constitutes a special case. Courts have responded differently to somewhat similar cases in this category. Two medicolegal examples involving severely mentally retarded patients were those of Storar and Saikewicz.[38,39] In the case of Storar, the New York court refused a request from the mother that life-prolonging blood transfusions be stopped. In the case of Saikewicz in Massachusetts, the court decided that, because uncomfortable treatments involving restraints for intravenous chemotherapy for myelogenous leukemia were proposed, such therapy was not warranted. In such cases, it is best to provide supportive therapy until or unless there are strong indications that such measures should be stopped. In the latter event, the attending physician is best advised to seek court approval.

Where there is no malice or negligence, physicians are not likely to be held liable for discontinuing life support on any patient, including victims of violence, who is in a PVS. The Barber case in California served as an important legal precedent. Mr Barber suffered severe hypoxic-ischemic encephalopathy secondary to cardiopulmonary arrest. After his physicians discontinued life support measures, the physicians involved were accused of homicide. The court held that because Mr Barber's condition was so poor, his physicians had no legal duty to maintain such life support.[40]

The law is interpreted in the context of current, accepted medical practice. To avoid problems, physicians should take the following measures: (1) comply with state/provincial/national laws, (2) follow hospital policies and bylaws, (3) communicate with the patient's family, (4) communicate with other medical staff, and (5) document decisions and the decision-making process carefully.[2]

QUALITY-ADJUSTED LIFE YEARS

Health economists have advanced the concept of quality-adjusted life years (QALYs) as a method of determining the cost-effectiveness and therefore an attempt to establish priorities for health care funding.[41] This was motivated by the high cost of health care, scarcity of resources, and a perceived need to ration medical dollars. Mathematical and engineering models cannot, however, be readily applied to individual cases because of the complexity of the various issues. There are serious methodological problems in establishing acceptable guidelines, measurement, and implementation. More importantly, such initiatives shift the emphasis of medicine from patient autonomy and beneficence to economic gate-keeping.[42]

Attempts at using age as the sole criterion for intensive therapy are unsound. There is ample evidence that many elderly survivors of critical illnesses enjoy a reasonable quality of life and may have lower expectations of life. Arguments that the elderly, compared with younger adults, have reduced duration and quality of life, and reduced likelihood of medical benefit are based on statistical generalities. In the individual case, the age factor alone may not be valid for management decisions.[43]

EUTHANASIA

The topic of euthanasia is not relevant to cases of acute, unexpected impairment of consciousness, but it is germane in situations of progressive, subacute, or chronic illnesses that affect brain function. In conditions such as inoperable brain tumors and neurodegenerative disorders, patients often become incapacitated before they die of their illnesses.[44]

There are four categories of euthanasia[45]:

1. *Physician-assisted suicide* (PAS or "assisted killing") requires that a physician, at the patient's request, performs an act that is necessary, but not sufficient in itself, to kill the patient. The deliberate (specifically for suicide) prescription of a lethal dose of a drug that the patient himself/herself then self-administers would be an example.

2. *Voluntary active euthanasia* (VAE) requires that the physician's deliberate act, at the patient's request and with consent, is both necessary and sufficient to result in the death of the patient. The physician intravenously administering the lethal dose of a drug, carrying out the wishes of the patient, would be an example.

3. *Nonvoluntary active euthanasia* involves the physician intentionally administering medications or other interventions to cause the patient's death while the patient is incompetent and mentally incapable of explicitly requesting this action.

4. *Involuntary active euthanasia* in which the physician deliberately ends the patient's life by administering medications or other interventions while the patient is still competent, but without the patient's request or informed consent.

Both PAS and VAE should be clearly differentiated from withdrawal of care, formerly erroneously called "passive euthanasia." In withdrawal of care, the patient is refusing medical therapy either by living will or by proxy. This recognizes the right of autonomy and must be respected. However, in PAS and VAE, the deliberate act of the physician is also required. Nonvoluntary and involuntary active euthanasia are widely regarded as unethical and immoral.

Euthanasia has drawn a great deal of media attention. Reasons for public interest include the following: (1) patients fear being helpless and losing control of their treatment and the course of the dying process; (2) patients fear their pain and suffering will not be adequately relieved; and (3) patients anticipate financial catastrophes for their families if their lives are artificially prolonged.

Advocates of euthanasia argue that legalizing such measures would allow self-determination, alleviate suffering, allow compassion or beneficence, minimize harm to the patient and others, and produce the same end as withdrawal of care, a more generally accepted practice.

Those opposed to euthanasia argue that (1) the autonomy argument is fallacious: in electing for mercy killing, the patient is, in fact, giving up self-control; (2) there is always another choice besides euthanasia to alleviate suffering effectively; (3) the dying process is not an altogether negative experience for the patient or the family in that richer understanding and insights are often experienced by both; (4) there is uncertainty of prognosis in some cases; and (5) the role of medicine becomes distorted into one of destruction and killing rather than one of healing and alleviating suffering.[2] Such opponents argue that legalization of VAE would create a "slippery slope" situation, in which the indications and controls may become indistinct or lax.

The Netherlands, which has legalized VAE, has attempted to safeguard against this "slippery slope" by insisting that three criteria are met before VAE is allowed: (1) the patient must take the initiative in requesting euthanasia, and must request it repeatedly; (2) the patient must be experiencing extreme suffering that cannot be relieved by any mechanism other than death; and (3) the physician must consult with another physician who must agree that euthanasia is acceptable in such case. However, some initial follow-up has shown that 40 percent of cases of euthanasia occurred without all three of the criteria being fulfilled and that fewer than 20 percent of euthanasia cases were reported to the authorities, which was a further condition of the enabling legislation.[46] The Dutch experience has shown that the law is not enforceable.[47] Thus, a slippery slope situation seems to be occurring in the Netherlands despite such legislation.

ACQUIRED IMMUNODEFICIENCY SYNDROME

The Ethics and Humanities Subcommittee of the American Academy of Neurology issued a statement regarding the treatment of human immunodeficiency virus (HIV)-infected patients and those with acquired immunodefiency syndrome (AIDS).[48] Physicians should:

1. Provide appropriate, compassionate care to such patients; i.e., they should not be abandoned, but should be given therapy to ease suffering and to reverse treatable complications when indicated. Also, the burden of care should be shared among the appropriate/necessary health care providers.

2. Endeavor to diminish public discrimination and erroneous concepts re modes of transmission.

3. Know the disease and practice appropriate precautions.

4. Promote advance directives.

5. Support public health measures to prevent spread of the virus, e.g., safe sex, nonsharing of needles.

6. Inform patients about the disease, obligations to report, advice re contacts. The legal obligation re partner notification has been a controversial area and is currently variable and in flux in various states and countries. However, physicians should urge the patient to inform his/her partner voluntarily. If the partner remains at risk because the patient has not informed him/her, the physician should take the necessary steps to notify a public official or, if that fails, to notify the partner directly.

PLACEBOS AND PROVOCATIVE TESTING

Although there is controversy regarding the use of placebos (e.g., injections of saline) or provocative suggestions to precipitate nonepileptic seizures, ethical principles should not be compromised.[49] Deception can be avoided by the clinician being honest about the differential diagnosis; provocative testing with standard measures used in electroencephalogram (EEG) recordings, e.g., hyperventilation and photic stimulation, can be used rather than contrived devices. The procedure should be explained, verbal consent should be obtained and the nature of the spell should be explained to the patient afterwards. In this way the trust of the patient is not betrayed and patients are more likely to co-operate in further therapeutic plans.

CLINICAL RESEARCH

In university medical centers, there are legal/ethical safeguards against research that is inherently or morally wrong, in which the risks are too great, or where there is a significant risk of undesirable applications of resultant technologies or procedures. Local ethics review boards are the main controlling bodies in the initiation of approval for projects.

However, in research involving critically ill patients with life-threatening diseases, the risks and costs of randomized clinical trials are often high. Some suggested principles include the following:

1. Randomized clinical trials that involve placebo treatment for life-threatening diseases are probably unethical.[50]

2. In the randomization, there should be equipoise or unbiased uncertainty in the medical community as to which of the competing therapies is better.[51]

3. Consents, including those obtained by proxy in this situation, should be fully informed.

4. The full procedures, risks, and benefits should be honestly described.

5. The research should be relevant for patient care and should address significant questions. The protocol should be scientifically constructed to properly address the issues.

6. The results should be accurately reported in the scientific literature before being released to the media.

7. There should not be a conflict of interest on the part of the involved physician: e.g., financial gain for enrollment of patients.

RESPONSIBILITIES AS AN EXPERT WITNESS

Physicians who serve as "expert witnesses" for medicolegal issues, usually decided upon in court by academic and practice qualifications, should act responsibly. They should not have a strong bias towards either side in an adversarial situation that allows contamination of their testimony. "The expert's sole allegiance is to the truth and the body of accepted knowledge and standards."[52] The witness should qualify statements as to the quality of the evidence, e.g., class I to V studies, and whether the statements represent opinion that is not grounded on hard evidence. The witness should also be aware of the difference between malpractice and maloccurrence. Malpractice refers to the failure to use an appropriate standard of judgment, diligence, or skill in the management of a patient. Maloccurrence is the less-than-ideal outcome of management. Most often, maloccurrence is not the result of malpractice, as revealed by the Harvard Malpractice Study.[53] Physicians have a responsibility to exercise fairness and their best judgment. We must reverse the trend for "hired gun" expert witnesses who have indirectly contributed to the litigious nature of our society.

REFERENCES

1. Pfaff DW (ed) *Ethical Questions in Brain and Behavior*. New York, Springer Verlag, 1981, p. 1.
2. Bernat KJ: *Ethical Issues in Neurology*. Boston, Butterworth-Heinemann, 1995, pp 3-22.
3. Rutledge-Harding S, Patrick J: Euthenasia: Principles and Observations from a Christian Perspective. Submitted to the Special Senate Committee on Mercy Killing and Assisted Suicide, 1994.
4. Gilligan T, Raffin TA: Whose death is it, anyway? *Ann Inter Med* 125: 137, 1996.
5. Beauchamp TL, Childress JF: *Principles of Biomedical Ethics*. New York, Oxford University Press, 1989, pp 68-69.
6. Gert B. Morality: *A New Justification of the Moral Rules?* New York, Oxford University Press, 1988, pp 160-162.
7. Lynoe N, Sanlund M, Dahlqvst G, Jacobsson L: Informed consent: study of quality of information given to participants in a clinical trail. *BMJ* 303:610m, 1991.
8. Hansot E: A letter from a patient's daughter. *Ann Intern Med* 125:149, 1996.
9. Trevor-Deutsch B, Nelson RF: Refusal of treatment, leading to death: towards optimization of informed consent. *Ann RCPSC* 29:487, 1996.
10. Smeidra NG, Evans BH, Grais LS, et al: Withholding and withdrawal of life support from the critically ill. *N Eng J Med* 322:309, 1990.
11. Christakis NA, Asch DA: Biases in how physicians choose to withdraw life support. *Lancet* 42:642, 1993.
12. Editorial: Ethical considerations in resuscitation. *JAMA* 268:2281, 1992.
13. Marshall SB, Marshall LF, Vos HR, Chesnut RM: *Neuroscience Critical Care*. Philadelphia, WB Saunders, 1990, pp 431-440.
14. Landi G: No to DNR orders in acute stroke. *Lancet* 347:848, 1996.

15. Alexandrov AV, Pullicino PM, Meslin EM, Norris JW: Agreement on disease-specific criteria for do-not-resuscitate orders in acute stroke. *Stroke* 27:232, 1996.

16. Cote R, Battista RN, Wolfson C, et al: The Canadian Neurological Scale: validation and reliability assessment. *Neurology* 39:638, 1989.

17. Wold JL: The living will: legal and ethical perspectives. *J Neurosci Nurs* 24:50-53, 1992.

18. Wold JL: The living will: legal and ethical perspectives. *J Neurosci Nurs* 24:50, 1992.

19. Brennan TA: Ethics committees and decisions to limit care. *JAMA* 260:803, 1988.

20. Cantor NL: The permanently unconscious patient, nonfeeding and euthanasia. *Am J Law Med* 15:381, 1989.

21. Lynn JL, Childress JF: Must patients always be given food and water. *Hastings Cent Rep* 13:17, 1983.

22. Steinbrook R, Lo B: Artificial feeding—solid ground, not a slippery slope. *N Eng J Med* 318:186, 1988.

23. American Medical Association Council on Scientific Affairs and Council on Ethical and Judicial Affairs: Persistent vegetative state and the decision to withold or withdraw life support. *JAMA* 263:426, 1990.

24. Hodges MO, Tolle SW, Stocking C, Cassel CK: Tube feeding: internists' attitudes regarding ethical obligations. *Arch Intern Med* 154:1013, 1994.

25. Miles SH: Informed demand for "non-beneficial" medical treatment. *N Eng J Med* 325:512, 1991.

26. Society for Critical Care Medicine. Consensus report on the ethics of forgoing life-sustaining treatments in the critically ill. *Crit Care Med* 18:1435, 1990.

27. Beresford HR: Moral, ethical, and legal issues raised by catastrophic brain injury, in Levin HS, Benton AL Muizelaar JP, Eisenberg HM (eds): *Catastropluc Brain Injury*. New York, Oxford University Press 1996, pp 153-173.

28. ANA Committee on Ethical Affairs: Persistent vegetative state: report of the American Neurological Association Committee on Ethical Affairs. *Ann Neurol* 33:386, 1993.

29. Levy DE, Caronna JJ, Singer BH, et al: Predicting coma from hypoxic-ischemic coma. *JAMA* 253:1420, 1985.

30. Braaktnan R, Jennett B, Minderhoud JM: Prognosis of a post-traumatic vegetative state. *Acta Neurochir* (Wien) 95:49, 1988.

31. Arts WF, van Dongen HR, Meulstee J: Unexpected improvement after prolonged post-traumatic vegetative state. *Acta Neurochir* (Wien) 95:78, 1988.

32. Shewmon DA, DeGiorgio CM: Early prognosis in anoxic coma. *Neurol Clin* 7:823, 1989.

33. Murray LS, Teasdale GM, Murray GD, et al: Does prediction of outcome alter patient management? *Lancet* 341:1487, 1993.

34. Andrews K: Misdiagnosis of the vegetative state. *BMJ* 313:13, 1996.

35. Cassell EJ: Clinical incoherence about persons: the problem of the persistent vegetative state. *Ann Intern Med* 125:146, 1996.

36. Grubb A, Walsh P, Lambe N, Murrells T, Robinson S: Survey of British clinicians' views on management of patients in persistent vegetative state. *Lancet* 348:35, 1996.

37. Rhoden NK: Litigating life and death. *Harvard Law Rev* 102:375, 1988.

38. New York State Court of Appeals opinions concerning: *In the matter of John Storar, in the matter of Father Philip K. Eichneer. NY Law J* 185:1, 1981.

39. *Superintendent of Belchertown State School v. Saikewicz*, 370, N.E. 2d 417, 1977.

40. *Barber v. Superior Court.* 147 Call App 3d 1006, 195 Cal Rptr 414, 1983.

41. LaPuma JL, Lawlor EF: Quality-adjusted life years: ethical implications for physicians and policymakers. *JAMA* 263:2917, 1990.

42. Kurtzke JF: Slippery slope in medicine. *Neurology* 44:1775, 1994.

43. Kilner JF: Age criteria in medicine. Are the medical justifications ethical. *Arch Intern Med* 149:2343, 1989.

44. McIntyre KM: Legal aspects of decision making in neurologic intensive care, in Ropper AH (ed): *Neurological and Neurosurgical Intensive Care*, 3rd ed, 1993, pp 467-479.

45. Emanuel EJ: Euthanasia: historical, ethical and empiric perspectives. *Arch Intern Med* 154:1890, 1994.

46. Van der Maas PJ, van Delen JJM, Pinjnenborg L, Looman CWN: Euthanasia and other medical decisions concerning the end of life. *Lancet* 338:669, 1991.

47. Van der Wal G, Onweuteana-Philipsen BD: Cases of euthanasia and assisted suicide reported to the public prosecutor in North Holland over 10 years. *BMJ* 312:612, 1996.

48. Report of the Ethics and Humanities Subcommittee of the American Academy of Neurology: The ethical role of the neurologist in the AIDS epidemic. *Neurology* 42:1116, 1992.

49. Devinsky O, Fisher R: Ethical use of placebos and provocative testing in diagnosing nonepileptic seizures. *Neurology* 47:866, 1996.

50. Levine RJ: Some ethical considerations in the use of placebos in randomized clinical trials, in Nicholas JM (ed): *Moral Priorities in Medical Research: The Second Hannah Conference.* Toronto, The Hannah Institute, 1984, 113-121.

51. Freedman B: Equipoise and the ethics of clinical research. *N Eng J Med* 317:141, 1987.

52. Weintraub MI: Expert witness testimony: a time for self-regulation? *Neurology* 45:855, 1995.

53. Harvard Malpractice Study: Patients, doctors and lawyers: medical injury, malpractice litigation and patient compensation in New York—the report of the Harvard Medical Practice Study to the State of New York. Cambridge, Mass., Harvard Medical Malpractice Study, 1990.

INDEX

INDEX

NOTES

NOTES

NOTES

NOTES

NOTES

ISBN 0-07-072371-0

90000

9 780070 723719